Treating Endocrine and Metabolic Disorders With Herbal Medicines

Arif Hussain
Manipal Academy of Higher Education, UAE

Shalini Behl
Manipal Academy of Higher Education, UAE

IGI Global
PUBLISHER of TIMELY KNOWLEDGE

A volume in the Advances in Medical Diagnosis, Treatment, and Care (AMDTC) Book Series

Published in the United States of America by
IGI Global
Medical Information Science Reference (an imprint of IGI Global)
701 E. Chocolate Avenue
Hershey PA, USA 17033
Tel: 717-533-8845
Fax: 717-533-8661
E-mail: cust@igi-global.com
Web site: http://www.igi-global.com

Library of Congress Cataloging-in-Publication Data

Names: Hussain, Arif, 1980- editor. | Behl, Shalini, 1983- editor.
Title: Treating endocrine and metabolic disorders with herbal medicines / [edited by] Arif Hussain, Shalini Behl.
Description: Hershey, PA : Medical Information Science Reference, [2021] | Includes bibliographical references and index. | Summary: "In order to provide the optimal care and counseling for patients who use herbal drugs, pharmacists/practitioners need to be well informed about the use and safety of herbs. This book will significantly help to spread awareness to the practicing pharmacists, Ayurveda practitioners and related scientific community by focusing on safety, potential harmful effects and rational use of herbal medicines"-- Provided by publisher.
Identifiers: LCCN 2020022599 (print) | LCCN 2020022600 (ebook) | ISBN 9781799848080 (hardcover) | ISBN 9781799848097 (ebook)
Subjects: MESH: Endocrine System Diseases--therapy | Obesity--therapy | Neoplasms--therapy | Phytotherapy
Classification: LCC RC649 (print) | LCC RC649 (ebook) | NLM WK 140 | DDC 616.4/061--dc23
LC record available at https://lccn.loc.gov/2020022599
LC ebook record available at https://lccn.loc.gov/2020022600

This book is published in the IGI Global book series Advances in Medical Diagnosis, Treatment, and Care (AMDTC) (ISSN: 2475-6628; eISSN: 2475-6636)

British Cataloguing in Publication Data
A Cataloguing in Publication record for this book is available from the British Library.

Advances in Medical Diagnosis, Treatment, and Care (AMDTC) Book Series

ISSN:2475-6628
EISSN:2475-6636

Mission

Advancements in medicine have prolonged the life expectancy of individuals all over the world. Once life-threatening conditions have become significantly easier to treat and even cure in many cases. Continued research in the medical field will further improve the quality of life, longevity, and wellbeing of individuals.

The **Advances in Medical Diagnosis, Treatment, and Care (AMDTC)** book series seeks to highlight publications on innovative treatment methodologies, diagnosis tools and techniques, and best practices for patient care. Comprised of comprehensive resources aimed to assist professionals in the medical field apply the latest innovations in the identification and management of medical conditions as well as patient care and interaction, the books within the AMDTC series are relevant to the research and practical needs of medical practitioners, researchers, students, and hospital administrators.

Coverage

- Cancer Treatment
- Emergency Medicine
- Disease Management
- Patient Interaction
- Diagnostic Medicine
- Critical Care
- Medical Procedures
- Internal Medicine
- Alternative Medicine
- Experimental Medicine

IGI Global is currently accepting manuscripts for publication within this series. To submit a proposal for a volume in this series, please contact our Acquisition Editors at Acquisitions@igi-global.com or visit: http://www.igi-global.com/publish/.

The Advances in Medical Diagnosis, Treatment, and Care (AMDTC) Book Series (ISSN 2475-6628) is published by IGI Global, 701 E. Chocolate Avenue, Hershey, PA 17033-1240, USA, www.igi-global.com. This series is composed of titles available for purchase individually; each title is edited to be contextually exclusive from any other title within the series. For pricing and ordering information please visit http://www.igi-global.com/book-series/advances-medical-diagnosis-treatment-care/129618. Postmaster: Send all address changes to above address.

Titles in this Series

For a list of additional titles in this series, please visit:
http://www.igi-global.com/book-series/advances-medical-diagnosis-treatment-care/129618

Handbook of Research on Disease Prediction Through Data Analytics and Machine Learning
Geeta Rani (Manipal University Jaipur, India) and Pradeep Kumar Tiwari (Manipal University Jaipur, India)
Medical Information Science Reference • © 2021 • 586pp • H/C (ISBN: 9781799827429) • US $395.00

Handbook of Research on Evidence-Based Perspectives on the Psychophysiology of Yoga and Its Applications
Shirley Telles (Patanjali Research Foundation, India) and Ram Kumar Gupta (Patanjali Research Foundation, India)
Medical Information Science Reference • © 2021 • 577pp • H/C (ISBN: 9781799832546) • US $345.00

New Developments in Diagnosing, Assessing, and Treating ADHD
Rejani Thudalikunnil Gopalan (Mahatma Gandhi Medical College and Hospital, India)
Medical Information Science Reference • © 2021 • 419pp • H/C (ISBN: 9781799854951) • US $265.00

Handbook of Research on Oncological and Endoscopical Dilemmas in Modern Gynecological Clinical Practice
Konstantinos Dinas (2nd Department of Obstetrics and Gynaecology, Aristotle University of Thessaloniki, Greece) Stamatios Petousis (2nd Department of Obstetrics and Gynaecology, Aristotle University of Thessaloniki, Greece) Matthias Kalder (Department of Obstetrics and Gynaecology, Philipps-University of Marburg, Germany) and George Mavromatidis (2nd Department of Obstetrics and Gynaecology, Aristotle University of Thessaloniki, Greece)
Medical Information Science Reference • © 2021 • 460pp • H/C (ISBN: 9781799842132) • US $385.00

Diagnostic Techniques and Therapeutic Strategies for Parotid Gland Disorders
Mahmoud Sakr (Alexandria University, Egypt)
Medical Information Science Reference • © 2021 • 362pp • H/C (ISBN: 9781799856030) • US $295.00

Evaluation and Management of High-Risk Pregnancies Emerging Research and Opportunities
Sapna Nanda (Panjab University, India)
Medical Information Science Reference • © 2021 • 216pp • H/C (ISBN: 9781799843573) • US $195.00

Noninvasive Ventilation Technologies and Healthcare for Geriatric Patients
César Fonseca (Universidade de Évora, Portugal) Manuel José Lopes (Universidade de Évora, Portugal) David Mendes (Universidade de Évora, Portugal) Jose Garcia-Alonso (University of Extremadura, Spain) and Felismina Mendes (Universidade de Évora, Portugal)
Medical Information Science Reference • © 2020 • 252pp • H/C (ISBN: 9781799835318) • US $245.00

IGI Global
PUBLISHER of TIMELY KNOWLEDGE

701 East Chocolate Avenue, Hershey, PA 17033, USA
Tel: 717-533-8845 x100 • Fax: 717-533-8661
E-Mail: cust@igi-global.com • www.igi-global.com

Table of Contents

Detailed Table of Contents

Diabetes mellitus is a chronic metabolic disorder which is at present rapidly growing to an alarming epidemic level. Various pathogenic processes are involved in the development of diabetes mellitus. This spectrums from autoimmune destruction of pancreatic beta cells with consequent deficiency of insulin to abnormalities that lead to resistance to the action of insulin. In the 21st century, the astounding rise in obesity, poor diet, and inactive lifestyles have increased the prevalence dramatically. Although several therapies are in use, Western medications are associated with adverse drug reactions and high cost of treatment. Therefore, there is currently a growing interest in herbal medicines to replace or supplement the Western medications. Extensive research is essential to enhance diagnoses, treatment, and to lessen healthcare expenditures. This chapter provides an overview of the classification, diagnosis, symptoms, complications, and economic burden of diabetes mellitus. Additionally, the authors discuss the current and upcoming therapies to treat this metabolic disorder.

The rapidly increasing incidence of diabetes mellitus as a chronic disease is becoming a serious threat to mankind health in all parts of the world. However, the currently available therapies are not of much use in prevention or reduction of disease. There are a large number of plants and natural biomolecules that have been discussed in the literature for their antidiabetic effects. Recently, the screening of many types of plant derived alpha-amylase, alpha-glucosidase inhibitors and other compounds that reduce the glucose level in the body and have fewer side effects has been successfully isolated. In this chapter, the mechanism of diabetes mellitus has been discussed. Also, the plants having anti-diabetic property along with its constituents has been presented summarized with the available literature resource. In addition to

Dysbiosis is characterized by an alteration in quantity and quality of intestinal microbiota composition. In the presence of dysbiosis, enterocytes will have difficulty in maintaining the integrity of the mucosal barrier, leading to increased intestinal permeability. These events are recognised to be linked to several chronic diseases. One of the consequences of dysbiosis is the manifestation of small intestinal bacterial overgrowth (SIBO), which is associated to a variety of chronic diseases. Single food nutrients and bioactive molecules, food additives, pre- and probiotics, and different dietary patterns may change the composition of the intestinal microbiota. Low FODMAPs diet has been a reference in SIBO treatment. This chapter intends to describe how the intestinal microbiota, dysbiosis, and SIBO can be related; to define dysbiosis food and nutrients influence; and to offer some nutritional therapy strategies for applying the low FODMAPs protocol, enabling better adherence by patients in order to increase their wellbeing.

Malnutrition is one of the major challenges for infants and children throughout the world. Breast feeding is a natural way of providing infants with the essential nutrients and is recommended as a perfect food for newborns. According to the WHO, breast feeding should be initiated within the first hour of birth and should be continued up to six months. Qilla al-Laban is a condition mentioned in Unani medicine in which breast milk production decreases or becomes scanty. It is due to the altered blood quality or quantity, Sū'-i-Mizāj and Ghalaba-i-Akhlat. Muwallid-i-Laban is an agent that promotes the secretion of milk. Synthetic drugs for augmentation of lactation have major safety concerns. Several galactogogues like Satawar, Musli safaid, etc. are being successfully prescribed by Unani physician since ancient times. This chapter describes various galactogogue mentioned in Unani system of medicine for promoting the production and secretion of milk. The dietary recommendations and drugs used to increase milk production are from natural source and chances of adverse effects are minimal.

Preface

Traditional medical systems have been the primary medical system in many countries all over the world. The use of plants and natural herbs for healing purposes predates recorded history and forms the origin of much of modern medicine. A number of conventional drugs have originated from plant sources. Few examples include aspirin (from willow bark), digoxin (from foxglove), quinine (from cinchona bark), and morphine (from the opium poppy).

In the present century, the use of herbal medicines and phytonutrients or nutraceuticals continues to expand rapidly across the world with many people now resorting to these products for treatment of various health challenges in different national healthcare settings (WHO, 2004). The past decade has witnessed a tremendous surge in acceptance and public interest in natural therapies both in developing and developed countries, with these herbal remedies being available not only in drug stores, but now also in food stores and supermarkets. It is estimated that up to four billion people (representing 80% of the world's population) living in the developing world rely on herbal medicinal products as a primary source of healthcare and traditional medical practice which involves the use of herbs is viewed as an integral part of the culture in those communities (Mukherjee, 2002; Bodeker et al., 2005; Bandaranayake, 2006).

CHALLENGES

Herbal medication has now become a popular form of healthcare owing to their ease of availability, lower side effects, clinical efficacy, and cost effectiveness. Although a number of therapies have shown promising potential with the efficacy of a good number of herbal products clearly established, many of them remain untested and their use are either poorly monitored or not even monitored at all. The public is often misled to believe that all-natural treatments are inherently safe, however, herbal medicines do carry risks. The consequence of this is an inadequate knowledge of their mode of action, potential adverse reactions, contraindications, and interactions with existing orthodox pharmaceuticals and functional foods to promote both safe and rational use of these agents. Since safety continues to be a major issue with the use of herbal remedies, it becomes imperative, therefore, that relevant regulatory authorities put in place appropriate measures to protect public health by ensuring that all herbal medicines are safe and of suitable quality. Objective understanding, neutral and fair interpretation, and publicity with regards to safety issues of herbal medicine are warranted.

Although scant literature has addressed selected issues such as informed consent and independent review related to traditional herbal medicine research, a practical, comprehensive and widely accepted ethical framework to international traditional herbal medicine research and acceptance is needed. Researchers all over the globe increasingly agree that it is important to establish a rational basis for dosing and standardization of biologically active compounds before conducting large-scale treatment trials. These efforts can improve investigators' ability to assess the risks and benefits of participation in large-scale herbal medicine trials. More rigorous monitoring of adverse events and standardized reporting of research results for both safety and efficacy data will improve long-term efforts to enhance risk–benefit ratio determination for trial participation.

ORGANIZATION OF THE BOOK

The book is organized into 16 chapters. A brief description of each of the chapters follows:

Chapter 1 reviews the pathophysiology, classification, symptoms and diagnosis of diabetes mellitus. It gives a comprehensive list of both conventional and traditional medications focusing on the various strategies for combating the disease. The chapter also addresses the complications associated with diabetes mellitus and concludes with future research directions.

Chapter 2 briefly discusses the therapeutic approaches to combat diabetes mellitus. It primarily focuses on some of the medicinal/herbal plants that possess anti-diabetic properties. The author lists out some of these plants along with their constituents and possible mechanism of action. Future opportunities and challenges pertaining to research in this area have also been proposed.

Chapter 3 aims to provide up-to-date information on potential medicinal herbs that have demonstrated anti-hyperglycemic activity through either increased secretion of insulin from pancreatic β-cells, reduction of insulin resistance with subsequent increase in insulin sensitivity, or inhibition of intestinal glucose absorption via decreased α-glucosidase activity.

Chapter 4 establishes a pathophysiological correlation between obesity and diabetes. The author analyses and summarizes the various bioactive phytochemical compounds and medicinal herbs that display both anti-diabetic and anti-obesity properties. Chemical structures for some of the active components are also presented.

Chapter 5 presents a mechanistic approach to tackle obesity using traditional herbal plants. It focuses and describes some of the leading causes of obesity, its prevalence and treatment strategies.

Chapter 6 provides an insight on one of the most common endocrine disorders in females-Polycystic Ovary Syndrome (PCOS). This syndrome has been known to increase the risk of several other metabolic disorders like type 2 diabetes, obesity, hypertension, cardiovascular disease etc. This chapter reviews several research studies that have been carried out on the management of PCOS. It addresses the use of complimentary and alternative medicinal therapy to treat PCOS.

Chapter 7 identifies the promises, practice and perspectives of treating infertility in males using plant based alternative medicines. Important herbs recommended by each of the most popular regimens (Ayurveda, Arab Traditional Medicine (ATM) and Chinese herbal medicine) is discussed in detail. Certain limitations associated with herbal treatment such as toxicity concerns, lack of sufficient data and absence of information regarding mode of action are reviewed and finally recommendations for overcoming these issues are suggested in the concluding part of the chapter.

Chapter 8 reviews and summarizes the recent advances in synergistic combinatorial therapies involving the interaction of dietary bioactive compounds with conventional, clinically used chemotherapeutic drugs. Combination therapy involving dietary agents and chemotherapeutic agents appear to be a promising therapeutic strategy for the treatment of cancer and several *in vitro* studies and a few *in vivo* studies documenting the immense scope of this strategy are detailed in this chapter. Although, the identification of novel bioactive agents with chemo preventive potential can be viewed as an important goal of cancer research as well as public health initiative to ensure population-wide chemoprevention strategies, the chapter concludes with an urgent need to assess the effect of combination of these phytochemicals with chemotherapeutic agents, so that pharmacologically safe and effective compositions that can act on all the stages of carcinogenesis.

Chapter 9 addresses the role of herbal medicine/phyto-therapy in cancer prevention by inhibiting Epithelial-Mesenchymal Transition (EMT) Pathways. A number of Medicinal plants or plant-derived drugs exhibiting potent bioactivities against various chronic diseases like cancer have been discussed.

Chapter 10 takes philosophical orientation and discusses the global regulations and standardization of herbal medicine. It recognizes metabolic syndrome as a multifactorial disease and its association with a cluster of pathologies. A detailed account on the treatment of these metabolic and endocrine disorder using pharmacological and herbal medications has been presented. Detection and assessment of adverse reactions by ayurvedic medicines has also been addressed. The chapter raises critical questions in regards to the standardization and clinical indications of herbals and emphasis on the implementation of modern technical experiments and clinical trial studies to answer these questions.

Chapter 11 provides an overview about the efficacy of different herbal medicines and scientific evidences that necessitates their usage for improving the thyroid functions. It also gives an insight on the various thyroid dysfunctions. The authors, however, warrant the need for a careful and routine follow-up as a mandatory parameter before establishing the herbal medicine as a global treatment approach. An integrated approach of combined efforts of the clinicians and scientists is required to make herbal medicine-based treatment approach a trustworthy and certified treatment option for disease management.

Chapter 12 highlights the importance of nutraceuticals as dietary supplements and their functional role in the prevention and treatment of various diseases. A brief account of the status of nutraceuticals in India as compared to other countries has been presented.

Chapter 13 documents the potential role of nutraceuticals such as flavonoids, polyphenols, flavones etc. in the treatment of various metabolic disorders. The author provides a brief description about the benefits and classification of phytonutrients with special emphasis on their selective biological properties in preventing health benefits.

Chapter 14 outlines some of the pharmacological effects of resveratrol as a preventive and therapeutic alternative for a wide range of diseases such as cancer, diabetes, cardiovascular etc. The interaction of SIRT1, AMPK pathway and ROS with resveratrol has been detailed.

Chapter 15 intends to provide a translational approach to describe how the intestinal microbiota, dysbiosis and SIBO can be related; to define dysbiosis food and nutrients influence; and to offer some nutritional therapy strategies for applying the Low FODMAPs protocol, enabling better adherence by patients in order to increase their wellbeing.

Chapter 16 describes various galactagogue mentioned in Unani system of medicine for promoting the production and secretion of milk. The author focuses on dietary recommendations, lifestyle modifications and drugs used to increase milk production from natural source, thereby minimalizing the chances of adverse effects.

REFERENCES

WHO. (2004). *WHO Guidelines on Safety Monitoring of Herbal Medicines in Pharmacovigilance Systems*. World Health Organization.

Mukherjee, P. W. (2002). *Quality Control of Herbal Drugs: An Approach to Evaluation of Botanicals*. Business Horizons Publishers.

Bodeker, C., Bodeker, G., Ong, C. K., Grundy, C. K., Burford, G., & Shein, K. (2005). *WHO Global Atlas of Traditional, Complementary and Alternative Medicine*. World Health Organization.

Bandaranayake, W. M. (2006). Quality control, screening, toxicity, and regulation of herbal drugs. In Modern Phytomedicine. Turning Medicinal Plants into Drugs. Weinheim:Wiley-VCH GmbH & Co. KGaA. doi:10.1002/9783527609987.ch2

Section 1

Diabetes and Obesity Management

Chapter 1
Diabetes Mellitus:
A Concise Review

Ruksar Salim Damji
UAE University, UAE

Shamiha Chowdhury
Manipal Academy of Higher Education, UAE

Zaib-Un-Nisa Munawar Hussain
Manipal Academy of Higher Education, UAE

ABSTRACT

Diabetes mellitus is a chronic metabolic disorder which is at present rapidly growing to an alarming epidemic level. Various pathogenic processes are involved in the development of diabetes mellitus. This spectrums from autoimmune destruction of pancreatic beta cells with consequent deficiency of insulin to abnormalities that lead to resistance to the action of insulin. In the 21st century, the astounding rise in obesity, poor diet, and inactive lifestyles have increased the prevalence dramatically. Although several therapies are in use, Western medications are associated with adverse drug reactions and high cost of treatment. Therefore, there is currently a growing interest in herbal medicines to replace or supplement the Western medications. Extensive research is essential to enhance diagnoses, treatment, and to lessen healthcare expenditures. This chapter provides an overview of the classification, diagnosis, symptoms, complications, and economic burden of diabetes mellitus. Additionally, the authors discuss the current and upcoming therapies to treat this metabolic disorder.

INTRODUCTION

Diabetes Mellitus (DM), is a chronic metabolic disorder characterized by hyperglycemia due to insulin resistance or insufficient insulin secretion (Blair, 2016). Diabetes is escalating at an alarming rate, reaching pandemic dimensions with massive economic, health and social consequences (Kaul, Tarr, Ahmad, Kohner & Chibber, 2012). Based on the (International Diabetes Federation, 2017) Atlas guideline reports,

DOI: 10.4018/978-1-7998-4808-0.ch001

in the year 2017, it was estimated that 425 million individuals were diagnosed with DM and this value is expected to increase to 629 million by the year 2045 (Salman, AlSayyad & Ludwig, 2019). One of the maximal prevalence of diabetes in the world is the United Arab Emirates (U.A.E), but in children, it has been considered as a rarity until recently (Pinhas-Hamiel & Zeitler, 2005).

Currently, the incidence of DM is increasing dramatically due to sedentary lifestyles, unhealthy diet, and a rise in obesity levels, imposing an immediate need for novel therapies to treat this condition. Besides, due to the progressive nature of this disorder, continual assessment of glucose via A1C test and individualized, tailored alterations of therapeutic regimens can improve the clinical outcome. Although they are currently several approaches to lessen the ill effects of DM and its associated complications, it is necessary to search for further efficacious agents with minimal side effects, to halt the rational usage of western drugs (Ekor, 2014). Herbal formulated medicines have a long history of usage to treat several diseases; and today, they are gaining attention to be used in treating DM. This chapter enumerates the pathophysiology, classification, symptoms, diagnosis, treatment, complications, prevention and economic burden associated with DM.

PATHOPHYSIOLOGY

Type 1 Diabetes Mellitus (T1DM) develops when the body's own immune system attacks and destroys the insulin producing β-cells of the pancreas. As β-cell mass declines, insulin secretion decreases up until the insulin available is insufficient to maintain normal blood glucose levels (absolute insulin deficiency). In the absence of insulin, sugar is accumulated in the bloodstream instead of entering the cells. As a result, the body is unable to utilize this glucose for energy (Figure 1 and Figure 2). Once 80-90% of β-cells are destroyed, hyperglycemia initiates to develop and diabetes may be diagnosed (Harvard, 2018).

Type 2 Diabetes Mellitus (T2DM) is commonly associated with certain environmental factors, genetic elements, lifestyle choices and the dynamic between these varied aspects. It involves the dysfunction of insulin producing pancreatic β-cells, insulin hormone resistance in body cells or a combination of both. This condition initiates with resistance to insulin that gradually worsens over time. The resistance and the inadequate production of insulin by β-cells ultimately lead to β-cell failure. Once the β-cells fail, endogenous insulin can no longer be secreted. The inability of cells to utilize the hormone insulin, which inhibits the cell's ability to absorb and utilize glucose in metabolic processes is known as insulin resistance. This is of primary matter in cells that are generally high in metabolic function such as: the liver, muscles and adipose tissues (Sun, 2014).

Majority of the type 2 diabetic patients, have abundant abdominal fat which can cause lipotoxicity. The abdominal fat is resistant to the antilipolytic effect of insulin thereby resulting in elevated levels of free fatty acids (FFAs). Raised free fatty acids exacerbates insulin resistance in the liver and muscle cells and thus increases the formation of glucose and impairs beta cell secretion. Excess fat tissues lead to enormous secretion of cytokines (adipokines and adipocytokines) associated with inflammation, endothelial dysfunction and thrombosis. Atherosclerosis due to insulin resistance is as a result of hypercoagulability, debilitated fibrinolysis and the combination of endothelial damage, oxidative stress and hyperglycemia. The pathophysiology of insulin dependent DM (type 1) and non-insulin dependent DM (type 2) is further portrayed in Figure 3 and Figure 4, respectively.

Figure 1. Glucose mechanism of action in a healthy individual

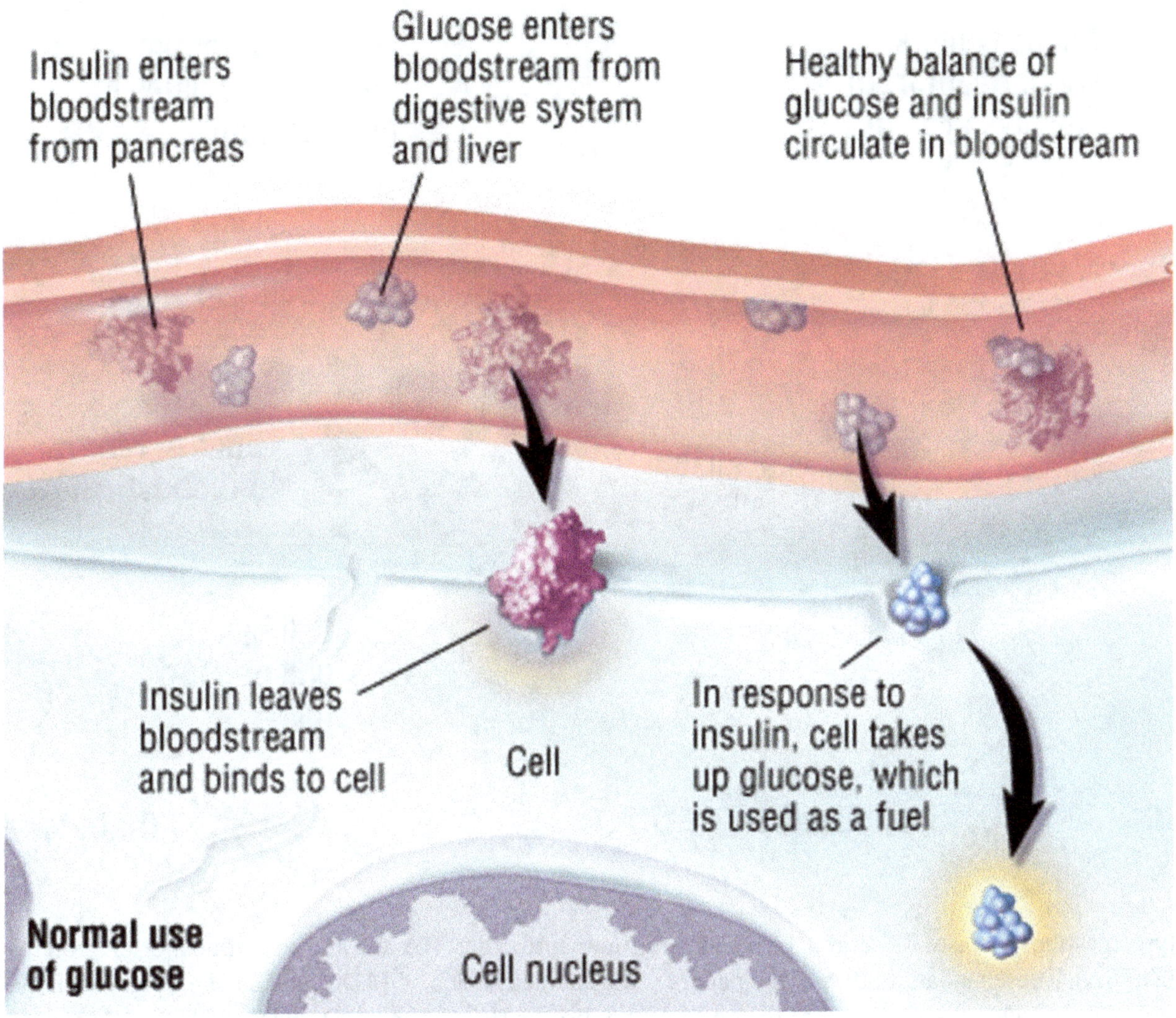

CLASSIFICATION

Majority of the diabetic patients are classified into two main categories: Type 1 Diabetes Mellitus (T1DM), which is caused due to the destruction of pancreatic β-cells predominantly by an autoimmune process. The body has either an absolute deficiency of insulin or produce very little insulin (Kharroubi & Darwish, 2015) or Type 2 Diabetes Mellitus (T2DM), which is represented by insulin resistance with an insufficient increase in the secretion of insulin. Additionally, the other classes of diabetes include Gestational Diabetes Mellitus (GDM), where women develop diabetes during their pregnancy and Monogenic Diabetes, which is a rare condition caused by a mutation in a single gene (Kaur, Mahajan & Goswami, 2018).

In T1DM, during the period of diagnosis, markers of immune destruction of β-cells are present in 90% of individuals. This includes antibodies of glutamic acid decarboxylase (GAD65), islet cells (ICAs),

Figure 2. Glucose mechanism of action in type 1 diabetic patient

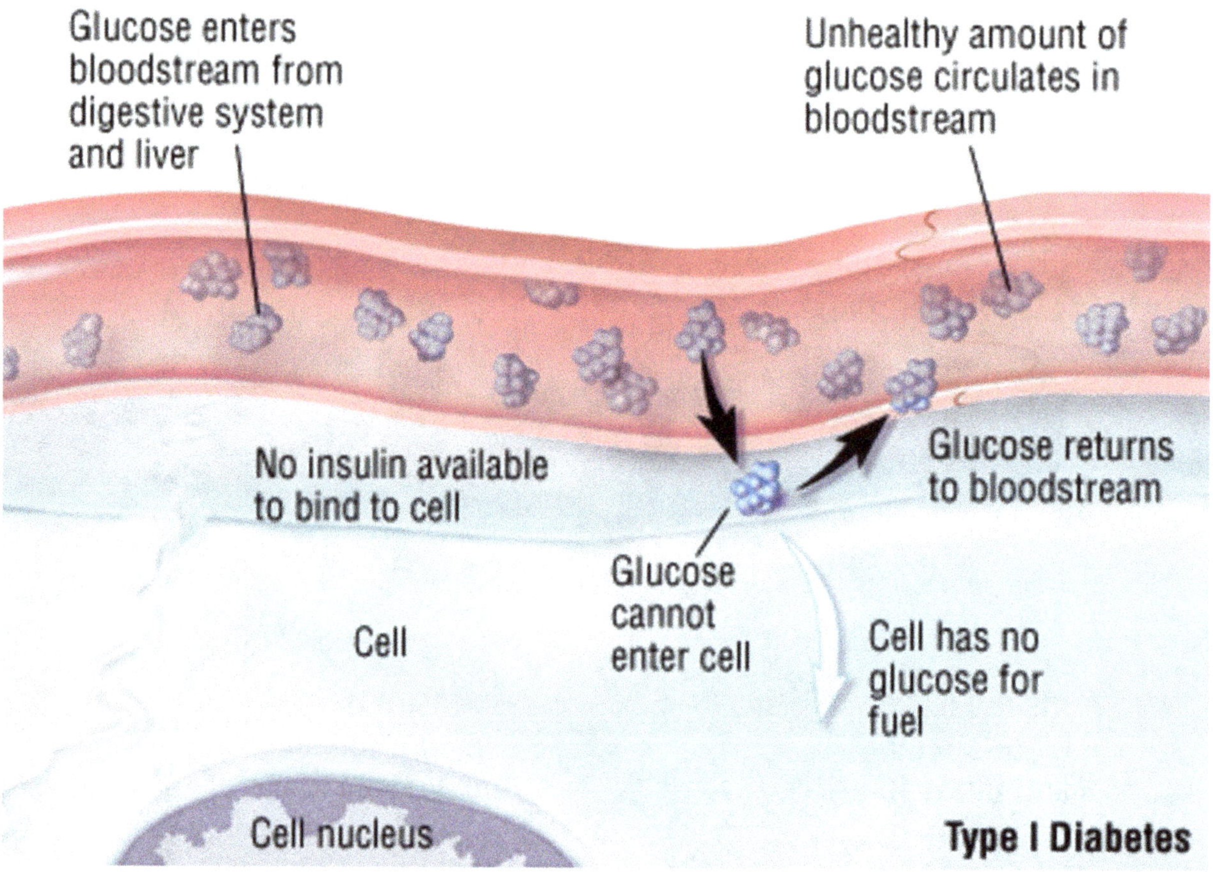

tyrosine phosphatases IA-2 and IA-2b, insulin autoantibodies (IAAs) and zinc transporter proteins (ZnT8A). These autoantibodies of the pancreas are characteristics of T1DM and can be observed in the serum of individual's years before the onset of the disease (Kharroubi & Darwish, 2015). The chances of developing T1DM increases according to the number of positive markers. Two positive antibodies can be interpreted as the individual having a 75% chance of acquiring diabetes in 10 years (Skyler et al., 2016). Children and adolescents are more likely to develop T1DM since they have a fast rate of β-cell destruction with the presence of ketoacidosis. Whereas, adequate insulin secretion to prevent ketoacidosis is maintained by adults (Krzewska& Ben-Skowronek, 2016).

T1DM is further subdivided into idiopathic and fulminant diabetes. Idiopathic is a rare form of type 1 diabetes with an unidentified origin. The severity is less in comparison to autoimmune type 1 diabetes. The majority of the patients with idiopathic diabetes are of Asian or African descent and experience a lack of insulin and episodic ketoacidosis. While, fulminant diabetes is a disparate form, which was first identified in the year 2000. It is distinguished by ketoacidosis straight after the onset of hyperglycemia, high levels of glucose (^{3} 288 mg/dL) along with unobservable serum C-peptide levels. Ultimately, to maintain normoglycemia, all T1DM patients will necessitate insulin therapy (Baynest, 2015).

Figure 3. Pathophysiology of T1DM (Hope, 2018)

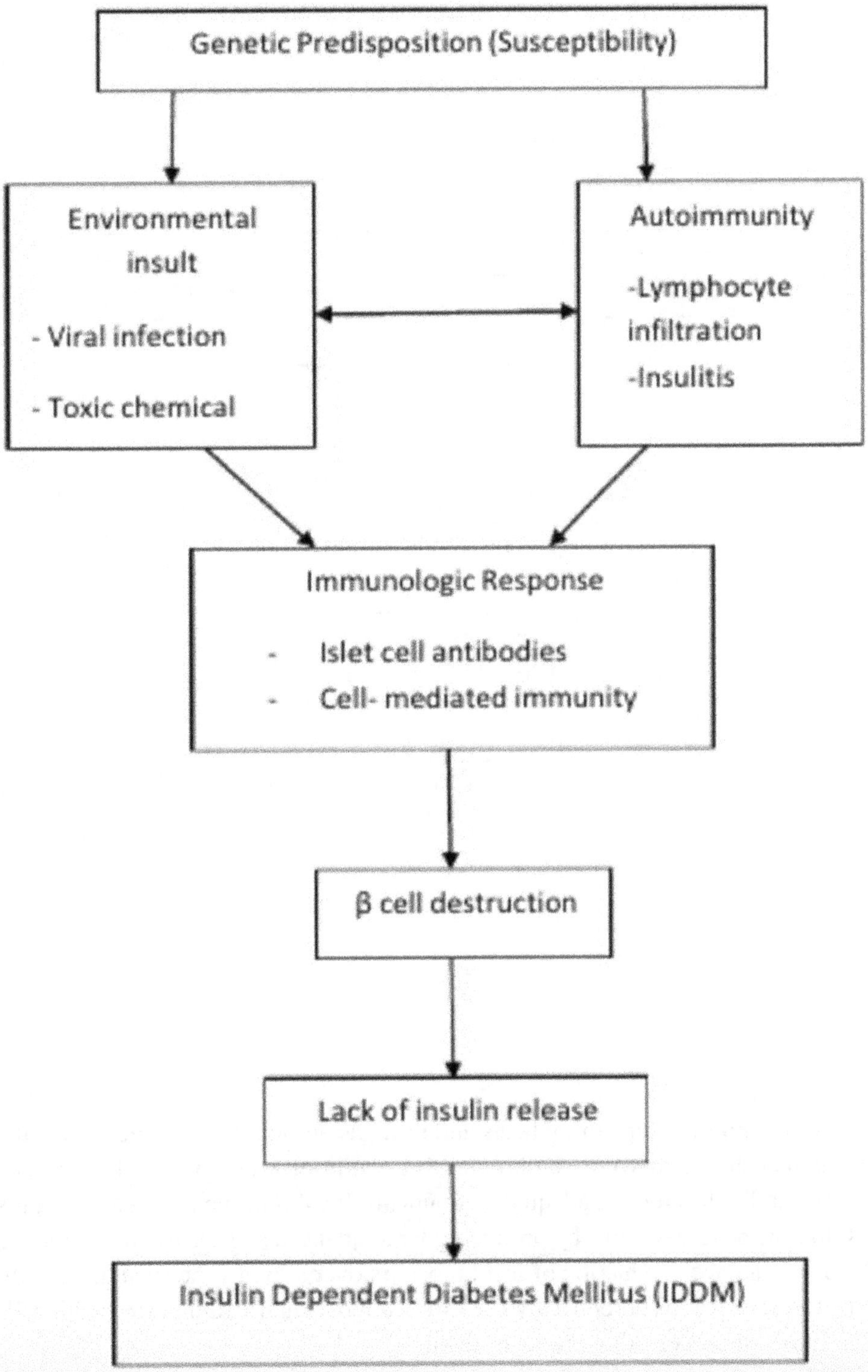

Figure 4. Pathophysiology of T2DM (Hope, 2018)

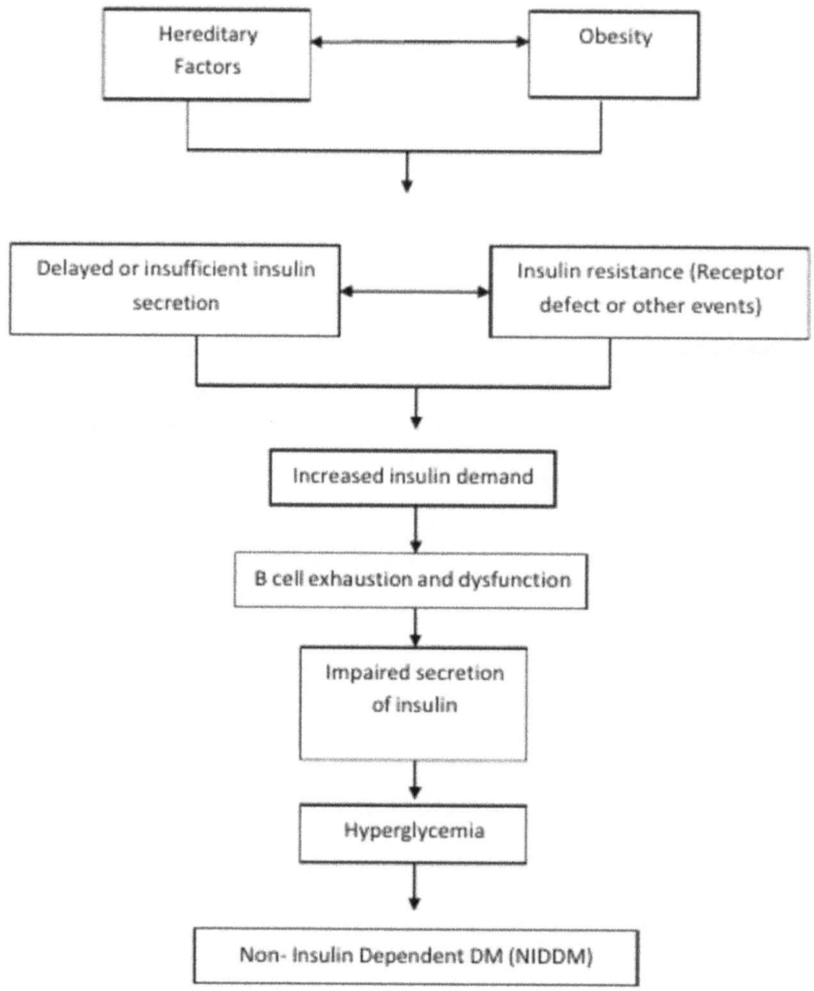

T2DM is the most common type of diabetes and remains among the chief health challenges around the globe (Al-Salameh et al., 2018). It is a progressive condition where the body becomes resistant to insulin or loses the ability to produce adequate amounts of insulin in the pancreas. As a result of being resistant to insulin, the pancreas retort by producing large quantities of insulin to try maintaining blood glucose levels. Since the overproduction of insulin occurs over a long-time span, the insulin-producing cells eventually get destroyed. Therefore, by the time an individual is diagnosed with T2DM, one has already lost 50-70% of their cells that produces insulin.

Several T2DM patients show intra-abdominal obesity, hypertension, vascular endothelial dysfunction, dyslipidemia and high plasminogen activator inhibitor 1 (PAI-1) levels (Cersosimo & DeFronzo, 2006). These mentioned abnormalities are known as "metabolic syndrome" or "insulin resistance syn-

Figure 5. A comparison between T1DM and T2DM (Rogal, Zbinden, Schenke-Layland & Loskill, 2019)

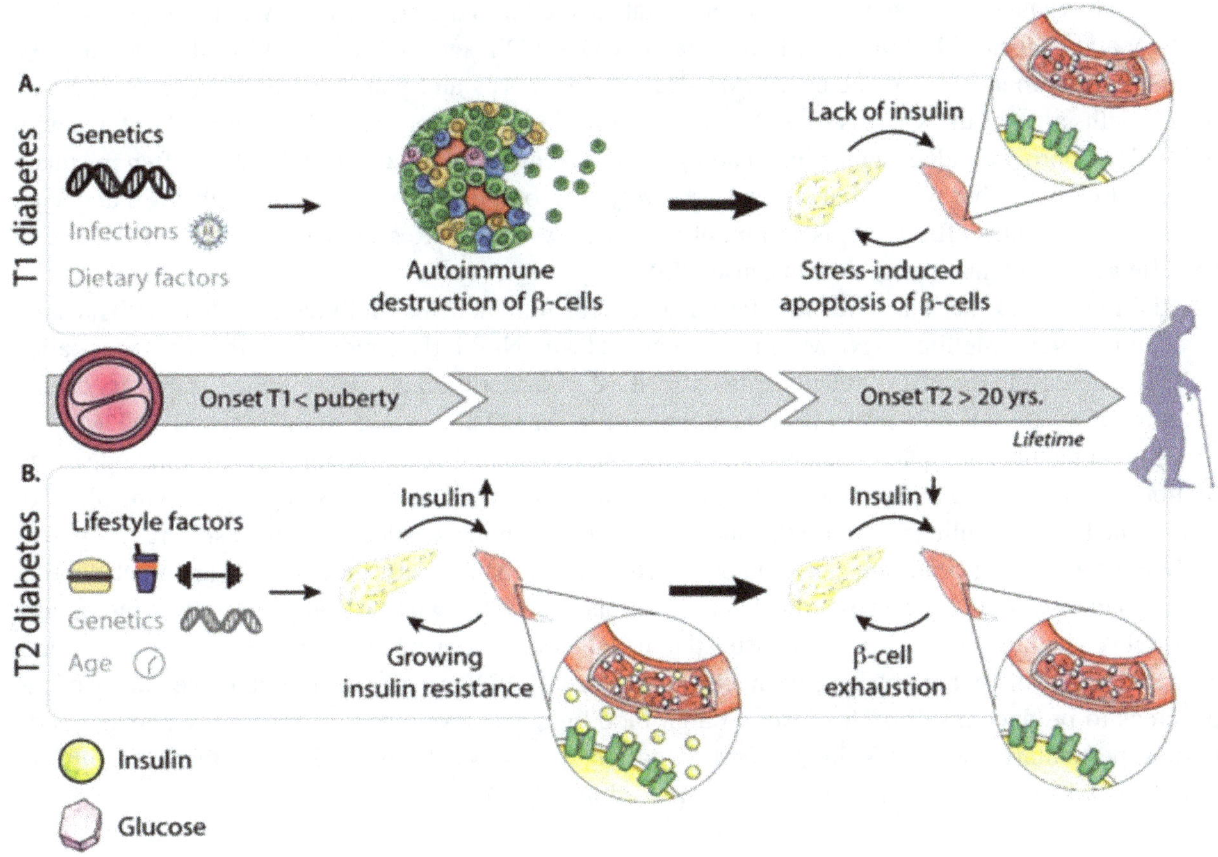

drome". Due to these abnormalities, T2DM patients are at higher risk of suffering from atherosclerotic cardiovascular disease (ASCVD) along with macrovascular complications (myocardial infection (MI) and stroke). This type of diabetes is more common in certain ethnic backgrounds, e.g. Latinos, African Americans, Mexican Americans, American Indians and is generally known to affect the women's gender (Kposowa, 2013). A comparison between the two types of DM is illustrated in Figure 5.

Diabetes diagnosed during pregnancy is referred to as Gestational Diabetes Mellitus (GDM). During pregnancy, a growing baby is provided with essential nutrients and oxygen via an organ called the placenta. The placenta also produces hormones such as estrogen, cortisol and lactogen, which blocks insulin and thereby, failing to effectively transport glucose into the cells. This leads to glucose accumulation in the blood. GDM is known to perplex approximately 8-9% of pregnancies and the onset of the disorder is primarily in the third trimester of pregnancies. Higher chances of morbidity and mortality exist for the mother, fetus and the following neonate. Thereupon, clinical tests, intensive monitoring, and treatment are required (Adapa& TK, 2020).

Monogenic Diabetes is a rare form of diabetes resulting from a mutation of a single gene. In the United States of America (USA), monogenic forms of diabetes account for 1-4% of all cases of diabetes. In the majority of the monogenic diabetes cases, the gene mutation is inherited either from one parent, both parents or gene mutation can develop spontaneously without acquiring it genetically from either of the parents. Most mutations that cause monogenic diabetes reduces the body's ability to produce insulin.

Neonatal Diabetes Mellitus (NDM) and Maturity Onset Diabetes of the Young (MODY) are the two main forms of monogenic diabetes. NDM occurs in newborns and young infants (occurs in the first 6-12 months after birth) whereas MODY usually occurs in adolescence or early adulthood. Infants with NDM do not produce adequate insulin, leading to an increase in blood glucose. NDM is often mistaken for type 1 diabetes, but type 1 diabetes is very rarely seen before 6 months of age. Diabetes that occurs in the first 6 months after birth, is commonly genetically caused. Researchers have identified several specific genes and mutations that can cause NDM.

NDM can be further classified into Permanent Neonatal Diabetes Mellitus (PNDM) and Transient Neonatal Diabetes Mellitus (TNDM). In some patients with NDM, the condition is lifelong and is called PNDM whereas, in the rest of the patients with NDM, the condition is transient and disappears during infancy. However, this may revert later during their life span. This type of NDM is called TNDM.

Clinical features of NDM depends on the individual's mutated genes. Symptoms may include dehydration, rapid breathing and polyuria. NDM can be diagnosed with high levels of glucose in the blood or urine. The lack of insulin may cause the body to produce chemicals called ketones, resulting in a potentially life-threatening condition called diabetic ketoacidosis. Most fetuses with NDM are much smaller in size than those of the same gestational age. This condition is known as intrauterine growth restriction.

MODY is a monogenic form of diabetes that usually occurs during adolescence or early adulthood. Many various gene mutations have been shown to cause MODY, all of which impede the ability of the pancreas to produce insulin. This leads to high blood glucose levels and, in time, may damage body tissues, particularly the eyes, kidneys, nerves, and blood vessels (Philipson, 2017). Clinical features of type 1, type 2 and monogenic diabetes are displayed in Table 1.

Table 1. Differentiating clinical features between Type 1, Type 2 and Monogenic Diabetes (Punthakee, Goldenberg & Katz, 2018)

	Type 1 diabetes	Type 2 diabetes	Monogenic diabetes
Onset Age	Commonly affects individuals less than 25 years old	More than 25 years old but incidence currently rising in adolescents and children	Less than 25 years old
Weight	Slim	More than 90% overweight	Similar to the general population
Islet autoantibodies	Usually present	Absent	Absent
C-peptide	Undetectable / Low	Normal / High	Normal
Production of insulin	Absent	Present	Usually present
First-line treatment	Insulin	Non-insulin antihyperglycemic agents. Gradually may depend on insulin	Depends on subtype
Family history of diabetes	Infrequent (5% - 10%)	Frequent (75% - 90%)	A multigenerational, autosomal pattern of inheritance
Diabetic ketoacidosis	Common	Rare	Rare

SYMPTOMS OF DIABETES MELLITUS

The severity of the symptoms associated with DM is dependent on the type and the duration since the diagnosis of diabetes. A minority of the diabetic patients are asymptomatic, particularly those with type 2 diabetes, during the initial stages of the disorder. The majority of the symptoms are similar between type 1 and type 2 diabetes, as shown in Table 2. However, the symptoms have shown to develop more rapidly in type 1. These symptoms include blurred vision, polyuria, polyphagia, polydipsia, weight loss, cramps, fatigue, and constipation. Chronic hyperglycemia is also accompanied by exposure to various infections and growth impairment. Supplementary warning signs include stomach pain, slow healing sores, nausea, vomiting, fatigue, dry and irritating skin, tingling and numbness in hands and feet.

DIAGNOSIS

Identifying individuals with pre-diabetes or diabetes by the process of screening, aids in early intervention along with probable reductions in future complications. Approximately 25% of the patients with T2DM are already experiencing microvascular complications during diagnosis, implying that they have had this disorder for longer than 5 years (Fowler, 2008). Resultantly, they are various approaches to diagnose diabetes as mentioned below:

Table 2. Symptoms of T1DM and T2DM (Kaur and Mahajan, 2018)

T1DM Symptoms	T2DM Symptoms
Xerostomia and polydipsia	Xerostomia and polydipsia
Sudden weight loss	Tingling and numbness of hand & feet
Blurry vision	Slow-healing wounds
Polyuria	Polyuria
Lack of energy	Extreme fatigue
Bedwetting	Recurring fungal infections in the skin

1. Random Plasma Glucose Test

It's the least complex test and doesn't necessitate fasting to take the test. If the blood glucose is 200 mg/dl or greater, it signifies diabetes. However, reconfirmation is required (Baynest, 2015).

2. Fasting Plasma Glucose Test

Fasting for 8 hours is mandatory before taking this test. A normal plasma glucose level after fasting is between 60 and 99mg/dl. Diabetes is not confirmed until 2 separate fasting plasma glucose tests each measure 126mg/dl or greater. Blood glucose of greater than 126 mg/dl assures the diagnosis of diabetes (Baynest, 2015).

3. Oral Glucose Tolerance Test

This test is only administered when the random plasma glucose test result is 160-200 mg/dl and the fasting plasma test result is 110-125 mg/dl. At least 8 hours (should not exceed 16 hours) of fasting is obligatory. This test is used to assess the body's response to glucose while fasting and then 75gm of glucose is given (100gm for pregnant women). The blood is then tested every 30 minutes to 1 hour repeatedly for 2/3 hours. The result of 140 mg/dl glucose level is considered normal. However, 126 mg/dl or more during fasting and 200 mg/dl or greater of glucose level for the 2-hour test reveals the diagnosis of diabetes (Baynest, 2015).

4. A1c Blood Test

Alternatively known as glycated haemoglobin test. This test determines an individual's average blood glucose level for the past 2 to 3 months, which is the presumed half-life of red blood cells. This test should only be performed in a lab utilizing a procedure that is certified by the National Glycohaemoglobin Standardization Program (NGSP) and regulated to Diabetes Control and Complications Trial (DCCT) assay. Fasting is not required for an A1c blood test. Glycated haemoglobin (A1C) levels over 6.5% are considered diagnostic of diabetes, values between 5.7-6.4% are diagnostic of pre-diabetes and test results less than 5.6% are normal (Sherwani, Khan, Ekhzaimy, Masood & Sakharkar, 2016).

TREATMENT

T1DM is treated with insulin along with a healthy lifestyle (dietary changes and physical activities). Whereas T2DM can be managed by lifestyle modifications and several oral hypoglycemic agents (OHAs). The medications utilized to manage T2DM can work in various ways to decrease blood glucose levels. This includes increasing excretion of glucose, increasing sensitivity of insulin or decreasing carbohydrates absorption from the digestive tract. The drugs that are currently used to treat T2DM include the following:

1. Metformin

This drug was approved by the FDA in 1994, for treating patients with T2DM. This drug is currently the first drug prescribed to patients with type 2 diabetes. Metformin boosts the sensitivity of the body cells to insulin, as well as reduces glucose production by the liver. Additionally, this drug suppresses one's appetite, which is beneficial to patients who are overweight. The side effects of metformin include diarrhoea and nausea which is often resolved with time. However, this drug is only prescribed with a combination of other medications (oral drugs or insulin) since it does not decrease blood glucose adequately alone (Horakova et al., 2019).

2. Sulfonylureas

The class of drugs that increases the output of insulin by the pancreas is known as sulfonylureas. Chlorpropamide (Diabinese) and tolbutamide are the older generation of sulfonylureas but was later neglected as it was highly associated with the risk of cardiovascular diseases. The recent sulfonylurea drugs include glipizide (Glucotrol), glyburide (DiaBeta) and glimepiride (Amaryl). These drugs lower blood sugar levels immediately but can cause abnormally low blood sugar levels, known as hypoglycemia. The side effect of these sulfonylurea drugs is weight gain (Costello & Shivkumar, 2019).

3. Meglitinides

This class of drugs promote insulin secretion from the pancreas. Meglitinides drugs include repaglinide (Prandin) and nateglinide (Starlix). These drugs act for a short time, showing peak effects within 1 hour. Therefore, they are prescribed to be consumed 3 times a day before meals. The side effect includes gaining weight (Luna &Feinglos, 2001).

4. Thiazolidinediones

This class of drugs includes pioglitazone (Actos) and rosiglitazone (Avandia), used to increase the sensitivity of the body's cells to insulin by lowering blood glucose. Thiazolidinediones drugs have major side effects such as the increased risk of heart failure and bone fractures and are, therefore, not prescribed as a first-line treatment but may be beneficial for some patients (Luna & Feinglos, 2001).

5. Alpha-Glucosidase Inhibitors

The availability of this class of drugs in the United States includes acarbose (Precose) and miglitol (Lexicomp). These drugs reduce the absorption of carbohydrates from the intestines. Enzymes present in the small intestine should break down carbohydrates such as glucose into smaller particles of sugar before being absorbed into the bloodstream. The enzymes involved in this process are known as alpha-glucosidase. Carbohydrates are not broken down thoroughly by inhibiting alpha-glucosidase and the absorption of glucose is deferred. The side effects of these drugs include abdominal pain, gas, and diarrhoea (Luna & Feinglos, 2001).

6. SGLT2 Inhibitors

The SGLT2 inhibitor, canagliflozin (Invokana), was approved by the Food and Drug Administration (FDA) in March 2013 and dapagliflozin (Farxiga), was approved in January 2014. These drugs are consumed orally and work by obstructing the kidney's reabsorption of glucose, resulting in increased excretion of glucose and reduction in blood sugar levels. SGLT2 medication is utilized as a single therapy as well as in combination with other drugs including pioglitazone, sulfonylurea, metformin and insulin (Hsia, Grove & Cefalu, 2017).

7. DPP-4 Inhibitors

Sitagliptin (Januvia), saxagliptin (Onglyza), alogliptin (Nusina) and linagliptin (Tradjenta) are members of this drug class. DPP-4 eliminates incretin (a natural hormone that informs the body to release insulin after meals) from your body. Inhibiting DPP-4 aids the incretin in the body to remain for a longer time. Thus, triggering the release of insulin which reduces blood sugar levels. Side effects include urinary tract infection (Godinho et al., 2015).

8. GLP-1 Receptor Agonists

GLP-1 is a hormone that provides signals to the body to release insulin after consuming meals. This class of drugs function in a similar way to the DPP-4 inhibitors but have a much stronger response. The first drug of this group was Exenatide (Byetta) followed by liraglutide (Victoza), albiglutide (Tanzeum) and dulaglutide (Trulicity). Since these drugs hinder the release of glucose from the liver and stomach emptying, they regulate the transfer of nutrients to the intestine for absorption. Side effects include weight loss, nausea and higher chances of pancreatitis. This group of drugs are prescribed in combination with other drugs (Heppner & Perez-Tilve, 2015).

9. Amylin Analogues-Pramlintide (Symlin)

Pramlintide was the first anti-hyperglycemic injectable medication for usage in addition to insulin. The usage of pramlintide along with insulin decreases blood sugar peaks after meals and lessens fluctuations of glucose throughout the day. Side effects include nausea and high chances of insulin-induced severe hypoglycemia, particularly in T1DM (Hoogwerf, Doshi & Diab, 2008).

10. Chitosan

Chitosan, a novel promising therapeutic agent and an effective drug carrier for DM. Chitosan is present in the endoskeletons of molluscs (examples: squid and octopus) and the cell walls of mushrooms. Chitosan oligosaccharides are the hydrolyzed products of chitin, which is abundant in the exoskeleton of crustaceans (examples: crab, crawfish, shrimps) and the cell walls of fungi (Sarkar et al., 2020). The consumption of chitosan oligosaccharide (GO2KA1) supplements with a meal can effectively reduce postprandial blood glucose levels. Chitosan supplementation can also improve altered lipid metabolism associated with DM (Jeong et al., 2019).

11. Novel Dual Aldose Reductase and Protein Tyrosine Phosphatase 1B Inhibitors

Aldose reductase and protein tyrosine phosphatase 1B enzymes have been identified as 2 novel molecular targets associated with the onset and progression of T2DM and related comorbidities. However, the data till date is yet limited (Kousaxidis et al., 2020).

TREATING DIABETES WITH INSULIN

Insulin remains as the backbone of treatment for T1DM patients. Besides, insulin is an essential therapy for T2DM patients when diet, oral medications, and weight loss does not aid in maintaining blood glucose levels. The various types of insulin are demonstrated below.

1. Rapid Acting Insulin

The effect begins 5 minutes post administration and lasts for 2 to 4 hours. The peak effect occurs 1 hour after administration.

2. Regular Insulin

The effect begins within 30 minutes of administration and lasts for 3 to 6 hours. Peak effect occurs 2 to 3 hours after injection.

3. Intermediate Acting Insulin

It lowers blood glucose levels 2 to 4 hours after administration and lasts for 12 to 18 hours. Peak effect occurs 4 to 12 hours after injection.

4. Long Acting Insulin

The effect begins within 6 to 10 hours of administration and lasts for 20 to 24 hours. Blood glucose levels are reduced uniformly for 24 hours without major peaks (Ahmad, 2014).

5. Insulin Pumps

In addition to syringes and pens, insulin pumps can also be used to deliver insulin. Pumps deliver insulin much more precisely than any available pen or syringe. They are small, computerized devices, about the size of a small cell phone. They can be worn on your belt, in your pocket, or under your clothes.

Insulin pumps deliver rapid-acting insulin 24 hours a day through a small flexible tube called a cannula. The cannula is inserted under the skin using a needle. The needle is removed, leaving only the flexible tube under the skin. The pump user replaces the cannula every 2-3 days. When using an insulin pump, you must check your blood sugar level at least 4 times a day. The pump delivers a continuous flow of insulin that can be adjusted if required. A pump user regularly enters information about their food intake and blood sugar levels so that the pump can help calculate insulin doses (Clinic, 2016). The pros and cons of utilizing insulin pumps are illustrated in Table 3.

A NOVEL DIAGNOSTIC GLUCOSE SENSING TECHNOLOGY

The Freestyle Libre Pro glucose monitoring was approved by the Food and Drug Administration (FDA) in September 2016. It is a continuous glucose monitoring (CGM) system for blinded healthcare professionals used in clinics whereas the Freestyle Libre, for personal use by patients was approved by the FDA in September 2017. The system's replaceable sensor is placed to the back of a patient' arm and can be worn for 10 days with the Freestyle Libre and approximately up to 14 days with the Freestyle Libre Pro version. To retrieve the blood sugar information stored in the sensor, providers and patients use a handheld device and thereafter the retrospective information can be utilized by the providers to read the glycemic control and amend the therapy accordingly. This aids patients to receive their glucose

Table 3. Advantages and disadvantages of utilizing insulin pumps (Joslin, 2020)

Advantages	Disadvantages
Having the flexibility to skip a meal or eat late (flexible lifestyle)	Cost
Precise insulin delivery	Technical difficulties
Fewer incidences of hypoglycemia; tighter blood glucose control	Risk of skin problems (skin irritation from the infusion set adhesive and skin infection if the infusion sets are worn too long or inserted incorrectly.
Convenience (pumps require only a needle stick once every 2-3 days to change the infusion set	Infusion set changes
Data Analysis	Checking blood glucose at least 4 times per day
Helps to manage the "dawn phenomenon" Dawn phenomenon: Abnormal increase in blood glucose levels typically between 2 am-8 am in diabetic patients	

reading without the need to perform a fingerstick for a glucose meter. The continuous glucose monitoring system is intended to detect blood glucose trends in patients $^{3}18$ years of age with type 1 or type 2 diabetes. The Freestyle Libre Pro and Freestyle Libre utilize a subcutaneous, wired enzyme glucose sensing technology to detect glucose levels in the interstitial fluid. The glucose is measured automatically and the readings are stored in 15 minutes intervals. The reader is held near the sensor when a glucose reading is required. The Libre reader device will then display 8 hours of glucose readings. The sensor device is factory calibrated and therefore patients do not have to calibrate it with blood sample glucose meter readings (Blum, 2018). The advantages and disadvantages of using Freestyle Libre sensors are demonstrated in Table 4.

Table 4. Advantages and disadvantages of using Freestyle Libre sensors (Blum, 2018)

Advantages	Disadvantages
The sensor does not need to be calibrated with blood glucose meter readings to maintain the accuracy	Inaccuracies of the system at lower glucose levels
The sensor is small and discreet. Therefore, patients can wear it for 10-14 days with minimal disturbance of their daily activities	Freestyle Libre does not have any alert functions for high or low glucose levels
	Freestyle Libre is not linked to phone applications and does not provide a channel for real-time sharing of glucose data

HERBAL TREATMENT FOR DIABETES MELLITUS

There has been a rapid growth in the sector of herbal medicines in the last few years. These drugs are attaining popularity in developing as well as developed countries due to their natural origin, minority side effects, and low cost. Studies have reported that 80% of individuals in developing countries solely depend on herbal medicines to treat various ailments. The World Health Organization (WHO) has revealed a list of 21,000 plants that are being utilized for medicinal purposes globally.

Herbs may not be used to cure diabetes as a standalone treatment. However, it can be combined with conventional treatment to provide relief from the symptoms of diabetes. Several herbs commonly used on a day-to-day basis are claimed to decrease blood glucose levels. The likelihood of not being very dependent on insulin injections and the chances of having better glycemic control simply by consuming herbal medications is undeniably appealing. Nonetheless, the variety of herbs used to treat DM may depend on various factors, including the availability and the stage of diabetes (Choudhury et al., 2018). Herbal plants with proven anti-diabetic effects are compiled and discussed below. Also, Table 5 displays other effective herbs and fruits extract used to maintain plasma glucose levels.

1. *Curcuma longa* (Curcumin)

The active component of turmeric, curcumin, has captured attention as a probable treatment for diabetes and its complications primarily due to its effectiveness in reducing glycemia and hyperlipidemia. The safety profile, low cost and high availability of curcumin also make it an excellent alternative in treating diabetes. A randomized double-blind placebo controlled clinical trial conducted by (Chuengsamarn, Rattanamongkolgul, Luechapudiporn, Phisalaphong & Jirawatnotai, 2012) exhibited promising results. This trial included 240 pre-diabetic subjects who were assigned randomly to either consume curcumin (250 mg) / day) or placebo capsules for 9 months. In the placebo group, 16.4% of the subjects were diagnosed with T2DM. Whereas, none of the subjects was diagnosed with diabetes in the group treated with curcumin. In addition, the function of β-cells, with high HOMA-β (homeostasis model assessment) and lower C-peptide was observed in the group treated with curcumin. Lower insulin resistance and higher adiponectin levels were also detected in the group treated with curcumin (Pivari, Mingione, Brasacchio & Soldati, 2019).

2. *Nigella sativa* (Fennel)

The usage of fennel has demonstrated to be equally effective as Metformin. A study was conducted to evaluate the anti-diabetic property of these seeds. A dose of 2gms/day significantly decreased haemoglobin subunit alpha 1 (HBA1), fasting blood glucose (FBG) and 2-hours-plasma glucose (2HPG) action without altering the body weight of the participants. The results obtained confirmed that this dose can be utilized as an adjuvant treatment for T2DM patients (Kooti, Farokhipour, Asadzadeh, Ashtary-Larky & Asadi-Samani, 2016).

3. *Urtica dioica* (Stinging nettle)

The hydroalcoholic extract from the leaves of UrticaDioica has shown to have hypoglycemic properties in Wistar male rats, with fructose-induced insulin resistance. Injecting differing dosages of the extracts for 2 weeks to the experimental rats showed an immense reduction in blood glucose levels and a reduction in the concentration of the serum insulin in comparison to the control group. The effects were nevertheless dependent on the dosage injected(Choudhury et al., 2018).

Moreover, a randomized double-blind placebo controlled clinical trial consisting of 46 patients and 46 placebo subjects were carried out. One nettle leaf extract capsule (500mg) was consumed every 8 hours for 3 months, in combination with the conventional anti-hyperglycemic oral medication on the fasting glucose blood levels, postprandial glucose, glycosylated haemoglobin, liver enzymes SGOT and

SGPT, systolic and diastolic blood pressure. As a result, the leaf extract reduced the fasting glucose blood levels, postprandial glucose and glycosylated haemoglobin significantly ($p < 0.001$, $p = 0.009$, $p = 0.006$, accordingly) without any major effects on the remaining parameters ($p > 0.05$) in comparison with the placebo group. Therefore, this reveals that nettle extracts have the potential of improving glycemic control in patients requiring insulin therapy (Kianbakht, Khalighi-Sigaroodi & Dabaghian, 2013).

4. *Cinnamomum verum* (Cinnamon)

Several studies have shown that adding cinnamon to our daily diet can aid in reducing glucose levels and is therefore currently marketed as a remedy in treating DM. A study was conducted by where 1 gram (g) of cinnamon was administered as a supplement to the usual care of diabetes in 109 T2DM patients for 90 days. The patients were allocated at random to either usual care with management changes by their physician or usual care with management plus consumption of 1g cinnamon daily. Patients consuming cinnamon showed a significant reduction in their HbA1c levels by 0.83% compared to 0.37% reduction in patients getting usual care only (Medagama, 2015).

5. *Momordica charantia* (Bitter gourd)

Several animal studies have illustrated hypoglycemic effects of the seeds, leaves and the whole plant of bitter gourd. Specifically, it enhances glucose tolerance, insulin sensitivity and lipolysis while suppressing postprandial hyperglycemia. Few studies have also claimed that the bitter gourd hypoglycemic effects were comparable to the oral drugs Chlorpropamide, Tolbutamide and Glibenclamide.

A clinical study was conducted by (Baldwa, Bhandari, Pangaria& Goyal, 1977) where 14 diabetics (T1DM and T2DM) patients and 5 healthy subjects were recruited to analyze the effects of bitter gourd in treating diabetes. 9 diabetic patients were administered with a subcutaneous injection. The remaining 5 diabetic patients together with 5 healthy subjects acted as controls and were given a placebo injection. There was a 21.5% reduction in blood glucose after 30 minutes and a 28% reduction after 12 hours. Whereas, those who received the placebo injection showed only a 5% reduction in glucose level regardless of whether they were healthy or diabetic. However, this was not a randomized trial and the subjects were not blinded(Leung, Birtwhistle, Kotecha, Hannah & Cuthbertson, 2009).

6. *Ocimum sanctum* (Basil)

Commonly known as Tulsi. These leaves are known for their diverse healing properties and numerous benefits. This includes strengthening the immune system in fighting viral and bacterial infections. It is said to enhance insulin secretion and pancreatic β-cell function as well as increase glucose uptake by the muscle cells. A study was carried out by Nottingham University where 60 T2DM patients were involved. 30 patients continued their usual medication whereas the other 30 patients consumed 250mg capsules of basil for 90 days. Significant improvement in glucose control was observed in patients who consumed the tulsi along with their usual medications. Spikes in blood glucose levels after consuming meals also showed major improvement.

7. *Eugenia jambolana* (Gooseberry)

Also known as Amla. It is an edible fruit that is eaten raw, pickled or cooked. Amla is served as a fruit as well as used to treat several disease conditions including diabetes. A clinical trial was conducted where 120 diabetic patients were recruited. The patients were assigned randomly into two groups: control or treatment. A supplement containing 5ml amla juice and other various hypoglycemic herbals (2.5g of ocimum sanctum leaves powder, aqueous extract of 60g of syzygiumcumini fruit, 10g seed powder of syzygiumcumini, 5g of momordicacharantia juice and 2g of gymnemasylvestre leaves) was consumed daily for 3 months by the treatment group. Whereas, a normal diet was given to the control group. The treatment group showed a significant reduction in fasting blood sugar whereas no changes were observed in the control group(Deng, 2012).

8. *Opuntia* (Prickly Pear Cactus)

It's a common cactus used as a herbal treatment for controlling glucose levels in Central and South America. The fruit and the fleshy stems are ingested as food and medicine. It contains high levels of pectin and soluble fibre that prevent sugar absorption. Promising results on dyslipidemia was observed in a pilot study of 24 non-diabetic male subjects. Particularly, prickly pear cactus reduced total cholesterol and triglycerides by 12%, LDL cholesterol by 15%, blood glucose and insulin levels by 11%. Two another controlled short term studies consisting of 14 and 22 human subjects reported a reduction in fasting glucose and insulin levels in patients with T2DM (Gouws, Georgousopoulou, Mellor, McKune & Naumovski, 2019).

HERBAL DRUGS MARKETED FOR TREATING DIABETES

Extensive research of herbal products for treating diabetes leads to the development of several antidiabetic medications in the market globally. Presently, there are various polyherbal formulated drugs for treating diabetes (Table 6). These formulations contain powders or aqueous extracts of many plant parts. They are commonly known as polyherbal formulation since they contain 3 to 25 herbs in the formula. The three most popular polyherbal drugs include; Glycoherb, Diabecon and Diabeta Plus.

Glycoherb is a polyherbal antihyperglycaemic formulation that has supplementary antioxidant and antihyperlipidemic properties. Whereas, Diabecon is known for promoting B-cell repair and regeneration, as well as secures the B-cell from oxidative stress. Diabecon mimics the action of insulin by decreasing HbA1c levels, regulating lipid profile and normalizing microalbuminuria. The herbal drug Diabeta Plus is an antidiabetic polyherbal formulation that contains extra properties of anti-stress, antihyperlipidemic and is hepatoprotective. Diabeta Plus relieves pain, pruritus, and polyuria which is caused by DM (Choudhury et al., 2018).

Table 5. Other effective herbs and fruits in managing plasma glucose levels (Choudhury et al., 2018; Nimesh, Tomar & Dhiman, 2019)

Herb / Fruit	Botanical Name	Result
Aloe vera	*Aloe barbadensis*	Increases insulin secretion and sensitivity
Fenugreek	*Trigonella foenum-graecum*	Alters secretion of insulin, decreases the pace of glucose absorption, aids in regenerating pancreatic B cells
Curry tree	*Murraya koenigii*	Increases insulin sensitivity, an inhibitor of alpha-glucosidase
Garlic	*Allium sativum*	Enhances plasma antioxidant activity and lipid metabolism
Onion	*Allium cepa*	Activates insulin secretion
Coriander	*Coriandrum sativum*	Increases B cells action, lowers blood sugar levels and synthesizes insulin
Guava	*Psidium guajava*	Improves blood sugar control
Mango	*Mangifera indica*	Reduces intestinal absorption of glucose
Papaya	*Carica papaya*	Lessens fasting blood sugar and total cholesterol levels
Castor	*Ricinus communis*	Raises levels of insulin and enhances lipid profile
Custard apple	*Annona squamosa*	Encourages insulin to be released from the pancreatic B cells
Pomegranate	*Punica granatum*	Lessens blood glucose and oxidative stress
White mulberry	*Morus alba*	Significantly decreases total blood glucose levels
Ginseng	*Panax ginseng*	Decrease blood glucose levels, improves insulin release from the pancreas and increases amount of insulin receptors
Chamomile	*Matricaria chamomilla*	Lowers blood sugar levels, prevents the progression of hyperglycemia and complications associated with diabetes
Dandelion	*Taraxacum officinale*	Helps our body to control and regulate blood sugar levels
Blueberry	*Vaccinium myrtillus*	Ability to get rid of excess sugar in the blood
Banaba	*Lagerstroemia speciosa*	Facilitates transport of glucose into cells and decreases the amounts of triglycerides

GENE THERAPY POTENTIAL IN TREATING DIABETES MELLITUS

Insulin injections and oral medications are essential therapeutic methods for treating T2DM. However, these agents have several adverse effects. Thus, novel alternative methods for treating T2DM including gene therapy have been examined.

Gene therapy is used to correct or compensate for the symptoms of diseases caused by abnormal or defective genes by introducing exogenous normal genes. The advantage of gene therapy is that diseases can possibly be cured only by a single treatment. Studies associated with genetics have found approximately 75 genetic loci linked to T2DM.

Table 6. Antidiabetic polyherbal formulations marketed

Brand	Dose Form	Ingredients	Mode of Action
Diacare	Powder	*Sanjeevanmool, himej, jambubeej, kadu, namejav, neem chal*	Lessens insulin resistance
Sharangdyab tea	Powder	*Green coffee beans, cinnamon, Boerhaviadiffusa*	Stimulates production of insulin
Pancreatic tonic	Liquid	*Tinosporacardifolia, Syzygiumcumini, Melia azadirachta, Momordicacharantia, Gymnenasylvestre, Aegle marmelos*	Regenerates pancreatic B cells
Stevia 33	Capsule	*Sudhshilajeet, syzygiumcumini, Tinosporacardifolia, Margosaindica, Gymnenasylvestre, Momordicacharantia, WithaniasomniferaKarela, jamun, chirayata, methi, kalijiri, indrayav, kutki*	Stimulates pancreas B cells
Diasulin	Tablet	*Cassia auriculata, Cocciniaindica, emblica officinalis, Gymnenasylvestre, Momordicacharantia, syzygiumcumini, Tinosporacardifolia, Trigonellafoenumgraecum*	Promotes secretion of insulin

Inhibiting the nucleotide-binding oligomerization domain-like receptor protein 3 (NLRP3) gene protects the pancreatic B-cells from apoptosis and prevents the development of T2DM. Moreover, glucose transporters (GLUTs) perform an essential role in liver and muscle glucose fluxes. The main targets for T2DM gene therapy are GLUT4 (*Slc2a4* gene) and GLUT2 (*Slc2a2* gene), since restoring the expressions of these genes in the liver and muscles enhance glycemic control. Sodium-glucose co-transporters (SGLTs) is accountable for the reabsorption of refining glucose from the kidneys into the bloodstream. Biopsy specimens taken from the human kidney displayed high expression of SGLT1 in patients with T2DM. SGLT1 mRNA is eminently correlated with HbA1c, fasting and postprandial plasma glucose. In comparison, SGLT2 and GLUT2 mRNA levels are down-regulated in patients with diabetes. Thence, a potent strategy to alleviate hyperglycemia in T2DM patients would be by inhibiting SGLT1 and enhancing SGLT2(Yue et al., 2019).

Fibroblast growth factors (FGFs), a class of potential targets are also examined concerning gene therapy. Various FGFs including FSF1, FGF19, and FGF21 have important roles in glucose homeostasis. Using mice models, FGF1 displayed diabetic phenotype with high blood glucose levels and insulin resistance. A single FGF1 injection intracerebroventricularly (ICV) brought glucose levels back to normal for relatively 18 weeks without any side effects such as weight gain or hypoglycemia in diabetic mice. The antidiabetic effect of FGF19 has been verified to be linked to the central nervous system. FF19 injection alleviate glycemia and increases insulin sensitivity by suppressing hypothalamic AGRP/NPY neuron activity. FGF21 plays a role in controlling lipid and glucose homeostasis. FGF21 is high in patients with impaired glucose tolerance and gradually rises in patients with T2DM. Therefore, targeting FGF21 has advantageous effects on glycemic control. Table 7 presents a list of genes categorized into different classes that hold potential for gene therapy.

Table 7. Genes categorized into distinct classes with capability for gene therapy

	Gene	Function
Genes that regulate glucose homeostasis	GLUTs	Re-absorption of filtered glucose from the kidney into the bloodstream
	SGLTs	An essential role in muscle and liver glucose fluxes
	FGFs	A significant role in glucose homeostasis
	SIRT6	Associated with GLUTs expression and increased glycolysis
Genes that enhance insulin secretion and sensitivity	GPGRs and their agonists	Stimulates secretion of GLP-1 and insulin
	GLP-1 and their analogues	Stimulates insulin secretion, gene expression and increases survival of β-cell
	CTB-APSL	Elevates insulin secretion and resistance
Genes that ameliorate diabetes-induced complications	ADPN	Improves diabetic nephropathy
	NLRP3	Improves diabetic cardiomyopathy
	MicroRNAs	Regulates diabetic microvasculature
	IL-1B	Linked with failure of β-cells

COMPLICATIONS ASSOCIATED WITH DIABETES MELLITUS

Diabetes is a disease strongly associated with both microvascular and macrovascular complications including retinopathy, nephropathy and neuropathy (microvascular) and ischemic heart disease, peripheral vascular disease and cerebrovascular disease (macrovascular), resulting in organ and tissue damage in approximately one-third to one-half of the patients with diabetes (Figure 6). Diabetic patients with cardiovascular and renal complications are the main cause of death globally which can be evaded through proper treatment (Salehi et al., 2019).

Chitotriosidase (CHIT 1), is a macrophage sourced enzyme which plays a role in immune response and is also high in diabetics. Studies have revealed, that chitotriosidase activity might be a marker for some diabetic complications (neuropathy and nephropathy) and is closely related to glycated haemoglobin (HBA1C) levels (Turan, Sozmen, Eltutan & Sozmen, 2017).

LIFESTYLE AND GENETICS

Various lifestyle factors lead to the development of T2DM. These include consumption of alcohol, poor diet, smoking cigarettes and lack of physical activities. Obesity is known to be responsible for approximately 55% of the cases. The rise in the rates of childhood obesity between the 1960s to 2000s has supposedly led to the growth of T2DM in adolescents and children. Therefore, it would be beneficial for patients to attain a medical nutrition evaluation and lifestyle advice according to their functional and physical abilities (Olokoba, Obateru & Olokoba, 2012). Consuming fresh fruits, vegetables, whole grains and limiting alcohol should also be encouraged. Gradual weight loss of approximately 5%-7% of the current body weight may decrease insulin resistance and other risk factors. This can be accomplished through calorie reduction and regular aerobic physical activities.

Figure 6. Major complications associated with diabetes (Jiang & Dutta, 2017)

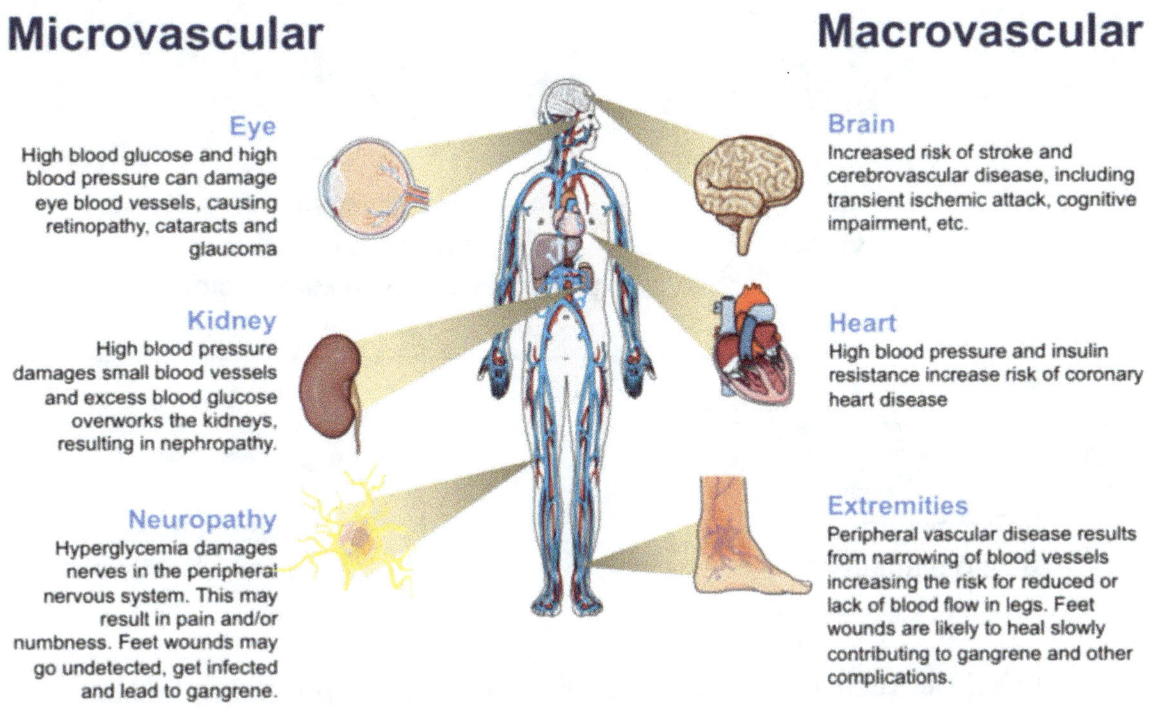

Moreover, there is a firm inheritable genetic connection to developing T2DM. Having relatives particularly first degree with type 2 diabetes raises the chances of developing it considerably. The genes identified to have a significant association in developing T2DM include PPARG, KCNJ11, TCF7L2, NOTCH2, CDKAL1, JAZF1, HHEX, KCNJ11, WFS1, and FTO. In an overview, genetic and environmental risk factors can impact insulin levels, as represented in Figure 7 (Sun, Yu & Hu, 2014).

GUT MICROBIOME AND TYPE 2 DIABETES MELLITUS

In the human body, the gut microbiome is known to be a large system. Eukaryotes, bacteria and archaea living in the gut are collectively called the gut microbiota. They are approximately more than 1000 types of the gut microbiome that protects us against pathogens by either fighting for nutrition and space or by enhancing our immune system. Probiotics (beneficial, live commensal bacteria) has been utilized for a long time to promote the growth of beneficial bacteria. However, despite the advantages of gut microbiomes, microbial imbalance also known as dysbiosis, can lead to various diseases as well as worsen the severity of diseases such as colorectal cancer, Crohn's disease and ulcerative colitis. Dysbiosis has also been associated with several metabolic disorders including diabetes. Recently, the association between the gut microbiome and T2DM has gained tremendous attention. Studies conducted have preliminarily confirmed that gut microbiome disorders are linked closely to the onset of T2DM and insulin resistance. However, can herbal medications be used to treat T2DM by gut microbiome regulation?

Figure 7. An illustration of how genetic and environmental risk factors lead to the development of diabetes (Skyler et al., 2016)

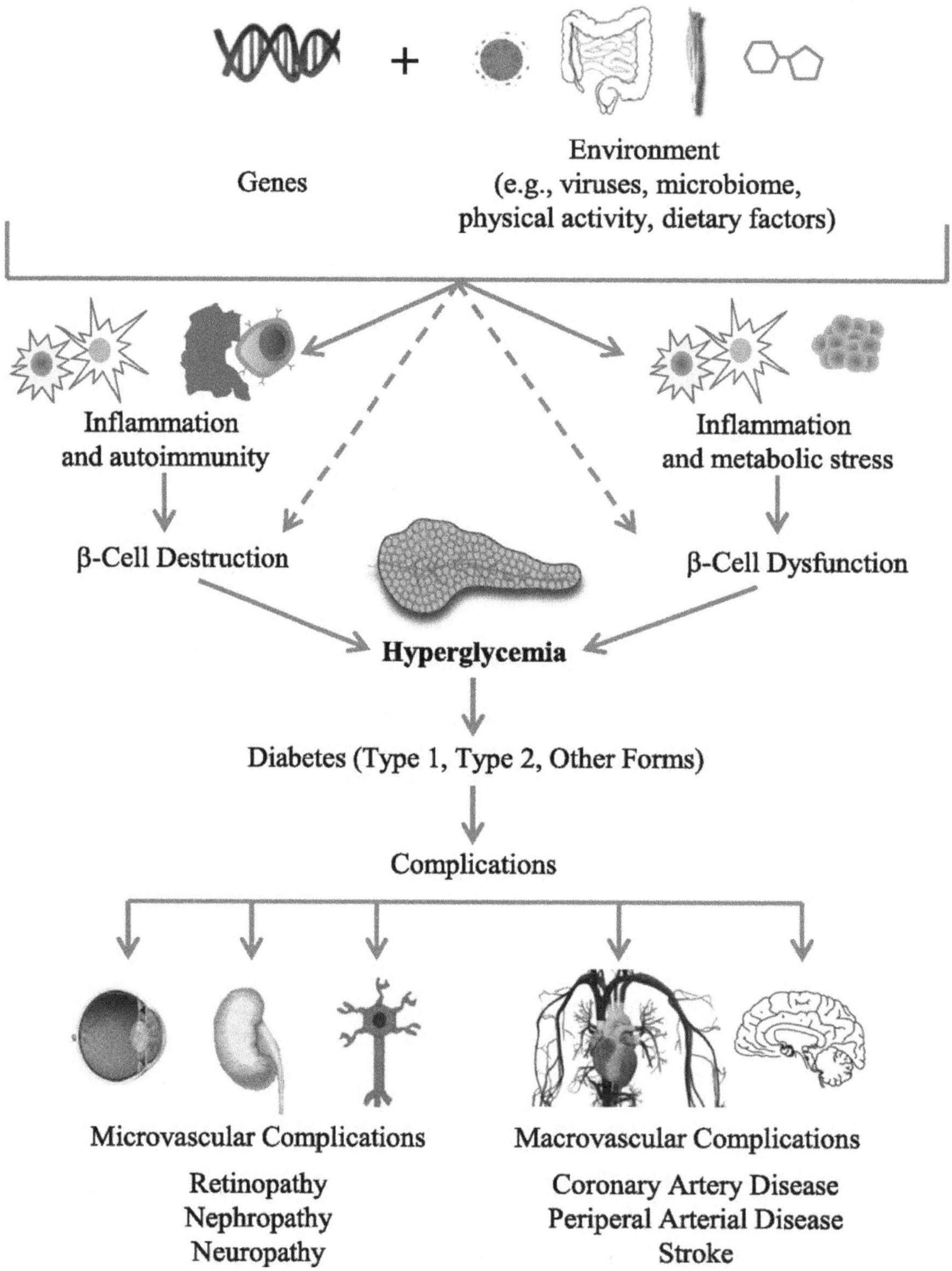

(Wang, Kim, Han & Kim, 2017) established that Ephedra sinica, an evergreen shrub, native to Mongolia, Russia, and northeastern China is highly effective in decreasing fasting blood glucose by amending the gut microbiome composition, particularly Blautia, Roseburia and Clostridium. Another herbal formulation mixture known as Qijian, is very rich in bacteroidetes and is demonstrated to be effective and a safe mixture in treating T2DM in a rat model. Moreover, the gut microbiome can be altered with several hosts or environmental conditions beginning from the genotype of the host, stress, diet or medications. A strictly controlled animal and human studies are warranted to further justify and explain these complicated issues and the interrelationship of microbiome and diseases (Sharma & Tripathi, 2019; Pang et al., 2019).

PREVENTION

The rise in the prevalence and the high economic costs of T2DM urges compelling circumstances for its prevention. The strategies that can be used to prevent or to delay the onset of T2DM include the following:

1. Annual monitoring for individuals with prediabetes is recommended. Prediabetes is the term utilized for individuals whose glucose levels are higher than the normal range but yet do not meet the criteria for the diagnosis of diabetes. Prediabetes must not be perceived as a clinical entity alone but rather as a greater risk for developing diabetes.
2. Bodyweight should be maintained by increasing the intensity of physical activities and reducing calorie intake. A low-fat meal plan and monitoring eating patterns may be beneficial.

In the Finnish Diabetes Prevention Study (FDPS), 522 males with a mean age of 55 years and 31kg/m2 mean body mass index (BMI) was enlisted. The participants with impaired glucose tolerance (IGT) were selected randomly to receive either a brief diet and exercise counselling (control group) or comprehensive guidelines on reducing weight (>5%), reducing food intake (<30%), increasing physical exercises (>150min/week) and received sessions with a dietician 7 times in the first year (intervention group). The number of participants progressing towards T2DM was 3.2% in the intervention group versus 7.8% in the control group.

3.2 years later, there was a risk reduction of developing DM by 58% in the intervention group in contrast to the control group. These results highlighted the importance of a healthy diet and an active lifestyle in preventing the development of T2DM (Younis, Soran & Farook, 2004).

A study conducted by (Oldroyd, Unwin, White, Mathers &Alberti, 2006) analyzed lifestyle amendments for improving an individual's health with IGT. 39 intervention participants were instructed to consume more vegetables and fruits, decrease sugar and fat intake. In addition, 30 minutes of aerobic activities (at least once a week) was necessitated. After 24 months, the improvement in the 2 hours of plasma glucose levels did not significantly vary between the control and the intervention group. Nevertheless, a greater number of participants (20%) from the intervention group reverted to normoglycaemia (normal glycaemic status) in contrast to the control group (13%) after 24 months.

These two studies conducted certainly affirmed the effects of lifestyle modifications concerning to T2DM. However, it is thus far unknown if these lifestyle modifications can be maintained in the long-term, whether the positive outcome described in the studies conducted will be replicated in clinical practice rather than in a research framework.

ECONOMIC BURDEN

The economic aspects of DM are at present attracting considerable attention and scrutiny as healthcare managements are going through a burden to attain more within confined resources. It poses a major economic threat with regards to direct health care costs and indirect costs emerging from the patient's disabilities and premature mortality. In addition, it is becoming a costly and dangerous biomedical task since the quantity of individuals suffering from this metabolic disorder has doubled over the last thirty years (Salehi et al., 2019). A major barrier in the treatment of diabetes is the cost of anti-hyperglycemic medications, specifically insulin (McEwen et al., 2017). In the United Kingdom, the cost of treating T2DM was estimated to be 21.8 billion pounds (direct cost 8.8 billion pounds and indirect cost 13.0 billion pounds) in the year 2010/2011. In the year 2035/2036, it is predicted to be 35.6 billion pounds (direct cost 15.1 billion pounds and indirect cost 20.1 billion pounds) (Alam, Islam, Kamal & Gan, 2019). Thence, immediate action is necessary to manage the tide of diabetes and to propose a cost-effective treatment strategy to overturn this trend (Rani Javalkar, 2019).

CONCLUSION

DM is a health problem that is causing significant distress globally. Lack of effective prevention and management programs will lead to an ongoing significant rise in diabetes, having crucial consequences on the lifespan and health of the population worldwide. This will, in turn, affect the world economy. To alleviate the incidence of DM, an active and healthy lifestyle including a dietary pattern with interventions against the increase in levels of obesity must be promoted and taken into consideration. In addition, the key to controlling this emerging epidemic disorder is to enhance education and screening for diabetic and prediabetic patients.

Herbal formulations containing anti-diabetic properties are now under scrutiny due to the complications associated with the usage of synthetic medications. The holistic quality of herbal medicines is superior and are, therefore, a preferable alternative for treating DM. However, the knowledge in this sector is still confined and further comprehensive study into identifying the active ingredients of various botanicals and their extracts, with affirmative anti-diabetic activity and revealing their mechanism of action is vital. In a nutshell, herbal medicines utilized as a primary treatment or as an adjunct therapy to synthetic medications is a hopeful therapy. Aggressive efforts are nevertheless earnestly necessary to lessen and ultimately cure this chronic metabolic disorder in the forthcoming years.

FUTURE RESEARCH DIRECTION

Regardless of the considerable advance in care, the management and treatment of DM yet remain elusive. Extensive research must be carried out consistently to formulate the most effective methods in managing and treating diabetic patients. The major techniques to look forward to in the near future include microchips, nanorobots, bionic pancreas and nano-herbal drugs.

A novel method of identifying T1DM symptoms earlier (warning signs) may prevent the disorder from developing. Scientists from the University of California and Stanford have constructed an inexpensive nanotech-based microchip that can identify T1DM antibodies much earlier in comparison to the current diagnostic methods. This microchip was put to test in six subjects who did not have diabetes. In two of the six subjects, the microchip recognized negative antibodies a year earlier whereas, in one of the subjects, they were recognized 4 years in advance. False positives were not identified in healthy subjects. This microchip has yet to be tested in larger clinical trials to confirm the findings.

Nanorobots are contemplated to be a new possibility in the near future to diagnose and treat diabetes. At present, diabetic patients take minuscule blood samples several times a day to control levels of glucose. This can get very bothersome and uncomfortable. Therefore, nanorobotics can be used to observe levels of sugar in the body via constant glucose monitoring. The size (2 micrometer) allows it to freely function inside the body. It utilizes an embedded chemosensor that involves modulation of hSGLT3 protein glucosensor activity. This nanorobot can efficiently determine when patients need to inject insulin or if any prescribed medicines need to be taken. A glucose level of around 130 mg/dl is maintained. The data obtained can be transferred to the patient's mobile phone automatically through RF signals. If the glucose reaches a critical level, an alarm is emitted to the phone (Kumar, Nasim & Abraham, 2018).

Several companies are in the process of developing non-invasive procedures to replace finger pricking. A device known as GlucoTrack measures glucose utilizing electromagnetic waves. It is at present already available in Europe. Another device known as GlucoSense (Figure 8) currently sold in London uses laser light to measure sugar levels (Fernández, 2018). Therefore, this may be utilized globally in the upcoming years.

Figure 8. GlucoseSense device (Fernández, 2018)

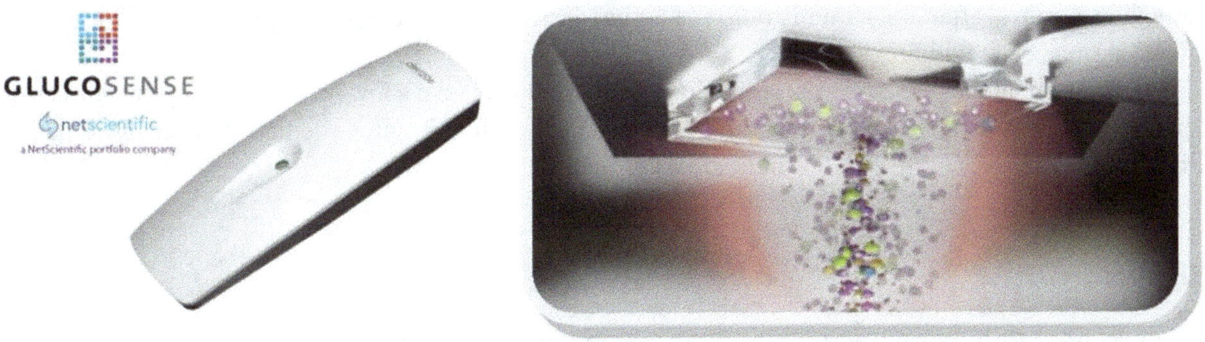

Bionic pancreas might be an alternative to aid T1DM patients in the future. A smartphone can be used to command a computer program that manages the artificial pancreas. It will be linked to a glucose monitor sensor and an insulin pump to determine blood sugar patterns and manage the delivery of insulin (Figure 9). Future bionic pancreas technology will be very effective if a closed-loop system algorithm functions as envisioned (Whelan, 2019).

Moreover, herbal medicines need to be further assessed in human subjects via a well-constructed, large-scale clinical trial. Considering that herbal formulas consist of various ingredients, it is challenging to precisely identify the active ingredients and the toxic ingredients. The quality and quantity of herbs in the final product should also be evaluated. Herbal medicines must be verified and certified specifically by the authorities of the country to boost the patient's assurance in the efficacy of these drugs (Guo-Ming et al., 2019).

Figure 9. Automated treatment with bionic pancreas (Fernández, 2016)

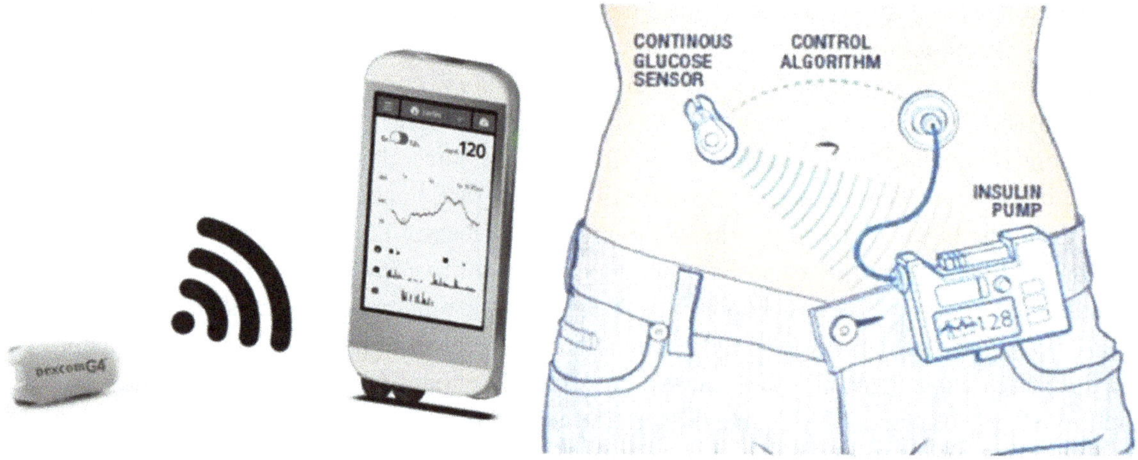

Furthermore, we should look forward to the development of nano-sized herbal drugs and their precise targeted delivery for treating diabetic patients in the future. This will aid in overcoming the limitations and complications associated with conventional drugs utilized to treat DM. In addition, the prospects of nanoformulation of herbal drugs include "smart drugs" which will only activate when required. This nanoformulation along with incorporating nanocarriers may increase the efficacy and absorption of certain herbal drugs which are at present considered to be mediocre. Poor solubility, permeability and immediate removal after oral administration of herbal drugs could be resolved in the near future (Amjad, Jafri, Sharma & Serajuddin, 2019).

All these techniques are currently still being refined and may take a few years until they are clinically beneficial. Nevertheless, regardless of what the future may bring, it will undeniably make an immense difference in the lives of millions of individuals globally.

REFERENCES

Adapa, D., & TK, S. (2020). A Review on Diabetes Mellitus: Complications, Management and Treatment Modalities. *Journal of Medical and Health Sciences*, *4*(3).

Ahmad, K. (2014). Insulin sources and types: A review of insulin in terms of its mode on diabetes mellitus. *Journal of Traditional Chinese Medicine*, *34*(2), 234–237. doi:10.1016/S0254-6272(14)60084-4 PMID:24783939

Al-Salameh, A., Bucher, S., Bauduceau, B., Benattar-Zibi, L., Berrut, G., Bertin, P., & … . (2018). Sex Differences in the Occurrence of Major Clinical Events in Elderly People with Type 2 Diabetes Mellitus Followed up in the General Practice. *Experimental and Clinical Endocrinology & Diabetes*, (2), 77–132. doi:10.1055/a-0662-5923 PMID:30134475

Alam, F., Islam, M., Kamal, M., & Gan, S. (2019). Updates on Managing Type 2 Diabetes Mellitus with Natural Products: Towards Antidiabetic Drug Development. *Current Medicinal Chemistry*, *25*(39), 5395–5431. doi:10.2174/0929867323666160813222436 PMID:27528060

Amjad, S., Jafri, A., Sharma, A., & Serajuddin, M. (2019). A novel strategy of nanotized herbal drugs and their delivery in the treatment of diabetes: Present status and future prospects. *Journal of Herbal Medicine*, *17-18*, 100279. doi:10.1016/j.hermed.2019.100279

Baldwa, V., Bhandari, C., Pangaria, A., & Goyal, R. (1977). Clinical Trial in Patients with Diabetes Mellitus of an Insulin-like Compound Obtained from Plant Source. *Upsala Journal of Medical Sciences*, *82*(1), 39–41. doi:10.3109/03009737709179057 PMID:20078273

Baynest, H. (2015). Classification, Pathophysiology, Diagnosis and Management of Diabetes Mellitus. *Journal of Diabetes & Metabolism*, *06*(05). Advance online publication. doi:10.4172/2155-6156.1000541

Blair, M. (2016). Diabetes Mellitus Review. *Urologic Nursing*, *36*(1), 27. doi:10.7257/1053-816X.2016.36.1.27 PMID:27093761

Blum, A. (2018). Freestyle Libre Glucose Monitoring System. *Clinical Diabetes*, *36*(2), 203–204. doi:10.2337/cd17-0130 PMID:29686463

Cersosimo, E., & DeFronzo, R. (2006). Insulin resistance and endothelial dysfunction: The road map to cardiovascular diseases. *Diabetes/Metabolism Research and Reviews*, *22*(6), 423–436. doi:10.1002/dmrr.634 PMID:16506274

Choudhury, H., Pandey, M., Hua, C., Mun, C., Jing, J., Kong, L., Ern, L. Y., Ashraf, N. A., Kit, S. W., Yee, T. S., Pichika, M. R., Gorain, B., & Kesharwani, P. (2018). An update on natural compounds in the remedy of diabetes mellitus: A systematic review. *Journal of Traditional and Complementary Medicine*, *8*(3), 361–376. doi:10.1016/j.jtcme.2017.08.012 PMID:29992107

Chuengsamarn, S., Rattanamongkolgul, S., Luechapudiporn, R., Phisalaphong, C., & Jirawatnotai, S. (2012). Curcumin Extract for Prevention of Type 2 Diabetes. *Diabetes Care*, *35*(11), 2121–2127. doi:10.2337/dc12-0116 PMID:22773702

Clinic, C. (2016). *Insulin Pumps*. Cleveland Clinic. Available at: https://my.clevelandclinic.org/health/articles/9811-insulin-pumps

Costello, R., & Shivkumar, A. (2019). *Sulfonylureas*. StatPearls Publishing.

Deng, R. (2012). A Review of the Hypoglycemic Effects of Five Commonly Used Herbal Food Supplements. *Recent Patents on Food, Nutrition & Agriculture*, *4*(1), 50–60. doi:10.2174/1876142911204010050 PMID:22329631

Ekor, M. (2014). The growing use of herbal medicines: Issues relating to adverse reactions and challenges in monitoring safety. *Frontiers in Pharmacology*, *4*, 177. doi:10.3389/fphar.2013.00177 PMID:24454289

Fernández, C. (2016). *The Future of Diabetes Treatment: Is A Cure Possible?* Available at: https://www.labiotech.eu/in-depth/diabetes-treatment-cure-review/

Fernández, C. (2018). *Needle-Free Diabetes Care: 8 Devices That Painlessly Measure Blood Glucose*. Available at: https://www.labiotech.eu/diabetes/needle-free-glucose-monitoring-for-diabetes-medtech/

Fowler, M. (2008). Microvascular and Macrovascular Complications of Diabetes. *Clinical Diabetes*, *26*(2), 77–82. doi:10.2337/diaclin.26.2.77

Godinho, R., Mega, C., Teixeira-de-Lemos, E., Carvalho, E., Teixeira, F., Fernandes, R., & Reis, F. (2015). The Place of Dipeptidyl Peptidase-4 Inhibitors in Type 2 Diabetes Therapeutics: A "Me Too" or "the Special One" Antidiabetic Class? *Journal of Diabetes Research, 2015*, 1–28. doi:10.1155/2015/806979 PMID:26075286

Gouws, C., Georgousopoulou, E., Mellor, D., McKune, A., & Naumovski, N. (2019). Effects of the Consumption of Prickly Pear Cacti (Opuntia spp.) and its Products on Blood Glucose Levels and Insulin: A Systematic Review. *Medicina*, *55*(5), 138. doi:10.3390/medicina55050138 PMID:31096667

Guo-Ming, P., Fang-Xu, L., Yong, Y., Yin, Z., Li-Li, K., Pu, Z., & … . (2019). Herbal medicine in the treatment of patients with type 2 diabetes mellitus. *Chinese Medical Journal*, *132*(1), 78–85. doi:10.1097/CM9.0000000000000006 PMID:30628962

Harvard, P. (2018). *Type 1 Diabetes Mellitus - Harvard Health*. Retrieved 27 August 2020, from https://www.health.harvard.edu/a_to_z/type-1-diabetes-mellitus-a-to-z

Heppner, K., & Perez-Tilve, D. (2015). GLP-1 based therapeutics: Simultaneously combating T2DM and obesity. *Frontiers in Neuroscience*, *9*. Advance online publication. doi:10.3389/fnins.2015.00092 PMID:25852463

Hinnen, D., Nielsen, L., Waninger, A., & Kushner, P. (2006). Incretin mimetics and DPP-IV inhibitors: New paradigms for the treatment of type 2 diabetes. *Journal of the American Board of Family Medicine*, *19*(6), 612–618. doi:10.3122/jabfm.19.6.612 PMID:17090794

Hoogwerf, B., Doshi, K., & Diab, D. (2008). Pramlintide, the synthetic analogue of amylin: Physiology, pathophysiology, and effects on glycemic control, body weight, and selected biomarkers of vascular risk. *Vascular Health and Risk Management*, *4*(2), 355–362. doi:10.2147/VHRM.S1978 PMID:18561511

Hope, I. (2018). *Diabetes Pathophysiology & Diseases Process (Diagram).* Retrieved 27 August 2020, from https://rnspeak.com/diabetes-pathophysiology-diseases-process-diagram/

Horakova, O., Kroupova, P., Bardova, K., Buresova, J., Janovska, P., Kopecky, J., & Rossmeisl, M. (2019). Metformin acutely lowers blood glucose levels by inhibition of intestinal glucose transport. *Scientific Reports*, *9*(1), 6156. Advance online publication. doi:10.103841598-019-42531-0 PMID:30992489

Hsia, D., Grove, O., & Cefalu, W. (2017). An Update on SGLT2 Inhibitors for the Treatment of Diabetes Mellitus. *Current Opinion in Endocrinology, Diabetes, and Obesity*, *24*(1), 73–79. PMID:27898586

International Diabetes Federation. (2017). *IDF Diabetes Atlas* (Eighth edition 2017). doi:10.1016/S0140-6736(16)31679-8

Jeong, S., Min Cho, J., Kwon, Y., Kim, S., Yeob Shin, D., & Ho Lee, J. (2019). Chitosan oligosaccharide (GO2KA1) improves postprandial glycemic response in subjects with impaired glucose tolerance and impaired fasting glucose and in healthy subjects: A crossover, randomized controlled trial. *Nutrition & Diabetes*, *9*(1), 31. Advance online publication. doi:10.103841387-019-0099-4 PMID:31685797

Jiang, J., & Dutta, S. (2017). *PDB101: Global Health: Diabetes Mellitus: Monitoring: Complications.* Retrieved 24 August 2020, from https://pdb101.rcsb.org/global-health/diabetes-mellitus/monitoring/complications

Joslin, D. (2020). *Advantages and disadvantages of insulin pump*. Retrieved 24 August 2020, from https://onlineclasses.joslin.org/info/the_advantages_and_disadvantages_of_an_insulin_pump.html

Kaul, K., Tarr, J., Ahmad, S., Kohner, E., & Chibber, R. (2012). Introduction to diabetes mellitus. *Advances in Experimental Medicine and Biology*, *771*, 1–11. PMID:23393665

Kaur, R., Mahajan, P., & Goswami, M. (2018). Diabetes mellitus: An emerging risk factor to public health. *World Journal of Pharmaceutical Research*, *7*(12), 257–281.

Kharroubi, A., & Darwish, H. (2015). Diabetes mellitus: The epidemic of the century. *World Journal of Diabetes*, *6*(6), 850–867. doi:10.4239/wjd.v6.i6.850 PMID:26131326

Kianbakht, S., Khalighi-Sigaroodi, F., & Dabaghian, F. (2013). Improved Glycemic Control in Patients with Advanced Type 2 Diabetes Mellitus Taking Urticadioica Leaf Extract: A Randomized Double-Blind Placebo-Controlled Clinical Trial. *Clinical Laboratory*, *59*(09+10/2013). Advance online publication. doi:10.7754/Clin.Lab.2012.121019 PMID:24273930

Kooti, W., Farokhipour, M., Asadzadeh, Z., Ashtary-Larky, D., & Asadi-Samani, M. (2016). The role of medicinal plants in the treatment of diabetes: A systematic review. *Electronic Physician*, *8*(1), 1832–1842. doi:10.19082/1832 PMID:26955456

Kousaxidis, A., Petrou, A., Lavrentaki, V., Fesatidou, M., Nicolaou, I., & Geronikaki, A. (2020). Aldose reductase and protein tyrosine phosphatase 1B inhibitors as a promising therapeutic approach for diabetes mellitus. *European Journal of Medicinal Chemistry*, *112742*. Advance online publication. doi:10.1016/j.ejmech.2020.112742 PMID:32871344

Kposowa, A. (2013). Mortality from Diabetes by Hispanic Groups: Evidence from the US National Longitudinal Mortality Study. *International Journal of Population Research*, *2013*, 1–12. doi:10.1155/2013/571306

Krzewska, A., & Ben-Skowronek, I. (2016). Effect of Associated Autoimmune Diseases on Type 1 Diabetes Mellitus Incidence and Metabolic Control in Children and Adolescents. *BioMed Research International*, *2016*, 1–12. doi:10.1155/2016/6219730 PMID:27525273

Kumar, S., Nasim, B., & Abraham, E. (2018). *Nanorobots a Future Device for Diagnosis and Treatment*. Retrieved 29 February 2020, from https://www.ommegaonline.org/article-details/NANOROBOTS-A-FUTURE-DEVICE-FOR-DIAGNOSIS-AND-TREATMENT/1815

Leung, L., Birtwhistle, R., Kotecha, J., Hannah, S., & Cuthbertson, S. (2009). Anti-diabetic and hypoglycaemic effects of Momordicacharantia (bitter melon): A mini review. *British Journal of Nutrition*, *102*(12), 1703–1708. doi:10.1017/S0007114509992054 PMID:19825210

Luna, B., & Feinglos, M. (2001). Oral Agents in the Management of Type 2 Diabetes Mellitus. *American Family Physician*, *63*(9), 1747–1757. PMID:11352285

McEwen, L., Casagrande, S., Kuo, S., & Herman, W. (2017). Why Are Diabetes Medications So Expensive and What Can Be Done to Control Their Cost? *Current Diabetes Reports*, *17*(9), 17. doi:10.100711892-017-0893-0 PMID:28741264

Medagama, A. (2015). The glycaemic outcomes of Cinnamon, a review of the experimental evidence and clinical trials. *Nutrition Journal*, *14*(1), 108. Advance online publication. doi:10.118612937-015-0098-9 PMID:26475130

Nimesh, S., Tomar, R., & Dhiman, S. (2019). Medicinal Herbal Plants and Allopathic Drugs to Treat Diabetes Mellitus: A glance. *Advances In Pharmacology And Clinical Trials*, *4*(1), 1–13.

Oldroyd, J., Unwin, N., White, M., Mathers, J., & Alberti, K. (2006). Randomised controlled trial evaluating lifestyle interventions in people with impaired glucose tolerance. *Diabetes Research and Clinical Practice*, *72*(2), 117–127. doi:10.1016/j.diabres.2005.09.018 PMID:16297488

Olokoba, A., Obateru, O., & Olokoba, L. (2012). Type 2 Diabetes Mellitus: A Review of Current Trends. *Oman Medical Journal*, *27*(4), 269–273. doi:10.5001/omj.2012.68 PMID:23071876

Pang, G., Li, F., Yan, Y., Zhang, Y., Kong, L., Zhu, P., Wang, K.-F., Zhang, F., Liu, B., & Lu, C. (2019). Herbal medicine in the treatment of patients with type 2 diabetes mellitus. *Chinese Medical Journal*, *132*(1), 78–85. doi:10.1097/CM9.0000000000000006 PMID:30628962

Philipson, L. (2017). *Monogenic Diabetes (Neonatal Diabetes Mellitus & MODY) | NIDDK*. Retrieved 22 August 2020, from https://www.niddk.nih.gov/health-information/diabetes/overview/what-is-diabetes/monogenic-neonatal-mellitus-mody

Pinhas-Hamiel, O., & Zeitler, P. (2005). The global spread of type 2 diabetes mellitus in children and adolescents. *The Journal of Pediatrics*, *146*(5), 693–700. doi:10.1016/j.jpeds.2004.12.042 PMID:15870677

Pivari, F., Mingione, A., Brasacchio, C., & Soldati, L. (2019). Curcumin and Type 2 Diabetes Mellitus: Prevention and Treatment. *Nutrients*, *11*(8), 1837. doi:10.3390/nu11081837 PMID:31398884

Punthakee, Z., Goldenberg, R., & Katz, P. (2018). Definition, Classification and Diagnosis of Diabetes, Prediabetes and Metabolic Syndrome. *Canadian Journal of Diabetes*, *42*, S10–S15. doi:10.1016/j.jcjd.2017.10.003 PMID:29650080

Rani Javalkar, S. (2019). The economic burden of health expenditure on diabetes mellitus among urban poor: A cross sectional study. *International Journal of Community Medicine And Public Health*, *6*(3), 1162. doi:10.18203/2394-6040.ijcmph20190604

Rogal, J., Zbinden, A., Schenke-Layland, K., & Loskill, P. (2019). Stem-cell based organ-on-a-chip models for diabetes research. *Advanced Drug Delivery Reviews*, *140*, 101–128. doi:10.1016/j.addr.2018.10.010 PMID:30359630

Salehi, B., Ata, A., Anil, V., Kumar, N., Sharopov, F., Ramírez-Alarcón, K., Ruiz-Ortega, A., & … . (2019). Antidiabetic Potential of Medicinal Plants and Their Active Components. *Biomolecules*, *9*(10), 551. doi:10.3390/biom9100551 PMID:31575072

Salman, R., AlSayyad, A., & Ludwig, C. (2019). Type 2 diabetes and healthcare resource utilisation in the Kingdom of Bahrain. *BMC Health Services Research*, *19*(1), 939. Advance online publication. doi:10.118612913-019-4795-5 PMID:31805932

Sarkar, S., Das, D., Dutta, P., Kalita, J., Wann, S., & Manna, P. (2020). Chitosan: A promising therapeutic agent and effective drug delivery system in managing diabetes mellitus. *Carbohydrate Polymers, 247*, 116594. doi:10.1016/j.carbpol.2020.116594 PMID:32829787

Sharma, S., & Tripathi, P. (2019). Gut microbiome and type 2 diabetes: Where we are and where to go? *The Journal of Nutritional Biochemistry, 63*, 101–108. doi:10.1016/j.jnutbio.2018.10.003 PMID:30366260

Sherwani, S., Khan, H., Ekhzaimy, A., Masood, A., & Sakharkar, M. (2016). Significance of HbA1c Test in Diagnosis and Prognosis of Diabetic Patients. *Biomarker Insights, 11. BMI, S38440*. Advance online publication. doi:10.4137/bmi.s38440 PMID:27398023

Skyler, J., Bakris, G., Bonifacio, E., Darsow, T., Eckel, R., Groop, L., Groop, P.-H., Handelsman, Y., Insel, R. A., Mathieu, C., McElvaine, A. T., Palmer, J. P., Pugliese, A., Schatz, D. A., Sosenko, J. M., Wilding, J. P. H., & Ratner, R. E. (2016). Differentiation of Diabetes by Pathophysiology, Natural History, and Prognosis. *Diabetes, 66*(2), 241–255. doi:10.2337/db16-0806 PMID:27980006

Sun, N. (2014). *Pathophysiology | Diabetes Mellitus Type 2*. Retrieved 27 August 2020, from https://u.osu.edu/diabetestype2/diagnosis/

Sun, X., Yu, W., & Hu, C. (2014). Genetics of Type 2 Diabetes: Insights into the Pathogenesis and Its Clinical Application. *BioMed Research International, 2014*, 1–15. doi:10.1155/2014/926713 PMID:24864266

Turan, E., Sozmen, B., Eltutan, M., & Sozmen, E. (2017). Serum chitotriosidase enzyme activity is closely related to HbA1c levels and the complications in patients with diabetes mellitus type 2. *Diabetes & Metabolic Syndrome, 11*, S503–S506. doi:10.1016/j.dsx.2017.03.044 PMID:28392356

Wang, J., Kim, B., Han, K., & Kim, H. (2017). Ephedra-Treated Donor-Derived Gut Microbiota Transplantation Ameliorates High Fat Diet-Induced Obesity in Rats. *International Journal of Environmental Research and Public Health, 14*(6), 555. doi:10.3390/ijerph14060555 PMID:28545248

Whelan, K. (2019). *Artificial Pancreas—The Future for Diabetes Treatment? – Medical Expo e-Magazine*. Retrieved 29 February 2020, from http://emag.medicalexpo.com/artificial-pancreas-the-future-for-diabetes-treatment/

Younis, N., Soran, H., & Farook, S. (2004). The prevention of type 2 diabetes mellitus: Recent advances. *QJM, 97*(7), 451–455. doi:10.1093/qjmed/hch077 PMID:15208433

Yue, Z., Zhang, L., Li, C., Chen, Y., Tai, Y., Shen, Y., & Sun, Z. (2019). Advances and potential of gene therapy for type 2 diabetes mellitus. *Biotechnology, Biotechnological Equipment, 33*(1), 1150–1157. doi:10.1080/13102818.2019.1643783

Chapter 2
Application of Some Medicinal Plants and Their Constituents in the Treatment of Diabetes Mellitus

Raghunath Satpathy
https://orcid.org/0000-0001-5296-8492
Gangadhar Meher University, India

ABSTRACT

The rapidly increasing incidence of diabetes mellitus as a chronic disease is becoming a serious threat to mankind health in all parts of the world. However, the currently available therapies are not of much use in prevention or reduction of disease. There are a large number of plants and natural biomolecules that have been discussed in the literature for their antidiabetic effects. Recently, the screening of many types of plant derived alpha-amylase, alpha-glucosidase inhibitors and other compounds that reduce the glucose level in the body and have fewer side effects has been successfully isolated. In this chapter, the mechanism of diabetes mellitus has been discussed. Also, the plants having anti-diabetic property along with its constituents has been presented summarized with the available literature resource. In addition to this, the common strategy that is followed for inhibition assay for an anti-diabetic compound has been discussed. Finally, future opportunities and challenges in this research area are proposed.

INTRODUCTION

Diabetes mellitus commonly known as diabetes, is a metabolic disorder characterized by enhanced blood glucose level due to inadequate amount of insulin hormone secretion from the pancreatic gland (Owolabi et al., 2014). The rapid increase in the numbers of diabetes patients throughout the globe is a great concern in recent times. As per a recent report, about 177 million of the global population live with diabetes and this figure is more likely to increase by 2030 (World Health Organisation, 2000; Ndarubu et al., 2019). Considering the severity of the disease, the diabetes mellitus, is considered as one of the

DOI: 10.4018/978-1-7998-4808-0.ch002

five leading causes of death in the world, also it affects the carbohydrate, fat, and protein metabolism and ultimately causes the disorder. A worldwide survey report says that the disease spreads progressively, that affects nearly 10% of the population in each year (Venkatachalam et al., 2017). If left untreated, diabetes mellitus can cause many more complications such as diabetic ketoacidosis and non-ketotic hyperosmolar coma (Kitabchi et al., 2009). Therapeutic point of view, the available synthetic drugs are associated with a large number of side effects, therefore continuous taking these medicine can create side effects. Therefore, the drugs that are of plant origin are preferred as it is associated with less or no side effects, hence increasing attention for all (Monday et al.,2013). Fortunately, so many of the plant extract has shown their significant anti-diabetic properties with more efficacy than oral hypoglycaemic agents that are currently used in clinical therapeutics. Several categories of diverse plant products are available called as antidiabetic *active compounds* used as alternatives for the treatment of diabetes. One of the basic mechanism of treating the disease is carbohydrate absorption in the body after food intake is to be reduced in case of diabetes patients. The theory behind the mechanism is that the complex polysaccharides are broken down to simpler form such as glucose and fructose (monosaccharide) by the enteric enzymes, like pancreatic α-amylase and α-glucosidases. Then these monosaccharides transported from the intestinal lumen to the bloodstream, thereby increasing the sugar level. Hence finding suitable inhibitor compounds (hypoglycemic agents) to the above enzymes is essential for the treatment of diabetes patient. Currently, most commonly practised treatment methods include different oral hypoglycaemic agents described in the below section (Gallaghe et al., 2015; Ortiz-Andrade RR et al., 2007).

Throughout the world, attempts have been made to discover as well as to isolate potential phytoconstituents from the plants those having a broader range of biological activities (Bailey & Day, 1989). However, the details about the major categories of phytochemicals responsible for the antidiabetic activity has not been studied so far. Hence, there exists a great opportunity to search for new antidiabetic drugs from plant-based natural compounds such as glycosides, alkaloids, terpenoids, flavonoids, carotenoids that exhibit anti-diabetic effect (Ahmad et al., 2003). The easy availability of the plant resources, least side effects and low cost of making the herbal medicine preparations can make the plant-based medicine as the key player of all available therapies against diabetes mellitus. As every plant has a natural habitat and, are restricted to particular areas on the globe so the preliminary requirement is for exploring the antidiabetic potentials of unexplored plants as well (Malviya et al., 2010; Bashir et al., 2015). In the traditional mode of practising the medicinal plants to control diabetes mellitus, many countries use the ethnobotanical information that reports about 800 documented plants worldwide and can be used for beneficial effects in the treatment of diabetes. These traditional antidiabetic plants require the proper scientific and medical evaluation for their ability to improve blood glucose control. However, a few comprehensive studies on traditional antidiabetic plants have been carried out, that causes an increase in the number of experimental and clinical investigations directed toward the validation of the antidiabetic properties, which are empirically attributed to these remedies. The antidiabetic activity of several plants has been confirmed along with their studies of mechanisms of hypoglycemic activity. Chemical studies directed to the isolation, purification and identification of the substances responsible for the hypoglycemic activity have also been conducted (Malviya et al., 2010; Kaur et al., 2013; Patil et al., 2014; Roman-Ramos et al, 1995; Sonkamble & Kamble 2015).

In this chapter, the basic aspects of some of the potential anti-diabetic plants, their available therapeutic molecules and the extraction process will be discussed by narrating the literature.

Diabetes Mellitus: Disease, Causes and Types

Diabetes mellitus is one of the common and very prevalent human diseases affecting the population of both developed and developing countries of the world. It is a metabolic disorder consist of multiple phenomena of occurrence and characterized by chronic hyperglycaemia with disturbances in carbohydrate, protein and fat metabolism. Ultimately causes defects in insulin secretion in the body. Similarly, the imbalance in the cortisol and testosterone hormone in men also causes diabetes. Prolonged hyperglycaemic condition in the body leads to glucose toxicity creates damage in β cell of pancreas thereby stopping the secretion of insulin hormone. Also, the inflammatory response may lead to the deficiency in the insulin causes the diabetes mellitus. Details of the factors responsible for the cause of diabetes mellitus has been shown in Figure 1. The effects include long term damage, dysfunction and failure of various organs including progressive development of specific complications of neuropathy with risk of foot ulcers, nephropathy leading to renal failure, retinopathy with potential blindness including sexual dysfunction. Individuals with diabetes are at increased risk of peripheral vascular, cardiovascular and cerebrovascular diseases. The severity of symptoms is due to the type and duration of diabetes. Some of the diabetes patients are asymptomatic especially those with type 2 diabetes during the early years of the disease. Uncontrolled diabetes may lead to stupor, coma and if not treated death, due to ketoacidosis or rarely from nonketotic hyperosmolar syndrome (Mellitus, 2005; American Diabetes Association 2014; Craig et al. 2009; Galtier, 2010; Kharroubi & Darwish, 2015; Giaccari et al., 209). In the late 1970s, both National Diabetic Data Group (1979) and World Health Organization (1980) recognized two major forms of diabetes which they termed as type 1 diabetes (previously termed juvenile onset diabetes) or Insulin Dependent Diabetes Mellitus (IDDM) and type 2 diabetes or Non-Insulin Dependent Diabetes Mellitus (NIDDM) (Ekoé, et al., 2013).

Therapeutic Approaches to Diabetes Mellitus

There are many key molecular mechanisms which can be exploited in diabetes treatment. The major mechanism is how to reduce the carbohydrate absorption in the body by inhibiting the α-amylase and α-glucosidase activity. In another way, enhancing the stimulation of insulin from the β pancreatic cells would be another one. In addition to this, some other indirect factors are also responsible as shown in Figure 2.

Two types of therapeutic approaches are used to treat diabetes mellitus.

1. Chemotherapy Approaches to Diabetes

Different types of synthetic drugs that are mainly hypoglycaemic in nature are used to treat the disease by different mechanism as described in the following sections (Lorenzati, et al., 2010; Bösenberg & Van 2008; Chaudhury, et al., 2017)

a. **Sulfonylureas (Sulpha group containing drug):** These categories of drug molecules act by stimulating insulin release from the pancreatic cells and slightly improve insulin resistance in peripheral target tissues such as muscle and fat. However, the hypoglycaemia is the most common side effect of these drugs.

Figure 1.

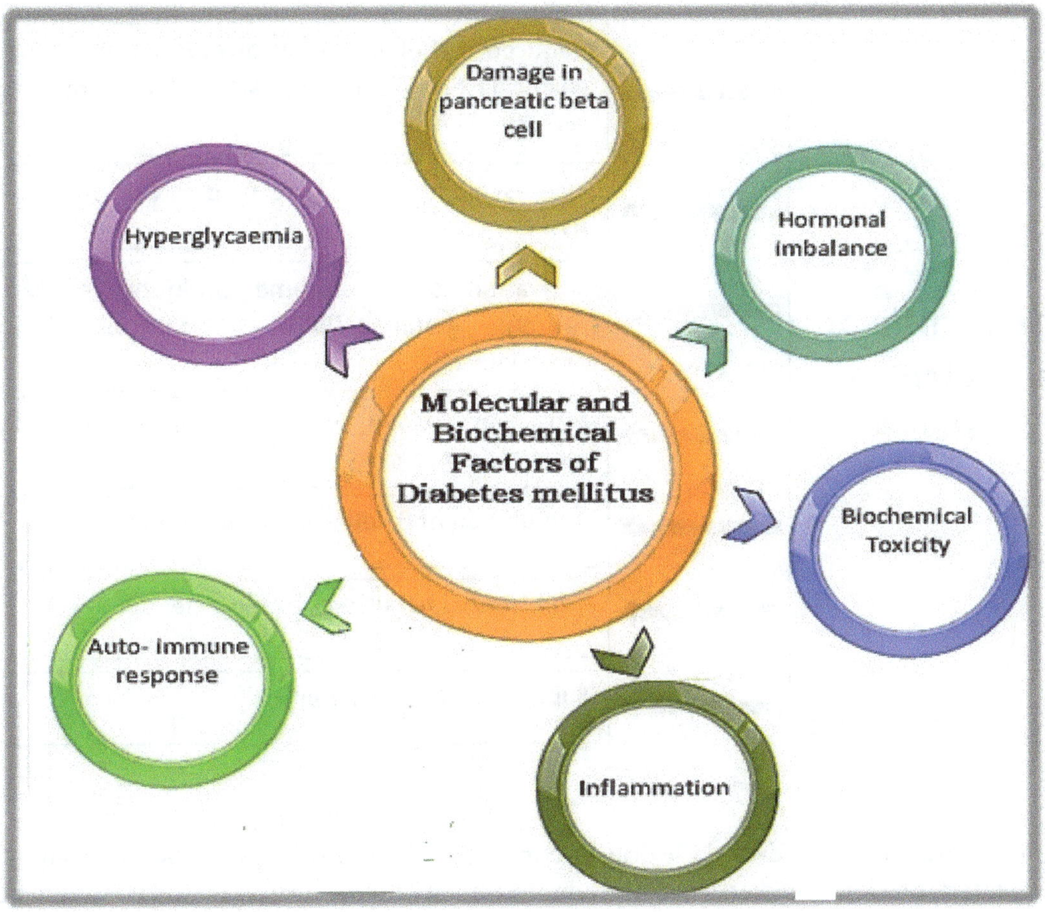

b. **Synthetic Biguanides:** This types of drug work by reducing hepatic glucose output and enhancing the insulin sensitivity in the peripheral tissues, also it reduces the plasma triglyceride levels and low-density lipoprotein (LDL) levels. The best example of this category drug is metformin having many side effects such as metallic taste, gastrointestinal discomfort and nausea as commonly reported only during the administration of the drug. Although the metformin is associated with a lack of weight gain and even weight loss in some overweight patients, the results from studies have shown that metformin also improves glycaemic control in patients who are not overweight.

c. **Thiazolidinediones:** The thiazolidinedione type drug work by enhancing insulin sensitivity in both muscle and adipose tissue to a lesser extent by inhibiting hepatic glucose production. In addition to this, these drug molecules have a significant effect on improving insulin resistance, especially whenever used in combination with other antidiabetic drugs. In addition to this, continuous intake of the drug is also associated with severe side effcts and may lead to diabetic macular edema, hepatotoxicity, bladder cancer, hormonal imbalance and teratogenic effect.

d. **α -glucosidase inhibitors:** These type of drugs usually act by inhibiting the enzyme activity of **α** -glucosidase found in the brush border cells in the small intestine. The enzyme functions by cleaving the complex carbohydrates (dextrins, maltose, sucrose and starch) into a simpler form of sugars

Figure 2.

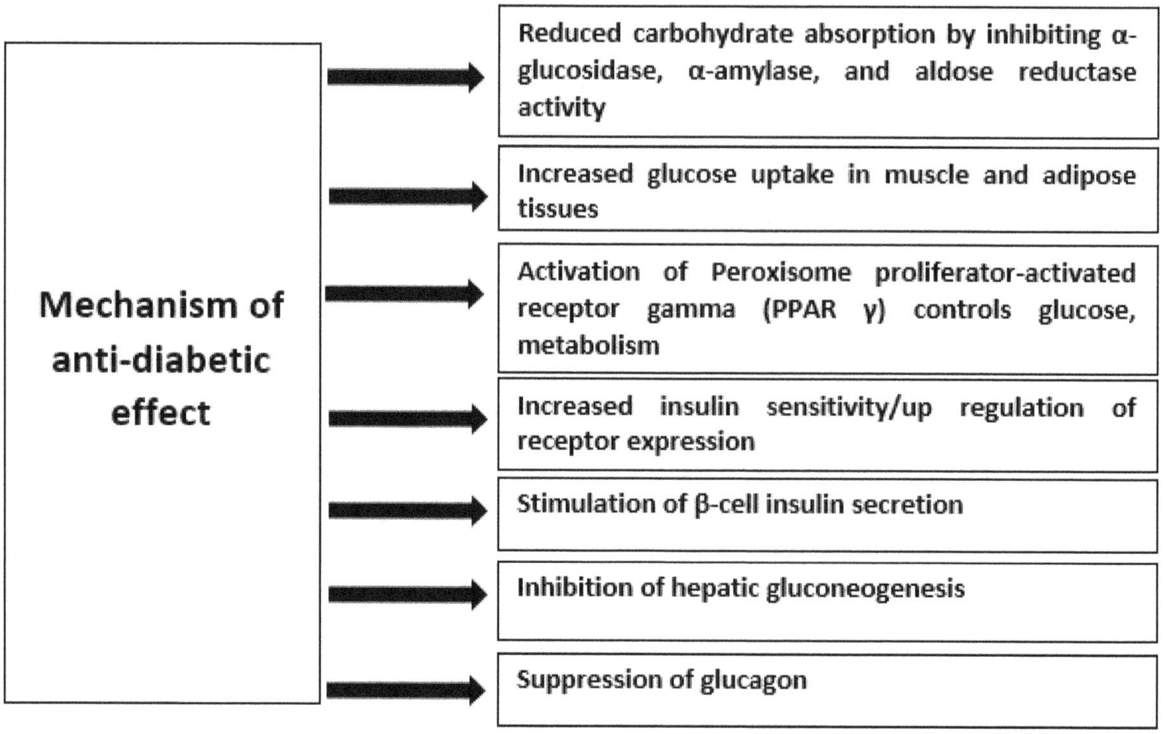

(glucose, fructose). However, these drugs having many types of side effects such as gastrointestinal discomfort, bloating and diarrhoea. The administration of these drugs also linked to enhancement in serum transaminase levels which may lead to liver cirrhosis in patients.

e. **Insulin** Insulin treatment has been successfully used in the case of IDDM to control hyperglycaemia occurs in the patient. Usually, the treatment is done by intravenous administration of insulin that decreases plasma glucose level in 30 minutes. Various forms of insulin are available commercially in the market as per their activities such as rapid-acting, intermediate and long-acting etc. The treatment of diabetes by administration of insulin is also associated with some side effects like hypoglycaemic shock, weight gain and an increased risk of atherogenesis.

2. Herbal therapy approaches

It is observed that all the above-mentioned classes of drugs exhibited major serious side effects if taken for a longer time, therefore as an alternative strategy, the herbal therapy is considered as the effective one. The plant-based preparations are the preferred antidiabetic agents in terms of their easy availability, economical point of view and having lesser or no side effects in comparison to other drugs as mentioned in the above section. Plants with proven hypoglycemic properties have been used as a part of traditional healing systems around the world. Many modern pharmaceuticals currently used are from natural plant origins. For example, the drug *metformin* was derived from the flowering plant *Galega officinalis* that was initially used as a common traditional remedy for the diabetic patient (Patade & Marita, 2014). A large number of medicinal plants are described for the treatment of diabetes of which only a few are being systematically evaluated. The ethno-botanical information reports about thousands of plants that may possess anti-diabetic potential. Therefore, there is a need for the development of a safe in terms of less side effects, cost effective phytopharmaceuticals that have antidiabetic potential. Among the major phytochemical constituents of plants credited with hypoglycemic action are saponins, glycosides, alkaloids, glycans, triterpenes, mucilages, polysaccharides, oils, vitamins, glycoproteins, peptides, amino acids and proteins. A list of plants with potent antidiabetic activity along with their beneficial effects is given in Table 1. Similarly, numerous protocols have been proposed for quantification of these plant extracts for their anti-diabetic nature by many researchers. However, in the majority of cases, very little is known about the mechanism of action of traditionally used antidiabetic plants, thus preventing them from being used in standard diabetes care. Recently, more research is being focused on elucidating the action of different natural compounds. Although the mentioned plants are used in traditional medicine to treat diabetes, the scientific evidence endorsing mechanism of action is not reported. Hence, it was planned to screen the plants for anti-diabetic activity and elucidate the anti-diabetic mechanism in the selected medicinal plant using reverse pharmacology approach. The methods used for screening were simple in-vitro and ex-vivo assays viz., glucose adsorption potency, amylolysis kinetics, glucose diffusion retardation index, α-amylase inhibition, α-glycosidase inhibition and sucrase inhibition assay (Moradi et al., 2028; Kumar et al., 2014; Bordoloi & Dutta, 2014; Saxena & Vikram, 2004).

Several online resources as well as the literature are available regarding the plants that contain anti-diabetic compounds. These resources include a specific database of the plants and their plant parts, taxonomy, active compound that they produce and so on. Some of the anti-diabetic plant resources are documented as the literature resources to encourage the researchers to research on isolation and identification of these compounds in many aspects. Some of these resources and their availability has been given in Table 2.

In vitro Measurement of Enzyme Inhibitor Activity of Plant Products

The proper product formulation of the medicinal plants is important for its promotion as their use as anti-diabetic drugs in the drug market. However, only a small fraction of medicinal plants have been explored and validated. In this context, there is scope for screening and development of unexplored medicinal plants and their components as antidiabetic agents are very crucial and challenging. In-vitro assays of the compounds having an anti-diabetic property are essential for the development of an anti-diabetic drug. Methods like enteric enzyme inhibition assays such as α-amylase inhibition, sucrase inhibition and α-glucosidase inhibition are popularly used as primary assays to screen the medicinal plants those having the anti-diabetic potential (Kazeem et al., 2013; Kwon et al., 2007; Matsui et al., 2006; Matsuda et al., 2002; Ogunwande et al., 2007; Kumar et al., 2015).Various steps are frequently used to quantify the action of the inhibitor of the phytoproduct leading to evaluate their antidiabetic potential of the plant shown in Figure 3.

Further, for more precise and concrete isolation and identification process, many modern methods of the screening process like high-pressure liquid chromatography (HPLC), Capillary Electrophoresis can be used. In addition to this high throughput screening pipeline methods such as high pressure liquid chromatography / Liquid chromatography-Mass spectrometry (HPLC/LC-MS) and various sensing strategies such as by using the fluorescence sensors, electrochemical sensors, and surface plasmon resonance (SPR) sensors may be used.

Table 1. Plants with their antidiabetic activities and beneficial effects

S. No	Compounds	Type of compound	Plant sources	Family	Mode of action	Reference
1	Trans-tiliroside	flavonoid	*Potentilla chinesis*	*Rosaceae*	decreased blood glucose level and total cholesterol, low density lipoprotein (LDL–C) and triglyceride	
2	Eleutherinoside A	Lignans	Eleutherine americana	Iridaceae	In vitro α-glucosidase inhibitory activity.	
3	Bergenin	glycoside	*Caesalpinia digyna*	Leguminosae	antidiabetic, hypolipidemic and antioxidant activity and regenerative effect on pancreatic β cells in Type 2 diabetic rats.	
4	5,7-dihydroxy-6,8-dimethyl-4¢ -methoxy flavone	flavonoid	*Callistemon lanceolatus* DC	Myrtaceae	exhibited blood glucose lowering effect in streptozotocin induced diabetic rats.	
5	Marrubiin	phenolic	*Leonotis leonurus*	Lamiaceae	Increased the insulin level and glucose transporter-2 gene expressions in INS-1 cells	
6	Alisol F and Alisol B	Triterpenoids	*Alismatis Rhizoma*	Alismataceae	*In vitro* α-glucosidase inhibitory activity.	Firdous, S. M. (2014).
7	Scrophuside	glycoside	*Scrophularia ningpoensis*	*Scrophulariaceae*	α-glucosidase inhibitory activity.	
8	Ningposide I and Ningposide II	glycosides	*Scrophularia ningpoensis* Hemsl.	*Scrophulariaceae*	α-glucosidase inhibitory activity.	
9	Chalcomoracin, Moracin C, Moracin D and Moracin N	flavonoids	*Morus alba*	Moraceae	α-glucosidase inhibitory activity.	
10	Malonyl ginsenosides	*ginsenosides*	*Panax ginseng*	Araliaceae	significantly lower fasting blood glucose level, improvement of insulin sensitivity	
11	mangiferin,	xanthonoid	*Mangifera indica*	Anacardiaceae	reduced the blood glucose levels in alloxan-induced diabetic rats	
12	Chicoric acid	hydroxycinnamic acid	*Ocimum gratissimum* L.	Lamiaceae	Reduced significantly the glycemic levels of diabetic mice.	
13	Vindogentianine	Alkaloid	Catharanthus roseus	Apocynaceae	Inducing higher glucose uptake and significant PTP1B inhibition in vitro	
14	Berberine	Alkaloid	Coptis chinensis	Ranunculaceae	Significantly decreased the levels of HbA1c, total cholesterol and triglyceride, and increased the secretion of insulin in diabetic rats	
15	Nigelladines A-C and nigellaquinomine	Alkaloid	Nigella glandulifera	Ranunculaceae	Exhibited potent PTP1B inhibitory activity	
16	Betulonic acid, betulone and spinasterol	Terpenoids	Buddleja saligna	Scrophulariaceae	Significant inhibition against α-glucosidase	(Teoh & Das, 2018)
17	lactucin	Terpenoids	Cichorium intybus L.	Asteraceae	Significant inhibition against α glucosidase	
18	Limonene	Terpenoids	Citrus sinensis (L.)	Rutaceae	Reduced high fat diet-induced increase inblood glucose levels	
19	Compound K16	Terpenoids	Momordica charantia L.	Cucurbitaceae	Significantly reduced blood glucose and blood lipid levels, while improving glucose tolerance in diabetic mice	
20	24-methylencycloartan-3-one	Terpenoids	Prosopis juliflora (Sw.)	Fabaceae	Reduced blood glucose significantly	
21	quercetrin	flavonoid	*Kalopanax pictum*	Araliaceae)	α-amylase inhibition	
22	astragalin	glucoside	*Polygala japonica*	Polygalaceae	α-amylase inhibition	
23	narcisin	flavonoid	*Sophora japonica* L.	Leguminosae	α-amylase inhibition	
24	kaempferol-3- O-[6"-O-(3-hydroxy-3-methylglutaroyl) glucoside	flavonoid	*Polygala japonica* Houtt.	Polygalaceae	α-amylase inhibition	(Sales et al., 2012)
25	Quercetagetin	flavonoid	*Allium cepa* L.	Liliaceae	α-amylase inhibition	
26	Luteolin	flavonoid	*Lonicera japonica* Thunb	Caprifoliaceae	α-amylase inhibition	
27	eupafolin	flavonoid	*Lonicera japonica* Thunb.	Caprifoliaceae	α-amylase inhibition	

a. α-Amylase Inhibition Assay

The most important digestive enzyme is pancreatic αamylase (EC 3.2.1.1), that catalyzes the hydrolysis of the α-1, 4 glycosidic linkages of the starch, amylose, amylopectin, glycogen, etc. and responsible for most of the starch digestion in case of humans. From the experiments, a positive correlation between human pancreatic α-amylase (HPA) activity and the increase in glucose levels has been established, that

Table 2. Resources of some anti-diabetic plants

S.No	Literature /Database/ on-line Resources	Web address	References
1	A database for anti-diabetic plants with clinical / experimental trials	http://www.biotechpark.org.in/antidia/index.html	Singh et al., 2009
2	A Database of Antidiabetic Plant Species of Family Asteraceae, Euphorbiaceae, Fabaceae, Lamiaceae and Moraceae	https://www.florajournal.com/archives/2013/vol1issue2/PartA/22.1.pdf	Sidhu & Tanu 2013
3	Database on antidiabetic indigenous plants of Tamil Nadhu, India.	http://www.ijpsr.info/docs/IJPSR12-03-02-001.pdf	Makheswari & Sudarsanam 2012
4	Indian medicinal plants for diabetes: text data mining the literature of different electronic databases for future therapeutics	https://www.biomedres.info/biomedical-research/indian-medicinal-plants-for-diabetes-text-data-mining-the-literature-of-different-electronic-databases-for-future-therapeutics.html	(Selvaraj & Periyasamy, 2016)
5	Phyto diab care: Phytoremedial database for antidiabetics.	http://www.gbpuat-cbsh.ac.in/departments/bi/database/phytodiabcare/HOME%20PAGE/Home%20page.html.	Luhach et al., 2013
6	Database on Anti-Diabetic Medicinal Plants (DADMP))	http://www.mkarthikeyan.bioinfoau.org/dadmp/	---
7	ADNCD: a compendious database on anti-diabetic natural compounds focusing on mechanism of action.	http://www.adncd.com/index.php	Khatoon et al., 2013
8	DiaMedBase	http://www.progenebio.in/DMP/DMP.htm	Babu et al., 2006
9	Antidiabetic Potency of Bangladeshi Medicinal Plants	http://www.ayurvedjournal.com/JAHM_201841_08.pdf	Hasan & Sultana,2018
10	Phytochemica	home.iitj.ac.in/~bagler/webservers/Phytochemica	Pathania et al., 2015
11	anti-diabetic plants in Iranian traditional medicine	https://academicjournals.org/journal/JDE/article-full-text-pdf/C43CFE31200	Dabaghian et al., 2012
12	Iranian Medicinal Plants for Diabetes Mellitus	https://scialert.net/fulltext/?doi=pjbs.2013.401.411	Rashidi et al., 2013
13	An overview on antidiabetic medicinal plants having insulin mimetic property	https://www.ncbi.nlm.nih.gov/pmc/articles/PMC3609288/	Patel et al., 2012
14	Plants used for the treatment of diabetes in Jordan: A review of scientific evidence	https://www.tandfonline.com/doi/full/10.3109/13880209.2010.501802	Al-Aboudi& Afifi 2011
15	Anti Diabetic Plants: Global Distribution, Active ingredients, Extraction Techniques and Acting Mechanisms	http://www.phcogrev.com/article/2012/6/11/1041030973-784795854	Chan et al., 2012
16	Indian Medicinal Plants, Phytochemistry And Therapeutics (IMPPAT)	https://cb.imsc.res.in/imppat/home	Mohanraj et al., 2018
17	DIA-DB web server	(http://bio-hpc.eu/software/dia-db/)	Pereira et al., 2019
18	InDiaMed	http://www.indiamed.info	Tota et al., 2013

demonstrate about the relevance of the enzymes in the treatment of type 2 diabetes. The phytochemicals for which the inhibitor activity for the enzyme is to be studied is usually following a common procedure as shown in the Figure 4.

Figure 3.

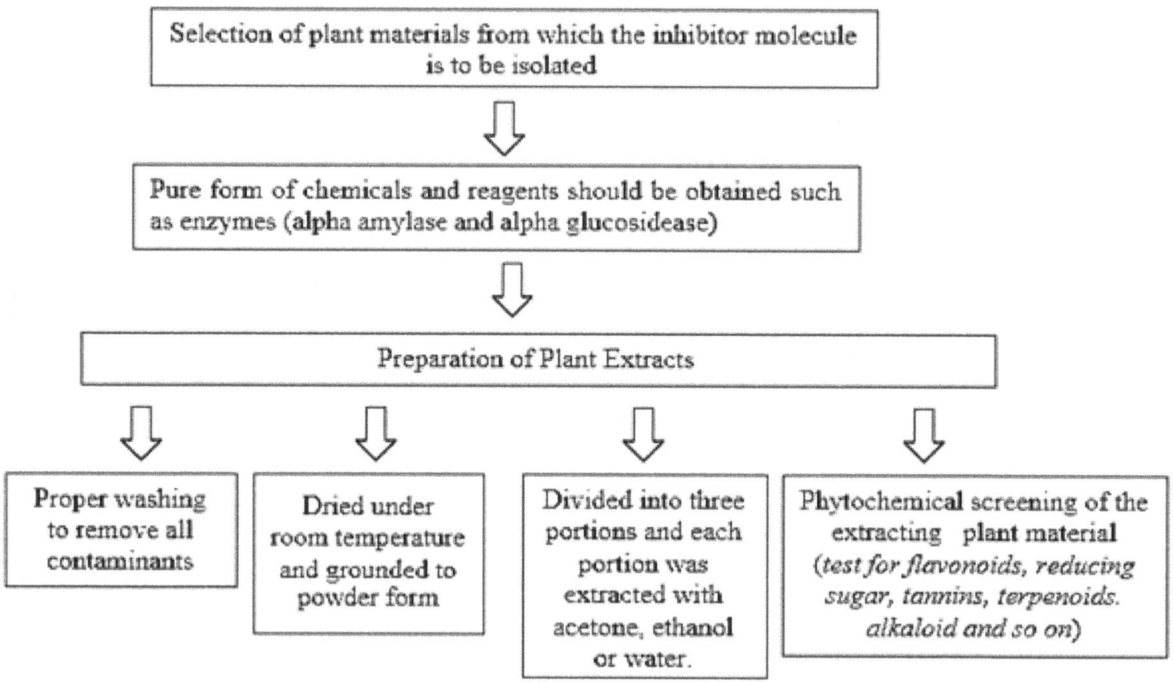

b. α -Glucosidase Inhibition Assay

Another enzyme is called as α-glucosidase or maltase (EC 3.2.1.20), that catalyzes the final step of the digestive process of carbohydrates acting upon 1, 4-α bonds. Since the carbohydrates are the major constituents of the human diet and play a major role in the energy supply, however, the complex components of carbohydrates should be broken down to monosaccharides. Only this form it can be absorbed from the intestinal lumen and transported into blood circulation. Delay of carbohydrate digestion by inhibition of enzymes such as **α** glucosidase would lead to blood glucose level reduction and hence could be considered as a therapeutic strategy for the treatment of diabetes. The basic procedure for biochemical quantification of the phytoextract as the **α** glucosidase inhibitor has been shown in Figure 5.

CONCLUSION

The continuous global prevalence of diabetes mellitus and treatment with oral hypoglycaemic drugs ends with numerous side effects as well as in terms of huge monetary expenditure causes a great concern now. Therefore, treating this disease using plant-derived compounds that possess less side effect and more potential nature is a suitable alternative therapeutic strategy. In this chapter, the plants and their product details, as well as the literature / online resources, are presented. In addition to this, the mechanism of plant-based inhibitors and their detail in vitro strategy has been explained. Although the process of isolation and screening is challenging and requires the collective efforts of ethnobotanists,

Figure 4.

A total of 250 μL of phyto extract (1.25–10 mg/mL) is to be placed in a tube and to it 250 μL of 0.02 M sodium phosphate buffer (pH 6.9) containing Alpha -amylase solution (0.5 mg/mL) is to be added.

⇩

This solution should be pre-incubated at 25°C for 10 min, after which 250 μL of 1% starch solution in 0.02 M sodium phosphate buffer (pH 6.9 is to be added at timed intervals and then further incubated at 25°C for 10 min.

⇩

The reaction is to be terminated by adding 500 μL of dinitrosalicylic acid (DNS) reagent followed by keeping the tubes under incubation in boiling water for 5 min and cooled to room temperature

⇩

The reaction is to be terminated by adding 500 μL of dinitrosalicylic acid (DNS) reagent followed by incubating the tubes in boiling water for 5 min and cooled to room temperature.

⇩

Then the reaction mixture is to be diluted with 5 ml of distilled water and the absorbance is to be measured at 540 nm using spectrophotometer

⇩

A control is to be prepared using the above procedure replacing the extract with distilled water. Then the amylase inhibitory activity is to be calculated as percentage inhibition as:

$$\%\text{Inhibition} = \left[\frac{\text{Abs}_{\text{control}} - \text{Abs}_{\text{extracts}}}{\text{Abs}_{\text{control}}}\right] \times 100.$$

⇩

Finally, the concentrations of extracts resulting in 50% inhibition of enzyme activity (IC_{50}) are determined graphically

phytochemists, pharmacognosist and pharmacologists for the proper evaluation of the compound. Also, not only challenges are there in case of large scale screening of the compounds but also exists in proving their efficacy and safety. Therefore, this opens the door for conducting research in plant-based drugs, developing standard bioassays protocols that would lead to their toxicological and pharmacological evaluation by using animal models. In this context, many indigenous medicinal plants are useful to succeed in managing the diabetes mellitus but many of them have not characterized yet. Plant extract or different folk plant preparations are being prescribed by the traditional practitioners and also accepted by the users for diabetes. Moreover, a compressive, unique and worldwide updated database of antidiabetic plants are essential, that would attract the scientific community to work in this emerging field and to uncover the potentiality of many of the novel compounds obtained from the plant.

Figure 5.

50 μL of the (5 mg/mL) plant extract is to be preincubated with 100 μL of α -glucosidase solution for 10 min at 25°C in one set of tubes.

⇩

In another set of tubes α glucosidase enzyme is to be preincubated with 50 μL of phosphate buffer (pH 6.9). 50 μL of 4-Nitrophenyl-β-D- glucopyranoside (PNPG) at increasing concentrations (0.63–2.0 mg/mL) and the same to be added both sets of reaction mixtures to start the reaction.

⇩

Then the mixture is to be incubated for 10 min at 25°C, and 500 μL of Na_2CO_3 is added to stop the reaction.

⇩

The amount of reducing sugars released is to be determined spectrophotometrically (405 nm)

⇩

A control is to be prepared using the same procedure replacing the extract with distilled water. The α glucosidase inhibitory activity is calculated as percentage inhibition as:

$$\%\text{Inhibition} = \left[\frac{\text{Abs}_{\text{control}} - \text{Abs}_{\text{extracts}}}{\text{Abs}_{\text{control}}}\right] \times 100.$$

⇩

Concentrations of extracts resulting in 50% inhibition of enzyme activity (IC_{50}) are determined graphically

REFERENCES

Ahmad, D. S., Jasra, W. A., & Imtiaz, A. (2003). Genetic diversity in Pakistani genotypes of Hypophae rhamnoides L. ssp. Turkestanica. *Int J Agric Biol Sci*, *5*(1), 10–13.

Al-Aboudi, A., & Afifi, F. U. (2011). Plants used for the treatment of diabetes in Jordan: A review of scientific evidence. *Pharmaceutical Biology*, *49*(3), 221–239. doi:10.3109/13880209.2010.501802 PMID:20979537

American Diabetes Association. (2014). Diagnosis and classification of diabetes mellitus. *Diabetes Care*, *37*(Supplement 1), S81–S90. doi:10.2337/dc14-S081 PMID:24357215

Babu, P. A., Suneetha, G., Boddepalli, R., Lakshmi, V. V., Rani, T. S., RamBabu, Y., & Srinivas, K. (2006). A database of 389 medicinal plants for diabetes. *Bioinformation*, *1*(4), 130–131. doi:10.6026/97320630001130 PMID:17597872

Bailey, C. J., & Day, C. (1989). Traditional plant medicines as treatments for diabetes. *Diabetes Care, 12*(8), 553–564. doi:10.2337/diacare.12.8.553 PMID:2673695

Bashir, L., Shittu, O. K., Sani, S., Busari, M. B., & Adeniyi, K. A. (2015). African Natural Products with Potential Antitrypanosoma Properties: A Review. *International Journal of Biochemistry Research & Review, 7*(2), 45–79. doi:10.9734/IJBCRR/2015/16039

Bordoloi, R., & Dutta, K. N. (2014). A review on herbs used in the treatment of diabetes mellitus. *J Pharm Chem Biol Sci, 2*(2), 86–92.

Bösenberg, L. H., & Van Zyl, D. G. (2008). The mechanism of action of oral antidiabetic drugs: A review of recent literature. *Journal of Endocrinology. Metabolism and Diabetes of South Africa, 13*(3), 80–88.

Chan, C. H., Ngoh, G. C., & Yusoff, R. (2012). A brief review on anti diabetic plants: Global distribution, active ingredients, extraction techniques and acting mechanisms. *Pharmacognosy Reviews, 6*(11), 22. doi:10.4103/0973-7847.95854 PMID:22654401

Chaudhury, A., Duvoor, C., Reddy Dendi, V. S., Kraleti, S., Chada, A., Ravilla, R., ... Sasapu, A. (2017). Clinical review of antidiabetic drugs: Implications for type 2 diabetes mellitus management. *Frontiers in Endocrinology, 8*, 6. doi:10.3389/fendo.2017.00006 PMID:28167928

Craig, M. E., Hattersley, A., & Donaghue, K. C. (2009). Definition, epidemiology and classification of diabetes in children and adolescents. *Pediatric Diabetes, 10*, 3–12. doi:10.1111/j.1399-5448.2009.00568.x PMID:19754613

Dabaghian, F. H., Kamalinejad, M., Shojaei, A., & Fard, M. A. (2012). Presenting anti-diabetic plants in Iranian traditional medicine. *Journal of Diabetes and Endocrinology, 3*(5), 70–76. doi:10.5897/JDE12.004

Ekoé, J. M., Punthakee, Z., Ransom, T., Prebtani, A. P., & Goldenberg, R. (2013). Screening for type 1 and type 2 diabetes. *Canadian Journal of Diabetes, 37*, S12–S15. doi:10.1016/j.jcjd.2013.01.012 PMID:24070932

Firdous, S. M. (2014). Phytochemicals for treatment of diabetes. *EXCLI Journal, 13*, 451. PMID:26417272

Gallagher, A. M., Flatt, P. R., Duffy, G. A. W. Y., & Abdel-Wahab, Y. H. A. (2003). The effects of traditional antidiabetic plants on in vitro glucose diffusion. *Nutrition Research (New York, N.Y.), 23*(3), 413–424. doi:10.1016/S0271-5317(02)00533-X

Galtier, F. (2010). Definition, epidemiology, risk factors. *Diabetes & Metabolism, 36*(6 Pt 2), 628–651. doi:10.1016/j.diabet.2010.11.014 PMID:21163426

Giaccari, A., Sorice, G., & Muscogiuri, G. (2009). Glucose toxicity: The leading actor in the pathogenesis and clinical history of type 2 diabetes–mechanisms and potentials for treatment. *Nutrition, Metabolism, and Cardiovascular Diseases, 19*(5), 365–377. doi:10.1016/j.numecd.2009.03.018 PMID:19428228

Hasan, T., & Sultana, M. (2018). Antidiabetic potency of Bangladeshi medicinal plants. *J Ayurvedic Herb Med, 4*(1), 35–42.

Kaur, J., Kaur, S., & Mahajan, A. (2013). Herbal medicines: Possible risks and benefits. *Am J Phytomed Clin Ther, 1*(2), 226–239.

Kazeem, M. I., Adamson, J. O., & Ogunwande, I. A. (2013). Modes of inhibition of α-amylase and α-glucosidase by aqueous extract of Morinda lucida Benth leaf. *BioMed Research International.* PMID:24455701

Kharroubi, A. T., & Darwish, H. M. (2015). Diabetes mellitus: The epidemic of the century. *World Journal of Diabetes*, *6*(6), 850. doi:10.4239/wjd.v6.i6.850 PMID:26131326

Khatoon, A., Rashid, I., Shaikh, S., Rizvi, S. M. D., Shakil, S., Pathak, N., ... Srivastava, P. (2018). ADNCD: a compendious database on anti-diabetic natural compounds focusing on mechanism of action. *3 Biotech, 8*(8), 361.

Kitabchi, A. E., Umpierrez, G. E., Miles, J. M., & Fisher, J. N. (2009). Hyperglycemic crises in adult patients with diabetes. *Diabetes Care*, *32*(7), 1335–1343. doi:10.2337/dc09-9032 PMID:19564476

Kumar, K., Fateh, V., Verma, B., & Pandey, S. (2014). Some herbal drugs used for treatment of diabetes. *International Journal of Research and Development in Pharmacy & Life Sciences*, *3*, 1116–1120.

Kumar, K. K., Jayaprakash, A. P., & Srinivasan, K. K. (2015). Antidiabetic evaluation of Hemionitis arifolia leaves by in vitro methods. *Manipal Journal of Pharmaceutical Sciences*, *1*(1), 13–20.

Kwon, Y.-I., Apostolidis, E., & Shetty, K. (2007). Evaluation of pepper (Capsicum annuum) for management of diabetes and hypertension. *Journal of Food Biochemistry*, *31*(3), 370–385. doi:10.1111/j.1745-4514.2007.00120.x

Lorenzati, B., Zucco, C., Miglietta, S., Lamberti, F., & Bruno, G. (2010). Oral hypoglycemic drugs: pathophysiological basis of their mechanism of actionoral hypoglycemic drugs: pathophysiological basis of their mechanism of action. *Pharmaceuticals*, *3*(9), 3005–3020. doi:10.3390/ph3093005 PMID:27713388

Luhach, S., Goel, A., Taj, G., Goyal, P., & Kumar, A. (2013). Phyto diab care: Phytoremedial database for antidiabetics. *Bioinformation*, *9*(7), 375–377. doi:10.6026/97320630009375 PMID:23750083

Makheswari, M. U., & Sudarsanam, D. (2012). Database on antidiabetic indigenous plants of Tamil Nadhu, India. *International Journal of Pharmaceutical Sciences and Research*, *3*(2), 287–293.

Malviya, N., Jain, S., & Malviya, S. (2010). Antidiabetic potential of medicinal plants Acta Pol Pharmaceutical. *Drug Research*, *67*, 113–118.

Malviya, N., Jain, S., & Malviya, S. A. P. N. A. (2010). Antidiabetic potential of medicinal plants. *Acta Poloniae Pharmaceutica*, *67*(2), 113–118. PMID:20369787

Matsuda, H., Morikawa, T., & Yoshikawa, M. (2002). Antidiabetogenic constituents from several natural medicines. *Pure and Applied Chemistry*, *74*(7), 1301–1308. doi:10.1351/pac200274071301

Matsui, T., Ogunwande, I. A., Abesundara, K. J., & Matsumoto, K. (2006). Anti-hyperglycemic Potential of Natural Products. *Mini-Reviews in Medicinal Chemistry*, *6*(3), 349–356. doi:10.2174/138955706776073484 PMID:16515474

Mellitus, D. (2005). Diagnosis and classification of diabetes mellitus. *Diabetes Care*, *28*(S37), S5–S10. PMID:15618111

Mohanraj, K., Karthikeyan, B. S., Vivek-Ananth, R. P., Chand, R. B., Aparna, S. R., Mangalapandi, P., & Samal, A. (2018). IMPPAT: A curated database of Indian Medicinal Plants, Phytochemistry And Therapeutics. *Scientific Reports*, *8*(1), 1–17. doi:10.103841598-018-22631-z PMID:29311619

Monday, O. M., & Uzoma, A. I. (2013). Histological changes and antidiabetic activities of Icacina trichantha tuber extract in beta–cells of alloxan induced diabetic rats. *Asian Pacific Journal of Tropical Biomedicine*, *3*(8), 628–633. doi:10.1016/S2221-1691(13)60127-6 PMID:23905020

Moradi, B., Abbaszadeh, S., Shahsavari, S., Alizadeh, M., & Beyranvand, F. (2018). The most useful medicinal herbs to treat diabetes. *Biomedical Research and Therapy*, *5*(8), 2538–2551. doi:10.15419/bmrat.v5i8.463

Ndarubu, T. A., Chiamaka, O. S., Alfa, S., Aishatu, M., Chinedu, O. E., Wenawo, D. L., ... Eustace, B. B. (2019). Phytochemicals, hypoglycemic and hypolipidemic effects of methanol leaf extract of Hibiscus sabdariffa in alloxan induced diabetic rats. *GSC Biological and Pharmaceutical Sciences, 8*(3), 070-078.

Ogunwande, I. A., Matsui, T., Fujise, T., & Matsumoto, K. (2007). α-Glucosidase inhibitory profile of Nigerian medicinal plants in immobilized assay system. *Food Science and Technology Research, 13*(2), 169–172. doi:10.3136/fstr.13.169

Ortiz-Andrade, R. R., Garcia-Jimenez, S., Castillo-Espana, P., Ramirez-Avila, G., Villalobos-Molina, R., & Estrada-Soto, S. (2007). α-Glucosidase inhibitory activity of the methanolic extract from Tournefortia hartwegiana: An anti-hyperglycemic agent. *Journal of Ethnopharmacology*, *109*(1), 48–53. doi:10.1016/j.jep.2006.07.002 PMID:16920301

Owolabi, O. J., Inninh, S. O., Anaka, O. N., & Iyamu, O. A. (2014). Antidiabetic and Hypolipidemic Effects of Methanol Leaf Extract of *Napoleona vogelii* (Lecythidaceae). *Hook and Planch on Alloxan–Induced Diabetes Mellitus in Rats Tropical Journal of Pharmaceutical Research, 13*(11), 1903–1909.

Patade, G. R., & Marita, A. R. (2014). Metformin: A Journey from countryside to the bedside. *Journal of Obesity and Metabolic Research*, *1*(2), 127. doi:10.4103/2347-9906.134435

Patel, D. K., Prasad, S. K., Kumar, R., & Hemalatha, S. (2012). An overview on antidiabetic medicinal plants having insulin mimetic property. *Asian Pacific Journal of Tropical Biomedicine*, *2*(4), 320–330. doi:10.1016/S2221-1691(12)60032-X PMID:23569923

Pathania, S., Ramakrishnan, S. M., & Bagler, G. (2015). Phytochemica: A platform to explore phytochemicals of medicinal plants. *Database (Oxford)*, *2015*, 2015. doi:10.1093/database/bav075 PMID:26255307

Patil, A., Jadhav, V., & Arvindekar Aand More, T. (2014). Antidiabetic Activity of Maesa indica (Roxb.) Stem Bark in Streptozotocin Induced Diabetic Rats. *American Journal of Phytomedicine and Clinical Therapeutics*, *2*(8), 957–962.

Pereira, A. S., den Haan, H., Peña-García, J., Moreno, M. M., Pérez-Sánchez, H., & Apostolides, Z. (2019). Exploring african medicinal plants for potential anti-diabetic compounds with the DIA-DB inverse virtual screening web server. *Molecules (Basel, Switzerland)*, *24*(10), 2002. doi:10.3390/molecules24102002 PMID:31137754

Rashidi, A. A., Mirhashemi, S. M., Taghizadeh, M., & Sarkhail, P. (2013). Iranian medicinal plants for diabetes mellitus: A systematic review. *Pakistan journal of biological sciences. PJBS, 16*(9), 401. PMID:24498803

Roman-Ramos, R., Flores-Saenz, J. L., & Alarcon-Aguilar, F. J. (1995). Anti-hyperglycemic effect of some edible plants. *Journal of Ethnopharmacology, 48*(1), 25–32. doi:10.1016/0378-8741(95)01279-M PMID:8569244

Saxena, A., & Vikram, N. K. (2004). Role of selected Indian plants in management of type 2 diabetes: A review. *Journal of Alternative and Complementary Medicine (New York, N.Y.), 10*(2), 369–378. doi:10.1089/107555304323062365 PMID:15165418

Selvaraj, B., & Periyasamy, S. (2016). *Indian medicinal plants for diabetes: text data mining the literature of different electronic databases for future therapeutics*. Academic Press.

Sidhu, M. C., & Tanu, S. (2013). A database of antidiabetic plant species of family Asteraceae, Euphorbiaceae, Fabaceae, Lamiaceae and Moraceae. *International Journal of Herbal Medicine, 1*(2), 187–199.

Singh, S., Gupta, S. K., Sabir, G., Gupta, M. K., & Seth, P. K. (2009). A database for anti-diabetic plants with clinical/experimental trials. *Bioinformation, 4*(6), 263–268. doi:10.6026/97320630004263 PMID:20975921

Sonkamble, V. V., & Kamble, L. H. (2015). Antidiabetic potential and identification of phytochemicals from Tinospora cordifolia. *American Journal of Phytomedicine and Clinical Therapeutics, 3*(1), 97-110.

Teoh, S. L., & Das, S. (2018). Phytochemicals and their effective role in the treatment of diabetes mellitus: A short review. *Phytochemistry Reviews, 17*(5), 1111–1128. doi:10.100711101-018-9575-z

Tota, K., Rayabarapu, N., Moosa, S., Talla, V., Bhyravbhatla, B., & Rao, S. (2013). InDiaMed: A comprehensive database of Indian medicinal plants for diabetes. *Bioinformation, 9*(7), 378–380. doi:10.6026/97320630009378 PMID:23750084

Venkatachalam, T., Kumar, V. K., Selvi, P. K., Maske, A. O., Anbarasan, V., & Kumar, P. S. (2011). Antidiabetic activity of Lantana camara Linn fruits in normal and streptozotocin-induced diabetic rats. *Journal of Pharmacy Research, 4*(5), 1550–1552.

World Health Organisation. (2000). *Global Strategy on Diet Physical Activity and Health*. World Health Organization.

KEY TERMS AND DEFINITIONS

Anti-Diabetic Plants: Plants having components used to treat diabetes mellitus disease.
Beta Cell: Cells present in the pancreas that secretes insulin.
Diabetes Mellitus: A metabolic disease occurs due to deficiency of insulin hormone secretion.
Herbal Therapy: Plant products that are used commercially to treat the disease.
Hyperglycaemia: A physiological condition in the body, where excess amount of sugar is available.
Insulin: A hormone, the presence of which reduces the glucose level.
Pancreas: An organ, that is responsible for secretion of enzymes as well as hormone like insulin.

Chapter 3
Medical Herbs and the Treatment of Diabetes Mellitus:
Mechanisms of Action

Donovan Anthony McGrowder
Department of Pathology, Faculty of Medical Sciences, The University of the West Indies, Jamaica

Fabian G. Miller
https://orcid.org/0000-0002-5821-1711
Faculty of Education, The Mico University College, Jamaica

Chukwuemeka Nwokocha
Department of Basic Medical Sciences, Faculty of Medical Sciences, The University of the West Indies, Jamaica

Cameil F. Wilson-Clarke
https://orcid.org/0000-0002-9475-9637
Department of Basic Medical Sciences, Faculty of Medical Sciences, The University of the West Indies, Jamaica

Melisa Anderson
School of Allied Health and Wellness, College of Health Sciences, University of Technology, Jamaica

Lennox Anderson-Jackson
https://orcid.org/0000-0002-9712-0214
Department of Pathology, Faculty of Medical Sciences, The University of the West Indies, Jamaica

Lowen Williams
Department of Biotechnology, Faculty of Science and Technology, The University of the West Indies, Jamaica

Ruby Alexander-Lindo
Department of Basic Sciences, Faculty of Medical Sciences, The University of the West Indies, Jamaica

ABSTRACT

Diabetes mellitus is a chronic metabolic disorder that affects millions of persons worldwide, and if uncontrolled may cause cardiovascular disease, retinopathy, or chronic kidney disease. Effective therapeutic management of diabetes mellitus involves the use of mainly oral hypoglycemic drugs whose mechanism of action includes improved insulin secretion, reduced insulin resistance, or increased glucose uptake. There is growing exploration of medicinal herbs as potential therapeutic sources for the management of type 2 diabetes mellitus and compared with conventional oral hypoglycemic drugs they have little

DOI: 10.4018/978-1-7998-4808-0.ch003

or no side effects. The aim of this review is to provide up-to-date information on potential medicinal herbs that have demonstrated anti-hyperglycemic activity through either increased secretion of insulin from pancreatic β-cells, reduction of insulin resistance with subsequent increase in insulin sensitivity, or inhibition of intestinal glucose absorption via decreased α-glucosidase activity.

INTRODUCTION

Diabetes mellitus

Diabetes mellitus is a chronic endocrine metabolic syndrome described by hyperglycemia (higher levels of blood glucose) and glucose intolerance due to deficiencies in insulin secretion or impairment in insulin's action (American Diabetes Association, 2009). It is classified into two main types, type 1 diabetes mellitus and type 2 diabetes mellitus.

Type 1 diabetes is caused by the destruction of insulin producing pancreatic islet β-cells with resultant insulin deficiency and increased tendency for ketoacidosis. Pancreatic islet β-cell destruction is largely attributable to an autoimmune process, but other unknown mechanisms have been described (Punthakee et al., 2018). Type 2 diabetes mellitus is defined by peripheral insulin resistance with relative insulin deficiency or impaired insulin secretion (Punthakee et al., 2018). Type 2 diabetes mellitus presents with increased demand for insulin. There is an inability of insulin target tissues to respond or progressive failure of pancreatic islet β-cells (Halban et al., 2014).

The chronic hyperglycemic milieu associated with diabetes mellitus can affect many vital organs in the body and cause considerable complications such as blindness, stroke, lower extremity amputations, kidney disease, heart failure and may lead to death (World Health Organization, 2018). Epidemiological data indicate that over 700 million people will be affected by diabetes mellitus in 2045, (International Diabetes Foundation, 2019). Global estimates suggest that the mortality burden of diabetes mellitus is over one million deaths annually (Khan et al., 2020). Diabetes mellitus was also ranked the seventh leading cause of death for the year 2016 (World Health Organization, 2018). As such, it is imperative to conduct more extensive research on the prevention and management of diabetes mellitus for improved patient outcomes.

In recent years, the pharmacologic armamentarium for the treatment of diabetes mellitus has considerably advanced but maintaining well controlled glucose levels is an ongoing challenge. The management of diabetes mellitus is largely dependent on the type of diabetes mellitus present. There are a number of oral antidiabetic conventional drugs that are employed in the control and management of diabetes mellitus. These include (i) Drugs that promote the release of insulin from pancreatic islet β-cells such as sulfonylurea-type (e.g. glibenclamide, glipizide, tolazamide and glimepiride), (ii) Drugs which improve insulin sensitivity by lowering resistance such as thiazolidinediones (e.g. pioglitazone and rosiglitazone), (iii) Drugs that reduce the production and release of glucose from the liver, and increase the sensitivity of peripheral tissues to insulin such as biguanides (e.g. metformin), (iv) Drugs that decrease glucose reabsorption via the intestine by inhibition of α-glucosidase (e. g. acarbose and miglitol) and (v) Drugs known as glucagon-like peptide 1 receptor agonists whose mechanism of action include the lowering of glucose via stimulation of insulin release from pancreatic islet β-cells, inhibition of glucagon and reducing glucose absorption into the bloodstream (e.g. liraglutide and exenatide) (Marre and Penfornis, 2011; Krentz and Bailey, 2005). There are other available pharmacological options such as amylinomimetics, meglitinide derivatives, selective sodium glucose transport-2 inhibitors, dipeptidyl peptidase IV inhibitors and dopamine agonists.

BACKGROUND

Medicinal herbs and their active principles for therapeutic purposes

In this modern era there is the continual use of plants for therapeutic purposes. Globally approximately 25% of prescription medicines are produced from plants (Yuan et al., 2016). Herbal medicine or phytomedicine is one of the subdivisions of complementary and alternative medicinal therapies. According to the World Health Organization herbs are utilized in traditional medicine to satisfy primary care needs in many countries (World Health Organization, 2002) possibly due to their lower costs, less adverse effects, and dissatisfaction of patients with outcomes from conventional therapies. However, medicinal herbs may be amalgamated with or used as an alternate to conventional allopathic medicines (Thompson et al., 2015).

There are thousands of medicinal herbs and each possess many biological constituents although only a few maybe therapeutically active (Tu et al., 2002). A large number of extraction methods have been employed in the past which have produced diverse active ingredients (Altemimi et al., 2017). Due to the bioactivities of the components and intricacies of the phytochemicals, medicinal plants are used alone or combined with other herbs producing multiple benefits as several essential metabolic pathways are targeted and modified resulting in the desired therapeutic outcome (Kennedy and Wightman, 2011). Moreover, the various parts of the plant such as the leaves, roots, berries, flowers, seeds, bark and fruits are utilized for therapeutic purposes (Herman, 2015). There are active ingredients residing in these parts of the herbs and are directed towards treating a wide range of disease conditions such as liver disorders, cardiovascular diseases including hypertension, tuberculosis, inflammatory disorders, gastrointestinal disorders, obesity, hyperlipidemia, dermatological infections, diseases associated with respiratory tract, urinary tract and central nervous system as well as diabetes mellitus (Choudhury et al., 2017).

Traditional medicine herbs used for therapeutic purposes have diverse bioactive compounds that are used in the management of diabetes mellitus (Governa et al., 2018). The hypoglycemic activity and their multiple mechanisms of actions involve insulin production from the pancreatic islet β-cells and insulin action, or both (Hui et al., 2009). In the last decade more research has concentrated on elucidating the mechanism of action of medicinal plants with anti-hyperglycemic effect and their bioactive components. This entails conducting investigations of glucose-lowing herbs and phytochemicals using experimental in vitro cell culture systems, in vivo animal models of mainly streptozotocin-induced diabetes mellitus, and clinical trials involving type 2 diabetic patients (Singh et al., 2011).

The aim of this review is to focus on potential medicinal herbs that have demonstrated anti-hyperglycemic activity through either increased secretion of insulin from pancreatic islet β-cells, reduction of insulin resistance thus increase in insulin sensitivity, or inhibition of intestinal glucose absorption by the small intestine via decreased activities of α-glucosidase.

MEDICINAL HERBS AND REGULATION OF INSULIN SECRETION

Mechanism of action (insulin secretion) - Preclinical In Vitro and In Vivo (Animal) Studies

Traditionally, medicinal herbs have been explored as hypoglycemic agents for the treatment of diabetes mellitus. Their antidiabetic properties have been described by many researchers using in vitro studies, in vivo animal models, as well as clinical studies (Salehi et al., 2019). There is growing evidence of the precise mechanisms of action of medicinal herbs that display hypoglycemic activity including improving insulin secretion in diabetic rats and patients with type 2 diabetes mellitus (Patel et al., 2012).

The anti-hyperglycemic effects of ginseng, a long-established Chinese medicine have been reported both in experimental animal models and clinical studies (Park et al., 2012; Vuksan et al., 2008). There are several species of ginseng and the two most widely consumed varieties are the American (*Panax quinquefolius L*) and Asian (*Panax ginseng*) ginseng. The antidiabetic efficacy of ginseng is due to the main constituents, triterpene β-glycoside, well-known as ginsenosides (Reeds et al., 2011).

In the last few years there are studies that have reported the antidiabetic effects of *Panax ginseng* in animal models of streptozotocin-induced diabetic rats and clinical studies of type 2 diabetic patients (Park et al., 2018; Abdelazimaf, et al., 2019). In a study by Park et al. (2012) berry extracts of *Panax ginseng* (100 or 200 mg/kg body weight) were administered to streptozotocin-induced diabetic mice daily for 10 weeks. There was significant improvement in glucose tolerance concomitant with an increased insulin secretion. The latter was probably due to increased proliferation of pancreatic islet β-cells (Park et al., 2012; Table 1). In another study that investigated the antidiabetic potential of *Panax ginseng* extract in type 1 diabetic rats, there was significant decrease in blood glucose concentrations and improved glucose challenge testing. The mechanism of action appeared to be protective of the pancreatic tissue from streptozotocin-induced destruction and restored insulin secretion (Hong et al., 2012). Likewise, an alcoholic extract of North American Ginseng (*Panax Quinquefolius*) administered 1 or 2 months decreased blood glucose and HbA1c levels in streptozotocin-induced diabetic mice and a type 2 (db/db) diabetic rat model. There was evidence of regeneration of pancreatic islet β-cells post-treatment and significant increase in C-peptide and plasma insulin levels in the streptozotocin-diabetic mice (Sen et al., 2013). The anti-hyperglycemic effect of components in ginseng radix in alloxan-induced diabetic mice was associated with an increase in blood insulin levels (Kimura et al., 1981). In a recent study, the ginsenosides of Korean red ginseng enhanced insulin secretion in response to glucose stimulation in a type 2 diabetic rat model (Park et al., 2019).

The effect of ginseng on glycemic control probably due to insulin secretion in diabetic rat models is encouraging. However, conclusive results in experimental diabetic rat models are limited and necessitates the need for further elucidation of the mechanism of ginseng.

Berberine is a quaternary ammonium isoquinoline alkaloid and the main active constituent of the Chinese herb *Coptis chinensis French* and *Scutellaria*. A number of studies have reported that berberine displays a therapeutic effect on type 2 diabetes mellitus as it lowers blood glucose levels and regulates lipid metabolism (Dong et al., 2012; Pang et al., 2015). Berberine controls glucose metabolism probably via numerous mechanisms and signal pathways including impeding gluconeogenesis in the liver, stimulating the secretion of intestinal glucagon-like protein-1, initiating adenosine monophosphate-activated protein kinase pathway and increasing the sensitivity of insulin (Vuddanda et al., 2010). Chueh and colleague (2011) investigated the effect of berberine on type 1 non-obese diabetic mice. The berberine supplementation administered over 14 weeks significantly improved glucose tolerance and increased the insulin levels as there were less damaged pancreatic islet β-cells. This finding suggests that berberine supplementation in vivo protects pancreatic islet β-cells in non-obese diabetic mice (Chueh et al., 2011; Table 1). In another study that sought to determine the underlying mechanism of action of berberine using a streptozotocin-induced diabetic rat model, the observed hypoglycemiac effect was demonstrated by lowered fasting blood glucose levels that was associated with the insulin-sensitizing effects during oral glucose tolerance testing (Wang et al., 2011). The antidiabetic effect of berberine may be due its ability to stimulate insulin secretion (Leung et al., 2004) and its insulin sensitizing and insulinotropic activities in diabetic rat models (Ko et al., 2005). Similar to berberine, *Cuminum cyminum* is known to have antidiabetic activity. The bioactive components cuminaldehyde and cuminol were found to possess insulinotrophic activities as they lowered blood glucose levels by increasing insulin secretion. The mechanism of action of the β-cell protective action of cuminaldehyde and cuminol involved the elevation of intracellular Ca^{2+} concentration and the closure of the ATP-sensitive K (K^+-ATP) channel (Patil et al., 2013).

Based on these findings, the anti-diabetic effect of berberine, which is associated with the stimulation of insulin secretion in diabetic animal models is an area of study that requires further investigation.

There are several other plant species that possess anti-hyperglycemic properties and whose mechanisms of action involves increased insulin secretion have been documented in the literature. *Chloroxylon swietenia* DC. (Family: *Rutaceae*) is an essential well-established folklore medicinal plant with chemical constituents such as terpenes, phenols, and alkaloids that are responsible for its biological action (Charanraj et al., 2019). Jayaprasad et al. (2016) investigated the antidiabetic potential of methanolic and aqueous extracts of *Chloroxylon swietenia* bark on streptozotocin-induced diabetic rats. The results indicated moderately controlled blood glucose levels in the treatment group equivalent to glibenclamide, concomitant with an increase in plasma insulin level (Jayaprasad et al., 2016; Table 1). Similarly, the fruit of *Forsythia Suspensa* (Thunb.) produced a dose-dependent decrease in blood glucose levels after 4 weeks of intervention in streptozotocin-induced diabetic mice, accompanied by a significant rise in plasma insulin levels (Zhang et al., 2016). Correspondingly, the therapeutic benefits of the leaf of *Coccinia grandis* as a hypoglycemic agent include significant reduction in blood glucose levels in streptozotocin-induced diabetic rats (Mohammed et al., 2016). The mechanism of action of the hypoglycemic activity of the ethanolic extract of the leaf of *Coccinia grandis* is due to increase insulin secretion as reflected by elevated plasma insulin levels (Mohammed et al., 2016). Other evidence of the antidiabetic properties of *Coccinia grandis* include an in vitro study where extracts from the plant demonstrated significant insulinotrophic property with increased insulin release in the treatment group (Meenatchi et al., 2017), and reduced blood glucose levels with concomitant statistically significant increase in serum insulin and C-peptide levels in streptozotocin-induced diabetic rats (Attanayake et al., 2015).

These medicinal plants with promising antidiabetic potential acts through enhancing the number of pancreatic β-cells in the islets of Langerhans with subsequent increased insulin secretion. Nevertheless, further investigation into the mechanism of action of these plants is warranted.

Mechanism of action (insulin secretion) – Clinical studies

The ability of ginseng extracts as a hypoglycemic agent have been well documented in animal models (Hong et al., 2012; Sen et al., 2013). However, only a limited number of randomized controlled clinical trials have evaluated the effectiveness of ginseng extract in type 2 diabetic patients (Vuksan et al.,

2000; Reeds et al., 2011). In a randomized controlled clinical trial comprised of nondiabetic subjects and patients with type 2 diabetes mellitus, American Ginseng (*Panax Quinquefolius L*) significantly reduced postprandial blood glucose levels in both groups (Vuksan et al., 2000; Table 1). In another randomized, double-blind, placebo-controlled clinical trial with 4-week intervention using red ginseng supplementation, there was significant decreased postprandial glucose levels in type 2 diabetic patients with concomitant increased plasma insulin levels (Oh et al., 2014). Similarly, the root of American ginseng attenuates hyperglycemia and its mechanism of action involves a reduction in pancreatic β-cell death with resulting increase in insulin production (Luo and Luo, 2009). This same plant combined with Konjac-mannan exhibited antidiabetic effect in type 2 diabetic patients. The mechanism of action of American ginseng was likely the enhancement of insulin secretion from pancreatic islet β-cells while that of Konjac-mannan increased insulin sensitivity (Vuksan et al., 2001). The same group of investigators performed a double-blind, randomized, crossover design study of 19 well-controlled type 2 diabetic patients using Korean red ginseng and observed good blood glycemic control with HbA1c inside normal limits post 12-week supplementation, and an associated increase insulin sensitivity (Vuksan et al., 2008). However, in a randomized controlled study of overweight or obese subjects with impaired glucose tolerance or newly diagnosed type 2 diabetes, ginseng or ginsenoside Re did not increase insulin secretion or β-cell function due to its poor systemic bioavailability (Reeds et al., 2011).

The effectiveness of ginseng-related antidiabetic therapy in clinical trials differ in variation in the species, dosage, formulations and duration of treatment. The clinical efficacy of ginseng could be improved with the implementation of a standardized treatment regimen and study duration for over three months.

Herbs have been used in the management of diabetes mellitus and the mechanism of action involved increased insulin secretion (Li et al., 2012). Extract from Rosemary, an evergreen shrub containing polyphenols has been shown to possess anti-hyperglycemic properties as it significantly reduced fasting blood glucose levels (Labban et al. 2014) via improved secretion in insulin from pancreatic islet β-cells (Naimi et al., 2017). There is evidence that the mechanism of action of hypoglycemic herbs such as bitter melon, banaba, *Gymnema sylvestre*, fenugreek and *Coptis chinensis* in clinical studies with diabetic patients involved increased insulin secretion and inhibition of intestinal glucose absorption (Prabhakar et al., 2011). There are also reports that Rutin a flavonoid, found in black and green tea demonstrates a pancreatic anti-hyperglycemic effect and its mode of action may include enhancing insulin release from pancreatic islet β-cells inhibiting gluconeogenesis and decreasing carbohydrate absorption from the small intestine (Ghorbani, 2017; Sattanathan et al., 2011).

The pharmacological activities of these herbs in clinical studies have emphasized their potential efficacy in the management of diabetes mellitus. However, their mechanistic pathways including improving insulin secretion require further elucidation. This requires conducting multicenter large-scale clinical trials to assess the therapeutic efficacy and safety of these medicinal herbs.

MEDICINAL HERBS AND REGULATION OF INSULIN RESISTANCE

Mechanism of action (insulin resistance) - Preclinical In Vitro and In Vivo (Animal) Studies

Insulin resistance is one of the chief contributors to the etiology and pathophysiology of type 2 diabetes mellitus (Olokoba et al., 2012) and poor control of blood glucose levels in type 1 diabetic patients is concomitant with hepatic insulin resistance (Kaul et al., 2015). The metabolic activity of berberine in regulating blood glucose concentrations has been extensively studied and evidenced in various animal models of type 1 and type 2 diabetes mellitus (Jianping and Jiaa, 2015). Zhou et al. (2009) investigated the protective effect of berberine against β-cell damage in streptozotocin- and high-carbohydrate/high-fat diet-induced diabetic rats and found increased insulin expression and pancreatic islet β-cell regeneration post 16 weeks intervention. In another study that investigated the effects of berberine on glycemic control and exploration of possible hypoglycemic mechanism, the herb ameliorates hyperglycemia via the upregulation of protein kinase B (Akt) signaling pathway (Xie et al. 2011). In a recent study, berberine significantly decreased fasting blood glucose levels and low-density lipoprotein in type 2 diabetic rats. Berberine improved insulin sensitivity and plasma insulin levels as well as reduced insulin resistance via elevated mRNA and protein expressions of glucose transporter 4 (GLUT4) in skeletal muscle (Mi et al., 2019; Table 1). Berberine reduced insulin resistance in animal models of type 2 diabetes mellitus via upregulation of insulin receptor mRNA expression that was associated with elevated protein kinase C activity in the liver (Kong et al., 2009). Other modes of action of the antidiabetic properties of berberine involved stimulation of AMP-activated protein kinase in type 2 diabetic and insulin-resistant states (Lee et al., 2006), and activation of transcriptional factors expression such as PPAR-γ that improved insulin sensitivity (Deng et al., 2014).

Although the findings support the antidiabetic effect of berberine via diminishing insulin resistance, more experimental *in vivo* and *in vitro* studies involving type 2 diabetic models are needed to elucidate the precise mechanism of action.

Garlic (*Allium sativum L.*) is reported to possess numerous biological properties including antibacterial, antihypertensive, antidiabetic and antioxidant due to the presence of sulfur phyto-constituents such as diallyl disulfide, alliin, allicin, S-allyl cysteine, allyl mercaptan, ajoene and flavonoids such as quercetin (Batiha et al., 2020). The antidiabetic activity of garlic and its active ingredients in experimentally induced or animal model of diabetes mellitus is well documented in the literature (Padiya and Banerjee, 2013; Brahmanaidu et al., 2017).

Brahmanaidu et al. (2017) investigated the effects of S-allylcysteine from garlic on glucose, insulin, insulin resistance, and other parameters in streptozotocin-nicotinamide-induced diabetic rats. There were reductions in plasma glucose levels, lipid peroxidation and insulin resistance by S-allylcysteine, signifying the mechanism by which garlic and its constituents alleviate the hyperglycemia in diabetic rats (Brahmanaidu et al., 2017). Garlic oil regulates glucose control, and improves insulin tolerance and insulin-stimulated use of glucose to produce glycogen in skeletal muscles of streptozotocin-induced diabetes mellitus (Chang et al., 2011). Garlic oil also improves insulin sensitivity and increased the expression of GLUT4 in skeletal muscle (Liu et al., 2012). There are also other reports of the efficacy of garlic extract in reducing insulin resistance (Padiya and Banerjee, 2013) and assisting in recovering of glucose homeostasis including decreased insulin resistance in rats with chronic intermittent hypoxia and diabetes mellitus (Peng and Hu, 2018).

The findings of these studies suggest that garlic and its constituents possess anti-hyperglycemic properties mediated through alteration in insulin resistance and improved insulin sensitivity. However, there are few studies conducted in this area, hence further investigations are warranted.

Resveratrol (3, 5, 4¢-trihydroxystilbene) is a naturally occurring polyphenol and potent antioxidant present in high levels red wine and grapes (Perrone et al., 2017). Resveratrol is commercially accessible as a dietary supplement in tablet form. There is evidence that it has anti-platelet, anti-inflammatory and anti-carcinogenic properties as well as anti-hyperglycemic activity in diabetic animal models

(González-Rodríguez et al., 2015; Rezaei Farimani et al., 2015). A study by González-Rodríguez et al. (2015) evaluated the effect of resveratrol in regulating insulin resistance in Irs2-deficient mice and streptozotocin-induced diabetic mice. It was found that resveratrol enhanced systemic insulin sensitivity of Irs2-deficient mice by protein tyrosine phosphatase 1B inhibition in muscle and liver. Also, resveratrol re-established hepatic insulin signaling and insulin sensitivity in streptozotocin-induced diabetic mice (González-Rodríguez et al., 2015; Table 2). Another study investigated the effect of resveratrol on the expressions soluble N-ethylmaleimide-sensitive factor attachment protein receptor (SNARE) complex proteins in streptozotocin- and nicotinamide-induced diabetic mice. There was increased expression of SNARE proteins resulting in reduced insulin resistance and hyperglycemia (Rezaei Farimani et al., 2015). Moreover, in a recent study, resveratrol (RES)-loaded solid lipid nanoparticle demonstrated improved glucose tolerance and decreased insulin resistance by targeting the expression of VAMP2, STX4 and SNAP23 in muscle and liver tissues (Mohseni et al., 2019). There are other studies that have reported that resveratrol exhibited anti-hyperglycemic effect and decreased insulin resistance via increasing the expression of GLUT4 (Vallianou et al., 2013) and improved plasma insulin level (Palsamy et al., 2008). However, it should be stated that in two in vivo experiments resveratrol did not decrease blood glucose levels in streptozotocin-induced diabetic rats (Schmatz et al., 2009; Schmatz et al., 2010).

The findings from these studies suggest that resveratrol ameliorates diabetes mellitus and improves insulin resistance via molecular mechanisms which include targeting SNARE proteins and PTP1B. Although significant work has been conducted in animal models of experimental diabetes mellitus using resveratrol, there is need to conduct more clinical trials.

Mechanism of action (insulin resistance) – Clinical studies

The antidiabetic activity, lowering of lipids and insulin-resistance improving actions of berberine have been established in a number of randomized clinical trials. Berberine decreased fasting and postprandial plasma glucose levels (Zhang et al., 2008; Li et al., 2017). In a randomized, double-blind, and placebo-controlled trial involving type 2 diabetic patients, there was reduction of fasting and postprandial plasma glucose levels three months post-treatment with berberine (Yin & Ye, 2008). Moreover, in a randomized control trial conducted by Zhang et al. (2010), berberine decreased fasting blood glucose in patients with chronic hepatitis and diabetes mellitus. The molecular mechanism of berberine in reducing insulin resistance in patients with diabetes mellitus involve: higher insulin receptor messenger RNA expression and increased insulin-stimulated phosphorylation of Akt (Zhang et al., 2008), increased GLUT-4 and retinol-binding protein-4 with subsequent improved glucose uptake into cells (Cicero et al., 1995) augmented glucagon-like peptide-1 levels, modified the peroxisome proliferator-activated receptor-γ molecular targets and phosphorylated insulin receptor substrate-1 (Cicero et al., 2016).

The antidiabetic action of berberine and its effect on the reduction of insulin resistance have been confirmed in many clinical studies with multiple molecular mechanisms proposed. However, safety issue is a concern as high doses is associated with gastrointestinal complaints.

There are a number of clinical studies that have investigated the hypoglycemic effect of cinnamon in type 2 diabetic patients (Khan et al., 2003; Imparl-Radosevich et al., 1998). Chuengsamarn et al. (2012) conducted a randomized, double-blinded, placebo- controlled trial comprising of 240 subjects with criteria of prediabetes who were evaluated for type 2 diabetes mellitus progression subsequent to curcumin treatments. The researchers found that 16.4% of the subjects in the placebo group were diagnosed with type 2 diabetes mellitus compared with none in the curcumin-treated group. The subjects in the curcumin-treated group demonstrated reduced insulin resistance and better overall β-cell function compared to the placebo group (Chuengsamarn et al., 2012). In an earlier study, cinnamon taken daily (1 – 3 g) by patients with type 2 diabetes mellitus decreased the mean fasting plasma glucose levels after 40 days (Khan et al., 2003). The researchers suggested that mechanism of action of cinnamon could be due to reduced insulin resistance, stimulation of glycogen synthase, improved glucose uptake, and reduced activity of glycogen synthase kinase-3β (Imparl-Radosevich et al., 1998). In a recent triple-blind placebo-controlled randomized clinical trial involving 140 type 2 diabetic patients, cinnamon supplement administered for 3 months improved glycemic control, total cholesterol and HDL-cholesterol as well as reduced insulin resistance (Zare et al., 2019; Table 2). Cinnamon was reported to decrease blood glucose concentration through the reduction of insulin resistance and elevated hepatic glycogenesis (Qin et al., 2010). However, in a study that examined the effects of cinnamon supplementation on glucose tolerance and insulin sensitivity in patients with type 2 diabetes mellitus, there was no improvement in oral glucose tolerance and whole-body insulin sensitivity (Vanschoonbeek et al., 2006). Likewise, another study reported that cinnamon supplementation fails to improve postprandial blood glucose and insulin resistance and only modified fasting glucose levels (Rafehi et al., 2012).

In some clinical studies the findings of the antidiabetic action of cinnamon and its mechanism of action involving improving insulin resistance are encouraging, but there are others that have shown no beneficial effect. Further investigations into the mechanism of action is warranted, employing large-scale randomized controlled clinical trials.

Nigella sativa is a yearly herbaceous plant that is a member of the Ranunculaceae family. It is well-known as "black seed" or "kalonji" and different forms of *Nigella sativa* have been used in traditional medicine to treat diarrhea, gastrointestinal diseases, bronchitis and diabetes mellitus (Ramadan, 2007). The antidiabetic effect of *Nigella sativa* have been described in different animal models where it lowered blood glucose levels, improved glucose uptake in peripheral tissues, and increased proliferation of pancreatic islet β-cells and the secretion of insulin (Benhaddou-Andaloussi et al., 2011; Fararh et al., 2004). In a randomized controlled trial, Kaatabi et al. (2015) investigated the glucose lowering effect of *Nigella sativa* (2 g/day capsule) over one year in patients with type 2 diabetes mellitus. They found that *Nigella sativa* significantly decreased fasting plasma glucose and HbA1c levels as well as insulin resistance which was associated with higher pancreatic β-cell activity over the treatment period (Kaatabi et al., 2015; Table 2). In another randomized controlled trial, *Nigella sativa* seeds (dose of 1, 2 and 3 gm/day for three months) were administered as an adjuvant therapy in patients with type 2 diabetes mellitus. Nigella *sativa* at a dose of 2 gm/day significantly reduced fasting and postprandial blood glucose levels as well as insulin resistance index, and improved β-cell function (Bamosa et al., 2010; Table 2). Likewise, in another study, *Nigella sativa* oil significantly reduced fasting blood glucose levels and increased insulin levels post-treatment for 40 days in type 2 diabetes mellitus patients (Ahmad et al., 2009). In addition, in a systematic review Hesmati et al. (2015) stated that *Nigella sativa* modulated hyperglycemia by decreasing insulin resistance in the intervention group, although this effect was not significant after adjusting for confounders.

The findings of these studies suggest that long-term *Nigella sativa* supplementation improves glucose homeostasis via a reduction in insulin resistance. However, further investigations into the diabetic properties of *Nigella sativa* are needed due to challenges in determining the effective dosage and types which give the best outcome.

MEDICINAL HERBS AND INHIBITION OF GLUCOSE ABSORPTION

Mechanism of action (inhibition of glucose absorption) - In vitro experimental studies

Numerous researches have established that herbal plants and their bioactive compounds in vitro inhibit α-amylase and α-glucosidase activities and some of them are noted here. The inhibition of α-amylase have been linked with the antihyperglycemic effect of medicinal herbs such as *Corchorus olitorius* whose leaf contain chlorogenic acid, isorhamnetin and caffeic acid (Oboh et al., 2012), *Phyllanthus urinaria* a wild plant in Indonesia that contains gallic acid, corilagin and and macatannin B (Guanawan-Puteri et al., 2012), and *Ocimum basilicum* whose aqueous extract contains tannins, glycosides, steroids, reducing sugars and flavonoids and in addition inhibit α-glucosidase activity (El-Beshbishy and Bahashwan, 2012). In vitro studies have also reported that some herbs are inhibitors of the carbohydrate digestive enzyme, α-glucosidase. These herbs include: *Holarrhena antidysenterica* where the methanolic extract of the seeds contain gallic acid and flavonoids [IC(50) of 0.52 mg/mL; Ali et al., 2011)], safflower (*Carthamus tinctorius* L.) that contains the serotonin derivatives N-feruloyl serotonin and N-p-coumaroyl serotonin (Takahashi et al., 2012), *Cassia Alata* of which the ethyl acetate and n-butanol fractions of the leaves contain kaempferol and kaempferol 3-O-gentiobioside (Varghese et al., 2013) and Chinese aloes that contain aloeresin A which demonstrated significant dose-dependent inhibition on the enzyme activity (Jong-Anurakkun et al., 2011).

In vitro enzyme inhibition studies indicate that these herbal medicines could possibly be effective natural α-amylase and *α*-glucosidase inhibitors used in the treatment of diabetes mellitus.

Medicinal plants are traditionally used as alternative therapies in many countries and regions and they are strongly linked to the cultural values of the people. These plants are good sources of α-glucosidase inhibitors and may be useful in the treatment of type 2 diabetes mellitus. In *vitro* enzyme inhibition studies demonstrated that flavonoids isolated from the leaves of *Nelumbo nucifera* inhibit α-glucosidase, and α-amylase activities (Liu et al., 2013). In Australia, extracts from *Petalostigma pubescens* and *Petalostigma banksia* that contain phenols and flavonoids significantly inhibited both α-amylase and α-glucosidase activities and the angiotensin converting enzyme (Deo et al., 2016). In Latin America, herbs such as *Chancapiedra* (*Phyllantus niruri* L.), *Huacatay* (*Tagetes minuta*) and *Zarzaparrilla* (*Smilax officinalis*) demonstrated significant antihyperglycemic effect and their mode of action involves the inhibition of α-glucosidase with no effect on α-amylase (Ranilla et al., 2010). Moreover, in Mexico extracts of herbs such as *Hintonia standleyana* (*Rubiaceae*), *Brickellia cavanillesii* (*Asteraceae*), *Hintonia latiflora* and *Ligusticum porteri* (*Apiaceae*) have been found to possess antihyperglycemic properties and inhibit α-glucosidase activity (Mata et al., 2013). In addition, Malaysia medicinal plants such as *Garcinia mangostana* (*mangosteen*), *Nephelium lappaceum*, *Barringtonia Racemosa* and *Phyllanthus Acidus* contain phytochemicals such as terpenoids, glycosides, alkaloids, flavonoids and phenolic compounds which exhibit significant inhibition of α-glucosidase activity (Mohd Bukhari et al., 2017).

These studies demonstrated that in vitro tests of α-glucosidase activities of the extracts from the medicinal plants give credence to their potential as antihyperglycemic agents.

Mechanism of action (inhibition of glucose absorption) - In vivo experimental animal models tudies

There are a number of in vivo studies that have investigated the effect of extracts from herbs with anti-hyperglycemic action on the inhibition of α-glucosidase activity. In a study by Mohamed et al. (2011), *Cinnamomum zeylanicum* commonly utilized in traditional medicine for managing diabetes mellitus was evaluated for its α-glucosidase inhibitory potential. The methanolic extract of the *Cinnamomum zeylanicum* bark ameliorated postprandial hyperglycemia in streptozotocin-induced diabetic rats mainly by α-glucosidase inhibition (Mohamed et al., 2011). In another study, berberine (100 or 200 mg/kg) was orally administered to streptozotocin-induced diabetic rats. Berberine significantly reduced post-prandial blood glucose levels in diabetic rats via suppression of intestinal disaccharide activities (Liu et al., 2010). Similarly, dietary administration of *Aloe Arborescens* Miller components (phenolic compounds) to streptozotocin-induced diabetic rats lowered blood glucose levels and exhibited inhibitory action on intestinal glucose absorption (Beppu et al., 2006). In an earlier study, Chung et al. (2001) investigated the mechanism of action of white ginseng radix and the rootlet in KKAy mice. White ginseng radix reduced fasting blood glucose levels and the hypoglycemic mechanism involved possibly delaying intestinal glucose absorption and inhibition of hepatic glucose-6-phosphatase (Chung et al., 2011). In addition, chronic oral administration of the seed of *Nigella sativa* (aqueous extract of 0.1 - 100 pg/mL) improved glucose tolerance in rats, and in vitro studies indicated inhibition of intestinal absorption of glucose (Meddah et al., 2009).

The medicinal herb *Ficus deltoidea* which belongs to the Moraceae family, have been reported as an alternative remedy for diabetes mellitus (Sulaiman et al., 2008). Ficus *deltoidea* decreased postprandial glucose levels and the mechanism of action involved increase basal and insulin-stimulated uptake of glucose into hepatocytes (Adam et a., 2009a) and reduced glucose uptake from the small intestine due to inhibition of sucrose activity (Adam et al., 2009b). Moreover, Choo et al. isolated vitexin and isoviten, two C-glycosyl bioflavonoids from leaf extracts of *Ficus deltoidea* which significantly reduced post-prandial blood glucose levels in sucrose loaded-induced diabetic rats via α-glucosidase inhibition (Choo et al., 2012). Huanglian Wan, a traditional herbal medicine used to treat diabetes mellitus in China was investigated for its antihyperglycemic effect in streptozotocin-induced diabetic rats. The Huanglian Wan extract lowered postprandial plasma glucose and exerted its action partly via the inhibition of intestinal disaccharidases and increasing the levels of insulin (Deng et al., 2012). Interestingly, there is a report of 13 out of 34 medicinal herbs in Chinese traditional medicine that significantly decreased plasma glucose levels in streptozotocin-induced diabetic rats. Zymologic assay indicated that *Anemarrhena asphodeloides* and *Pueraria lobata* demonstrated the highest inhibition against α-glucosidase (He et al., 2011). Furthermore, the ethyl acetate fraction containing butyl-isobutyl-phthalate from the rhizoid of *Laminaria japonica*, a medicinal plant widely utilized in traditional Chinese medicine for managing diabetes mellitus demonstrated significant hypoglycemic effect in streptozotocin-induced diabetic mice via α-glucosidase inhibition (Bu et al., 2010).

The findings of these in vivo studies demonstrated the potential of medicinal herbs in treating diabetes mellitus and their influence on intestinal glucose absorption through the inhibition of α-glucosidase activity.

Mechanism of action ((inhibition of glucose absorption) – Clinical studies

In vitro and in vivo animal studies presented have revealed that medicinal herbs possess hypoglycemic properties and the mechanism of action involves the inhibition of α-glucosidase. There are only a few clinical studies that examine the potential benefits of medicinal herbs that are antidiabetic and act by inhibiting disaccharidases. Hussain et al. 2012 conducted a randomized, blinded crossover study designed to assess the potential of quercetin to lower postprandial blood glucose level in type 2 diabetic patients after maltose and glucose loading. Quercetin ameliorated postprandial blood glucose levels particularly after the maltose loading compared with placebo. The mode of action may be ascribed to α-glucosidase inhibition (Hussain et al., 2012). Likewise, a randomized controlled clinical trial of 70 type 2 diabetic patients was conducted to investigate the effect of cinnamon (*Cinnamomum cassia*) on fasting blood glucose levels and HbA1c. Cinnamon, one month post-treatment decreased the fasting blood glucose levels, although there was no difference between the intervention and placebo groups (Hasanzade et al., 2013). The major mechanism of action of cinnamon is through the inhibition of α-glucosidase (Mohamed et al., 2011).

It is clear from these findings that the mechanism of action of herbal plants involving α-glucosidase inhibition in randomized controlled clinical trials warrants further investigation.

CONCLUSION AND RECOMMENDATIONS

Medicinal herbs and their bioactive components which include potent phytochemicals significantly possess antidiabetic potential and continue to be explored for the management and treatment of type 2 diabetes mellitus. Herbs have been used in alternative and complementary medicines for over decades and an understanding of the mechanism of action through which they mitigate type 2 diabetes mellitus is evolving. Findings from research as presented in this review have shown that the efficacy of hypoglycemic herbs and their active principles is achieved through multiple mechanisms such as: stimulation of insulin secretion from pancreatic islet β-cells and improvement in β-cell function, reduction of insulin resistance and enhancement in insulin sensitivity, inhibition of intestinal glucose absorption via decrease activities of α-glucosidase and α-amylase, increasing the uptake of glucose by muscle and adipose tissues, decrease in gluconeogenesis or glycogenolysis and regulation of different aspects of the insulin signaling pathway such as inducing protein and gene expression.

From this review, it has been demonstrated that medicinal herbs have enormous potential as pharmaceutical agents for the treatment of diabetes mellitus and are used as adjuvants to conventional therapy due to their affordability and possibly less adverse effects. However, although much progress has been made particularly in vitro and in vivo studies using experimental animal models of diabetes mellitus where different herbs have shown varying degree of hypoglycemic activity, the number of clinical studies is woefully inadequate and only few translated to clinical use. Moreover, appropriate methods should be established to define the active constituents of these hypoglycemic herbs in order to provide assurance of stable pharmaceutical and clinical effects.

In this rapidly growing ethnopharmaceutical field where there is also a shift from monotherapy to combination therapy as more formulations comprising of two or more herbs are employed, there is an urgent need for the implementation of validated testing protocols. This will enable the evaluation of the quality and quantity of active drugs present in the final products that should be tested in well-designed

Table 1. Medicinal herbs that display antihyperglycemic effects with mechanism of action involving the regulation of insulin secretion

Medicinal herbs	Experimental model/Clinical study	Effective dose and duration	Molecular mechanisms	References
Panax ginseng (Red and green berry extracts)	STZ-induced diabetic mice	Administered orally (100 or 200 mg/kg BW) for 10 weeks	Improved glucose tolerance and increased insulin secretion; likely due to increased proliferation of β-cells	Park et al., 2012
Panax ginseng	STZ-induced diabetic mice	250-350 mg/dL for two weeks	Decreased blood glucose levels; protection of pancreatic β-cells and increased insulin secretion	Hong et al., 2012
North American Ginseng (*Panax Quinquefolius*)	STZ-induced & type 2 (db/db) diabetic mice	200 mg/kg BW/ day, oral gavage for 1 or 2 months	Decreased blood glucose and HbA1c levels; regeneration of pancreatic β-cells with increased C-peptide and plasma insulin levels	Sen et al., 2013
Coptis chinensis French (Berberine)	Non-obese diabetic mice	50, 150 & 500 mg/ kg BW over 14 weeks	Improved glucose tolerance and increased insulin levels; protects pancreatic β-cells	Chueh et al., 2011
Chloroxylon swietenia	STZ-induced diabetic rats	Methanolic and aqueous extracts - 250 mg/kg B.W. for 45 days	Moderate reduction in blood glucose with associated increased plasma insulin levels	Jayaprasad et al., 2016
Coccinia grandis	STZ-induced diabetic rats	0.75 gm/kg daily for 30 days	Reduction in HbA1c and concomitant increased serum insulin and C-peptide concentrations; increase in number of pancreatic β-cells	Attanayake et al., 2015
Red Ginseng	Randomized, double-blind, placebo-controlled clinical trial; 42 subjects with IFG or type 2 diabetes	3 times per day for four weeks	Significant decrease in postprandial glucose levels and associated increase in plasma insulin levels	Oh et al., 2014
Panax ginseng [Korean Red Ginseng (rootlets)]	Double-blind, randomized, crossover design; 19 type 2 diabetic patients	6 gm/day for 12 weeks	Improved glucose tolerance and HbA1c levels; increased insulin sensitivity	Vuksan et al., 2008
American ginseng (Panax quinquefolius L)	Clinical trial of 9 subjects with type 2 diabetes	3 gm ginseng 40 minutes before a 25 gm oral glucose challenge	Improved glucose tolerance; no mechanism given	Vuksan et al., 2000

clinical trials. Favorable outcomes of these clinical trials and oversight by regulatory authorities in different countries will build consumer confidence particularly in the efficacy and safety of herbs used as monotherapy or herbal formulations.

Table 2. Medicinal herbs display antihyperglycemic effects with mechanism of action involving the regulation of insulin resistance

Medicinal herbs	Experimental model/ Clinical study	Effective dose and duration	Molecular mechanism	References
Rhizoma coptidis (Berberine)	STZ-induced diabetic rats	200 mg/kg once a day for 4 weeks	Decreased insulin resistance with increased insulin sensitivity and levels; elevated mRNA and protein expressions of GLUT4	Mi et al., 2019
Allium sativum (Garlic oil)	STZ-induced diabetic rats	Garlic oil (10, 50, or 100 mg/kg BW for 3 weeks	Dose-dependently reduction in insulin resistance; elevated the expression of GLUT4 in skeletal muscle	Liu et al., 2012
Resveratrol	Irs2-deficient mice and STZ-induced diabetic mice	-	Decreased insulin resistance via inhibition of PTP1B	González-Rodríguez et al., 2015
Red ginseng (protopanaxadiol (PPD) and protopanaxatriol (PPT)-type saponins	STZ-induced diabetic rats	50 mg/kg BW PPD or 150 mg/kg BW PPT	Improved glucose tolerance and reduced insulin resistance; suppressed expression of PGC-1α and glucose-6-phosphatase	Deng et al., 2017
Rhizoma coptidis (Berberine)	Randomized control trial of 36 adults with type 2 diabetes mellitus	0.5 gm/3 times a day for 3 months	Reduced fasting and post-prandial blood glucose levels; decreased insulin resistance index	Yin et al., 2008
Curcumin	Randomized, double-blinded, placebo-controlled trial of 240 pre-diabetic subject	Curcumin capsules for 9 months	Decreased insulin resistance and better overall pancreatic β-cell function compared with the placebo group	Chuengsamarn et al. 2012
Cinnamon	Randomized controlled clinical trial involving 140 type 2 diabetic patients	Cinnamon bark powder in 500 mg capsules twice daily for 3 months	Improved glycemic control, total cholesterol and HDL-cholesterol as well as reduced insulin resistance	Zare et al., 2019
Nigella sativa	Randomized controlled trial of 114 type 2 diabetic patients on standard oral hypoglycemic drugs	Capsules of 500 mg (2 g/day for 3 months)	Decreased fasting blood glucose levels and HbA1c levels; reduced insulin resistance and higher β-cell activity	Kaatabi et al. 2015
Nigella sativa (seeds)	Randomized controlled trial of 94 type 2 diabetic patients	Capsules administered orally in doses of 1, 2 and 3 gm/day for 3 months	Significant reductions in fasting, postprandial glucose and HbA1c levels; reduced insulin resistance index and increased β-cell function	Bamosa et al., 2010

Table 3. Medicinal herbs that display antihyperglycemic effects with mechanism of action involving the inhibition of glucose absorption

Medicinal herbs	Experimental model/Clinical study	Effective dose and duration	Molecular mechanisms	References
Methanol extract of *Cinnamomum zeylanicum* (bark)	Streptozotocin (STZ)-induced diabetic rats	200 mg/kg BW cinnamon extract (oral)	Reduced postprandial hyperglycemia by 78.2% and 52.0% in maltose and sucrose loaded STZ- induced diabetic rats due to α-glucosidase inhibition	Mohamed et al. 2011
Berberine	Streptozotocin-induced diabetic rats	Berberine (100 or 200 mg/kg) orally once daily	Berberine significantly decreased the disaccharidase activities and sucrase-isomaltase complex mRNA expression of diabetic rats in a concentration-dependent manner	Liu et al., 2010
Aloe arborescens Miller components	Streptozotocin-induced diabetic rats	Basal diets supplemented with Aloe arborescens Miller components from 31 days before to 73 days after streptozotocin administration	Decreased blood glucose levels and inhibitory action on intestinal glucose absorption	Beppu et al., 2006
White ginseng radix (Ginseng Radix Alba)	Diabetic KKAy mice	Four week oral administration of white ginseng radix	Reduced fasting blood glucose levels, delaying intestinal glucose absorption and inhibition of hepatic glucose-6-phosphatase activity	Chung et al., 2011
Ficus deltoidea	Sucrose-induced diabetic rats	Partitioned extracts, sub-fractions and pure bioactive constituents of Ficus deltoidea	C-glycosyl bioflavonoids, vitexin and isovitexin exhibited in vivo α-glucosidase inhibition	Choo et al., 2012
34 Medicinal herbs in Chinese traditional medicine	Streptozotocin-induced diabetic rats	Oral administrated of herbal solution once a day for 4 weeks	Herbs such as Pueraria lobata and Anemarrhena asphodeloides showed the highest inhibition against α-glucosidase activity	He et al., 2011
Rhizoid of *Laminaria japonica*	Streptozotocin-induced diabetic rats	Administration of pure active compound, butyl-isobutyl-phthalate to rats	Significant hypoglycemic effect via α-glucosidase inhibition	Bu et al., 2010
Quercetin	Randomized, blinded crossover study of group of 12 type 2 diabetic patients	Single oral dose (400 mg) of quercetin administered 30 min. before loading with either maltose (2g/kg) or glucose (100g)	Significant reduction of postprandial glucose levels in type 2 diabetic patients loaded with maltose due to α-glucosidase inhibition	Hussain et al., 2012
Cinnamomum cassia	Randomized controlled clinical trial of 70 type 2 diabetic patients	Patients were treated with capsules of cinnamon for one month	Decreased the fasting blood glucose levels post-treatment probably due to inhibition of α-glucosidase activity	Hasanzade et al., 2013

REFERENCES

Jianping, J.Y., & Jiaa, Y. W. (2012). Effects and mechanisms of berberine in diabetes treatment. *Acta Pharmaceutica Sinica B*, *2*(4), 327-334.

Abdelazim, A., Khater, S., & Ali, H. (2019). Panax ginseng improves glucose metabolism in streptozotocin-induced diabetic rats through 5¢ adenosine monophosphate kinase up-regulation. *Saudi Journal of Biological Sciences, 26*(7), 1436-1441.

Abu-helalah, M., Al-hanaqta, M., Alshraideh, H., & Hijazeen, J. (2014). Quality of life and psychological well-being of breast cancer survivors in Jordan. *Asian Pacific Journal of Cancer Prevention*, *15*(14), 5927–5936. doi:10.7314/APJCP.2014.15.14.5927 PMID:25081724

Adam, Z., Hamid, M., Ismail, A., & Khamis, S. (2009a). Effect of Ficus deltoidea extracts on hepatic basal and insulin-stimulated glucose uptake. *The Journal of Biological Sciences*, *9*(2), 9–16.

Adam, Z., Hamid, M., Ismail, A., & Khamis, S. (2009b). Effect of Ficus deltoidea extracts on hepatic basal and insulin-stimulated glucose uptake. *The Journal of Biological Sciences*, *9*(8), 796–803. doi:10.3923/jbs.2009.796.803

Ahmad, B., Tariq, M., Uppal, A. M., & Naveed, A. K. (2009). Effects of *Nigella sativa* oil on some blood parameters in type 2 diabetes mellitus patients. *Asian Journal of Chemistry*, *21*, 5373–5381.

Ali, K. M., Chatterjee, K., De, D., Jana, K., Bera, T. K., & Ghosh, D. (2011). Inhibitory effect of hydro-methanolic extract of seed of Holarrhena antidysenterica on alpha-glucosidase activity and postprandial blood glucose level in normoglycemic rat. *Journal of Ethnopharmacology*, *135*(1), 194–196. doi:10.1016/j.jep.2011.02.034 PMID:21385604

Altemimi, A., Lakhssassi, N., Baharlouei, A., Watson, D. G., & Lightfoot, D. A. (2017). Phytochemicals: Extraction, isolation, and identification of bioactive compounds from plant extracts. *Plants (Basel, Switzerland)*, *6*(4), 42.

American Diabetes Association. (2009). Diagnosis and classification of diabetes mellitus. *Diabetes Care*, *32*(Suppl 1), S62–S67. doi:10.2337/dc09-S062 PMID:19118289

Attanayake, A. P., Jayatilaka, K. A., Pathirana, C., & Mudduwa, L. K. (2015). Antihyperglycemic activity of Coccinia grandis (L.) Voigt in streptozotocin induced diabetic rats. *Indian Journal of Traditional Knowledge*, *14*(3), 376–381.

Bamosa, A. O., Kaatabi, H., Lebdaa, F. M., Elq, A. M., & Al-Sultanb, A. (2010). Effect of *Nigella sativa* seeds on the glycemic control of patients with type 2 diabetes mellitus. *Indian Journal of Physiology and Pharmacology*, *54*, 344–354. PMID:21675032

Benhaddou-Andaloussi, A., Martineau, L., Vuong, T., Meddah, B., Madiraju, P., Settaf, A., & Haddad, P. S. (2011). The *in vivo* antidiabetic activity of *Nigella sativa* is mediated through activation of the AMPK Pathway and increased muscle Glut4 Content. *Evidence-Based Complementary and Alternative Medicine*, *2011*, 1–9. doi:10.1155/2011/538671 PMID:21584245

Beppu, H., Shimpo, K., Chihara, T., Kaneko, T., Tamai, I., Yamaji, S., Ozaki, S., Kuzuya, H., & Sonoda, S. (2006). Antidiabetic effects of dietary administration of Aloe arborescens Miller components on multiple low-dose streptozotocin-induced diabetes in mice: Investigation on hypoglycemic action and systemic absorption dynamics of aloe components. *Journal of Ethnopharmacology, 103*(3), 468–477. doi:10.1016/j.jep.2005.10.034 PMID:16406411

Brahmanaidu, P., Uddandrao, V. V. S., Sasikumar, V., Naik, R. R., Pothani, S., Begum, M. S., Rajeshkumar, M. P., Varatharaju, C., Meriga, B., Rameshreddy, P., Kalaivani, A., & Saravanan, G. (2017). Reversal of endothelial dysfunction in aorta of streptozotocin-nicotinamide-induced type-2 diabetic rats by S-Allylcysteine. *Molecular and Cellular Biochemistry, 432*(1-2), 25–32. doi:10.100711010-017-2994-0 PMID:28258439

Bu, T., Liu, M., Zheng, L., Guo, Y., & Lin, X. (2010). α-Glucosidase inhibition and the in vivo hypoglycemic effect of butyl-isobutyl-phthalate derived from the Laminaria japonica rhizoid. *Phytotherapy Research, 24*(11), 1588–1591. doi:10.1002/ptr.3139 PMID:21031613

Chang, S. H., Liu, C. J., Kuo, C. H., Chen, H., Lin, W.-Y., Teng, K.-Y., Chang, S.-W., Tsai, C.-H., Tsai, F.-J., Huang, C.-Y., Tzang, B.-S., & Kuo, W.-W. (2011). Garlic oil alleviates MAPKs- and IL-6-mediated diabetes-related cardiac hypertrophy in STZ-induced DM rats. *Evidence-Based Complementary and Alternative Medicine, 950150*, 1–11. Advance online publication. doi:10.1093/ecam/neq075 PMID:21792366

Chang, S. H., Liu, C. J., Kuo, C. H., Chen, H., Lin, W.-Y., Teng, K.-Y., Chang, S.-W., Tsai, C.-H., Tsai, F.-J., Huang, C.-Y., Tzang, B.-S., & Kuo, W.-W. (2011). Garlic oil alleviates MAPKs- and IL-6-mediated diabetes-related cardiac hypertrophy in STZ-induced DM rats. *Evidence-Based Complementary and Alternative Medicine, 2011*, 1–11. Advance online publication. doi:10.1093/ecam/neq075 PMID:21792366

Charanraj, N., Venkateswararao, P., Vasudha, B., & Narender, B. (2019). Phytopharmacology of Chloroxylon swietenia: A review. *Journal of Drug Delivery and Therapeutics, 9*(1), 273–278. doi:10.22270/jddt.v9i1.2188

Choo, C. Y., Sulong, N. Y., Man, F., & Wong, T. W. (2012). Vitexin and isovitexin from the Leaves of Ficus deltoidea with in-vivo?? -glucosidase inhibition. *Journal of Ethnopharmacology, 142*(3), 776–781. doi:10.1016/j.jep.2012.05.062 PMID:22683902

Choudhury, H., Pandey, M., Hua, C. K., Mun, C. S., Jing, J. K., Kong, L., Ern, L. Y., Ashraf, N. A., Kit, S. W., Yee, T. S., Pichika, M. R., Gorain, B., & Kesharwani, P. (2017). An update on natural compounds in the remedy of diabetes mellitus: A systematic review. *Journal of Traditional and Complementary Medicine, 8*(3), 361–376. doi:10.1016/j.jtcme.2017.08.012 PMID:29992107

Chueh, W.-H., & Lin, J.-Y. (2011). Berberine, an isoquinoline alkaloid in herbal plants, protects pancreatic islets and serum lipids in nonobese diabetic mice. *Journal of Agricultural and Food Chemistry, 59*(14), 8021–8027. doi:10.1021/jf201627w PMID:21696141

Chuengsamarn, S., Rattanamongkolgul, S., Luechapudiporn, R., Phisalaphong, C., & Jirawatnotai, S. (2012). Curcumin extract for prevention of type 2 diabetes. *Diabetes Care, 35*(11), 2121–2127. doi:10.2337/dc12-0116 PMID:22773702

Chung, S. H., Choi, C. G., & Park, S. H. (2001). Comparisons between white ginseng radix and rootlet for antidiabetic activity and mechanism in KKAy mice. *Archives of Pharmacal Research, 24*(3), 214–218. doi:10.1007/BF02978260 PMID:11440080

Cicero, A. F., & Baggioni, A. (2016). Berberine and its role in chronic disease. *Advances in Experimental Medicine and Biology, 928*, 27–45. doi:10.1007/978-3-319-41334-1_2 PMID:27671811

Deng, J., Liu, Y., Duan, Z., Zhu, C., Hui, J., Mi, Y., Ma, P., Ma, X., Fan, D., & Yang, H. (2017). Protopanaxadiol and protopanaxatriol-type saponins ameliorate glucose and lipid metabolism in type 2 diabetes mellitus in high-fat Diet/Streptozocin-induced mice. *Frontiers in Pharmacology, 8*, 506. doi:10.3389/fphar.2017.00506 PMID:28824430

Deng, X. W., & Xie, N. (2014). Progress of berberine for treatment of type 2 diabetes. *Zhongguo Zhongyao Zazhi, 39*(8), 1374–1378. PMID:25039167

Deng, Y. X., Zhang, X. J., Shi, Q. Z., Chen, Y. S., Qiu, X. M., & Chen, B. (2012). Anti-hyperglycemic effects and mechanism of traditional Chinese medicine Huanglian Wan in streptozocin-induced diabetic rats. *Journal of Ethnopharmacology, 144*(2), 425–432. doi:10.1016/j.jep.2012.09.039 PMID:23036812

Deo, P., Hewawasam, E., Karakoulakis, A., Claudie, D. J., Nelson, R., Simpson, B. S., Smith, N. M., & Semple, S. J. (2016). In vitro inhibitory activities of selected Australian medicinal plant extracts against protein glycation, angiotensin converting enzyme (ACE) and digestive enzymes linked to type II diabetes. *BMC Complementary and Alternative Medicine, 16*(1), 435. doi:10.118612906-016-1421-5 PMID:27809834

Dong, H., Wang, N., Zhao, L., & Lu, F. (2012). Berberine in the treatment of type 2 diabetes mellitus: a systemic review and meta-analysis. *Evidence-based Complementary and Alternative Medicine: eCAM*, 591654. . doi:10.1155/2012/591654

El-Beshbishy, H., & Bahashwan, S. (2012). Hypoglycemic effect of basil (Ocimum basilicum) aqueous extract is mediated through inhibition of α-glucosidase and α-amylase activities: An in vitro study. *Toxicology and Industrial Health, 28*(1), 42–50. doi:10.1177/0748233711403193 PMID:21636683

El-Saber Batiha, G., Magdy Beshbishy, A. G., & Wasef, L. (2020). Chemical constituents and pharmacological activities of garlic (*Allium sativum* L.): A review. *Nutrients, 12*(3), 872. doi:10.3390/nu12030872 PMID:32213941

Fararh, K. M., Atoji, Y., Shimizu, Y., Shiina, T., Nikami, H., & Takewaki, T. (2004). Mechanisms of the hypoglycaemic and immunopotentiating effects of Nigella sativa L. oil in streptozotocin-induced diabetic hamsters. *Research in Veterinary Science, 77*(2), 123–129. doi:10.1016/j.rvsc.2004.03.002 PMID:15196902

Ghorbani, A. (2017). Mechanisms of antidiabetic effects of flavonoid rutin. *Biomedicine and Pharmacotherapy, 96*, 305–312. doi:10.1016/j.biopha.2017.10.001 PMID:29017142

González-Rodríguez, Á., Santamaría, B., Mas-Gutierrez, J. A., Rada, P., Fernández-Millán, E., Pardo, V., Álvarez, C., Cuadrado, A., Ros, M., Serrano, M., & Valverde, Á. M. (2015). Resveratrol treatment restores peripheral insulin sensitivity in diabetic mice in a sirt1-independent manner. *Molecular Nutrition & Food Research, 59*(8), 1431–1442. doi:10.1002/mnfr.201400933 PMID:25808216

Governa, P., Baini, G., Borgonetti, V., Cettolin, G., Giachetti, D., Magnano, A. R., Miraldi, E., & Biagi, M. (2018). Phytotherapy in the management of diabetes: A review. *Molecules (Basel, Switzerland)*, *23*(1), 105. doi:10.3390/molecules23010105 PMID:29300317

Gunawan-Puteri, M. D., Kato, E., & Kawabata, J. (2012). α-Amylase inhibitors from an Indonesian medicinal herb, Phyllanthus urinaria. *Journal of the Science of Food and Agriculture*, *92*(3), 606–609. doi:10.1002/jsfa.4615 PMID:22095704

Halban, P. A., Polonsky, K. S., Bowden, D. W., Hawkins, M. A., Ling, C., Mather, K. J., Powers, A. C., Rhodes, C. J., Sussel, L., & Weir, G. (2014). Beta-cell failure in type 2 diabetes: Postulated mechanisms and prospects for prevention and treatment. *Diabetes Care*, *37*(6), 1751–1758. doi:10.2337/dc14-0396 PMID:24812433

Hasanzade, F., Toliat, M., Emami, S. A., & Emamimoghaadam, Z. (2013). The effect of cinnamon on glucose of type II diabetes patients. *Journal of Traditional and Complementary Medicine*, *3*(3), 171–174. doi:10.4103/2225-4110.114900 PMID:24716174

He, K., Li, X., Chen, X., Ye, X., Huang, J., Jin, Y., Li, P., Deng, Y., Jin, Q., Shi, Q., & Shu, H. (2011). Evaluation of antidiabetic potential of selected traditional Chinese medicines in STZ-induced diabetic mice. *Journal of Ethnopharmacology*, *137*(3), 1135–1142. doi:10.1016/j.jep.2011.07.033 PMID:21798327

Herman, L. (2015). *Herb and spice companion: the complete guide to over 100 herbs & spices*. Wellfleet Press.

Hong, Y. J., Kim, N., Lee, K., Hee Sonn, C., Eun Lee, J., Tae Kim, S., Ho Baeg, I., & Lee, K.-M. (2012). Korean red ginseng (Panax ginseng) ameliorates type 1 diabetes and restores immune cell compartments. *Journal of Ethnopharmacology*, *144*(2), 225–233. doi:10.1016/j.jep.2012.08.009 PMID:22925946

Hui, H., Tang, G., & Go, V. L. (2009). Hypoglycemic herbs and their action mechanisms. *Chinese Medicine*, *4*(1), 11. doi:10.1186/1749-8546-4-11 PMID:19523223

Hussain, S., Ahmed, A. A., Mahwi, T. O., & Aziz, T. A. (2012). Postprandial hyperglycemia in type 2 diabetic patients challenged with carbohydrates load. *International Journal of Experimental Diabetes Research*, *1*(3), 32–35. doi:10.5923/j.diabetes.20120103.01

Imparl-Radosevich, J., Deas, S., Polansky, M. M., Baedke, D. A., Ingebritsen, T. S., Anderson, R. A., & Graves, D. J. (1998). Regulation of PTP-1 and insulin receptor kinase by fractions from cinnamon: Implications for cinnamon regulation of insulin signalling. *Hormone Research*, *50*(3), 177–182. doi:10.1159/000023270 PMID:9762007

International Diabetes Foundation. (2019). *Diabetes: facts and figures*. Available from: https://www.idf.org/WDD15-guide/facts-and-figures.html

Jayaprasad, B., Sharavanan, P. S., & Sivaraj, R. (2016). Antidiabetic effect of *Chloroxylon swietenia* bark extracts on streptozotocin induced diabetic rats. *Beni-Suef Univ. Journal of Basic and Applied Sciences*, *5*(1), 1–9.

Jong-Anurakkun, N., Bhandari, M. R., Hong, G., & Kawabata, J. (2008). α-Glucosidase inhibitor from Chinese aloes. *Fitoterapia*, *79*(6), 456–457. doi:10.1016/j.fitote.2008.02.010 PMID:18508205

Kaatabi, H., Bamosa, A. O., Badar, A., Al-Elq, A., Abou-Hozaifa, B., Lebda, F., Al-Khadra, A., & Al-Almaie, S. (2015). *Nigella sativa* improves glycemic control and ameliorates oxidative stress in patients with type 2 diabetes mellitus: Placebo controlled participant blinded clinical trial. *PLoS One*, *10*(2), e0113486. doi:10.1371/journal.pone.0113486 PMID:25706772

Kaul, K., Apostolopoulou, M., & Roden, M. (2015). Insulin resistance in type 1 diabetes mellitus. *Metabolism, 64*(12), 1629-1639.

Kennedy, D. O., & Wightman, E. L. (2011). Herbal extracts and phytochemicals: Plant secondary metabolites and the enhancement of human brain function. *Advances in Nutrition (Bethesda, Md.)*, *2*(1), 32–50. doi:10.3945/an.110.000117 PMID:22211188

Khan, A., Safdar, M., Khan, M. A., Khattak, K. N., & Anderson, R. A. (2003). Cinnamon improves glucose and lipids of people with type 2 diabetes. *Diabetes Care*, *26*(12), 3215–3218. doi:10.2337/diacare.26.12.3215 PMID:14633804

Khan, M. A. B., Hashim, J. M., King, J. K., Govender, R. D., Mustafa, H., & Kaabi, J. A. (2020). Epidemiology of type 2 diabetes-global burden of disease and forecasted trends. *Journal of Epidemiology and Global Health*, *10*(1), 107–111. doi:10.2991/jegh.k.191028.001 PMID:32175717

Kimura, M., Waki, I., Chujo, T., Kikuchi, T., Hiyama, C., Yamazaki, K., & Tanaka, O. (1981). Effects of hypoglycemic components in ginseng radix on blood insulin level in alloxan diabetic mice and on insulin release from perfused rat pancreas. *Journal of Pharmacobio-Dynamics*, *4*(6), 410–417. doi:10.1248/bpb1978.4.410 PMID:7026762

Ko, B.-S., Choi, S. B., Park, S. K., Jang, J. S., Kim, Y. E., & Park, S. (2005). Insulin sensitizing and insulinotropic action of berberine from Cortidis rhizoma. *Biological & Pharmaceutical Bulletin*, *28*(8), 1431–1437. doi:10.1248/bpb.28.1431 PMID:16079488

Kong, W.-J., Zhang, H., Song, D.-Q., Xue, R., Zhao, W., Wei, J., Wang, Y.-M., Shan, N., Zhou, Z.-X., Yang, P., You, X.-F., Li, Z.-R., Si, S.-Y., Zhao, L.-X., Pan, H.-N., & Jiang, J.-D. (2009). Berberine reduces insulin resistance through protein kinase C-dependent up-regulation of insulin receptor expression. *Metabolism: Clinical and Experimental*, *58*(1), 109–119. doi:10.1016/j.metabol.2008.08.013 PMID:19059538

Krentz, A. J., & Bailey, C. J. (2005). Oral antidiabetic agents: Current role in type 2 diabetes mellitus. *Drugs*, *65*(3), 385–411. doi:10.2165/00003495-200565030-00005 PMID:15669880

Labban, L., Mustafa, U. E.-S., & Ibrahim, Y. M. (2014). The effects of Rosemary (Rosmarinus officinalis) leaves powder on glucose level, lipid profile and lipid perodoxation. *International Journal of Clinical Medicine*, *5*(06), 297–304. doi:10.4236/ijcm.2014.56044

Lee, Y. S., Kim, W. S., Kim, K. H., Yoon, M. J., Cho, H. J., Shen, Y., Ye, J.-M., Lee, C. H., Oh, W. K., Kim, C. T., Hohnen-Behrens, C., Gosby, A., Kraegen, E. W., James, D. E., & Kim, J. B. (2006). Berberine, a natural plant product, activates AMP-activated protein kinase with beneficial metabolic effects in diabetic and insulin-resistant states. *Diabetes*, *55*(8), 2256–2264. doi:10.2337/db06-0006 PMID:16873688

Leng, S. H., Lu, F. E., & Xu, L. J. (2004). Therapeutic effects of berberine in impaired glucose tolerance rats and its influence on insulin secretion. *Acta Pharmacologica Sinica*, *25*(4), 496–502. PMID:15066220

Li, C., He, J. Z., Zhou, X. D., & Xu, X. (2017). Berberine regulates type 2 diabetes mellitus related with insulin resistance. *Zhongguo Zhongyao Zazhi*, *42*(12), 2254–2260. PMID:28822177

Li, G. Q., Kam, A., Wong, K. H., Zhou, X., Omar, E. A., Alqahtani, A., Li, K. M., Razmovski-Naumovski, V., & Chan, K. (2012). Herbal medicines for the management of diabetes. *Advances in Experimental Medicine and Biology*, *771*, 396–413. doi:10.1007/978-1-4614-5441-0_28 PMID:23393692

Liu, C.-T., Hsu, T.-W., Chen, K.-M., Tan, Y.-P., Lii, C.-K., & Sheen, L.-Y. (2012). The antidiabetic effect of garlic oil is associated with ameliorated oxidative stress but not ameliorated level of pro-inflammatory cytokines in skeletal muscle of streptozotocin-induced diabetic rats. *Journal of Traditional and Complementary Medicine*, *2*(2), 135–144. doi:10.1016/S2225-4110(16)30087-6 PMID:24716126

Liu, L., Yu, Y. L., Yang, J. S., Li, Y., Liu, Y.-W., Liang, Y., Liu, X.-D., Xie, L., & Wang, G.-J. (2010). Berberine suppresses intestinal disaccharidases with beneficial metabolic effects in diabetic states, evidences from in vivo and in vitro study. *Naunyn-Schmiedeberg's Archives of Pharmacology*, *381*(4), 371–381. doi:10.100700210-010-0502-0 PMID:20229011

Liu, S., Li, D., Huang, B., Chen, Y., Lu, X., & Wang, Y. (2013). Inhibition of pancreatic lipase, α-glucosidase, α-amylase, and hypolipidemic effects of the total flavonoids from Nelumbo nucifera leaves. *Journal of Ethnopharmacology*, *149*(1), 263–269. doi:10.1016/j.jep.2013.06.034 PMID:23811214

Luo, J. Z., & Luo, L. (2009). Ginseng on hyperglycemia: Effects and mechanisms. *Evidence-Based Complementary and Alternative Medicine*, *6*(4), 423–427. doi:10.1093/ecam/nem178 PMID:18955300

Marre, M., & Penfornis, A. (2011). GLP-1 receptor agonists today. *Diabetes Research and Clinical Practice*, *93*(3), 317–327. doi:10.1016/j.diabres.2011.01.004 PMID:21767888

Mata, R., Cristians, S., Escandón-Rivera, S., Juárez-Reyes, K., & Rivero-Cruz, I. (2013). Mexican antidiabetic herbs: Valuable sources of inhibitors of α-glucosidases. *Journal of Natural Products*, *76*(3), 468–483. doi:10.1021/np300869g PMID:23398496

Meddah, B., Ducroc, R., El Abbes Faouzi, M., Eto, B., Mahraoui, L., Benhaddou-Andaloussi, A., Martineau, L. C., Cherrah, Y., & Haddad, P. S. (2009). Nigella sativa inhibits intestinal glucose absorption and improves glucose tolerance in rats. *Journal of Ethnopharmacology*, *121*(3), 419–424. doi:10.1016/j.jep.2008.10.040 PMID:19061948

Meenatchi, P., Purushothaman, A., & Maneemegalai, S. (2017). Antioxidant, antiglycation and insulinotrophic properties of Coccinia grandis (L.) in vitro: Possible role in prevention of diabetic complications. *Journal of Traditional and Complementary Medicine*, *7*(1), 54–64. doi:10.1016/j.jtcme.2016.01.002 PMID:28053889

Mi, J., He, W., Lv, J., Zhuang, K., Huang, H., & Quan, S. (2019). Effect of berberine on the HPA-axis pathway and skeletal muscle GLUT4 in type 2 diabetes mellitus rats. *Diabetes, Metabolic Syndrome and Obesity*, *12*, 1717–1725. doi:10.2147/DMSO.S211188 PMID:31564939

Mohamed Sham Shihabudeen, H., Hansi Priscilla, D., & Thirumurugan, K. (2011). Cinnamon extract inhibits α-glucosidase activity and dampens postprandial glucose excursion in diabetic rats. *Nutrition & Metabolism*, *8*(1), 46. doi:10.1186/1743-7075-8-46 PMID:21711570

Mohammed, S. I., Chopda, M. Z., Patil, R. H., Vishwakarma, K. S., & Maheshwari, V. L. (2016). In vivo antidiabetic and antioxidant activities of Coccinia grandis leaf extract against streptozotocin induced diabetes in experimental rats. *Asian Pacific Journal of Tropical Disease*, *6*(4), 298–304. doi:10.1016/S2222-1808(15)61034-9

Mohd Bukhari, D. A., Siddiqui, M. J., Shamsudin, S. H., Rahman, M. M., & So'ad, S. Z. M. (2017). α-Glucosidase inhibitory activity of selected Malaysian plants. *Journal of Pharmacy & Bioallied Sciences*, *9*(3), 164–170. doi:10.4103/jpbs.JPBS_35_17 PMID:28979070

Mohseni, R., ArabSadeghabadi, Z., Ziamajidi, N., Abbasalipourkabir, R., & RezaeiFarimani, A. (2019). Oral administration of resveratrol-loaded solid lipid nanoparticle improves insulin resistance through targeting expression of SNARE Proteins in adipose and muscle tissue in rats with type 2 diabetes. *Nanoscale Research Letters*, *14*(1), 227. doi:10.118611671-019-3042-7 PMID:31290033

Naimi, M., Vlavcheski, F., Shamshoum, H., & Tsiani, E. (2017). Rosemary extract as a potential anti-hyperglycemic agent: Current evidence and future perspectives. *Nutrients*, *9*(9), 968. doi:10.3390/nu9090968 PMID:28862678

Oboh, G., Ademiluyi, A. O., Akinyemi, A. J., Henle, T., Saliu, J. A., & Schwarzenbolz, U. (2012). Inhibitory effect of polyphenol-rich extracts of jute leaf (Corchorus olitorius) on key enzyme linked to type 2 diabetes (α-amylase and α-glucosidase) and hypertension (angiotensin I converting) in vitro. *Journal of Functional Foods*, *4*(2), 450–458. doi:10.1016/j.jff.2012.02.003

Oh, M. R., Park, S. H., Kim, S. Y., Back, H.-I., Kim, M.-G., Jeon, J.-Y., Ha, K.-C., Na, W.-T., Cha, Y.-S., Park, B.-H., Park, T., & Chae, S.-W. (2014). Postprandial glucose-lowering effects of fermented red ginseng in subjects with impaired fasting glucose or type 2 diabetes: A randomized, double-blind, placebo-controlled clinical trial. *BMC Complementary and Alternative Medicine*, *14*(1), 237. doi:10.1186/1472-6882-14-237 PMID:25015735

Olokoba, A. B., Obateru, O. A., & Olokoba, L. B. (2012). Type 2 diabetes mellitus: A review of current trends. *Oman Medical Journal*, *27*(4), 269–273. doi:10.5001/omj.2012.68 PMID:23071876

Padiya, R., & Banerjee, S. K. (2013). Garlic as an anti-diabetic agent: Recent progress and patent reviews. *Recent Patents on Food, Nutrition & Agriculture*, *5*(2), 105–127. doi:10.2174/18761429113059990002 PMID:23270395

Palsamy, P., & Subramanian, S. (2008). Resveratrol, a natural phytoalexin, normalizes hyperglycemia in streptozotocin-nicotinamide induced experimental diabetic rats. *Biomedicine and Pharmacotherapy*, *62*(9), 598–605. doi:10.1016/j.biopha.2008.06.037 PMID:18675532

Pang, B., Zhao, L.-H., Zhou, Q., Zhao, T.-Y., Wang, H., Gu, C.-H., & Tong, X.-L. (2015). Application of berberine on treating type 2 diabetes mellitus. *International Journal of Endocrinology*, *905749*, 1–12. Advance online publication. doi:10.1155/2015/905749 PMID:25861268

Park, E. Y., Kim, H. J., Kim, Y. K., Park, S. U., Choi, J. E., Cha, J. Y., & Jun, H. S. (2012). Increase in insulin secretion induced by Panax ginseng berry extracts contributes to the amelioration of hyperglycemia in streptozotocin-induced diabetic mice. *Journal of Ginseng Research*, *36*(2), 153–160. doi:10.5142/jgr.2012.36.2.153 PMID:23717115

Park, H. S., Cho, J. H., Kim, K. W., Chung, W. S., & Song, M. Y. (2018). Effects of Panax ginseng on obesity in animal models: A Systematic review and meta-analysis. *Evidence-based Complementary and Alternative Medicine: eCAM,* 2719794.

Park, S. J., Nam, J., Ahn, C. W., & Kim, Y. (2019). Anti-diabetic properties of different fractions of Korean red ginseng. *Journal of Ethnopharmacology*, *236*, 220–230. doi:10.1016/j.jep.2019.01.044 PMID:30849506

Patel, D. K., Prasad, S. K., Kumar, R., & Hemalatha, S. (2012). An overview on antidiabetic medicinal plants having insulin mimetic property. *Asian Pacific Journal of Tropical Biomedicine*, *2*(4), 320–330. doi:10.1016/S2221-1691(12)60032-X PMID:23569923

Patil, S. B., Takalikar, S. S., Joglekar, M. M., Haldavnekar, V. S., & Arvindekar, A. U. (2013). Insulinotropic and β-cell protective action of cuminaldehyde, cuminol and an inhibitor isolated from Cuminum cyminum in streptozotocin-induced diabetic rats. *British Journal of Nutrition*, *110*(8), 1434–1443. doi:10.1017/S0007114513000627 PMID:23507295

Peng, Y., & Hu, K. (2018). Effect of garlic on rats with chronic intermittent hypoxia combined with diabetes mellitus. *Molecular Medicine Reports*, *17*(4), 6174–6184. doi:10.3892/mmr.2018.8568 PMID:29436658

Perrone, D., Fuggetta, M. P., Ardito, F., Cottarelli, A., De Filippis, A., Ravagnan, G., De Maria, S., & Lo Muzio, L. (2017). Resveratrol (3,5,4¢-trihydroxystilbene) and its properties in oral diseases. *Experimental and Therapeutic Medicine*, *14*(1), 3–9. doi:10.3892/etm.2017.4472 PMID:28672886

Prabhakar, P. K., & Doble, M. (2011). Mechanism of action of natural products used in the treatment of diabetes mellitus. *Chinese Journal of Integrative Medicine*, *17*(8), 563–574. doi:10.100711655-011-0810-3 PMID:21826590

Punthakee, Z., Goldenberg, R. & Katz, P. (2018). Definition, classification and diagnosis of diabetes, prediabetes and metabolic syndrome. *Can. J. Diabetes, 42*(Suppl 1), S10-S15. doi:. doi:10.1016/j.jcjd.2017.10.003

Qin, B., Panickar, K. S., & Anderson, R. A. (2010). Cinnamon: Potential role in the prevention of insulin resistance, metabolic syndrome, and type 2 diabetes. *Journal of Diabetes Science and Technology*, *4*(3), 685–693. doi:10.1177/193229681000400324 PMID:20513336

Rafehi, H., Ververis, K., & Karagiannis, T. C. (2012). Controversies surrounding the clinical potential of cinnamon for the management of diabetes. *Diabetes, Obesity & Metabolism*, *14*(6), 493–499. doi:10.1111/j.1463-1326.2011.01538.x PMID:22093965

Ramadan, M. F. (2007). Nutritional value, functional properties and nutraceutical applications of black cumin (*Nigella sativa* L.): An overview. *International Journal of Food Science & Technology*, *42*(10), 1208–1218. doi:10.1111/j.1365-2621.2006.01417.x

Ranilla, L. G., Kwon, Y. I., Apostolidis, E., & Shetty, K. (2010). Phenolic compounds, antioxidant activity and in vitro inhibitory potential against key enzymes relevant for hyperglycemia and hypertension of commonly used medicinal plants, herbs and spices in Latin America. *Bioresource Technology*, *101*(12), 4676–4689. doi:10.1016/j.biortech.2010.01.093 PMID:20185303

Reeds, D. N., Patterson, B. W., Okunade, A., Holloszy, J. O., Polonsky, K. S., & Klein, S. (2011). Ginseng and ginsenoside Re do not improve beta-cell function or insulin sensitivity in overweight and obese subjects with impaired glucose tolerance or diabetes. *Diabetes Care*, *34*(5), 1071–1076. doi:10.2337/dc10-2299 PMID:21411505

Rezaei Farimani, A., Saidijam, M., Goodarzi, M. T., Yadegar Azari, R., Asadi, S., Zarei, S., & Shabab, N. (2015). Effect of resveratrol supplementation on the SNARE Proteins expression in adipose tissue of streptozotocin-nicotinamide induced type 2 diabetic rats. *Iranian Journal of Medical Sciences*, *40*(3), 248–255. PMID:25999625

Sattanathan, K. C., Dhanapal, R., & Umarani, R. (2011). ManavalanBeneficial health effects of rutin supplementation in patients with diabetes mellitus. *Journal of Applied Pharmaceutical Science*, *1*(8), 227–231.

Schmatz, R., Mazzanti, C. M., Spanevello, R., Stefanello, N., Gutierres, J., Maldonado, A., Correa, M., da Rosa, C. S., Becker, L., Bagatini, M., Gonçalves, J. F., Jaques, J. D. S., Schetinger, M. R., & Morsch, V. M. (2010). Ectonucleotidase and acetylcholinesterase activities in synaptosomes from the cerebral cortex of streptozotocin-induced diabetic rats and treated with resveratrol. *Brain Research Bulletin*, *80*(6), 371–376. doi:10.1016/j.brainresbull.2009.08.019 PMID:19723569

Schmatz, R., Schetinger, M. R., Spanevello, R. M., Mazzanti, C. M., Stefanello, N., Maldonado, P. A., Gutierres, J., Corrêa, M. C., Girotto, E., Moretto, M. B., & Morsch, V. M. (2009). Effects of resveratrol on nucleotide degrading enzymes in streptozotocin-induced diabetic rats. *Life Sciences*, *84*(11-12), 345–350. doi:10.1016/j.lfs.2008.12.019 PMID:19166862

Sen, S., Querques, M. A., & Chakrabarti, S. (2013). North American Ginseng (Panax quinquefolius) prevents hyperglycemia and associated pancreatic abnormalities in diabetes. *Journal of Medicinal Food*, *16*(7), 587–592. doi:10.1089/jmf.2012.0192 PMID:23875898

Singh, J., Cumming, E., Manoharan, G., Kalasz, H., & Adeghate, E. (2011). Medicinal chemistry of the anti-diabetic effects of momordica charantia: Active constituents and modes of actions. *The Open Medicinal Chemistry Journal*, *5*(supplement 2), 70–77. doi:10.2174/1874104501105010070 PMID:21966327

Sulaiman, M. R., Hussain, M. K., Zakaria, Z. A., Somchit, M. N., Moin, S., Mohamad, A. S., & Israf, D. A. (2008). Evaluation of the antinociceptive activity of Ficus deltoidea aqueous extract. *Fitoterapia*, *79*(7-8), 557–561. doi:10.1016/j.fitote.2008.06.005 PMID:18672036

Takahashi, T., & Miyazawa, M. (2012). Potent α-glucosidase inhibitors from safflower (Carthamus tinctorius L.) seed. *Phytotherapy Research*, *26*(5), 722–726. doi:10.1002/ptr.3622 PMID:22021176

Thomford, N. E., Dzobo, K., Chopera, D., Wonkam, A., Skelton, M., Blackhurst, D., Chirikure, S., & Dandara, C. (2015). Pharmacogenomics implications of using herbal medicinal plants on African populations in health transition. *Pharmaceuticals (Basel, Switzerland)*, *8*(3), 637–663. doi:10.3390/ph8030637 PMID:26402689

Tu, P. F., Guo, H. Z., & Guo, D. A. (2002). Researches on active constituents of natural and traditional medicine and development of new drugs. *J. Peking Univ. Health Sci.*, *34*, 513–518.

Vallianou, N. G., Evangelopoulos, A., & Kazazis, C. (2013). Resveratrol and diabetes. *The Review of Diabetic Studies; RDS*, *10*(4), 236–242. doi:10.1900/RDS.2013.10.236 PMID:24841877

Vanschoonbeek, K., Thomassen, B. J., Senden, J. M., Wodzig, W. K., & van Loon, L. J. (2006). Cinnamon supplementation does not improve glycemic control in postmenopausal type 2 diabetes patients. *The Journal of Nutrition*, *136*(4), 977–980. doi:10.1093/jn/136.4.977 PMID:16549460

Varghese, G. K., Bose, L. V., & Habtemariam, S. (2013). Antidiabetic components of Cassia alata leaves: Identification through α-glucosidase inhibition studies. *Pharmaceutical Biology*, *51*(3), 345–349. doi:10.3109/13880209.2012.729066 PMID:23137344

Vuddanda, P. R., Chakraborty, S., & Singh, S. (2010). Berberine: A potential phytochemical with multispectrum therapeutic activities. *Expert Opinion on Investigational Drugs*, *19*(10), 1297–1307. doi:10.1517/13543784.2010.517745 PMID:20836620

Vuksan, V., Sievenpiper, J. L., Koo, V. Y., Francis, T., Beljan-Zdravkovic, U., Xu, Z., & Vidgen, E. (2000). American ginseng (Panax quinquefolius L) reduces postprandial glycemia in nondiabetic subjects and subjects with type 2 diabetes mellitus. *Archives of Internal Medicine*, *160*(7), 1009–1013. doi:10.1001/archinte.160.7.1009 PMID:10761967

Vuksan, V., Sievenpiper, J. L., Xu, Z., Wong, E. Y. Y., Jenkins, A. L., Beljan-Zdravkovic, U., Leiter, L. A., Josse, R. G., & Stavro, M. P. (2001). Konjac-mannan and American ginseng: Emerging alternative therapies for type 2 diabetes mellitus. *Journal of the American College of Nutrition*, *20*(5, supplement), 370S–380S. doi:10.1080/07315724.2001.10719170 PMID:11603646

Vuksan, V., Sung, M. K., Sievenpiper, J. L., Stavro, P. M., Jenkins, A. L., Di Buono, M., Lee, K.-S., Leiter, L. A., Nam, K. Y., Arnason, J. T., Choi, M., & Naeem, A. (2008). Korean red ginseng (Panax ginseng) improves glucose and insulin regulation in well-controlled, type 2 diabetes: Results of a randomized, double-blind, placebo-controlled study of efficacy and safety. *Nutrition, Metabolism, and Cardiovascular Diseases*, *18*(1), 46–56. doi:10.1016/j.numecd.2006.04.003 PMID:16860976

Wang, Y., Campbell, T., Perry, B., Beaurepaire, C., & Qin, L. (2011). Hypoglycemic and insulin-sensitizing effects of berberine in high-fat diet- and streptozotocin-induced diabetic rats. *Metabolism: Clinical and Experimental*, *60*(2), 298–305. doi:10.1016/j.metabol.2010.02.005 PMID:20304443

World Health Organisation. (2000). *General guidelines for methodologies on research and evaluation of traditional medicine*. World Health Organisation.

World Health Organization. (2018). *Diabetes*. Available from [https://www.who. int/news-room/fact-sheets/detail/diabetes

Xie, X., Li, W., Lan, T., Liu, W., Peng, J., Huang, K., Huang, J., Shen, X., Liu, P., & Huang, H. (2011). Berberine ameliorates hyperglycemia in alloxan-induced diabetic C57BL/6 mice through activation of Akt signaling pathway. *Endocrine Journal*, *58*(9), 761–768. doi:10.1507/endocrj.K11E-024 PMID:21705841

Yin, J., Xing, H., & Ye, J. (2008). Efficacy of berberine in patients with type 2 diabetes mellitus. *Metabolism: Clinical and Experimental*, *57*(5), 712–717. doi:10.1016/j.metabol.2008.01.013 PMID:18442638

Yuan, H., Ma, Q., Ye, L., & Piao, G. (2016). The traditional medicine and modern medicine from natural products. *Molecules (Basel, Switzerland)*, *21*(5), 559. doi:10.3390/molecules21050559 PMID:27136524

Zare, R., Nadjarzadeh, A., Zarshenas, M. M., Shams, M., & Heydari, M. (2019). Efficacy of cinnamon in patients with type II diabetes mellitus: A randomized controlled clinical trial. *Clinical Nutrition (Edinburgh, Lothian)*, *38*(2), 549–556. doi:10.1016/j.clnu.2018.03.003 PMID:29605574

Zhang, H., Wei, J., Xue, R., Wu, J.-D., Zhao, W., Wang, Z.-Z., Wang, S.-K., Zhou, Z.-X., Song, D.-Q., Wang, Y.-M., Pan, H.-N., Kong, W.-J., & Jiang, J.-D. (2010). Berberine lowers blood glucose in type 2 diabetes mellitus patients through increasing insulin receptor expression. *Metabolism: Clinical and Experimental*, *59*(2), 285–292. doi:10.1016/j.metabol.2009.07.029 PMID:19800084

Zhang, Y., Feng, F., Chen, T., Li, Z., & Shen, Q. W. (2016). Antidiabetic and antihyperlipidemic activities of Forsythia suspensa (Thunb.) Vahl (fruit) in streptozotocin-induced diabetes mice. *Journal of Ethnopharmacology*, *192*, 256–263. doi:10.1016/j.jep.2016.07.002 PMID:27377336

Zhang, Y., Li, X., Zou, D., Liu, W., Yang, J., Zhu, N., Huo, L., Wang, M., Hong, J., Wu, P., Ren, G., & Ning, G. (2008). Treatment of type 2 diabetes and dyslipidemia with the natural plant alkaloid berberine. *The Journal of Clinical Endocrinology and Metabolism*, *93*(7), 2559–2565. doi:10.1210/jc.2007-2404 PMID:18397984

Zhou, J., Zhou, S., Tang, J., Zhang, K., Guang, L., Huang, Y., Xu, Y., Ying, Y., Zhang, L., & Li, D. (2004). Protective effect of berberine on beta cells in streptozotocin- and high-carbohydrate/high-fat diet-induced diabetic rats. *European Journal of Pharmacology*, *606*(1-3), 262–268. doi:10.1016/j.ejphar.2008.12.056 PMID:19374872

KEY TERMS AND DEFINITIONS

Diabetes Mellitus: A chronic disorder of carbohydrate metabolism associated with unusually elevated levels of glucose in the blood due to insufficient insulin production or failure of the body to respond to insulin.

Herbs: Herbaceous plants with parts that possess bioactive ingredients that are of medicinal value.

Hypoglycemia: A decrease in blood glucose concentrations in the blood which may result in symptoms such as confusion, feeling of hunger, sweating, seizures, loss of conscious or death.

In Vitro: Studies regarding the testing of different biological entities on individual parts of cells.

In Vivo: Studies regarding the testing of different biological entities on the whole living organism e.g. animals.

Insulin: A peptide hormone made by pancreatic islet β-cells that regulates the blood glucose levels in the body as well as metabolism of protein and fats.

Mechanism of Action: Precise biochemical interaction resulting in functional changes at the cellular level.

Chapter 4
Role of Herbal Supplements in the Treatment of Obesity and Diabetes

Sonia Singh
https://orcid.org/0000-0003-1503-2745
GLA University, Mathura, India

Bhupesh C. Semwal
GLA University, Mathura, India

Yogesh Murti
https://orcid.org/0000-0002-5278-0681
Institute of Pharmaceutical Research, India

ABSTRACT

Around the world, the prevalence of obesity and diabetes are high raising multiple severe diseases. Some of the common disorders associated with obesity are diabetes, heart diseases, and hypertension. These disorders have a tremendous effect on social lifestyles of every individual. However, another lifestyle disorder is diabetes, which can also be called hyperglycemia. Uncontrolled diabetes has the potential to cause serious complications in the body including kidney disease, loss of vision, and cardiovascular disease, which contribute towards morbidity and mortality. Though various allopathic drugs are available in the market, the herbal products and their derivatives have enough potential to treat such diseases with little or no side effects. This chapter is concerned and focuses on the application of herbal drugs along with proven mechanisms of action.

DOI: 10.4018/978-1-7998-4808-0.ch004

INTRODUCTION

Obesity, as well as diabetes mellitus, is considered an important health issue worldwide. Their increasing high rate of incidence might be producing numerous social costs (Desai, 2006). Obesity is the most commonly seen factor in those individuals who had high profile lifestyles, consuming fast foods or either suffer from genetic diseases. Some factors such as insulin resistance, oxidative stress and enhanced inflammation are responsible to generate a complex disease, Obesity. According to International Obesity Taskforce, it is analyzed that around more than 300 million individuals have a BMI index higher than 30 kg/m^2, called obese. In developing countries, the cases of obese-born children are increasing rapidly, as the number of obese adults in developed countries (Sharma,2012). It is calculated that in the current century, 1-in -3 children born would be expected to have obesity-related diabetic problems (Mokdad,2001; Ogden,1999-2004).

Obesity, considered as one of the major cause of developing metabolic dysfunctions including diabetes mellitus, cardiovascular diseases, hypertension, and so on (Devendra, 2004). Research findings reported that in upcoming years approximately 600 million people will develop diabetic related issues, due to their increasing obesity incidence, living standards. Incoming 20 years nearly 600 million individuals will become diabetic, due to high obesity prevalence, ageing, increased living standards, enhanced urbanization, and fast food (Guariguata, 2014). As the rate of incidence of obesity increased, the number of diabetic patients also increased proportionally (Shi Y, 1948). Diabetes mellitus is defined as a metabolic dysfunction with enhanced levels of blood glucose for a prolonged duration, due to destruction in the regulation of insulin-secreting pancreatic β cells (WHO, 2014; Kawser, 2016). It is responsible for causing several vascular complications in the body (Fowler, 2008). The treatment of diabetes includes a well-defined healthy diet, exercise and mediation. A healthy nutritious diet is important for those who have diabetic complications (Patel, 2012). Numerous allopathic drugs are available in the market for the treatment of obesity and diabetes, but with many adverse side effects. Therefore, identification of phytoconstituents and dietary supplements for proper regulation and function of accumulated body fat and elevated blood sugar level. Such supplements have some potential to enhance antioxidant activity, insulin secretion (Sandborn, 2000).

Flavonoids are originated from the Latin word *'flavus'*, which means yellow colour, and are abundantly present in numerous plants. Such components are polyphenolic, commonly found present in the human diet (Prasad, 2010; Castellarin, 2007). Chemically, they have a 15 carbon skeleton structure with a heterocyclic ring and two phenyl rings; they are even regarded as secondary metabolites of plants. More than 5000 flavonoids have been isolated till now, among which only selected ones are possessing beneficiary effects over chemically synthesized compounds. These compounds contain a tremendous mechanism of action in controlling and regulating obesity and diabetes.

Mechanism linked between Obesity and Diabetes with related pathophysiology

Obesity is closely concerned with the low level of inflammation, showing a close relationship between immunity and metabolism (as shown in Figure 1) (Xie B, 2012; Al-Goblan, 2014). Adipocytes, a kind of fat cells secrete product that links obesity with diabetes. In obese individuals, Macrophage infiltration is prominently present in their adipose tissues (Weisberg SP, 2003; Xu HY, 2003). The adipose tissue-derived MCP-1 plays an important role in inducing macrophage infiltration into adipose tissue and it also exhibits the chemotactic action in inflammatory cells. MCP-1 activates the macrophage infiltration, which subsequently releases inflammatory mediator TNF-α (Maury, 2007). This hampers insulin signalling and however triggers the lipolysis in adipocytes. The pro-inflammatory cytokines such as IL-6, IL-1β and TNF- α are associated with chronic inflammation and insulin resistance (Fain,2004; Yu, 2006). It is reported that such inflammatory cytokines suppressed triglyceride synthesis through downregulation of PPARγ, LPL, and even glucose transporter, such as GLUT4 (Fain, 2004; Guilherme, 2008). Besides this, TNF-α regulates various process such as it helps in reducing the insulin-mediated attenuation of lipolysis, downregulating the PLIN, in which all these increases the release of free fatty acid (FFA) release (Khorami, 2015). The increased level of FFA thereby decreases the IRS-1 expression which reduces the PI3K-AKT (Bouzakri, 2003; Khorami, 2015) expression in liver and skeletal muscles; and increases the expression of JNK signalling in the pancreas (Cheon H, 2010). The reduced expression of PI3K-AKT causes insulin resistance and the increased expression of JNK activates apoptosis. The insulin resistance may increase glucose production and decrease the glucose uptake, this would ultimately cause hyper-insulinemia. Both factors, the apoptosis of pancreatic β cell and insulin resistance lead to diabetes (Guilherme A, 2008).

HERBAL SUPPLEMENTS IN CURING OBESITY AND DIABETES

Figure 1. The correlation between the mechanism of action of obesity and diabetes

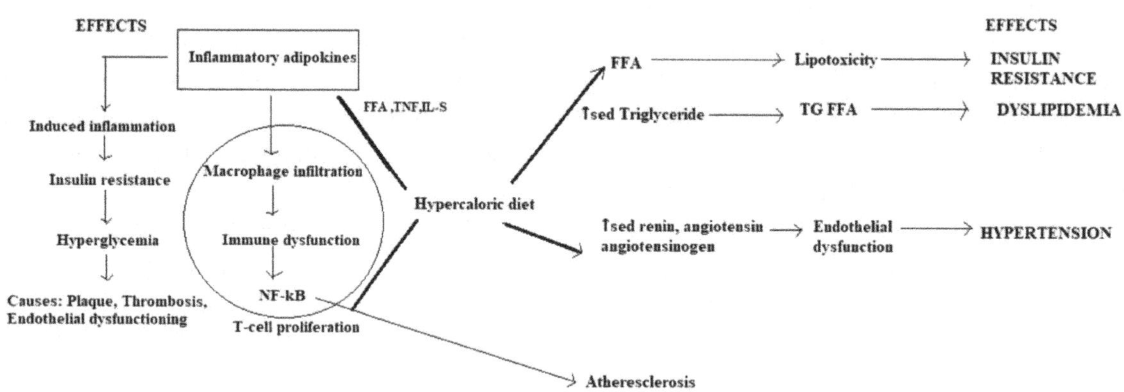

Flavonoids and their functions

Flavonols

It is the most common subclass of flavonoid distributed in the plant kingdom. The main herbal supplements such as kaempferol, myricetin and quercetin (Crozier A, 2009). Among all these components, Quercetin is considered as dietary nutrition present in numerous foods like apples, berries, grapes, pepper, coriander, citrus fruits. It has a wide range of pharmacological properties like reduction in body weight

(Yamamoto,2006), blood pressure in humans and animal models (Edwards, 2007; Yamamoto,2006). The compound was investigated to lower the blood pressure in hypertensive individuals (Edwards, 2007). Even its antioxidative property suppresses the increased blood pressure level in high fat diet-induced obesity animals (Yamammoto, 2006).

Rutin present in oranges, grapes, lemon, peaches, berries and citrus fruits, was reported to possess anti-obesity as well as anti-diabetic activities (Kreft S, 1999; Huang WY, 2012). It is reported that oral administration of rutin to diabetic induced mice showed consequent deduction of blood glucose levels, and enhanced the levels of insulin along with re-establishment of metabolic activities of carbohydrate enzyme and even of glycogen content (Prince P, 2006).

Isorhamnetin is abundantly present in herbs such as *Ginkgo biloba*, *Oenanthe javanica* (Yokozawa,2002). It contains several biological activities, including anti-obesity and anti-diabetic properties. From the literature survey, it has reported that the oral administration of the compound significantly inhibited the concentration of serum glucose level, and reduced the sorbitol accumulation in red blood cells, sciatic nerves in STZ-induced diabetic animal models (Lee YS, 2005).

Kaempferol is commonly found in grapes, apple, tomato, tea, potato, spinach and berries (Hakkinen, 1999; Nirmala P, 2011). It has the potency to reduce hyperglycemia and enhance the glucose uptake in the rat (Jorge AP,2004).

Myricetin is found in wines, berries, fruits and vegetables and possess various beneficiary effects (Hiermann A,1998; Hertog, 1993). It is reported that the myricetin treatment to diabetic obese rats showed augmentation of GLUT4 expression (Tzeng, 2011; Liu, 2007), and enhanced the AKT phosphorylation (Tzeng, 2011; Liu, 2007; Kandasamy, 2014).

Flavanones

Naringenin and hesperidin, are major flavanones present in most of the citrus fruits. They have reported containing antidiabetic, anti-obesity, antioxidant, lipid-lowering and anti-inflammatory properties (Hasanein, 2014; Jung, 2004; Kim, 2004; Zygmunt, 2010). Naringenin was found to reduce the mass of adipose tissue and suppress preadipocyte proliferation. It repressed the glucose uptake (Harmon, 2003) and simultaneously suppressed the PI3K and AKT phosphorylation in 3T3-L1 adipocytes (Koch, 2013).

Hesperidin is abundantly found in lemons and most of the citrus fruits show lipid-lowering effects (Choe, 2001). The flavonoid reported having a beneficial effect in lowering the blood glucose levels by upregulating hepatic glucokinase, PPARγ, and adipocyte GLUT4(Jung,2006; Agrawal, 2014). On administration of hesperidin as nutrient supplement decreased the glucose-6-phosphate and increased the glucokinase which ultimately declining the glucose export in STZ induced diabetic animal models (Akiyama,2010).

Isoflavones

Isoflavones are found in legume plants, such as soybean. Daidzein and genistein, are the major compounds found in soy food supplements (Crozier, 2009). Such compounds may affect the glucose homeostasis, lipid metabolism, insulin secretion and adiposity (Park 2011). They do possess some beneficial effects on life-threatening diseases such as cardiovascular disease, diabetes, and obesity. It reduced the deposition of adipose tissue, and another *in vitro* studies revealed that both the components enhanced lipolysis pathway via suppressing the expression of cAMP-specific PDE (Szkudelska,2000; Szkudelska,2002).

Flavones

It is found abundantly in celery, and several different herbs (Panda,2007). Apigenin is widely distributed in chamomile, and have been claimed to cure a wide variety of diseases. Previous studies reported that the oral administration of such compound reversed the reduction of antioxidant properties in alloxan-induced diabetic mice (Zang,2006). The compound was 200 times more potent and effective than metformin, and also known as AMPK activator, involved in the treatment of chronic diseases including diabetes and dyslipidemia (Neuhouser,2004).

Luteolin is present in cabbage, celery, onion, peppers, apple peel (Miean,2004; Gates,2007; Ding,2010). In adipose cells and 3T3-L1 adipocytes mouse model, luteolin reported to enhance the insulin action and even activate the expression of PPARγ target genes (Liu, 2014). It has a beneficial role in the metabolism of insulin resistance and diabetes mellitus pathophysiology via suppressing the circulating levels of inflammatory molecules, resistin (Yang,1998).

Flavan-3-ols

Flavan-3-ols are present in fruits, teas, grapes and cocoa (Sartippour,2002). Some of the flavanols such as catechin, epicatechin, ECG, gallocatechin, EGC, and EGCG. The components of tea contain anti-obesity and anti-diabetic properties (Kavanagh,2001; Osada,2001; Kao,2000; Wolfram,2007). The administration of EGCG has been proved to show an effective result in preventing cardiovascular diseases and metabolic disorders (Takikawa,2010).

Anthocyanidins

Anthocyanidins are broadly distributed in the human diet in several fruits, vegetables, and berries (Galvano,2007). It has been used for its anti-inflammatory, anti-obesity, antidiabetic and antioxidant effects (Ghosh,2007). Around 635 anthocyanin components have been isolated and identified, including delphinidin, cyaniding, peonidin, and malvidin (Tsuda,2004). Researchers reported the therapeutic effects of cyanidin 3-glucoside as antidiabetic and anti-obesity properties. Oral administration of such flavonoid component to the high diet-fed rats suppressed the body weight, decreased adipose tissue mass, and increased the hyperinsulinemia through regulating the enzyme expression associated in the synthesis of fatty acid and triacylglycerol (Bak, 2014).

Wogonin was reported to contain anti-obesity and antidiabetic action, (Ku SK,2015) as they help in modulating the lipid metabolism, blood glucose level and activating PPARα and AMPK. It effectively attenuated monocyte adhesion, molecular expression of cell adhesion, ROS synthesis, and activation of NF-κB (Gupta,2015) (as summarized in Figure 2, 3 and detailed in Table 1).

Phytosterols

Phytosterols are those compounds which are structurally similar to cholesterol and are commonly called sterols or stanols, obtained naturally from plants. They are available in higher concentration in edible oils including soybean, corn and sunflower oils (Rideout, 2010) They have proved to block the absorption of fatty acid through the intestine and capable of reducing the body weight in animal models (Trigueros, 2013).

Alkaloids

These are the basic organic compounds containing nitrogen in their heterocyclic ring structure. Alkaloidal components such as caffeine have reported to significantly enhance energy utilization, reduce the appetite, and also inhibit the adipocyte differentiation and pancreatic lipase.

Polyunsaturated Fatty Acids

Such components play an important role in balancing between energy uptake and energy utilization, neuroendocrine system, adipocytes condition and lipid metabolism (Janovska, 2013). It helps in reducing the enzymatic activities involved in lipid synthesis (Poudyala, 2005). Therefore, they might prevent the entry of free fatty acids in adipocytes for lipogenesis pathway and also improve the lipid oxidation (Slavin, 2005).

Dietary Fiber

Some of the examples of dietary fibre such as gum, pectin, and cellulose showed anti-obesity effects (Papathanasopoulos, 2010). Several soluble dietary fibres such as pectins, β-glucans compose thick solution when mixed with liquids. However, viscosity plays an important role in contributing to the physiological aspects of the small intestine. With an increase in viscosity of the formulation may act as a barrier to reduce the gastric emptying and conventionally reduce the nutrient absorption (Van der Klaauw, 2013).

Dietary fiber enhances the glucagon-like peptide-1, known as a gut hormone employed in the control of satiety, gastric emptying and even in small intestine transit. Additionally, the fiber is fermented in the large intestine with the aid of intestinal bacteria which influences the microbiota composition of microbiota. The short-chain fatty acids (SCFAs) obtained from intestinal bacteria such as acetic acid, propionic acid and butyric acid would significantly influence body weight regulation through various mechanisms such as reducing gastric emptying, delaying satiety, improving insulin and modulating glucose level and lipid oxidation. In addition to this, the dietary fibre may increase the number of *Bacteroidetes* and *Actinobacteria*, dominant in lean persons, and decline the prevalence of *Firmicutes* and *Proteobacteria*, which are dominant in obese individuals (Ulrich, 2011).

Protein Supplement

Previous research works stated that high protein intake may enhance the plasma protein level which plays a key role of inhibitor in the food intake (Zemel, 2005). Protein is comparatively more satiating when compared to carbohydrate. This is associated mainly with a highly composed diet-induced thermogenesis (Chu, 2016). Several protein supplements including whey, casein and soy protein have been marketed as anti-obese products. Therefore, such a high protein diet would help individuals to reduce their weight (Zemel, 2005).

Dietary Calcium Supplement

It is an important supplement in the maintenance of skeletal bone integrity, calcium level, and regulation of chronic diseases. High intake of calcium might increase fat excretion and energy utilization (Janovska, 2013). Even it also plays an important role in regulating the metabolism of adipocyte (Delzenne, 2011).

Probiotics

From the literature survey, it is reported that gut microbes are responsible for the development of diabetes and obesity (Fei, 2013). The lipopolysaccharide found in the gram-negative bacterial cell wall such as Escherichia coli may have the possibility to cause HFD obesity (Kadooka, 2010). Some probiotics are capable to reduce the body weight and fat mass in obese patients (Minami, 2015; Delzenne, 2013). The mechanism of action of such probiotics may include regulation of metabolism, appetite, suppression of lipid absorption (Jensen, 1995). Combination of both probiotics and prebiotics might produce better results in preventing obesity problems.

Psyllium tends to absorb water in the stomach and ultimately declined the appetite. It has also some beneficiary effects on treating diabetes by decreasing the cholesterol level. Level (Di-lorenzo, 1988; Frati-Munari,1983; Desmet, 1993; Leite-Silva, 2007). Some other examples of natural bulk producers including Laminaria, chitosans, agar (Desmet, 1993)

Natural Laxative Stimulants

Herbal formulations used in the treatment of obesity containing anthraquinones as a phytocomponents such as Cascara, Senna, Rhubarb, Aloe. Such herbs have the potential to act as a laxative which rapidly excretes out the foods and water, may lead to cause weight reduction (Desmet, 1993). The laxative effect of anthraquinones leads to rapid excretion of foods and water loss which can aid in weight reduction (Tapas, 2017).

Natural Sweeteners

Currently, neohesperidin-DHC synthesized from Seville oranges has been found to have great potential in food applications. Naringin isolated from *Citrus paradisi* is converted to naringin dihydrochalcone which is 1000 times sweeter than sucrose and is used to reduce body weight (Leite-Silva, 2007).

The Mohd-Radzman, et al has reviewed on the significant role of stevia in controlling insulin resistance and diabetes in the animal model. Results revealed a reduction in lipid peroxidation when pre-fed with stevia and an increase in the insulin secretion, supporting the reduced progression of diabetic co-morbid complications. In randomized studies, there was a decrease in postprandial glucose levels when fed meals supplemented with stevioside, as compared with sucrose and aspartame, respectively (Nabilatul, 2013).

Natural Products Obtained From Marine Source

Lipase inhibition is one of the main targets of anti-obesity drugs. Orlistat approved anti-obesity drug can act by this mechanism. Chemically, it is a hydrogenated derivative of lipstatin, acts as a potent, efficient long-acting reversible inhibitor of both pancreatic and gastric lipases. Lipstatin isolated from the

Figure 2. Bioactive components used in the treatment of obesity and diabetes

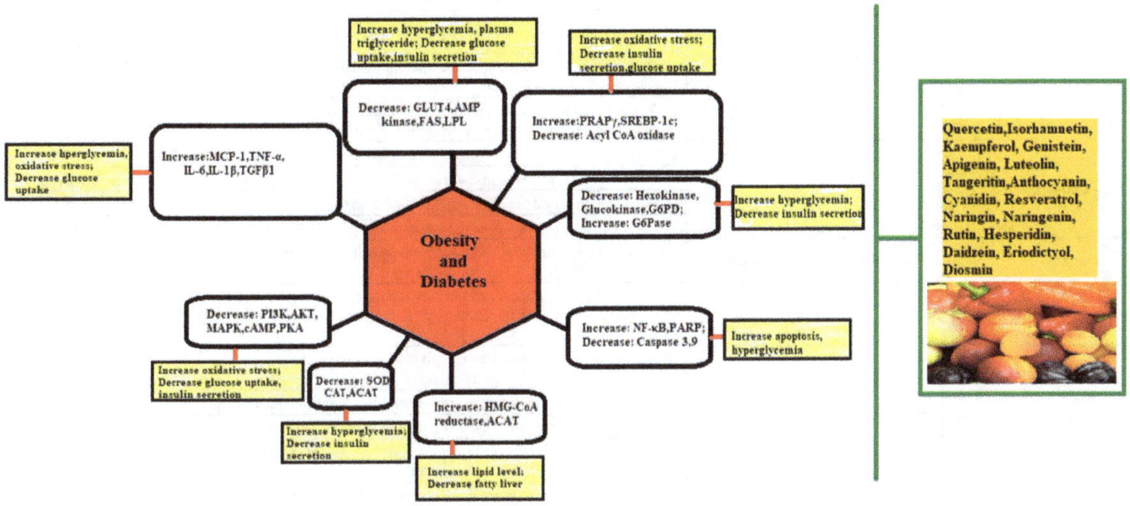

Figure 3. Flavonoids used in the prevention and treatment of obesity and diabetes

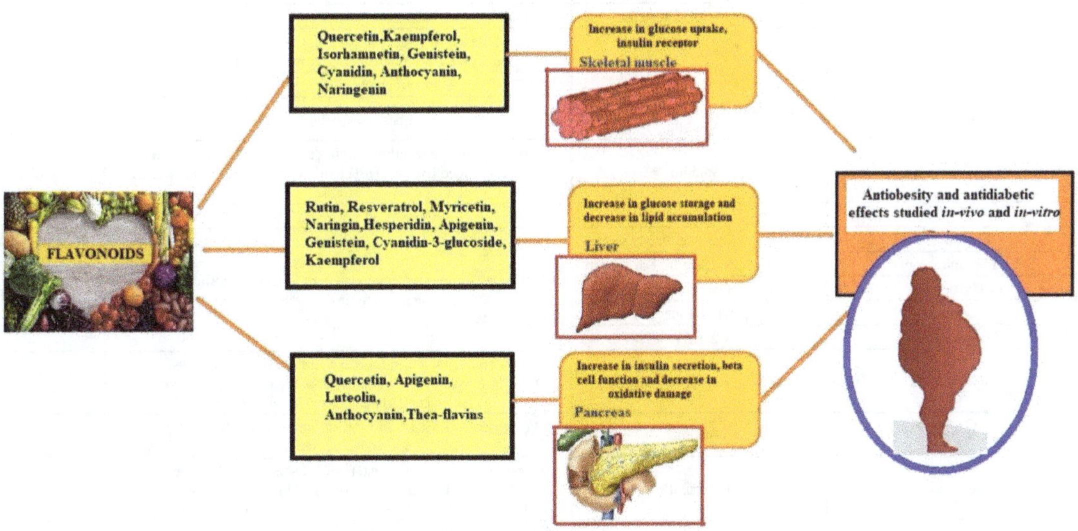

Table 1. Bio-active phytochemical compounds with anti-obesity and antidiabetic property.

Groups	Bio-active chemicals	Biological effects	References
Polyphenols	Ferulic acid	Hypolipidemic effect; reduced the serum cholesterol.	(Son, 2010)
	Stilbenes (resveratrol)	Downregulation effect on adipocyte transcription factors, thus significantly decreased the adipogenesis.	(Baile, 2015)
		Reduced the gained body weight and body fat.	(Bureau, 2008;Nelson-Dooley, 2005;Ramprasath, 2010)
		Antioxidant effect as preventing the lipid peroxidation; reduced the LDL cholesterol.	(Bureau,2008)
		Reduced the lipogenesis and lipid accumulation; enhanced the lipolysis and induced the apoptosis in the mature adipocytes cells.	(Fischer-Posovszky,2010)
Curcuminoids	Curcumins	Inhibited the lipid accumulation	(Pongchaidecha, 2009)
		Involved in energy metabolism.	(Alappat, 2010)
		Suppressed the angiogenesis in adipose tissues.	(Ejaz,2009)
		Regulated the adipocyte and lipogenesis transcription factors.	(Aggarwal, 2010)
Lignans	Secoisolariciresinol, matairesinol	Converted into enterodiol and enterolactone that reduced the high risk of obesity.	(Adlercreutz,2007)
Flavonoids (Flavonols)	Quercetin	Decreased the adipogenesis expression factors; attenuated in adipogenesis via activating AMPK signaling pathway in preadipocytes.	(Ahn, 2008)
Alkaloids	Capsaicin	Effective against inflammation-related diseases such as obesity and inflammation.	(Reyes-Escogido, 2011)
		Reduced food intake, increases energy expenditure and lipid oxidation	(Kang, 2010)
	Ephedrine	Enhanced norepinephrine, thereby inducing appetite suppression.	(Kaufinan, 1999)
		Produced thermogenic effect (increase basal metabolic rate) and energy expenditure.	(Astrup, 1995)
	Caffeine	Stimulated the breakdown of fat, potentiated the anorectic and thermogenic effects along with its diuretic effect	(Astrup, 1995; Astrup, 1992)
	Nicotine	Decreased the diet intake; increased fat oxidation and regulate the energy metabolism.	(Jensen, 1995;Tucci, 2010)
Terpenoids	Abscisic acid	Found effective against inflammation-related diseases such as obesity and inflammation.	(Guri, 2007)
	Carotenoids	Protect against obesity and atherosclerosis.	(Vivekananthan, 2003)
	Lycopene	Inhibited lipid peroxidation and LDL oxidation; lowered the risk of cardiovascular diseases.	(Agarwal, 2000)
Organosulfur compound	Ajoene	Decreased cholesterol synthesis, lowered the blood pressure, and stimulated the non-specific immunity.	(Cartea, 2008)
		Reduced body fat.	(Yang, 2006)
Phytosterols	Diosgenin, Campesterol,	Reduced LDL cholesterol level and act against atherosclerosis.	(Schonfeld, 2010)
	Brassicasterol, Sitosterol	Inhibited the cholesterol absorption in the intestinal lumen.	(Izar, 2011)
	Protodioscin	Reduced the triglyceride, cholesterol, LDL levels in the blood and increased the high-density lipoprotein levels in the body.	(Wang, 2010)
	Diosgenin	Inhibited triglyceride accumulation.	(Uemura, 2011)
Anthocyanins	Cyanidins, Delphinidins, Malvidins, Pelargonidins, Peonidins, Petunidins,	Ameliorated obesity-associated chronic diseases.	(Lee,2017;Azzini,2017)
	Cyanidin	Inhibited high-fat diet-induced lipid deposition and inflammation in the liver; inhibited liver NADPH oxidase upregulation and oxidative stress.	(Daveria,2018)
	Catechins, Caffeine, Theanine	Significantly reduced triglyceride level in the liver.	(Zheng, 2004)
Flavonols	Quercetin, Kaempferol, Myricetin	Antioxidant properties; regulated carbohydrate digestion, adipose deposition, insulin release.	(Mohammed, 2016)
Flavanones	Eriodictyol, Hesperetin, Naringenin		
Isoflavonoids	Daidzein, Genistein, Glycitein		
Flavones	Apigenin, Luteolin		
Flavans-3-ol	Catechin		
Phenolic acids	Caffeic acid, Chlorogenic acid	Prevented fatty acid synthase, 3-hydroxy-3-methylglutaryl CoA reductase and acyl-CoA: cholesterol acyltransferase activities, enhanced fatty acid β-oxidation activity.	(Cho, 2010)
Flavones	Luteolin	Possessed antioxidant and anti-inflammatory action; inhibited metabolic alterations.	(Gentile, 2018)
Isoflavone	Genistein	Effective against obesity and type 2 diabetes; ameliorated effect on adipocyte life-cycle, obesity-related low-grade inflammation, oxidative stress; Significant protective effect on pancreatic β cells.	(Behloul, 2013)
Polyphenols and phenolic acids	Rutin and o-Coumaric acid	Suppressed action on dyslipidemia, hepatosteatosis, and oxidative stress.	(Hsu, 2009)
	Sesamol obtained from sesame oil	Protective effect against both lipid accumulation and adipogenesis.	(Go G, 2017)

actinobacterium *Streptomyces toxytricini*. It contains a ß-lactone basic structure accounts for the irreversible lipase inhibition. Seaweed marine drugs like alginates, fucoidans, and phlorotannins have been

Figure 4. Structures of some chemical components containing anti-obesity and antidiabetic activity

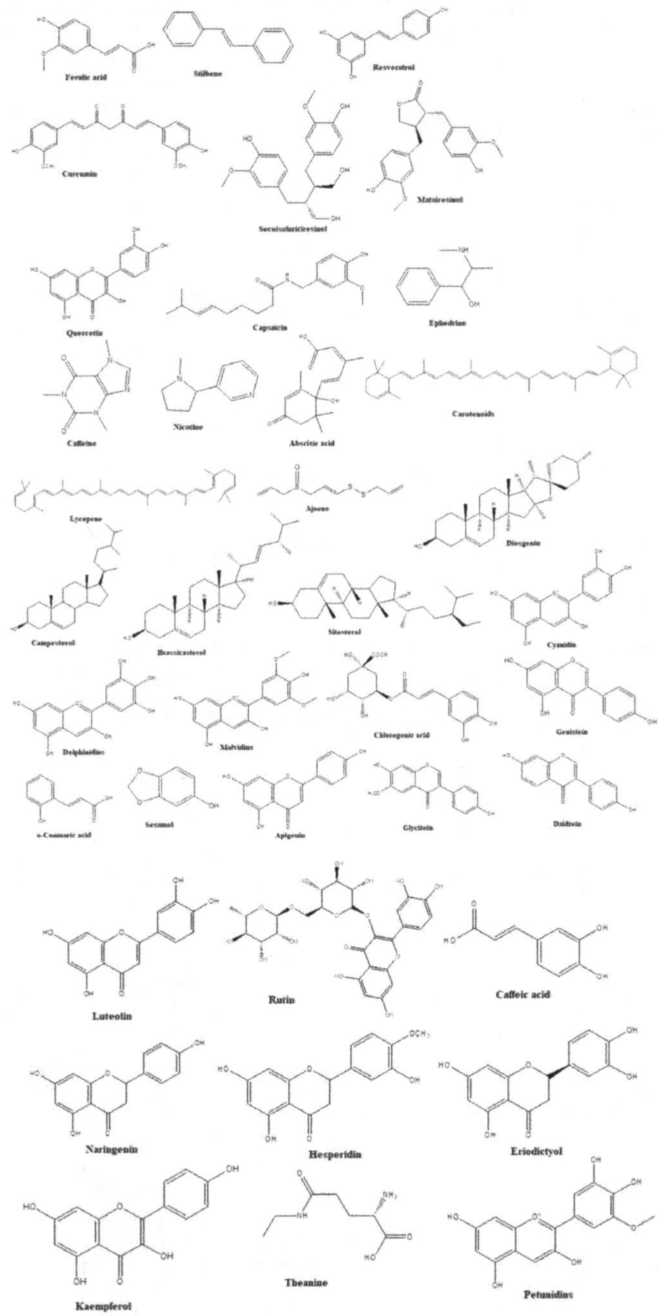

considered as the most potent agents for controlling obesity. Methanol extracts obtained from *Caulerpa taxifolia* and *Asparagopsis tociformis* revealed high activity along with 100% inhibition. In addition to this, similar extracts obtained from other marine seaweeds like *Codium latum*, *Hypnea charoides*, *Sargassum muticum*, *Gloiopeltis tenax* and *Dictyopteris latiuscula* possessed to contain anti-obesity properties.

Table 2. Medicinal herbs with anti-obesity property

Sl.no	Herbs	Part used	Solvent used for extraction	Animal model used	Effects observed	Mechanism of action	References
1	***Achyranthes aspera***	Seed	Ethanol	Swiss albino mice	Potentially inhibited body weight, liver weight, and serum levels such as total cholesterol, total triglyceride, and LDL-cholesterol.	Decreased the absorption of dietary fat.	(Rani,2012)
2	***Achyranthes bidentata***	Root	Aqueous	3T3-L1 adipocyte, a high-fat diet-fed obese rats	Reduced the body weight and triglyceride level, inhibited 3T3-L1 adipocyte differentiation, decreased the revealed that phospho-Akt expression.	Regulated the body weight and inhibited the adipogenesis.	(Oh,2014)
3	***Adenophora triphylla***	Root	Ethyl acetate	HFD mice	Declined the cholesterol levels in the plasma and hepatic region.	Possessed antioxidant property, protective effects on hypercholesterolaemia increased the LDL receptor and cholesterol 7α-hydroxylase expression.	(Hyun-Jin,2010)
4	***Aegle marmelos***	LeaF	Dichloromethane, ethyl acetate and n-butanol	HFD induced obese rats	Reduced body weight, total triglyceride, total cholesterol and glucose level.	Umbelliferone and esculetin regulated obesity through lipolysis.	(Karmase,2013)
5	***Bauhinia variegata***	Stem, root bark	Methanol	HFD induced obese female rats	Decreased the total cholesterol, triglyceride, LDL; significantly increased the serotonin level.	Bio-active component-sitosterol reduced the lipid content and enhanced the serotonin level in the brain.	(Balamurugan,2010)
6	***Brassica campestris***	Root	Ethanol	HFD mice, 3T3-L1 adipocytes	Suppressed body weight gain and fat accumulation.	Inhibited the lipid accumulation in the adipocyte.	(An,2010)
7	***Camellia sinensis***	Flower bud	Methanol	HFD mice	Reduced body weight gain and food intake.	Saponin component inhibited the appetite signals in the brain by stimulating the capsaicin-sensitive sensory nerves.	(Hamao,2011)
8	***Dioscoreae Tokoronis***	Rhizome	Aqueous	HFD mice	Significantly decreased the triglyceride, total plasma cholesterol, and LDL-cholesterol.	Suppressed the SREBP-1-dependent lipogenic pathway.	(Song,2009)
9	***Garcinia cambogia***	Fruit rind	-	Sprague-Dawley rats	Inhibited the lipogenesis,	Flavonoids possessed antioxidant and regulated obesity.	(Altiner,2012)
10	***Gymnema sylvestre***	Leaf	Ethanol	HFD induced Wistar rats	Enhanced the arterial blood pressure, heart rate, serum leptin, insulin, LDH, total cholesterol, triglycerides, apolipoprotein-B levels; decreased the serum HDL-C, apolipoprotein-A1 levels, cardiac Na $^{+}$K $^{+}$ ATPase.	-	(Kumar,2012)

continued on following page

Table 2. Continued

Sl.no	Herbs	Part used	Solvent used for extraction	Animal model used	Effects observed	Mechanism of action	References
11	***Hibiscus cannabinus***	Leaf	Ethanol	HFD female albino rats	Significantly decreased the serum cholesterol, triglycerides, LDL cholesterol level; decreased the levels of SGOT and SGPT.	-	(Karthik,2013)
12	***Laminaria japonica***	-	Ethanol	HFD rats	Effectively decreased the body weight gain, fat content and serum lipid levels.	Regulated the gene expression and proteins involved in lipolysis and lipogenesis.	(Jang,2013)
13	***Morinda citrifolia***	-	-	HFD mice	Regulated body mass and fat content.	-	(Saminathan,2013)
14	***Murraya koenigii***	Leaf	Dichloromethane, ethyl acetate	HFD obese rats	Significantly decreased the body weight gain, plasma total cholesterol and triglyceride levels.	-	(Birari,2010)
15	***Nelumbo nucifera***	Leaf	-	-	-	Inhibited the pancreatic lipase.	(Ahn,2013)
16	***Orthosiphon stamineus***	-	Betulinic acid isolated from Saussurea lappa ethanol	HFD mice	Decreased body weight significantly	-	(Choi,2013)
17	***Panax ginseng***	-	vinegar	Obese insulin-resistant rat	Beneficial effects on glucose metabolism and body weight control	Changing the expression of genes involved in glucose and fatty acid metabolism.	(Lim,2009)
18	***Premna integrifolia***	-	Chloroform: methanol	Female Swiss albino mice fed with cafeteria diet	Significantly decreased the body weight, and the levels of serum glucose, triglyceride, total cholesterol, LDL and VLDL	-	(Mali,2013)
19	***Sapindus emariganatus***	Leaf	Methanol	Monosodium glutamate-induced model in rats	Decreased the bodyweight	-	(Suneetha,2013)
20	***Schisandra chinensis***	-	-	3T3-L1 cells and high fat diet-induced obese rats	Decreased body weight and fat tissue mass	Inhibited preadipocyte differentiation and adipogenesis in cultured cells	(Park,2012)

'-': not known

Although another active inhibitor named as caulerpenyne isolated from ethyl acetate extract of *Caulerpa taxifolia* showed the promising effect. Oral administration of corn oil along with caulerpenyne exhibited reduced and delayed peak plasma triacylglycerol concentration in rodents (Chu, 2016).

Another marine source, *Undaria pinnatifida* contains fucoxanthinol, fucoxanthin. Fucoxanthin reduced the triglyceride level in plasma and hepatic region. It also reduced the activities involved in the adipocyte synthesis, triglyceride synthesis, whereas potentially increased the HDL-cholesterol level, fatty acid oxidation enzyme activity (Maeda, 2005).

The structures of various bioactive components are detailed in Figure 4; and Table 2, 3 showed the list of herbs used in the treatment of obesity and diabetes.

Table 3. Medicinal herbs with anti-diabetic property

Sl.no	Herbs	Part used	Solvent used for extraction	Animal model used	Mechanism of action./effects observed	References
1	***Zingiber officinalis***	Rhizome	Fresh Juice	-	Increased insulin level	(Akhani, 2004)
2	***Trigonella foenum graecum***	Seed	Aqueous	-	Increased serum insulin level possibly through β-cell regeneration or stimulation of insulin release from existing β cells of islets;	(Bera, 2013)
3	***Tinospora cardifolia***	Stem	Aqueous, alcoholic	STZ-induced diabetic rats	Increased the glycogen storage in the liver and decreased the glucose release from the liver	(Puranik, 2010)
4	***Terminalia catappa***	Fruit	Petroleum ether, methanol, and aqueous	Alloxan induced diabetic rats	Regeneration takes place by pancreatic beta cells	(Nagappa, 2003)
5	***Terminelia Arjuna***	Stem	Ethanol	Alloxan induced diabetic rats	Enhanced the peripheral utilization of glucose and kidney glycolysis by limiting its gluconeogenic formation	(Ragavan, 2006)
6	***Swertia chirata***	Entire herb	Aqueous Ethanol	*In vitro*	Lowered the blood glucose level; inhibited α-glucosidase and 2,2-diphenyl-1-picrylhydrazyl radical activity	(Kalhotra, 2020)
7	***Punica grantum***	Flower	Ethanol	STZ/ HFD rat	Improved insulin resistance activation of Akt-GSK3β signalling pathway	(Tang, 2018)
8	***Phyllanthus emblica***	Fruit	Methanol	STZ-induced diabetes	Stimulated insulin secretion	(Fatima, 2015)
9	***Panax ginseng***	-	-	Type II diabetes C57BKS -db/db mice	Up-regulated the expression of GLUT2 in liver and GLUT4 in muscle	(Kang, 2017
10	***Ocimum sanctum***	Entire herb	Hexane	STZ induced diabetes rats	Decreased oxidative stress, regulated the glucose and lipid level	(Suanarunsawat., 2016)
11	***Musa paradisiaca***	Flower	Aqueous	STZ induced diabetes	Decreased the fasting blood glucose level	(Vilhena, 2020)
12	***Berberis aristata***	Root	Ethanol	Alloxan induced diabetes	Decreased blood glucose and lipid level	(Semwal, 2009)
13	***Berberis asiatica***	Stem	Ethanol	Alloxan induced diabetes	Decrease the blood glucose level and improve the hepatic enzyme	(Semwal, 2007)
14	***Aloe barbadensis***	Leaf pulp	-	*In vitro*	Inhibit DDP-4 enzyme	(Prasannaraja, 2020)
15	***Andrographis paniculata***	Plant	Ethanol	-	Significantly decreased the blood glucose level	(Dandu, 2009)
16	***Annona squamosa***	Leaf	Hexane	STZ- induced diabetes	Inhibited the alpha-glucosidase enzyme activity and increase the secretion of Insulin	(Ranjana, 2014)
17	***Azadirachta indica***	Bark	Butanol, ethyl acetate fractions	*In vivo and in vitro*	Enhanced the glucose uptake in muscle	(Sanni, 2019)
18	***Brassica juncea***	Seed	Aqueous	STZ -induced diabetes	Increase insulin secretion from β cells	(Thirumalai, 2011)
19	***Cajanus cajan***	Leaf	Ethanol	*In vitro*	Significantly reduced the serum glucose level through activation of PPARγ .	(Schuster, 2016)
20	***Carica papaya***	Leaf	Hexane, ethyl acetate	HFD, STZ-induced diabetes	Increased insulin-sensitizing effect in the adipose tissue	(Irudayaraj, 2016)

'-': not known

CONCLUSIONS

Use of herbal supplements is one of the oldest traditions, which is being imposed a satisfactory effect on current society as an important need to evaluate their mechanism of action along with their associated benefits and less adverse effects. The utilization of natural anti-obesity products would be considered as an important and even supportive tool that help obese individuals to achieve their weight-loss goals. Furthermore, the multiple combinations of natural products may confer a synergistic effect with enhanced anti-obesity property along with multiple merits over chemical treatments. Such natural products are also associated with some other health benefits such as antidiabetic, anti-hyperlipidemic. Herbal medicines are used for wellbeing, prevention and treatment of obesity and diabetes. The commercially produced herbal products are widely derived from plants and form the mainstream way of modern medicine.

REFERENCES

Adlercreutz, H. (2007). Lignans and human health. *Critical Reviews in Clinical Laboratory Sciences*, *44*(5-6), 483–525. doi:10.1080/10408360701612942 PMID:17943494

Agarwal, S., & Rao, A. V. (2000). Tomato lycopene and its role in human health and chronic diseases. *Canadian Medical Association Journal*, *163*(6), 739–744. PMID:11022591

Aggarwal, B. B. (2010). Targeting inflammation-induced obesity and metabolic diseases by curcumin and other nutraceuticals. *Annual Review of Nutrition*, *30*(1), 173–199. doi:10.1146/annurev.nutr.012809.104755 PMID:20420526

Agrawal, Y. O., Sharma, P. K., Shrivastava, B., Ojha, S., Upadhya, H. M., Arya, D. S., & Goyal, S. N. (2014). Hesperidin produces cardioprotective activity via PPAR-γ pathway in ischemic heart disease model in diabetic rats. *PLoS One*, *9*(11), 1–13. doi:10.1371/journal.pone.0111212 PMID:25369053

Ahn, J., Lee, H., Kima, S., Parka, J., & Taeyoul, H. (2008). The anti-obesity effect of quercetin is mediated by the AMPK and MAPK signaling pathways. *Biochemical and Biophysical Research Communications*, *373*(4), 545–549. doi:10.1016/j.bbrc.2008.06.077 PMID:18586010

Ahn, J. H., Kim, E. S., Lee, C., Kim, S., Cho, S. H., Hwang, B. Y., & Lee, M. K. (2013). Chemical constituents from *Nelumbo nucifera* leaves and their anti-obesity effects. *Bioorganic & Medicinal Chemistry Letters*, *23*(12), 3604–3608. doi:10.1016/j.bmcl.2013.04.013 PMID:23642481

Akhani, S. P., Vishwakarma, S. L., & Goyal, R. K. (2004). Anti-diabetic activity of *Zingiber officinale* in streptozotocin-induced type I diabetic rats. *The Journal of Pharmacy and Pharmacology*, *56*(1), 101–105. doi:10.1211/0022357022403 PMID:14980006

Akiyama, S., Katsumata, S., Suzuki, K., Ishimi, Y., Wu, J., & Uehara, M. (2010). Dietary hesperidin exerts hypoglycemic and hypolipidemic effects in streptozotocin-induced marginal type 1 diabetic rats. *Journal of Clinical Biochemistry and Nutrition*, *46*(1), 87–92. doi:10.3164/jcbn.09-82 PMID:20104270

Al-Goblan, A. S., Al-Alfi, M. A., & Khan, M. Z. (2014). Mechanism linking diabetes mellitus and obesity. *Diabetes, Metabolic Syndrome and Obesity*, *7*, 587–591. doi:10.2147/DMSO.S67400 PMID:25506234

Alappat, L., & Awad, A. B. (2010). Curcumin and obesity: Evidence and mechanisms. *Nutrition Reviews*, *68*(12), 729–738. doi:10.1111/j.1753-4887.2010.00341.x PMID:21091916

Altiner, A. (2012). Effect of the antiobesity agent garcinia cambogia extract on serum lipoprotein (a), apolipoproteins a1 and b, and total cholesterol levels in female rats fed atherogenic diet. *The Journal of Animal and Plant Sciences*, *22*, 872–877.

An, S., Han, J. I., Kim, M. J., Park, J. S., Han, J. M., Baek, N. I., Chung, H. G., Choi, M. S., Lee, K. T., & Jeong, T. S. (2010). Ethanolic extracts of *Brassica campestris* spp. rapa roots prevent high-fat diet-induced obesity via beta(3)-adrenergic regulation of white adipocyte lipolytic activity. *Journal of Medicinal Food*, *13*(2), 406–414. doi:10.1089/jmf.2009.1295 PMID:20132043

Astrup, A., Breum, L., & Toubro, S. (1995). Pharmacological and clinical studies of ephedrine and other thermogenic agonists. *Obesity Research*, *3*(S4), 537S–540S. doi:10.1002/j.1550-8528.1995.tb00224.x PMID:8697055

Astrup, A., Toubro, S., Christensen, N., & Quade, F. (1992). Pharmacology of thermogenic drugs. *The American Journal of Clinical Nutrition*, *55*(1), 246S–248S. doi:10.1093/ajcn/55.1.246s PMID:1345887

Azzini, E., Giacometti, J., & Russo, G. L. (2017). Antiobesity effects of anthocyanins in preclinical and clinical studies. *Oxidative Medicine and Cellular Longevity*, *2017*(2740364), 1–11. doi:10.1155/2017/2740364 PMID:28785373

Baile, C. A., Yang, J. Y., Rayalam, S., Hartzell, D. L., Lai, C. Y., Andersen, C., & Della-Fera, M. A. (2011). Effect of resveratrol on fat mobilization. *Annals of the New York Academy of Sciences*, *1215*(1), 40–47. doi:10.1111/j.1749-6632.2010.05845.x PMID:21261640

Bak, E. J., Kim, J., Choi, Y. H., Kim, J. H., Lee, D. E., Woo, G. H., Cha, J. H., & Yoo, Y. J. (2014). Wogonin ameliorates hyperglycemia and dyslipidemia via pparα activation in db/db mice. *Clinical Nutrition (Edinburgh, Lothian)*, *33*(1), 156–163. doi:10.1016/j.clnu.2013.03.013 PMID:23623334

Balamurugan, G., & Muralidharan, P. (2010). Antiobesity effect of *Bauhinia variegata* bark extract on female rats fed on hypercaloric diet. *Bangladesh Journal of Pharmacology*, *5*(1), 8–12. doi:10.3329/bjp.v5i1.4310

Behloul, N., & Wu, G. (2013). Genistein: A promising therapeutic agent for obesity and diabetes treatment. *European Journal of Pharmacology*, *698*(1-3), 31–38. doi:10.1016/j.ejphar.2012.11.013 PMID:23178528

Bera, T. K., Ali, K. M., Jana, K., Ghosh, A., & Ghosh, D. (2013). Protective effect of aqueous extract of seed of *Psoralea corylifolia* (Somraji) and seed of *Trigonella foenum-graecum* L. (Methi) in streptozotocin-induced diabetic rat: A comparative evaluation. *Pharmacognosy Research*, *5*(4), 277–285. doi:10.4103/0974-8490.118840 PMID:24174822

Birari, R., Javia, V., & Bhutani, K. K. (2010). Antiobesity and lipid lowering effects of *Murraya koenigii* (L.) Spreng leaves extracts and mahanimbine on high fat diet induced obese rats. *Fitoterapia*, *81*(8), 1129–1133. doi:10.1016/j.fitote.2010.07.013 PMID:20655993

Bouzakri, K., Roques, M., Gual, P., Espinosa, S., Guebre-Egziabher, F., Riou, J. P., Laville, M., le Marchand-Brustel, Y., Tanti, J. F., & Vidal, H. (2003). Reduced activation of phosphatidylinositol-3 kinase and increased serine 636 phosphorylation of insulin receptor substrate-1 in primary culture of skeletal muscle cells from patients with type 2 diabetes. *Diabetes*, *52*(6), 1319–1325. doi:10.2337/diabetes.52.6.1319 PMID:12765939

Bureau, G., Longpré, F., & Martinoli, M. G. (2008). Resveratrol and quercetin, two natural polyphenols, reduce apoptotic neuronal cell death induced by neuroinflammation. *Journal of Neuroscience Research*, *86*(2), 403–410. doi:10.1002/jnr.21503 PMID:17929310

Cartea, M. E., & Velasco, P. (2008). Glucosinalates in Brasscia foods: Bioavailability in food and significance for human health. *Phytochemistry Reviews*, *7*(2), 213–229. doi:10.100711101-007-9072-2

Castellarin, S. D., & Di Gaspero, G. (2007). Transcriptional control of anthocyanin biosynthetic genes in extreme phenotypes for berry pigmentation of naturally occurring grapevines. *BMC Plant Biology*, *7*(1), 1–10. doi:10.1186/1471-2229-7-46 PMID:17760970

Cheon, H., Cho, J. M., Kim, S., Baek, S. H., Lee, M. K., Kim, K. W., Yu, S. W., Solinas, G., Kim, S. S., & Lee, M. S. (2010). Role of JNK activation in pancreatic beta-cell death by streptozotocin. *Molecular and Cellular Endocrinology*, *321*(2), 131–137. doi:10.1016/j.mce.2010.02.016 PMID:20176078

Cho, A. S., Jeon, S. M., Kim, M. J., Yeo, J., Seo, K. I., Choi, M. S., & Lee, M. K. (2010). Chlorogenic acid exhibits anti-obesity property and improves lipid metabolism in high-fat diet-induced-obese mice. *Food and Chemical Toxicology*, *48*(3), 937–943. doi:10.1016/j.fct.2010.01.003 PMID:20064576

Choe, S. C., Kim, H. S., Jeong, T. S., Bok, S. H., & Park, Y. B. (2001). Naringin has an antiatherogenic effect with the inhibition of intercellular adhesion molecule-1 in hypercholesterolemic rabbits. *Journal of Cardiovascular Pharmacology*, *38*(6), 947–955. doi:10.1097/00005344-200112000-00017 PMID:11707699

Choi, Y. J., Park, S. Y., Kim, J. Y., Won, K. C., Kim, B. R., Son, J. K., Lee, S. H., & Kim, Y. W. (2013). Combined treatment of betulinic acid, a PTP1B inhibitor, with *Orthosiphon stamineus* extract decreases body weight in high-fat-fed mice. *Journal of Medicinal Food*, *16*(1), 2–8. doi:10.1089/jmf.2012.2384 PMID:23256448

Chojnacka, K., Saeid, A., Witkowska, Z., & Tuhy, L. (2012). Biologically active compounds in seaweed extracts-the prospects for the application. *The Open Conference Proceedings Journal*, *3*(1), 20–28. doi :10.2174/1876326X01203020020

Chu, W., & Phang, S. (2016). Marine algae as a potential source for Anti-Obesity Agents. *Marine Drugs*, *14*(12), 222. doi:10.3390/md14120222 PMID:27941599

Crozier, A., Jaganath, I. B., & Clifford, M. N. (2009). Dietary phenolics: Chemistry, bioavailability and effects on health. *Natural Product Reports*, *26*(8), 1001–1043. doi:10.1039/b802662a PMID:19636448

Dandu, A. M., & Inamdar, N. M. (2009). Evaluation of beneficial effects of antioxidant properties of aqueous leaf extract of *Andrographis paniculata* in STZ-induced diabetes. *Pakistan Journal of Pharmaceutical Sciences*, *22*(1), 49–52. PMID:19168420

Daveri, E., Cremonini, E., Mastaloudis, A., Hester, S. N., Wood, S. M., Waterhouse, A. L., Anderson, M., Fraga, C. G., & Oteiza, P. I. (2018). Cyanidin and delphinidin modulate inflammation and altered redox signaling improving insulin resistance in high fat-fed mice. *Redox Biology*, *18*, 16–24. doi:10.1016/j.redox.2018.05.012 PMID:29890336

Delzenne, N. M., Neyrinck, A. M., Bäckhed, F., & Cani, P. D. (2011). Targeting gut microbiota in obesity: Effects of prebiotics and probiotics. *Nature Reviews. Endocrinology*, *7*(11), 639–646. doi:10.1038/nrendo.2011.126 PMID:21826100

Delzenne, N. M., Neyrinck, A. M., & Cani, P. D. (2013). Gut microbiota and metabolic disorders: How prebiotic can work? *British Journal of Nutrition*, *109*(S2), S81–S85. doi:10.1017/S0007114512004047 PMID:23360884

Desai, M. Y., Dalal, D., Santos, R. D., Carvalho, J. A., Nasir, K., & Blumenthal, R. S. (2006). Association of body mass index, metabolic syndrome, and leukocyte count. *The American Journal of Cardiology*, *97*(6), 835–838. doi:10.1016/j.amjcard.2005.10.021 PMID:16516585

Desmet, P., Keller, K., Hansel, R., & Chandler, R. (1993). *Adverse effects of herbal drugs 2*. Spriger-Verlag. doi:10.1007/978-3-642-48906-8

Devendra, D., Liu, E., & Eisenbarth, G. S. (2004). Type 1 diabetes: Recent developments. *British Medical Journal*, *328*(7442), 750–754. doi:10.1136/bmj.328.7442.750 PMID:15044291

Di-lorenzo, C., Williams, C., Hainal, F., & Valenzuela, J. (1988). Pectin delays gastric emptying and increases satiety in obese subjects. *Gastroenterology*, *95*(5), 1211–1215. doi:10.1016/0016-5085(88)90352-6 PMID:3169489

Ding, L., Jin, D., & Chen, X. (2010). Luteolin enhances insulin sensitivity via activation of PPARγ transcriptional activity in adipocytes. *The Journal of Nutritional Biochemistry*, *21*(10), 941–947. doi:10.1016/j.jnutbio.2009.07.009 PMID:19954946

Edwards, R. L., Lyon, T., Litwin, S. E., Rabovsky, A., Symons, J. D., & Jalili, T. (2007). Quercetin reduces blood pressure in hypertensive subjects. *The Journal of Nutrition*, *137*(11), 2405–2411. doi:10.1093/jn/137.11.2405 PMID:17951477

Ejaz, A., Wu, D., Kwan, P., & Meydani, M. (2009). Curcumin inhibits adipogenesis in 3T3-L1 adipocytes and angiogenesis and obesity in C57/BL mice. *The Journal of Nutrition*, *139*(5), 919–925. doi:10.3945/jn.108.100966 PMID:19297423

Fain, J. N., Madan, A. K., Hiler, M. L., Cheema, P., & Bahouth, S. W. (2004). Comparison of the release of adipokines by adipose tissue, adipose tissue matrix, and adipocytes from visceral and subcutaneous abdominal adipose tissues of obese humans. *Endocrinology*, *145*(5), 2273–2282. doi:10.1210/en.2003-1336 PMID:14726444

Fatima, N., Hafizur, R. M., Hameed, A., Ahmed, S., Nisar, M., & Kabir, N. (2015). Ellagic acid in *Emblica officinalis* exerts anti-diabetic activity through the action on β-cells of pancreas. *European Journal of Nutrition*, *56*(2), 591–601. doi:10.100700394-015-1103-y PMID:26593435

Fei, N., & Zhao, L. (2013). An opportunistic pathogen isolated from the gut of obese human causes obesity in germfree mice. *The ISME Journal*, *7*(4), 880–884. doi:10.1038/ismej.2012.153 PMID:23235292

Fischer-Posovszky, P., Kukulus, V., Tews, D., Unterkircher, T., Debatin, K. M., Fulda, S., & Wabitsch, M. (2010). Resveratrol regulates human adipocyte number and function in a Sirt1-dependent manner. *The American Journal of Clinical Nutrition*, *92*(1), 5–15. doi:10.3945/ajcn.2009.28435 PMID:20463039

Frati-Munari, A., Fernandez, J., Becerril, M., Chavez, A., & Banles, M. (1983). Decrease in serum lipids, glycemia and body weight by *Plantago psyllium* in obese and diabetic patients. *Archivos de Investigacion Medica*, *14*, 259–268. PMID:6322713

Galvano, F., La Fauci, L., Vitaglione, P., Fogliano, V., Vanella, L., & Felgines, C. (2007). Bioavailability, antioxidant and biological properties of the natural free-radical scavengers cyanidin and related glycosides. *Annali dell'Istituto Superiore di Sanita*, *43*, 382–393. PMID:18209272

Gates, M. A., Tworoger, S. S., Hecht, J. L., de Vivo, I., Rosner, B., & Hankinson, S. E. (2007). A prospective study of dietary flavonoid intake and incidence of epithelial ovarian cancer. *International Journal of Cancer*, *121*(10), 2225–2232. doi:10.1002/ijc.22790 PMID:17471564

Gentile, D., Fornai, M., Pellegrini, C., Colucci, R., Benvenuti, L., Duranti, E., Masi, S., Carpi, S., Nieri, P., Nericcio, A., Garelli, F., Virdis, A., Pistelli, L., Blandizzi, C., & Antonioli, L. (2018). Luteolin prevents cardiometabolic alterations and vascular dysfunction in mice with HFD-induced obesity. *Frontiers in Pharmacology*, *9*, 1094–1107. doi:10.3389/fphar.2018.01094 PMID:30319424

Ghosh, D., & Konishi, T. (2007). Anthocyanins and anthocyanin-rich extracts: Role in diabetes and eye function. *Asia Pacific Journal of Clinical Nutrition*, *16*(2), 200–208. PMID:17468073

Go, G., Sung, J. S., Jee, S. C., Kim, M., Jang, W. H., Kang, K. Y., Kim, D. Y., Lee, S., & Shin, H. S. (2017). In vitro anti-obesity effects of sesamol mediated by adenosine monophosphate-activated protein kinase and mitogen-activated protein kinase signaling in 3T3-L1 cells. *Food Science and Biotechnology*, *26*(1), 195–200. doi:10.100710068-017-0026-1 PMID:30263528

Guariguata, L., Whiting, D., Hambleton, I., Beagley, J., Linnenkamp, U., & Shaw, J. (2014). Global estimates of diabetes prevalence for 2013 and projections for 2035. *Diabetes Research and Clinical Practice*, *103*(2), 137–149. doi:10.1016/j.diabres.2013.11.002 PMID:24630390

Guilherme, A., Virbasius, J. V., Puri, V., & Czech, M. P. (2008). Adipocyte dysfunctions linking obesity to insulin resistance and type 2 diabetes. *Nature Reviews. Molecular Cell Biology*, *9*(5), 367–377. doi:10.1038/nrm2391 PMID:18401346

Gupta, V. K., Tuohy, M. G., O'Donovan, A., & Lohani, M. (2015). *Biotechnology of bioactive compounds: Sources and applications*. Wiley-Blackwell. doi:10.1002/9781118733103

Guri, A. J., Hontecillas, R., Si, H., Liu, D., & Bassaganya-Riera, J. (2007). Dietary abscisic acid ameliorates glucose tolerance and obesity-related inflammation in db/db mice fed high-fat diets. *Clinical Nutrition (Edinburgh, Lothian)*, *26*(1), 107–116. doi:10.1016/j.clnu.2006.07.008 PMID:17000034

Häkkinen, S. H., Kärenlampi, S. O., Heinonen, I. M., Mykkänen, H. M., & Törrönen, A. R. (1999). Content of the flavonols quercetin, myricetin, and kaempferol in 25 edible berries. *Journal of Agricultural and Food Chemistry*, *47*(6), 2274–2279. doi:10.1021/jf9811065 PMID:10794622

Hamao, M., Matsuda, H., Nakamura, S., Nakashima, S., Semura, S., Maekubo, S., Wakasugi, S., & Yoshikawa, M. (2011). Anti-obesity effects of the methanolic extract and chakasaponins from the flower buds of *Camellia sinensis* in mice. *Bioorganic & Medicinal Chemistry*, *19*(20), 6033–6041. doi:10.1016/j.bmc.2011.08.042 PMID:21925888

Harmon, A. W., & Patel, Y. M. (2003). Naringenin inhibits phosphoinositide 3-kinase activity and glucose uptake in 3T3-L1 adipocytes. *Biochemical and Biophysical Research Communications*, *305*(3), 229–234. doi:10.1016/S0006-291X(03)00720-4 PMID:12745063

Hasanein, P., & Fazeli, F. (2014). Role of naringenin in protection against diabetic hyperalgesia and tactile allodynia in male wistar rats. *Journal of Physiology and Biochemistry*, *70*(4), 997–1006. doi:10.100713105-014-0369-5 PMID:25407136

Hertog, M. G. L., Hollman, P. C., & van de Putte, B. (1993). Content of potentially anticarcinogenic flavonoids of tea infusions, wines, and fruit juices. *Journal of Agricultural and Food Chemistry*, *41*(8), 1242–1246. doi:10.1021/jf00032a015

Hiermann, A., Schramm, H., & Laufer, S. (1998). Anti-inflammatory activity of myricetin-3-O-β-d-glucuronide and related compounds. *Inflammation Research*, *47*(11), 421–427. doi:10.1007000110050355 PMID:9865500

Hossain, M. K., Dayem, A. A., Han, J., Yin, Y., Kim, K., Saha, S. K., Yang, G. M., Choi, H. Y., & Cho, S. G. (2016). Molecular mechanisms of the anti-obesity and anti-diabetic properties of flavonoids. *International Journal of Molecular Sciences*, *17*(4), 569–601. doi:10.3390/ijms17040569 PMID:27092490

Hsu, C. L., Wu, C. H., Huang, S. L., & Yen, G. C. (2009). Phenolic compounds rutin and o-coumaric acid ameliorate obesity induced by high-fat diet in rats. *Journal of Agricultural and Food Chemistry*, *57*(2), 425–431. doi:10.1021/jf802715t PMID:19119847

Huang, W. Y., Zhang, H. C., Liu, W. X., & Li, C. Y. (2012). Survey of antioxidant capacity and phenolic composition of blueberry, blackberry, and strawberry in nanjing. *Journal of Zhejiang University. Science. B.*, *13*(2), 94–102. doi:10.1631/jzus.B1100137 PMID:22302422

Hyun-Jin, C., Mi Ja, C., & Seung-Shi, H. (2010). Antiobese and hypocholesterolaemic effects of an *Adenophora triphylla* extract in HepG2 cells and high fat diet-induced obese mice. *Food Chemistry*, *119*(2), 437–444. doi:10.1016/j.foodchem.2009.06.039

Irudayaraj, S. S., Stalin, A., Sunil, C., Duraipandiyan, V., Al-Dhabi, N. A., & Ignacimuthu, S. (2016). Antioxidant, antilipidemic and antidiabetic effects of ficusin with their effects on GLUT4 translocation and PPARγ expression in type 2 diabetic rats. *Chemico-Biological Interactions*, *256*, 85–93. doi:10.1016/j.cbi.2016.06.023 PMID:27350165

Izar, M. C., Tegani, D. M., Kasmas, S. H., & Fonseca, F. A. (2011). Phytosterols and phytosterolemia: Gene-diet interactions. *Genes & Nutrition*, *6*(1), 17–26. doi:10.100712263-010-0182-x PMID:21437027

Jang, W. S., & Choung, S. Y. (2013). Antiobesity effects of the ethanol extract of *Laminaria japonica* Areshoung in high-fat-diet-induced obese rat. *Evidence-Based Complementary and Alternative Medicine, 2013*, 492807. doi:10.1155/2013/492807 PMID:23365609

Janovskà, P., Flachs, P., Kazdova, L., & Kopecký, J. (2013). Anti-obesity effect of n-3 polyunsaturated fatty acids in mice fed high-fat diet is independent of cold-induced thermogenesis. *Physiological Research, 62*, 153–161. doi:10.33549/physiolres.932464 PMID:23234412

Jensen, E. X., Fusch, C., Jaeger, P., Peheim, E., & Horber, F. F. (1995). Impact of chronic cigarette smoking on body composition and fuel metabolism. *The Journal of Clinical Endocrinology and Metabolism, 80*(7), 2181–2185. PMID:7608276

Jorge, A. P., Horst, H., de Sousa, E., Pizzolatti, M. G., & Silva, F. R. (2004). Insulinomimetic effects of kaempferitrin on glycaemia and on 14C-glucose uptake in rat soleus muscle. *Chemico-Biological Interactions, 49*(2-3), 89–96. doi:10.1016/j.cbi.2004.07.001 PMID:15501431

Jung, U. J., Lee, M. K., Jeong, K. S., & Choi, M. S. (2004). The hypoglycemic effects of hesperidin and naringin are partly mediated by hepatic glucose-regulating enzymes in C57BL/KsJ-*db/db* mice. *The Journal of Nutrition, 134*(10), 2499–2503. doi:10.1093/jn/134.10.2499 PMID:15465737

Jung, U. J., Lee, M. K., Park, Y. B., Kang, M. A., & Choi, M. S. (2006). Effect of citrus flavonoids on lipid metabolism and glucose-regulating enzyme mRNA levels in type-2 diabetic mice. *The International Journal of Biochemistry & Cell Biology, 38*(7), 1134–1145. doi:10.1016/j.biocel.2005.12.002 PMID:16427799

Kadooka, Y., Sato, M., Imaizumi, K., Ogawa, A., Ikuyama, K., Akai, Y., Okano, M., Kagoshima, M., & Tsuchida, T. (2010). Regulation of abdominal adiposity by probiotics (*Lactobacillus gasseri* SBT2055) in adults with obese tendencies in a randomized controlled trial. *European Journal of Clinical Nutrition, 64*(6), 636–643. doi:10.1038/ejcn.2010.19 PMID:20216555

Kalhotra, P., Chittepu, V.C.S.R., Osorio-Revilla, G. & Gallardo-Velazquez, T. (2020). Phytochemicals in garlic extract inhibit therapeutic enzyme DPP-4 and induce skeletal muscle cell proliferation: A possible mechanism of action to benefit the treatment of diabetes mellitus. *Biomolecules, 10*(2), 305.

Kandasamy, N., & Ashokkumar, N. (2014). Protective effect of bioflavonoid myricetin enhances carbohydrate metabolic enzymes and insulin signaling molecules in streptozotocin-cadmium induced diabetic nephrotoxic rats. *Toxicology and Applied Pharmacology, 279*(2), 173–185. doi:10.1016/j.taap.2014.05.014 PMID:24923654

Kang, J. H., Tsuyoshi, G., Han, I. S., Kawada, T., Kim, Y. M., & Yu, R. (2010). Dietary capsaicin reduces obesity-induced insulin resistance and hepatic steatosis in obese mice fed a high-fat diet. *Obesity (Silver Spring, Md.), 18*(4), 780–787. doi:10.1038/oby.2009.301 PMID:19798065

Kang, O. H., Shon, M. Y., Kong, R., Seo, Y. S., Zhou, T., Kim, D. Y., Kim, Y. S., & Kwon, D. Y. (2017). Anti-diabetic effect of black ginseng extract by augmentation of AMPK protein activity and upregulation of GLUT2 and GLUT4 expression in db/db mice. *BMC Complementary and Alternative Medicine, 17*(1), 341–352. doi:10.118612906-017-1839-4 PMID:28662663

Kao, Y. H., Hiipakka, R. A., & Liao, S. (2000). Modulation of endocrine systems and food intake by green tea epigallocatechin gallate. *Endocrinology*, *141*(3), 980–987. doi:10.1210/endo.141.3.7368 PMID:10698173

Karmase, A., Birari, R., & Bhutani, K. K. (2013). Evaluation of anti-obesity effect of *Aegle marmelos* leaves. *Phytomedicine*, *20*(10), 805–812. doi:10.1016/j.phymed.2013.03.014 PMID:23632084

Karthik, M., & Gayathri, C. (2013). Effect of ethanolic extract of *Hibiscus cannabinus* leaf on high cholesterol diet induced obesity in female albino rats. *Asian Journal of Pharmaceutical and Clinical Research*, *6*(4), 65–67.

Kaufinan, P., Cseke, L., Warber, S., Duke, J., & Brielmann, H. (1999). *Natural products from plants.* CRC Press.

Kavanagh, K. T., Hafer, L. J., Kim, D. W., Mann, K. K., Sherr, D. H., Rogers, A. E., & Sonenshein, G. E. (2001). Green tea extracts decrease carcinogen-induced mammary tumor burden in rats and rate of breast cancer cell proliferation in culture. *Journal of Cellular Biochemistry*, *82*(3), 387–398. doi:10.1002/jcb.1164 PMID:11500915

Kawser Hossain, M., Abdal Dayem, A., Han, J., Kumar Saha, S., Yang, G. M., Choi, H. Y., & Cho, S. G. (2016). Recent advances in disease modeling and drug discovery for diabetes mellitus using induced pluripotent stem cells. *International Journal of Molecular Sciences*, *17*(2), 256–273. doi:10.3390/ijms17020256 PMID:26907255

Khorami, S. A. H., Movahedi, A., Khaza'ai, H., Mutalib, A., & Sokhini, M. (2015). PI3K/AKT pathway in modulating glucose homeostasis and its alteration in diabetes. *Annals of Medical and Biomedical Sciences*, *1*(2), 46–55.

Kim, H. J., Oh, G. T., Park, Y. B., Lee, M. K., Seo, H. J., & Choi, M. S. (2004). Naringin alters the cholesterol biosynthesis and antioxidant enzyme activities in ldl receptor-knockout mice under cholesterol fed condition. *Life Sciences*, *74*(13), 1621–1634. doi:10.1016/j.lfs.2003.08.026 PMID:14738906

Koch, C. E., Ganjam, G. K., Steger, J., Legler, K., Stohr, S., Schumacher, D., Hoggard, N., Heldmaier, G., & Tups, A. (2013). The dietary flavonoids naringenin and quercetin acutely impair glucose metabolism in rodents possibly via inhibition of hypothalamic insulin signalling. *British Journal of Nutrition*, *109*(6), 1040–1051. doi:10.1017/S0007114512003005 PMID:22850125

Kreft, S., Knapp, M., & Kreft, I. (1999). Extraction of rutin from buckwheat (*Fagopyrum esculentummoench*) seeds and determination by capillary electrophoresis. *Journal of Agricultural and Food Chemistry*, *47*(11), 4649–4652. doi:10.1021/jf990186p PMID:10552865

Ku, S. K., & Bae, J. S. (2015). Baicalin, baicalein and wogonin inhibits high glucose-induced vascular inflammation *in vitro* and *in vivo*. *BMB Reports*, *48*(9), 519–524. doi:10.5483/BMBRep.2015.48.9.017 PMID:25739393

Kumar, V., Bhandari, U., Tripathi, C. D., & Khanna, G. (2012). Evaluation of antiobesity and cardioprotective effect of *Gymnema sylvestre* extract in murine model. *Indian Journal of Pharmacology*, *44*(5), 607–613. doi:10.4103/0253-7613.100387 PMID:23112423

Lee, Y. M., Yoon, Y., Yoon, H., Park, H. M., Song, S., & Yeum, K. J. (2017). Dietary anthocyanins against obesity and inflammation. *Nutrients, 9*(10), 1089–1104. doi:10.3390/nu9101089 PMID:28974032

Lee, Y. S., Lee, S., Lee, H. S., Kim, B. K., Ohuchi, K., & Shin, K. H. (2005). Inhibitory effects of isorhamnetin-3-O-β-d-glucoside from *Salicornia herbacea* on rat lens aldose reductase and sorbitol accumulation in streptozotocin-induced diabetic rat tissues. *Biological & Pharmaceutical Bulletin, 28*(5), 916–918. doi:10.1248/bpb.28.916 PMID:15863906

Leite-Silva, C., Gusmão, C. L. S., & Takahashi, C. S. (2007). Genotoxic and antigenotoxic effects of *Fucus vesiculosus* extract on cultured human lymphocytes using the chromosome aberration and Comet assays. *Genetics and Molecular Biology, 30*(1), 105–111. doi:10.1590/S1415-47572007000100019

Lim, S., Yoon, J. W., Choi, S. H., Cho, B. J., Kim, J. T., Chang, H. S., Park, H. S., Park, K. S., Lee, H. K., Kim, Y. B., & Jang, H. C. (2009). Effect of ginsam, a vinegar extract from *Panax ginseng*, on body weight and glucose homeostasis in an obese insulin-resistant rat model. *Metabolism: Clinical and Experimental, 58*(1), 8–15. doi:10.1016/j.metabol.2008.07.027 PMID:19059525

Liu, I. M., Tzeng, T. F., Liou, S. S., & Lan, T. W. (2007). Myricetin, a naturally occurring flavonol, ameliorates insulin resistance induced by a high-fructose diet in rats. *Life Sciences, 81*(21-22), 1479–1488. doi:10.1016/j.lfs.2007.08.045 PMID:17976658

Liu, Y., Fu, X., Lan, N., Li, S., Zhang, J., Wang, S., Li, C., Shang, Y., Huang, T., & Zhang, L. (2014). Luteolin protects against high fat diet-induced cognitive deficits in obesity mice. *Behavioural Brain Research, 267*, 178–188. doi:10.1016/j.bbr.2014.02.040 PMID:24667364

Lutgarda, B., Giuseppina, C., Giuseppe, D. P., Paola, C., Claudia, V., Marilena, V., Angela, A. R., & Giovanni, A. (2018). Dietary Fibre as a Unifying Remedy for the Whole Spectrum of Obesity-Associated Cardiovascular Risk. *Nutrients, 10*(7), 943. doi:10.3390/nu10070943 PMID:30037123

Maeda, H., Hosokawa, M., Sashima, T., Funayama, K., & Miyashita, K. (2005). Fucoxanthin from edible seaweed, *Undaria pinnatifida*, shows antiobesity effect through UCP1 expression in white adipose tissues. *Biochemical and Biophysical Research Communications, 332*(2), 392–397. doi:10.1016/j.bbrc.2005.05.002 PMID:15896707

Malekshahi, H., Bahrami, G., Miraghaee, S., Ahmadi, S. A., Sajadimajd, S., Hatami, R., Mohammadi, B., & Keshavarzi, S. (2019). *Momordica charantia* reverses type II diabetes in rat. *Journal of Food Biochemistry, 43*(11), e13021. doi:10.1111/jfbc.13021 PMID:31441956

Mali, P. Y., Bigoniya, P., Panchal, S. S., & Muchhandi, I. S. (2013). Anti-obesity activity of chloroform-methanol extract of *Premna integrifolia* in mice fed with cafeteria diet. *Journal of Pharmacy & Bioallied Sciences, 5*(3), 229–236. doi:10.4103/0975-7406.116825 PMID:24082700

Maury, E., Ehala-Aleksejev, K., Guiot, Y., Detry, R., Vandenhooft, A., & Brichard, S. M. (2007). Adipokines oversecreted by omental adipose tissue in human obesity. *American Journal of Physiology. Endocrinology and Metabolism, 293*(3), E656–E665. doi:10.1152/ajpendo.00127.2007 PMID:17578888

Michael, J., & Fowler, M. D. (2008). Microvascular and macrovascular complications of diabetes. *Clinical Diabetes, 26*(2), 77–82. doi:10.2337/diaclin.26.2.77

Miean, K. H., & Mohamed, S. (2001). Flavonoid (myricetin, quercetin, kaempferol, luteolin, and apigenin) content of edible tropical plants. *Journal of Agricultural and Food Chemistry*, *49*(6), 3106–3112. doi:10.1021/jf000892m PMID:11410016

Minami, J. I., Kondo, S., Yanagisawa, N., Odamaki, T., Xiao, J. Z., Abe, F., Nakajima, S., Hamamoto, Y., Saitoh, S., & Shimoda, T. (2015). Oral administration of Bifidobacterium breve B-3 modifies metabolic functions in adults with obese tendencies in a randomised controlled trial. *Journal of Nutritional Science*, *4*, e1–e7. doi:10.1017/jns.2015.5 PMID:26090097

Mirfeizi, M., Tourzani, Z. M., Mirfeizi, S. Z., Jafarabadi, M. A., Rezvani, H. R., & Afzali, M. (2015). Controlling type 2 diabetes mellitus with herbal medicines: A triple-blind randomized clinical trial of efficacy and safety. *Journal of Diabetes*, *8*(5), 647–656. doi:10.1111/1753-0407.12342 PMID:26362826

Mokdad, A. H., Bowman, B. A., Ford, E. S., Vinicor, F., Marks, J. S., & Koplan, J. P. (2001). The continuing epidemics of obesity and diabetes in the United States. *Journal of the American Medical Association*, *286*(10), 1195–1200. doi:10.1001/jama.286.10.1195 PMID:11559264

Nabilatul, H. M., Ismail, W. I. W., Zainah, A., Siti, S. J., & Aishah, A. (2013). Potential roles of *Stevia rebaudiana* Bertoni in arogating insulin resistance and diabetes: A review. *Evidence-Based Complementary and Alternative Medicine*, *2013*, 718049. PMID:24324517

Nagappa, A. N., Thakurdesai, P. A., Venkat Rao, N., & Singh, J. (2003). Antidiabetic activity of *Terminalia catappa* Linn fruits. *Journal of Ethnopharmacology*, *88*(1), 45–50. doi:10.1016/S0378-8741(03)00208-3 PMID:12902049

Nelson-Dooley, C., Della-Fera, M. A., Hamrick, M., & Baile, C. A. (2005). Novel treatments for obesity and osteoporosis: Targeting apoptotic pathways in adipocytes. *Current Medicinal Chemistry*, *12*(19), 2215–2225. doi:10.2174/0929867054864886 PMID:16178781

Neuhouser, M. L. (2004). Dietary flavonoids and cancer risk: Evidence from human population studies. *Nutrition and Cancer*, *50*(1), 1–7. doi:10.120715327914nc5001_1 PMID:15572291

Nirmala, P., & Ramanathan, M. (2011). Effect of kaempferol on lipid peroxidation and antioxidant status in 1,2-dimethyl hydrazine induced colorectal carcinoma in rats. *European Journal of Pharmacology*, *654*(1), 75–79. doi:10.1016/j.ejphar.2010.11.034 PMID:21172346

Ogden, C. L., Carroll, M. D., Curtin, L. R., McDowell, M. A., Tabak, C. J., & Flegal, K. M. (2006). Prevalence of overweight and obesity in the United States, 1999-2004. *Journal of the American Medical Association*, *295*(13), 1549–1555. doi:10.1001/jama.295.13.1549 PMID:16595758

Oh, S. D., Kim, M., Min, B. I., Choi, G. S., Kim, S. K., Bae, H., Kang, C., Kim, D. G., Park, B. J., & Kim, C. K. (2014). Effect of *Achyranthes bidentata* blume on 3T3-L1 adipogenesis and rats fed with a high-fat diet. *Evidence-Based Complementary and Alternative Medicine*, *2014*(158018), 1–8. PMID:24963319

Osada, K., Takahashi, M., Hoshina, S., Nakamura, M., Nakamura, S., & Sugano, M. (2001). Tea catechins inhibit cholesterol oxidation accompanying oxidation of low density lipoprotein *in vitro*. *Comparative Biochemistry and Physiology-Part C*, *128*(2), 153–164. doi:10.1016/S1532-0456(00)00192-7 PMID:11239828

Panda, S., & Kar, A. (2007). Apigenin (4¢,5,7-trihydroxyflavone) regulates hyperglycaemia, thyroid dysfunction and lipid peroxidation in alloxan-induced diabetic mice. *The Journal of Pharmacy and Pharmacology*, *59*(11), 1543–1548. doi:10.1211/jpp.59.11.0012 PMID:17976266

Papathanasopoulos, A., & Camilleri, M. (2010). Dietary fiber supplements: Effects in obesity and metabolic syndrome and relationship to gastrointestinal functions. *Gastroenterology*, *138*(1), 65–72. doi:10.1053/j.gastro.2009.11.045 PMID:19931537

Park, H. J., Cho, J.-Y., Kim, M. K., Koh, P.-O., Cho, K.-W., Kim, C. H., Lee, K.-S., Chung, B. Y., Kim, G.-S., & Cho, J.-H. (2012). Anti-obesity effect of *Schisandra chinensis* in 3T3-L1 cells and high fat diet-induced obese rats. *Food Chemistry*, *134*(1), 227–234. doi:10.1016/j.foodchem.2012.02.101 PMID:23265481

Park, H. Y., Kim, M., & Han, J. (2011). Stereospecific microbial production of isoflavanones from isoflavones and isoflavone glucosides. *Applied Microbiology and Biotechnology*, *91*(4), 1173–1181. doi:10.100700253-011-3310-7 PMID:21562980

Patel, D. K., Kumar, R., Laloo, D., & Hemalatha, S. (2012). Diabetes mellitus: An overview on its pharmacological aspects and reported medicinal plants having antidiabetic activity. *Asian Pacific Journal of Tropical Biomedicine*, *2*(5), 411–420. doi:10.1016/S2221-1691(12)60067-7 PMID:23569941

Pongchaidecha, A., Lailerd, N., Boonprasert, W., & Chattipakorn, N. (2009). Effects of curcuminoid supplement on cardiac autonomic status in high-fat-induced obese rats. *Nutrition (Burbank, Los Angeles County, Calif.)*, *25*(7-8), 870–878. doi:10.1016/j.nut.2009.02.001 PMID:19398300

Poudyala, H., Panchald, S. K., Waandersb, J., Wardc, L., & Browna, L. (2012). Lipid redistribution by α-linolenic acid-rich chia seed inhibits stearoyl-CoA desaturase-1 and induces cardiac and hepatic protection in diet-induced obese rats. *The Journal of Nutritional Biochemistry*, *23*(2), 153–162. doi:10.1016/j.jnutbio.2010.11.011 PMID:21429727

Prasad, S., Phromnoi, K., Yadav, V. R., Chaturvedi, M. M., & Aggarwal, B. B. (2010). Targeting inflammatory pathways by flavonoids for prevention and treatment of cancer. *Planta Medica*, *76*(11), 1044–1063. doi:10.1055-0030-1250111 PMID:20635307

Prasannaraja, C., Kamalanathan, A. S., Vijayalakshmi, M. A., & Venkataraman, K. A. (2020). A dipyrrole derivative from *Aloe vera* inhibits an anti-diabetic drug target dipeptidyl peptidase (DPP)-IV *in vitro*. *Preparative Biochemistry & Biotechnology*, *8*(5), 1–10. doi:10.1080/10826068.2019.1710712 PMID:31910723

Prince, P., & Kamalakkannan, N. (2006). Rutin improves glucose homeostasis in streptozotocin diabetic tissues by altering glycolytic and gluconeogenic enzymes. *Journal of Biochemical and Molecular Toxicology*, *20*(2), 96–102. doi:10.1002/jbt.20117 PMID:16615078

Puranik, N., Kammar, K. F., & Devi, S. (2010). Anti-diabetic activity of *Tinospora cordifolia* (Willd.) in streptozotocin diabetic rats; does it act like sulfonylureas? *Turkish Journal of Medical Sciences*, *40*(2), 265–270.

Ragavan, B., & Krishnakumari, S. (2006). Antidiabetic effect of *T. arjuna* bark extract in alloxan induced diabetic rats. *Indian Journal of Clinical Biochemistry*, *21*(2), 123–128. doi:10.1007/BF02912926 PMID:23105628

Rani, N., Sharma, S. K., & Vasudeva, N. (2012). Assessment of antiobesity potential of *Achyranthes aspera* Linn. seed. *Evidence-Based Complementary and Alternative Medicine*, *2012*(715912), 1–7. doi:10.1155/2012/715912 PMID:22919417

Ranjana, & Tripathi, Y.B. (2014). Insulin secreting and alpha-glucosidase inhibitory activity of hexane extract of *Annona squamosa* Linn. in streptozotocin (STZ) induced diabetic rats. *Indian Journal of Experimental Biology, 52*, 623-629.

Reyes-Escogido, M. L., Gonzalez-Mondragon, E. G., & Vazquez-Tzompantzi, E. (2011). Chemical and pharmacological aspects of capsaicin. *Molecules (Basel, Switzerland)*, *16*(2), 1253–1270. doi:10.3390/molecules16021253 PMID:21278678

Rideout, T. C., Harding, S. V., & Jones, P. J. H. (2010). Consumption of plant sterols reduces plasma and hepatic triglycerides and modulates the expression of lipid regulatory genes and de novo lipogenesis in C57BL/6J mice. *Molecular Nutrition & Food Research*, *54*(S1), S7–S13. doi:10.1002/mnfr.201000027 PMID:20333723

Saminathan, M., Rai, R. B., Dhama, K., Tiwari, R., & Chakraborty, S. (2013). Systematic review on anticancer potential and other health beneficial pharmacological activities of novel medicinal plant *Morinda citrifolia* (Noni). *International Journal of Pharmacology*, *9*(8), 462–492. doi:10.3923/ijp.2013.462.492

Sandborn, W. J., & Faubion, W. A. (2000). Clinical pharmacology of inflammatory bowel disease therapies. *Current Gastroenterology Reports*, *2*(6), 440–445. doi:10.100711894-000-0005-0 PMID:11079044

Sanni, O., Erukainure, O. L., Chukwuma, C. I., Koorbanally, N. A., Ibeji, C. U., & Islam, M. S. (2019). *Azadirachta indica* inhibits key enzyme linked to type 2 diabetes *in vitro*, abates oxidative hepatic injury and enhances muscle glucose uptake *ex vivo*. *Biomedicine and Pharmacotherapy*, *109*, 734–743. doi:10.1016/j.biopha.2018.10.171 PMID:30551526

Sartippour, M. R., Shao, Z. M., Heber, D., Beatty, P., Zhang, L., Liu, C., Ellis, L., Liu, W., Go, V. L., & Brooks, M. N. (2002). Green tea inhibits vascular endothelial growth factor (VEGF) induction in human breast cancer cells. *The Journal of Nutrition*, *132*(8), 2307–2311. doi:10.1093/jn/132.8.2307 PMID:12163680

Schonfeld, G. (2010). Plant sterols in atherosclerosis prevention. *The American Journal of Clinical Nutrition*, *92*(1), 3–4. doi:10.3945/ajcn.2010.29828 PMID:20519556

Schuster, R., Holzer, W., Doerfler, H., Weckwerth, W., Viernstein, H., Okonogi, S., & Mueller, M. (2016). *Cajanus cajan* - A source of PPARγ activators leading to anti-inflammatory and cytotoxic effects. *Food & Function*, *7*(9), 3798–3806. doi:10.1039/C6FO00689B PMID:27603115

Semwal, B., Shah, K., Chauhan, N., Badhe, R., & Divakar, K. (2008). Anti-diabetic activity of stem bark of *Berberis aristata* D.C. in alloxan induced diabetic rats. *International Journal of Pharmacology*, *6*(1), 1–8.

Semwal, B. C., Gupta, J., Singh, S., Kumar, Y., & Giri, M. (2009). Antihyperglycemic activity of root of *Berberis aristata* DC in alloxan-induced diabetic rats. *International Journal of Green Pharmacy*, *3*(3), 259–262. doi:10.4103/0973-8258.56288

Sharma, N. K., Ahirwar, D., Jhade, D., & Jain, V. K. (2012). *In-vitro* anti-obesity assay of alcoholic and aqueous extracts of *Camellia sinensis* leaves. *International Journal of Pharmaceutical Sciences and Research*, *3*(1), 863–1866.

Shi, Y., & Hu, F. B. (2014). The global implications of diabetes and cancer. *Lancet*, *383*(9933), 1947–1948. doi:10.1016/S0140-6736(14)60886-2 PMID:24910221

Slavin, J. L. (2005). Dietary fiber and body weight. *Nutrition (Burbank, Los Angeles County, Calif.)*, *21*(3), 411–418. doi:10.1016/j.nut.2004.08.018 PMID:15797686

Son, M. J., Rico, C. W., Nam, S. H., & Kang, M. Y. (2010). Influence of oryzanol and ferulic acid on the lipid metabolism and antioxidative status in high fat-fed mice. *Journal of Clinical Biochemistry and Nutrition*, *46*(2), 150–156. doi:10.3164/jcbn.09-98 PMID:20216948

Song, M. Y., Lv, N., Kim, E. K., Kwon, K. S., Yoo, Y. B., Kim, J. H., Lee, S. W., Song, J. H., Lee, J. H., Lee, S. K., Shin, B. C., Ryu, D. G., Park, B. H., & Kwon, K. B. (2009). Antiobesity activity of aqueous extracts of rhizoma *Dioscoreae tokoronis* on high-fat diet-induced obesity in mice. *Journal of Medicinal Food*, *12*(2), 304–309. doi:10.1089/jmf.2008.1010 PMID:19459730

Suanarunsawat, T., Anantasomboon, G., & Piewbang, C. (2016). Anti-diabetic and anti-oxidative activity of fixed oil extracted from *Ocimum sanctum* L. leaves in diabetic rats. *Experimental and Therapeutic Medicine*, *11*(3), 832–840. doi:10.3892/etm.2016.2991 PMID:26998000

Suneetha, D. S., Divya, T. B., & Ali, F. (2013). Antiobesity values of methanolic extract of *Sapindus emariganatus* on monosodium glutamate induced model in rats. *International Journal of Pharmacognosy and Phytochemical Research*, *5*(4), 267–270.

Szkudelska, K., Nogowski, L., & Szkudelski, T. (2000). Genistein affects lipogenesis and lipolysis in isolated rat adipocytes. *The Journal of Steroid Biochemistry and Molecular Biology*, *75*(4-5), 265–271. doi:10.1016/S0960-0760(00)00172-2 PMID:11282281

Szkudelska, K., Szkudelski, T., & Nogowski, L. (2002). Daidzein, coumestrol and zearalenone affect lipogenesis and lipolysis in rat adipocytes. *Phytomedicine*, *9*(4), 338–345. doi:10.1078/0944-7113-00148 PMID:12120815

Takikawa, M., Inoue, S., Horio, F., & Tsuda, T. (2010). Dietary anthocyanin-rich bilberry extract ameliorates hyperglycemia and insulin sensitivity via activation of AMP-activated protein kinase in diabetic mice. *The Journal of Nutrition*, *140*(3), 527–533. doi:10.3945/jn.109.118216 PMID:20089785

Tang, D., Liu, L., Ajiakber, D., Ye, J., Xu, J., Xin, X., & Aisa, H. A. (2018). Anti-diabetic effect of *Punica granatum* flower polyphenols extract in type 2 diabetic rats: Activation of Akt/GSK-3β and inhibition of IRE1α-XBP1 pathways. *Frontiers in Endocrinology*, *9*(586), 1–11. doi:10.3389/fendo.2018.00586

Tapas, P., Suraj, V., & Dr.Deepak, D. (2017). A herbal approach to obesity management: A review. *Asian Journal of Pharmaceutical Education and Research*, *6*(3), 1–15.

Thirumalai, T., Therasa, S. V., Elumalai, E. K., & David, E. (2011). Hypoglycemic effect of *Brassica juncea* (seeds) on streptozotocin induced diabetic male albino rat. *Asian Pacific Journal of Tropical Biomedicine, 1*(4), 323–325. doi:10.1016/S2221-1691(11)60052-X PMID:23569784

Trigueros, L., Peña, S., Ugidos, A., Sayas-Barberá, E., Pérez-Álvarez, J., & Sendra, E. (2013). Food ingredients as anti-obesity agents: A review. *Critical Reviews in Food Science and Nutrition, 53*(9), 929–942. doi:10.1080/10408398.2011.574215 PMID:23768185

Tsuda, T., Ueno, Y., Aoki, H., Koda, T., Horio, F., Takahashi, N., Kawada, T., & Osawa, T. (2004). Anthocyanin enhances adipocytokine secretion and adipocyte-specific gene expression in isolated rat adipocytes. *Biochemical and Biophysical Research Communications, 316*(1), 149–157. doi:10.1016/j.bbrc.2004.02.031 PMID:15003523

Tucci, S. A. (2010). Phytochemicals in the control of human appetite and body weight. *Pharmaceuticals, 3*(3), 748–763. doi:10.3390/ph3030748 PMID:27713277

Tzeng, T. F., Liou, S. S., & Liu, I. M. (2011). Myricetin ameliorates defective post-receptor insulin signaling via beta-endorphin signaling in the skeletal muscles of fructose-fed rats. *Evidence-Based Complementary and Alternative Medicine, 2011*(150752), 1–19. doi:10.1093/ecam/neq017 PMID:21785619

Uemura, T., Goto, T., Kang, M. S., Mizoguchi, N., Hirai, S., Lee, J. Y., Nakano, Y., Shono, J., Hoshino, S., Taketani, K., Tsuge, N., Narukami, T., Makishima, M., Takahashi, N., & Kawada, T. (2011). Diosgenin, the main aglycon of fenugreek, inhibits LXRα activity in HepG2 cells and decreases plasma and hepatic triglycerides in obese diabetic mice. *The Journal of Nutrition, 141*(1), 17–23. doi:10.3945/jn.110.125591 PMID:21106928

Ulrich, K. (2011). Dietary Proteins in Obesity and in Diabetes. *Int. J. Vitam. Nutr. Res., 81*(2 – 3), 125 – 133.

Van der Klaauw, A., Keogh, J., Henning, E., Trowse, V., Dhillo, W., Ghatei, M., & Farooqi, I. S. (2013). High protein intake stimulates postprandial GLP1 and PYY release. *Obesity (Silver Spring, Md.), 2013*(21), 1602–1607. doi:10.1002/oby.20154 PMID:23666746

Vilhena, R. O., Figueiredo, I. D., Baviera, A. M., Silva, D. B., Marson, B. M., Oliveira, J. A., Peccinini, R. G., Borges, I. K., & Pontarolo, R. (2020). Antidiabetic activity of *Musa x paradisiaca* extracts in streptozotocin-induced diabetic rats and chemical characterization by HPLC-DAD-MS. *Journal of Ethnopharmacology, 254*, 112666. doi:10.1016/j.jep.2020.112666 PMID:32084552

Vivekananthan, D. P., Penn, M. S., Sapp, S. K., Hsu, A., & Topol, E. J. (2003). Use of antioxidant vitamins for the prevention of cardiovascular disease: Meta-analysis of randomized trials. *Lancet, 361*(9374), 2017–2023. doi:10.1016/S0140-6736(03)13637-9 PMID:12814711

Wang, T., Choi, R. C., Li, J., Li, J., Bi, C. W., Zang, L., Liu, Z., Dong, T. T., Bi, K., & Tsim, K. W. (2010). Antihyperlipidemic effect of protodioscin, an active ingredient isolated from the rhizomes of Dioscorea nipponica. *Planta Medica, 76*(15), 1642–1646. doi:10.1055-0030-1249960 PMID:20509104

Weisberg, S. P., McCann, D., Desai, M., Rosenbaum, M., Leibel, R. L., & Ferrante, A. W. Jr. (2003). Obesity is associated with macrophage accumulation in adipose tissue. *The Journal of Clinical Investigation, 112*(12), 1796–1808. doi:10.1172/JCI200319246 PMID:14679176

WHO. (2014). *About Diabetes*. World Health Organization.

Wolfram, S. (2007). Effects of green tea and EGCG on cardiovascular and metabolic health. *Journal of the American College of Nutrition, 26*(4), 373S–388S. doi:10.1080/07315724.2007.10719626 PMID:17906191

Xie, B., Waters, M. J., & Schirra, H. J. (2012). Investigating potential mechanisms of obesity by metabolomics. *BioMed Research International, 2012*(805683), 1–10. PMID:22665992

Xu, H. Y., Barnes, G. T., Yang, Q., Tan, Q., Yang, D. S., Chou, C. J., Sole, J., Nichols, A., Ross, J. S., Tartaglia, L. A., & Chen, H. (2003). Chronic inflammation in fat plays a crucial role in the development of obesity-related insulin resistance. *The Journal of Clinical Investigation, 112*(12), 1821–1830. doi:10.1172/JCI200319451 PMID:14679177

Yamamoto, Y., & Oue, E. (2006). Antihypertensive effect of quercetin in rats fed with a high-fat high-sucrose diet. *Bioscience, Biotechnology, and Biochemistry, 70*(4), 933–939. doi:10.1271/bbb.70.933 PMID:16636461

Yang, C. S., Chen, L., Lee, M. J., Balentine, D., Kuo, M. C., & Schantz, S. P. (1998). Blood and urine levels of tea catechins after ingestion of different amounts of green tea by human volunteers. *Cancer Epidemiology, Biomarkers & Prevention, 7*(4), 351–354. PMID:9568793

Yang, J. Y., Della-Fera, M. A., Nelson-Dooley, C., & Baile, C. A. (2006). Molecular mechanisms of apoptosis induced by ajoene in 3T3-L1 adipocytes. *Obesity (Silver Spring, Md.), 14*(3), 388–397. doi:10.1038/oby.2006.52 PMID:16648609

Yokozawa, T., Kim, H. Y., Cho, E. J., Choi, J. S., & Chung, H. Y. (2002). Antioxidant effects of isorhamnetin 3,7-di-O-β-d-glucopyranoside isolated from mustard leaf (*Brassica juncea*) in rats with streptozotocin-induced diabetes. *Journal of Agricultural and Food Chemistry, 50*(19), 5490–5495. doi:10.1021/jf0202133 PMID:12207497

Yu, R., Kim, C. S., Kwon, B. S., & Kawada, T. (2006). Mesenteric adipose tissue-derived monocyte chemoattractant protein-1 plays a crucial role in adipose tissue macrophage migration and activation in obese mice. *Obesity (Silver Spring, Md.), 14*(8), 1353–1362. doi:10.1038/oby.2006.153 PMID:16988077

Zang, M., Xu, S., Maitland-Toolan, K. A., Zuccollo, A., Hou, X., Jiang, B., Wierzbicki, M., Verbeuren, T. J., & Cohen, R. A. (2006). Polyphenols stimulate amp-activated protein kinase, lower lipids, and inhibit accelerated atherosclerosis in diabetic ldl receptor-deficient mice. *Diabetes, 55*(8), 2180–2191. doi:10.2337/db05-1188 PMID:16873680

Zemel, M. B. (2005). The role of dairy foods in weight management. *Journal of the American College of Nutrition, 24*(6), 537S–546S. doi:10.1080/07315724.2005.10719502 PMID:16373953

Zheng, G., Sayama, K., Okubo, T., Juneja, L. R., & Oguni, I. (2004). Anti-obesity effects of three major components of green tea, catechins, caffeine and theanine, in mice. *In Vivo (Athens, Greece)*, *18*(1), 55–62. PMID:15011752

Zygmunt, K., Faubert, B., MacNeil, J., & Tsiani, E. (2010). Naringenin, a citrus flavonoid, increases muscle cell glucose uptake via AMPK. *Biochemical and Biophysical Research Communications*, *398*(2), 178–183. doi:10.1016/j.bbrc.2010.06.048 PMID:20558145

LIST OF ABBREVIATIONS

MCP-1 monocyte-chemo-attractant protein-1
TNF-α tumor necrosis factor-alpha
IL interleukins
PPAR γ peroxisome proliferator-associated receptor γ
GLUT4 glucose transport type 4
LPL plasma lipoprotein lipase
PLIN lipid droplet-associated protein perilipin
FFA free fatty acid
IRS insulin Receptor Substrates
PI3K phosphoinositide-3-kinase
AKT protein kinase B,
JNK c-Jun N-terminal kinase
STZ streptozotocin-induced
cAMP-specific PDE 3 ¢,5¢-cyclic-AMP phosphodiesterase
AMPK AMP-activated kinase
ECG epicatechingallate
EGC epigallocatechin
EGCG epigallocatechin gallate
ROS reactive oxygen species
NF-κB nuclear factor kappa-light-chain-enhancer of activated B cells
HFD high fat diet
HDL-C high-density lipoprotein cholesterol
SREBP-1 sterol regulatory element binding proteins
LDH lactate dehydrogenase
VLDL very-low density lipoproteins
T2DM Type 2 diabetes mellitus
DDP-4 dipeptidyl-peptidase 4
pAKT phosphorylated Protein kinase B
HbA1c gylcated hemoglobin A1c
GLP-1 glucagon-like peptide-1
GIP glucose dependent insulinotrophic polypeptide

Chapter 5
The Mechanistic Approach to Tackle Obesity Using Traditional Herbal Plants

Saniyah Saleem Khan
Zayed University, UAE

ABSTRACT

Obesity is a medical metabolic condition where a person accumulates excess body fat that might affect their health. Obesity is a prevalent global health problem linked with other life-threatening chronic diseases like cardiovascular, certain types of cancer, diabetes, renal, cerebrovascular, bone, and muscle-related diseases. According to the World Health Organization (WHO), obesity is the fifth foremost cause of global deaths. Many allopathic drugs and surgical treatments for managing obesity are available in the market. However, these conventional methods have adverse side effects and chances of recurrence. For more than 2,000 years, herbal medicines have been used for the treatment of many diseases efficiently. This chapter addresses the current progress in the effectiveness of several herbal medications used for the treatment of obesity without causing side effects. The possible effects and mechanisms of using these herbaceous plants in the treatment of obese and overweight humans and animals are covered extensively.

INTRODUCTION

The obese and overweight population is growing around the world. It is affecting people of all age groups and sex. Obesity leads to many chronic diseases, which is rising morbidity and mortality all across the globe. The increase in fat accumulation can be because of more fat absorption, increased lipogenesis, reduced lipolysis, or any combination of these three processes. The primary treatment for overweight and obese people is increasing exercise and decreasing the number of calories per meal. But this method is very time consuming and challenging to adhere mostly for unmotivated individuals. Hence, numerous methods for eliminating obesity are being used all over the world. Several medicines are being produced, and many are still undergoing research. These medicines are worked on, keeping four main actions of energy balance in mind, including appetite suppressants, fat absorption (i.e., Orlistat), stimulators of

DOI: 10.4018/978-1-7998-4808-0.ch005

thermogenesis, and fat mobilization stimulators. Some of these are allopathic medications (Padwal and Majumdur 2007), different types of aesthetic surgeries (Fried et al. 2007), and various kinds of nutrient specific diets (Yannakoulia, Poulimeneas, Mamalaki & Anastasiou 2019) which are used to cure obesity. But most of the synthetic medicines used for treating obesity have several adverse side effects (Al-Tahami et al. 2017). Quite the same happens with the surgeries where weight maintenance becomes a problem, especially after surgeries like liposuction (Liposuction - Mayo Clinic, 2020). Other bariatric surgeries have strict restrictions on several types of food, deficiencies of vitamins and minerals, and scars as a conscience of operation (Fried et al. 2007). Due to problems in pharmacotherapy and years of significant concern with the modern medicinal system and also difficulties in sustaining lifestyle modification, additional attention has been paid to herbal medicine as a practical, healthy and inexpensive alternative for reducing body weight and body fat (Ranjbar, Jouyandeh, Abdollahi and Systematic 2013). Isolated compounds extracted from herbal plants and their parts (Karri et al. 2019) have become popular as the raw material for the production of obesity treatments (Amin and Nagy 2009).

Although numerous research have been conducted worldwide to study the treatment and management of obesity, it remains a challenging issue (Cheng, 2006). This chapter focusses on prevalence, influencing factors, cause, risk, and treatments of obesity. Different strategies to tackle the epidemics of obesity will include non-medical and medical approaches. Positive and negative effects of using the allopathic and in-depth study of efficacy, safety, effectiveness, and potential mechanism of herbal medicine are discussed in this chapter.

OBESITY

WHO measures obesity by using the Body mass index(BMI) scale. An individual with BMI between 25-29.9 is scaled to be overweight and equal to or above 30 is considered obese. This index is for both male and female adults (Obesity and overweight, 2020). Obesity can be characterized as excessive increased adipose tissue to the extent that it can cause adverse health effects in the human body.

The leading cause of obesity is an imbalance in energy between calories consumed (Verma, 2014) and burned. This imbalance can be due to many factors, including inherited gene, hormonal imbalance, side effects of medicines taken for some other diseases, etc. as suggested by the authors Darbre (2017), Verhaegen (2017).

According to WHO, obesity is related to cardiovascular diseases, hypertension, diabetes mellitus, gallbladder disease, cancer, endocrine and metabolic disturbances, osteoarthritis, Gout, pulmonary diseases, as well as psychological issues, including social bias, prejudice, discrimination, and overeating (Obesity and overweight, 2020). Obesity is now one of the most prevalent health problems in all populations and age groups globally, resulting in substantial mortality and morbidity increases (Fleming and Robinson, 2013).

Researcher like Harvey & Ogden (2014) claim that in reducing obesity, at least about 5% or more weight loss should be viewed as a healing agent. Studies have shown that weight loss of 5% to 10% can make people vulnerable to some diseases such as type 2 diabetes mellitus, cardiovascular disorders can minimize and reduce other complications linked to obesity (Harvey and Ogden 2014).

Obesity can be caused by the following factors and can have many health risks, as summarized in Figure.1. Furthermore, the prevalence of obesity and its treatment and their limitations are also discussed in this chapter.

1. Factors causing obesity:

a) Energy intake and expenditure

An average person generally has an energy expenditure of 10–15 M.J./day or 3650–5475 MJ/ year. A weight change of 1 kg, equals to 30 M.J., suggests an annual discrepancy of around 0.6–0.8% between intake and expenditure. The energy consumption corresponds closely to the weekly energy expenditure (Leibel, Rosenbaum, & Hirsch 1995). Amongst the three elements of energy expenditure - 50–70% of the total energy consumption is dedicated to the size and composition of the body, which decide the basic metabolic rate (BMR) of the body. The second component is body movement or physical activity, which is the most variable part of the overall daily energy expenditure. The third part, diet-induced energy expenditure, is generally assumed to account for 10% of total daily energy expenditure in subjects who eat the average mixed diet and have an energy balance (Westerterp, 2004).

i. Basic metabolic rate (BMR)

It can be considered the sum of the energy expenditure of tissues and organs in fasting and resting-state and **neutral temperature** (26.2 °C). It depends on the mass and metabolic rate of tissues and organs. Organs like the liver, brain, heart, kidney, and digestive tract account for only around 7% of body weight, but they contribute approximately 60% of BMR. In comparison, skeletal and adipose tissues account for 35–40% of body weight but only 18–22% and 3–4% of BMR. Generally, BMR depends on body composition expressed by fat-free mass (FFM) and fat mass (F.M.) and on gender, age, physical activity, and nutritional status. The primary determinant of BMR is FFM in normal people, whereas F.M. is significant only in obese subjects .M..M.(Lazzer, S., Bedogni, G., Lafortuna, C. L., Marazzi, N., Busti, C., Galli, R., ... & Sartorio, A. 2010).

ii. Physical activity and Sedentary lifestyle

A considerable amount of the population worldwide is less physically active. Around 60% of the total population lacks in operation due to increased use of motorized transportation and unprecedented work-saving predominance at home (Abramof and Apovia 2006). Active people use more calories than sedentary people in their daily routines. Being physically active manages weight by decreasing BMI.

iii. Diet

Obesity can mainly be influenced by the kind of food eaten (i.e., high sugar and fat-containing food). The defective management mechanism of calories contributes to Obesity. Proper management of macronutrients is presented in table 1. Several routes that trigger obesity are habitual diet and changes in lifestyle (Blundell and Cooling 2000).

Controlling appetite sometimes improves the nourishment of the body. After any meal, the following hormones are released from the small intestine and pancreas, which help manage food and hence control of obesity.

- Cholecystokinin (CCK) - facilitating digestion, stimulation of gallbladder contraction and pancreatic and gastric acid secretion, slowing of gastric emptying, and suppression of energy intake (Little, Horowitz and Feinle 2005).
- Bombesin - stimulates the release of gastrin and pancreatic enzymes and causes contraction of the gallbladder.
- Enterostatin - restricts fat intake by preventing the overconsumption of fat (Berger, Winzell, Mei, and Erlanson, 2004).
- Somatostatin - suppressing beta-cell insulin secretion (Tzotzas, Papazisis, Perros, and Krassas, 2008).
- Glucagon and glucagon-like peptide-1 (GLP-1) are evolutionarily related to anorectic hormones. Glucagon also increases energy expenditure (Parker *et al.* 2013).

b) Genetics

Genes run in families causing the transfer of etiological traits from parents to their children and their grandchildren, and their cousins. In humans, around 250 genetic variants are found in connection with obesity. Research shows that genetic influences can be linked to 40% out of 80% of the BMI variation. It is estimated that for factors related to the energy balance such as body fat distribution, resting metabolic rate, energy consumption after overeating, heritability is as high as 30 to 40%. Gene plays a crucial role in the development of obesity in an individual at any stage of his life. Genetic and environmental factors influence the expression of these genes. Consideration of genetic causes and epigenetic changes affecting the emerging epidemic of obesity provide the clinician with useful resources for tackling the abundance of obesity (Thaker, 2017). More than 50 genes and their variants are said to be associated with obesity. Obesity is usually multifactorial, which is a result of interactions among these genes and environmental factors.

c) Medical and Psychiatric illness

Drugs of Certain physical and restorative sicknesses like antidepressants, anticonvulsants, antipsychotics, medicines for diabetes, hormones, and most corticosteroids can have side effects of increasing weight (Mizutani, Suzuki, Kondo and Yamagata, 2007). These medications lead to a lazy lifestyle or stimulate appetite to increase hunger leading to increased intake of calories, resulting in weight gain. Some antidepressants may make people want high-energy or sucrose rich foods. Patients suffering from mental health problems are two to three times more likely than the general population to experience obesity. An analysis of the therapeutic impact of medication on weight shows that ~70 percent of patients may experience some weight gain during the course of treatment (Serretti and Mandelli 2010). Weight gain of a few kilograms to an increase of 10% or more of initial body weight has been described (Verhaegen and Gaal 2017).

d) Age and gender

Obesity can also be observed in young children of any age. But hormonal shifts and a less healthy lifestyle are increasing the possibility of obesity as we age. Moreover, our body'" s muscle mass also decreases with age causing metabolism to diminish. These improvements often minimize energy needs and can make it more challenging to hold the extra weight off.

Overall, obesity is found more prevalent in women than in men. These gender disparities in overweight and obesity are exacerbated among women in developing countries. However, in developed countries, more men are observed to be overweight than women. (Kanter, R., & Caballero, B. 2012).

e) Social and environmental influence

The prevalence of obesity is substantially linked to age, racial, ethnic origin, and socioeconomic status, generating dynamic associations between each of these characteristics. Food availability is a significant factor related to obesity that connects with discrepancies in prevalence seen across geographic areas and higher obesity levels among individuals with low socioeconomic status. Easy availability of high calorie, energy-dense affordable food choices that are more accessible in conjunction with reductions in physical activity related to work and transportation has also led to a sustained positive energy balance. Furthermore, conditions experiencing poverty, depression, or high crime are seen to be associated with higher probabilities of obesity, which may occur more frequently in individuals with low social status. Both objective and subjective social status and inequality factors are correlated with increased energy consumption and reduced energy expenditure, which may place individuals with low social status at higher risk of developing obesity (Brehm and Alessio, 2014).

f) Cultural factor

Cultural susceptibility to obesity is usually found in the countries with an emerging economy, which tends to introduce more variety and availability of food and a relaxing lifestyle. In some cultures, a bigger body shape/size is considered perfect. Cultural faith about food, its ethnicity, the components of the food, way of cooking, consumption amount etc. all these factors lead to cultural predispositions to obesity. Cross-cultural comparison can help to explain the prevalence of obesity in some modern affluent societies (Brown, 1991).

g) Inadequate sleep

Short-term or sleep suppression is related to impaired glucose metabolism, appetite dysregulation, and elevated blood pressure. Observational studies have reported associations between short sleep periods (usually less than six h/night) and increased BMI or Obesity, diabetes, and hypertension prevalence. A few retrospective studies showed a substantially increased risk of weight gain, diabetes, and hypertension incident correlated with inadequate sleep (Knutson, 2012).

h) Endocrine disruptors

Endocrine-disrupting chemicals, known as "obesogens", can contribute to adipogenesis and weight gain. The human population is exposed to these compounds in everyday life. These compounds are found in pesticides/herbicides, industrial and household goods, plastics, detergents, flame retardants, and as ingredients in personal care items (Darbre, 2017).

2. Risk factors of obesity:

People with Obesity have high rates of getting many chronic medical conditions as follows.

i. Type 2 diabetes

In type 2 diabetes, blood sugar levels increase because body cells start resisting insulin produced by the pancreas. It is a genetic disorder involving a sedentary lifestyle, bad daily eating habits, and heavy Bodyweight. n the United States, it is increasingly common among Blacks, Latinos, and American Indians compared with whites (Nelson and Papakostas 2009).

ii. High blood cholesterol

Obesity inhibits the response of the body to change the type of fat that you eat. This tends to increase the level of triglycerides, low-density lipoprotein (LDL), and decreases high-density lipoprotein (HDL) levels.. This can further lead to risks of cardiovascular disease, hypertension, diabetes, and other metabolic disorders. (*Cholesterol Test* - Mayo Clinic, 2020).

iii. Hypertension

Obesity is a significant risk for arterial hypertension and other morbidities that develops kidney disease since this primarily increases tubular reabsorption to inhibit the natriuresis pressure, renin-angiotensin framework, and mismanages sodium maintenance. (Blood pressure test - Mayo Clinic, 2020).

iv. Cardiovascular disease

Obesity leads to atherosclerosis and Coronary Heart Disease (CHD)(Lavle, Milani, and Cardiac, 2005) and stroke (Poirier et al., 2006). Obesity leads to an increase in hypertension, increases triglycerides, LDL cholesterol. Untreated hypertension and hypercholesterolemia increase the chances of atherosclerosis, which may leads to a heart attack or stroke in some cases. For every 1 unit increase in BMI (»7 pounds for a human of average height), the risk for ischemic stroke increases »5%, and the risk seems to be nearly linear starting with a still-normal BMI of »20 kg/m2. (Kernan, Inzucchi, Sawan, Macko and Furie, 2013). obesity is more likely predicted to get a stroke (Hu et al. 2007).

v. Gout

In Gout, uric acid accumulates in the blood and form Urate crystals, which amasses in the joints causing inflammation and severe pain. Gout is commonly seen in overweight people; sudden increases in weight can cause a gout attack (Richette and Bardin 2010)

vi. Sleep apnea

An overweight person may have fat accumulated around his / her neck. This can make the path to aviation narrower, leading to noisy breathing or even stop breathing for a short time frame causing sleepless nights (Trollo and Rogers,1996).

vii. Complication in pregnancy

An overweight, and obese pregnant lady raises the possibility of medical issues for both mom and child (Haslam and James, 2005). Pregnant ladies who are overweight may have more risk for the following.

- Needing a C-section and, consequently, taking more time to recover from it.
- Having preeclampsia (hypertension during pregnancy that can cause severe issues for both mother and child if left untreated)
- Developing gestational diabetes (high glucose during pregnancy)

(Ravi and Krishnamurthy, 2019)

3. Prevalence of Obesity

Obesity has increased spectacularly worldwide (almost tripled) between the years 1975 and 2014. Globally, 13% of adults (18 years and older) were obese in 2016. There were over 1.9 billion adults, and over 650 million were obese. That means 39% of adults were overweight in the entire population, and 13% were obese. And about 340 million children and adolescents 5-19 years of age are overweight or obese. Roughly 40 million children (under five years) were overweight or obese in 2018 (Obesity and overweight, 2020).

As shown in (figure 2) data collected by the World Health Organization (WHO) until 2016, the small Pacific Island states, despite their income level, they have very high obesity rates – 61% in Nauru and 55% in Palau. On the other hand, Japan, South Korea, and Singapore show deficient levels of Obesity, although they are high-income countries.

As the Consequence of fast industrialization and urbanization, prompting ascend in expectations for everyday comforts, the prevalence of obesity is quickly rising. More than one in three adults (36%) in the U.S. were found to be obese. This share was about ten times lower in India (3.9%). But obesity has increased in India in the 21st century, now affecting 5% of the 'nation's population. (Ravi, and Krishnamurthy, 2019).

Genetic, epigenetic, metabolic, behavioral, and environmental variables are the etiological risk factors that account for obesity. The significant rise in obesity is one of the most preventable risk factors for morbidity and mortality. (Valizadeh, Ghalichi, and Ostadrahimi, 2016).

4. Treatment of Obesity

Obesity prevention has great meaning. Prevention of Obesity will start at the youth. Adolescence and pre-adult obesity give the weight of adulthood a back story. This will inform school, family, and community about well-adjusted sustenance and physical action. The treatment of Obesity is critical, long, and unceasing, in which the patient should be included in a viable and determined manner. Numerous essential ethological distinguishing elements make obesity avoidance and care highly tricky and confusing. To treatment obesity, individuals should focus on a realistic weight loss, decrease the risk of associated grimness and mortality, give people a good tendency to eat routine, and improve personal satisfaction. Indeed, even a 10% reduction in weight in a half-year can forestall much of the medical problem that Obesity has brought about (World Health Organization. Obesity, 2000).

a) Nutrition and Dietary approaches:

Clinical Nutrition (Diet) Therapy plays a significant part in treating obesity. The nutritional recommendations shown in table 2 are advised with medical nutrition (Diet) treatment. Everyday energy intake should be reduced to ensure 0.5-1.0 kg/1 to 2 pounds weight reduction per week. Shedding weight should be done gradually. But enough energy should be available to keep up the excellent metabolism rate of the body (Makris, & Foster, 2011). Three thousand five hundred calories make up to 1 pound, and 7,700 calories make up to 1 kilogram of fat. It is estimated that by burning 3,500 calories, 1 pound can be lost, or by burning 7,700 calories in one kilogram can be lost. Therefore, in general, 1 -2 pounds can be lost in a week if 500 -1,000 calories per day is reduced from a typical diet (The best ways to cut calories from your diet, 2020). As compared with healthy weight people, obese individuals have higher energy expenditure as they have a large body and higher resting metabolic rates. As demonstrated by Leibel et al. (1995), a 10% gain in weight may increases daily energy consumption from 370 to 530 kcal. This implies that the amount of energy consumed is proportional to body metabolism.

When fat consumption is increased, it is correlated with higher calorie consumption leading to weight gain, but this is mainly related to changes in food energy density and not to caloric fat intake. Given that a 'macronutrient's dietary contribution is declining, it is essential by what it is being substituted because increasing transition can lead to different metabolic effects and nutritional deficiencies. Dietary approaches can lead to a substantial loss of weight if energy is restricted. Some of the universal deity plans. Low-Fat diet, Low carbohydrate diets, Keto diet, High protein diets, and more are outlined in table 4 (Yannakoulia et al. 2019).

b) Physical exercise

It is a fact that obesity is an epidemic on the planet and continuing to rise. A significant way to manage this situation is to indulge individuals in regular physical activity. Exercising helps in the prevention of weight- and obesity-related medical problems. Efficient physical activity plays an essential role in balancing body energy levels and decreasing the risk of obesity and its consequences (Jakicic & Otto 2005).

World Health Organization and The United States Department of Health and Human Services recommend that every adult should be indulged in physical activity for at least two and a half hours of moderate to intense workout per week for good health (Health.gov. 2011; WHO | Global recommendations on physical activity for health, 2020). And children should spend even more time, at least one hour every day. Physical exercise appears to be an essential part of the weight loss and maintenance of lifestyle strategies. While the effects of physical exercise on weight loss may seem small, a dose-response relationship between physical activity and weight loss does exist. Physical exercise also tends to be a significantly necessary action to support weight loss in the long term and weight regains prevention. The benefits of physical activity can be observed in obese patients (BMI ³ 35 kg/m^2) lose weight and in individuals who have undergone bariatric or plastic surgery to maintain weight.

c) Medicinal Treatment

The medications used in treating obesity are appropriate for low and moderate weight individuals. It is crucial for the medicines used to have a safe decision in terms of well-being, to show an effect that is ideally suited to weight etiology is to have no noticeable impact in the short and long time and to have no fixation. These kinds of drugs should be used only with the recommendation and under the guidance of the medical expert (Snow et al., .2005).

Some of the medicines used in the treatment of obesity are Sibutramine, Orlistat, Rimonabant, and Pramlintide, etc. on the one hand, these medicines have presented a great success rate, but on the other hand, they have also shown to have many acute and chronic side effects. Some of the medicines are even banned in many countries because of the type of side effects they have on the patient. (Hollander et al. 2004; Akbas, Gasteyger, Sjodin, Astrup, and Larsen 2009; Tahami et al. 2017)

d) Surgical Treatment

Surgical approach to Obesity is differentiated into two options. The bariatric medical technique is used to decrease food admission vitality and gastrointestinal assimilation of foods. This type of surgery is only done on patients aged 18-60 years with BMI ³40 kg/m^2. Exceptions are made for patients (BMI 35-40 kg/m^2) with metabolic disorders, cardio-respiratory disease, severe joint disease. One option of surgery is the Bariatric medical method includes strategies such as bypass, gastrectomy, gastric banding, and biliopancreatic diversion (Fried et al. 2007) are outlined in table 5. The second option proposed a reconstructive medical procedure (table 6) where the present fat tissue is removed, confining in different body parts. Some of the body parts where aesthetic surgery is performed include the abdomen, face, breast, etc. (Gupta et al. 2016).

e) Herbal management for Obesity

Multiple treatments are used for treating obesity. Nature is the most valuable source leading to novel drugs to combat various pharmacological diseases. Treatment using herbal medicine is evolving immensely. Medicines from herbs are proved to provide more phytochemicals, antioxidants, nutrition, and multitargeting actions. They effectively treat cardiovascular disease, decreased risk of cancer, diabetes, along with obesity.

Obesity can be regulated either by suppressing the appetite or by raising the expenditure of calories. The appetite can be restricted by controlling the signals of hormones and receptors accountable for hunger and satiety. Additionally, a rise in physical activity also prevents white adipocyte accumulation. Such approaches should help combat obesity and avoid its effects.

Obesity is said to be multifactorial for the reason that it can be caused by downregulation or upregulation of several hormones and factors. For example, excess of fatty acids and tri-glycerol in the blood can cause accumulation of adipocytes all over the body leading to atherosclerosis. This leads to an increase in oxidative stress, hypertriglyceridemia, lipotoxicity, diabetes, and various metabolic syndromes. Thus, the reduction in levels of circulating fat and stored fat are the key factors in the management of obesity. Therefore, the reduction of oxidative stress, which is the common etiological factor in many pathological conditions, may helpful for counteracting the vulnerable consequences of obesity and other complications. The adipocytes are also responsible for stimulating the release of adipocytokine, which in turn releases three hormones, namely lectin, adiponectin, and visfatin. The adiponectin may induce cytotoxic autophagy in breast, colon, prostate, and female-specific carcinogenesis. Hence, the suppression of adiponectin can minimize the risk of obesity-associated carcinogenesis. These three hormones also stimulate the release of insulin, which maintains blood glucose levels and helps in the regulation of body fat. Thus, dysregulation of any sequence in this physiological format leads to imbalance and results in obesity. This indicates the role of insulin in the management of obesity and its correlation with diabetes (Karri et al. 2019).

The dopamine regulates adipose tissue, pancreas, and gastrointestinal tract to secret their respective hormones. These hormones maintain hunger, satiety, blood glucose levels, energy expenditure, and body fat, while its dysregulation may lead to obesity. Therefore, in the development of new anti-obesity agents, these factors and their role plays a crucial role. Figure 3 showcases the mechanism of action of traditional herbal plants to treat obese patients.

There are around 54 families of the plants (figure 4) such as *Solanaceae, Celastraceae, Zingiberaceae Theaceae, Magnoliaceae* that contributes a large number of anti-obesity agents. These plants are reported to have 11 different parts with anti-obesity potential, as shown in figure 5. It has been demonstrated that the leaves are possessing maximum therapeutic potential against obesity, followed by fruits, roots, seeds, etc. (Karri et al. 2019). Figure 6 represents several mechanisms of action posed by numerous agents present in diverse species of herbal plants. The figure is based on the abundance of the mechanism posed by these agents. The most common mechanism is the lowering of plasma lipid levels shown by around 41 plants, and the second being the inhibition of pancreatic lipase activity shown by approximately 31 plants (Karri et al. 2019).

Some of the plants from these Families are discussed below.

i. Araliaceae Family
   - ***Eleutherococcus*** – several species of *Eleutherococcus* are found in eastern Asia, especially in China, Korea, Japan, and Manchuria. These plants are usually small, woody shrub commonly called Siberian Ginseng. The entire plant of Acanthopanax senticosus, is used for preparing medicines to combat several diseases, including obesity. This plant contains chemical content like Carnitine, Triterpenoid saponins - acanthopanaxoside E, silphioside F, copteroside B, hederagenin 3-O-beta-D-glucuronopyranoside '6'-O-methyl ester and gypsogenin 3-O-beta-D- glucuronopyranoside and Chikusetsusaponins, which helps in reducing serum LDL-Cholesterol, inhibition pancreatic lipase, and liver Triglycerides and hence help eliminating obesity. Leaves of another species, namely *Eleutherococcus sessiliflorus* reduces plasma GTG levels, inhibit pancreatic lipase, and increase of undigested GTG in lumen, - Saponins. The main chemical components coming from leaves of *Eleutherococcus sessiliflorus* are lupane-type triterpene triglycosides chiisanoside, 11-deoxyisochiisanoside, isochiisanoside and sessiloside, Chiisanoside.
   - ***Panax*** – these plants are usually found in east Asia and east North America. Several species of the Panax genus help in fighting obesity. *Panax ginseng* contains Ginseng crude saponins (protopanaxadiol, protopanaxatriol). This chemical component extracted from the *Panax ginseng* plant controls the of obesity by inhibiting energy gain, regulating hypothalamic

neuropeptides and serum biochemical, reducing food intake, control plasma triglycerols by regulating pancreatic lipase. Unique components extracted from the rhizome of *Panax japonicas* Inhibits pancreatic lipase activity hence regulating body weight. Stems and leaves of *Panax quinquefolium* contain Saponin, which decreases GTG levels in plasma and increased in the faecal matter may be due to inhibiting pancreatic lipase activity. Hence help to combat obesity.

ii. Asteraceae Family

- ***Cosmos caudatus Kunth*** – these plants are native of Latin America and the West Indies. But they are also found in tropical parts of Asia, Africa, and Australia. Leaves of *Cosmos caudatus Kunth* contains Catechin, quercetin, rutin, kaempferol, and chlorogenic acid. These components help reduce body weight gain by improving lipid profile, adiponectin levels, and plasma ghrelin concentrations and by decreasing leptin levels.
- ***Eclipta alba*** – also known as a false daisy. The whole plant of *Eclipta alba* contains chemical components that perform Lipolytic, anti-dyslipidemic, anti-adipogenic activities. It also inhibits adipocyte differentiation in 3T3-L1 pre-adipocytes, finally helping in managing weight.
- ***Cirsium setidens*** – this plant is usually found in Korea, where it is commonly known as gondre or Korean thistle. Dried leaves of *Cirsium setidens* contain Pectolinarin, which helps fighting obesity by suppressing the expression of lipogenic genes and increasing the expression of lipolytic genes. It also alters the expression of PPARγ, C/EBPα, fatty acid-binding protein 4 (FABP4), sterol regulatory element-binding protein-1c (SREBP-1c), and fatty acid synthase (FAS) along with upregulating the adiponectin and carnitine palmitoyltransferase-1 (CPT-1).

iii. Brassicaceae Family

- ***Wasabia japonica Matsum*** – basically found in Japan. *Wasabia japonica Matsum* leaves are used for medicinal purposes. The leaves of this plant have the capability of lowering body weight gain by reducing liver weight, epididymal WAT by altering gene expression, enhancing levels of adiponectin and PPARα. It also suppresses SREBP-1C and expression of leptin PPARγ &C/EBPα.

iv. Celastraceae Family

- ***Salacia reticulata*** – is a flowering plant grown in Sri Lanka. Its root and stem consist of Mangiferin, (-)-epicatechin, (-)-epigallocatechin, which regulates HFD induced Bodyweight by controlling WAT and mesenteric fat accumulation. Improves glucose metabolism, suppress intracellular triacylglycerol accumulation, enhances lipogenesis genes, and suppress lipolysis genes through activation of AMPkα in the adipocyte. Inhibits adipocytes maturation & differentiation, and expression of metabolic genes & proteins like PPARγ & CCAAT-enhancer, effects binding protein (C/EBP)α, GPDH, and also acts through adiponectin, increase adiponectin levels in plasma, mRNA expression of hormone-sensitive lipase and increases adiponectin.
- ***Catha edulis*** – is commonly called Khat or qat. It is a native African plant and the Arabian Peninsula. Leaves of *Catha edulis* contain cathinone, which decreases the feeling of hunger hence helping in reducing weight.
- ***Tripterygium wilfordii Celastrus reqelii*** – it is found in Korea, Japan, and Manchuria. Roots of *Tripterygium regalii* consist of Celastrol – triterpene, which manages leptin sensitization,

suppress food intake, enhances energy expenditure, heat shock factor 1 (HSF1), Increases mitochondrial function in fat & muscle.

v. Clusiaceae Family
   - ***Garcinia*** – *Garcinia* genus consists of many species of plants. *Garcinia cambogia (GC)* - is abundantly found in southeast Asia. Dried fruit of GC contains Hydroxicitric acid (HCA), a fiber composed of β 1,4-linked D mannose and D-glucose monomers. This compound is responsible for the regulation of lipid biosynthesis, inhibition of lipogenesis impairing hydrocarbon conversion in lipids, and produces the inhibition of ATP- citrate lyase, an enzyme that is required for the first step in lipogenesis process. HCA action also increments glycogen hepatic deposit, decrease appetite and reduces weight gain, Glucomannan (GNN) is capable of absorbing 50 times its weight in water volume, this fiber will fill the stomach resulting in a delayed stomach emptying that induces a feeling of satiety and reduces appetite.
   - ***Clusia nemorosa*** – an evergreen tree found in Latin America. These plants consist of Pentacyclic triterpene - betulinic acid (BA), which reduces blood glucose, total cholesterol by elevating hormones like insulin and leptin. It eduction in activity if amylase and lipase. All these regulations managed by BA helps in reducing weight

vi. Fabaceae Family
   - ***Phaseolus vulgaris*** – known as common beans, are found all over the world. Phytohemagglutinin in these beans helps in inhibition of α amylase, modulation of cholecystokinin, and glucagon peptides, which decreases appetite. It lowers the increments in glucose, reduces C-peptide, and lowers ghrelin secretion.
   - ***Glycine hispida*** - commonly called soybean. They are suitable antioxidant and pancreatic lipase inhibitors. *Glycine hispida* consists of flavonoids and phenolic compounds that help combat obesity.

vii. Lamiaceae Family
   - ***Rosmarinus officinalis*** – a flowering fragrant herb native of the Mediterranean region, commonly known as rosemary. Leaves of *Rosmarinus officinalis* consist of carnosic acid and carnosol, which Inhibit 3T3-L1 adipocyte differentiation process accomplished by blockade of mitotic clonal expression. They also blockers the PPARγ & FABP4 expression, promotes the subnuclear de-localization of C\EBPβ, regulates serum triglycerides, leptin, cholesterol, and insulin, Inhibit pancreatic lipase hence reduce body weight gain.

viii. Moraceae Family
   - ***Morus alba*** – found in India, Pakistan, and Thailand. Leaves and root barks of this plant consist of Polyphenols, xanthines, purine alkaloids, and flavonoids carnosol and carnosic acid. These chemical compounds help to suppress apatite and hence to decrease body weight.
   - ***Morusaustrails poir*** – commonly known as mulberry. Fruits and leaves consist of Anthocyanins. This compound Inhibit body weight gain by reducing serum cholesterol, liver lipid peroxidation levels and adipocyte size, fasting plasma glucose levels, insulin resistance, lipid accumulation. It also maintains leptin secretion, improves hepatic steatosis, and controls stress-induced obesity by reducing protein levels of oxidative stress markers leading to a decrease in body weight gain.

ix. Rubiaceae Family
   - ***Coffea arabica*** – also known as Arabian coffee. Found in Africa, Latin America, Southeast Asia, and China. Seeds of *Coffea arabica* contain polyphenols and caffeine, which increases

energy expenditure, lowers mRNA levels of SREBP proteins like acetyl CoA carboxylase-1 & 2- stearoyl – CoA desaturase-1, pyruvate dehydrogenase kinase – 4 in the liver. These components also play an essential role in reducing weight gain by decreasing leptin levels, inhibit fatty acid absorption, reduce the IL-6 & TNF-α expression, and increases anti-oxidants.

x. Rutaceae Family
   - ***Citrus*** – has many species. *Citrus unshiu,* also called as mandarin. They are grown in Japan, Spain, central China, Korea, the U.S., South Africa, South America, New Zealand. Dried peels of *Citrus unshiu* contains flavonoids and phenolic compounds. These components reduce serum triacylglycerol, total cholesterol levels, and visceral fat through pancreatic lipase inhibition.
   - *Citrus depressa Hayata*, also called thin-skinned flat lemon, is a native to Taiwan and Japan. Fruits of *Citrus depressa* consist of several compounds like CoA-carboxylase 1, fatty acid transport protein, and diacylglycerol acyltransferase 1. These compounds decrease the body-weight gain by reducing white adipose tissue, plasma triglyceride, leptin levels, mRNA levels of lipogenesis-related genes, such as activating protein 2, stearoyl-CoA desaturase 1, acetyl.

xi. Solanaceae Family
   - ***Capsicum*** **–** it has many species. They are native of north and northern South America but are now grown all over the world. One of its species, namely, *Capsicum annuum*, is effective against fighting obesity. Flowers, seeds, and fruits of *Capsicum annuum* consist of capsaicin, Flavonoids and phenolic and capsicoside – G compounds. These compounds upregulated the expression of PPARα, PPARγ, UCP2 & adiponectin, adipocyte differentiation regulators, including peroxisome proliferator-activated receptor γ, CCAAT/enhancer-binding protein α, sterol regulatory element-binding protein 1c, and their target genes. Inhibit antioxidant and pancreatic lipase, epididymal adipose tissue weight, and adipocyte hypertrophy. All these alterations lead to lowering body weight and food efficiency ratio.
   - ***Curcuma longa*** – commonly known as turmeric, native to Indian continents and southeast Asia. The rhizome of *Curcuma longa* comprises of curcumin and curcumin polyphenols. These compounds lower the body fat by showing anti-angiogenic activity, suppression of adipogenesis in 3T3-L1 cells. They also cause Alteration in mRNA expression of AP2, which is a marker of adipocyte maturation, Increase Hepatic acyl-CoA oxidase activity and lower the lipid levels.
   - ***Alpinia officinarum*** – is found in Southeast Asia. Rhizome of *Alpinia officinarum* 1-phenyl-3-heptanone (HPH) - 3-Methylethergalangin, 5-hydroxy-7-(49-hydroxy-39-methoxyphenyl)- 1-phenyl-3-heptanone. These components are responsible for the reduction of serum total cholesterol, triacylglycerol, LDL cholesterol, pancreatic lipase inhibition, and increases HDL cholesterol.

5. Limitations of using herbal medicine:

Worldwide, herbal medicines are used to treat a wide variety of disorders and diseases. Herbal plant extracts are considered to be safer than synthetic drugs, but they are not entirely free of toxicity or adverse effects. There is little scientific evidence available on the potential effects and adverse interactions of many of their components with prescription drugs. Pharmaceutical companies mislead people with less medical awareness by advertising that herbal medicine originates from nature and has no toxicity or side effects, and people can take it in the long run. On the one hand, misuse of herbal medicine can lead to several serious adverse effects, and on the other hand, it can cause fear and anxiety in the people due to specific reports of adverse events.

Herbal preparations" content and quality are not tightly checked, with some ingredients either not listed or their concentrations inaccurately measured or documented on labels. Herbal products may also contain illegal ingredients such as ephedra, *Asarum europaeum* (European wild ginger), and endangered animal species like snow leopard (Byard, R. W. 2017, February 6).

Herbal medicines can cause intrinsic or external toxicity. Intrinsic toxicity of some herb can be in case of therapeutic dosage and course of treatment. For example, adverse reactions associated with Ephedra, *Aristolochia*, *Aconitum*, and toxicity of *Radix Bupleuri Chinensis*. Research on the quantity-toxin relation indicates that the toxic dose of *Radix Bupleuri Chinensis* (192 g/60 kg) is much greater than the standard clinical dose (9 g/60 kg). However, high-dose and long-term use may also cause an adverse event. (Lv, L., Huang, W., Yu, X., Ren, H., & Sun, R. 2009). Whereas external toxicity can result from contamination of herbal medicines with toxic metals, adulteration, misidentification or substitution of herbal ingredients, or improperly processed products. For example, *Caulis Akebiae* replaced by *Caulis Aristolochiae Manshuriensis* and *Stephania tetrandra* replaced by *Aristolochia fangchi* have led to the serious problem of "" "aristolochic acid nephropathy (Zhang, J., Wider, B., Shang, H., Li, X., & Ernst, E. 2012). Some herbal formulations contain heavy metals, toxic chemicals, and organic toxins that occur naturally. These drugs may have devastating consequences, including acute hepatic and kidney failure, exacerbating pre-existing conditions and diseases, and even death. (Byard, R. W. 2017, February 6).

Herbal drugs that are used for weight loss may directly or indirectly be dangerous and fatal for overweight patients. These side effects may range from acute symptoms like drying of the mouth, insomnia, and headache to chronic disease, and even death. As shown in one of the case studies of an obese 19-year-old male who lost 30kg after two months of consuming 15 cups of green tea per day and following an intensive dietary regimen. And one day after the usual exercise, he suddenly lost consciousness due to left ventricular fibrillation. Severe and rapid weight loss is also not safe. In some cases, herbal medicine, the risk is sufficient to shift the risk-beneðt balance against medicine (Najafian, J., Abdar-Esfahani, M., Arab-Momeni, M., & Akhavan-Tabib, A. 2014).

CONCLUSION

Obesity is escalating at an alarming rate all around the world. The underlying pathogenesis of obesity involves either up-regulation or down-regulation of calorie utilization by governing cellular functions, physical activity, etc. This dysregulation leads to life-threatening complications associated with hyperlipidemia, cardiovascular abnormalities, and atherosclerosis. Thus, many countries are involved in the research activities to find out the new entity for the management of obesity. It is a doubtless fact that various plants from different families and several phytochemical constituents are responsible for the anti-obesity activity.

One specific plant can be active in more than one pathway or mechanism, such as P. ginseng. Some active constituents are present or incorporated into food for daily consumption, such as Capsaicin, Glycine hispida, Morus, and Curcumin. The recently expanded metabolomics approach, along with multivariate data analysis, could be a valuable tool in obesity herbal discovery as it offers the potential of studying efficacy and safety in a holistic approach and thus would also reveal the presence of pro-drugs or synergy.

It is also essential for the quality control of herbal medicines. Nevertheless, the anti-obesity activity's probable mechanism is not enough to understand the pharmacological and therapeutic potential in a scientific discipline. The anticipation is that researchers have ample room for further contributions to establish the molecular mechanism of new natural anti-obesity agents. It will be of particular interest and an attention-grabbing subject for future research.

Herbal medicine has many beneficial effects on the treatment of obese patients. It has fewer adverse effects (Liu et al. 2017) than chemical agents, potentially herbal medicine mechanisms for obesity. More standardized procedures and clinical trials and a of herbal medicine producing are needed to confirm the safety and anti-obesity effect of herbal medicine and finally prevent/reduce obesity by herbal medicine consumption in humans. Also, all the variables that mark a plant as an alternative therapy for the treatment of diseases must be rigorously assessed to guarantee robust, safe, and reliable results.

Based on the current situation, global research on herbal medicine protection is still not broad enough. Future studies into the toxicity and herbal-drug interaction of widely used herbal medicines are the most critical and urgent work given greater attention. For clinical safety, accidental reporting or active pharmacovigilance should effectively detect therapeutically significant safety problems. Even in countries where herbal medicinal products are regularly assessed before market authorization, pharmacovigilance is a critical activity to promote herbal medicines' safe use throughout their life cycle.

To ensure herbal medicines' quality and safety, the WHO should propose global unified planning, including global management standards and quality standards, radical sources of herbs, seed and seedling breeding, planting, harvesting and storage, rational proceeding, manufacture, and quality standards. Moreover, a safety guarantee system comprised of rational clinical practice and risk monitoring should be established to improve herbal medicine safety and play a more critical role in maintaining human health.

REFERENCES

Akbas, F., Gasteyger, C., Sjodin, A., Astrup, A., & Larsen, T. M. (2009). A critical review of the cannabinoid receptor as a drug target for obesity management. *Obesity Reviews*, *10*(1), 58–67. doi:10.1111/j.1467-789X.2008.00520.x PMID:18721231

Al-Tahami, B. A. M., Ab, A. A. S. I., Sanip, Z., Yusoff, Z., Shihabudin, T. M. T., Singh, T. S. P., & Rasool, A. H. G. (2017). Metabolic and Inflammatory Changes with Orlistat and Sibutramine Treatment in Obese Malaysian Subjects. *Journal of Nippon Medical School*, *84*(3), 125–132. doi:10.1272/jnms.84.125 PMID:28724846

Amin, K. A., & Nagy, M. A. (2009). Effect of Carnitine and herbal mixture extract on obesity induced by high fat diet in rats. *Diabetology & Metabolic Syndrome*, *1*(1), 17. doi:10.1186/1758-5996-1-17 PMID:19835614

Berger, K., Winzell, M. S., Mei, J., & Erlanson-Albertsson, C. (2004). Enterostatin and its target mechanisms during regulation of fat intake. *Physiology & Behavior*, *83*(4), 623–630. doi:10.1016/j.physbeh.2004.08.040 PMID:15621068

Blundell, J. E., & Cooling, J. (2000). Routes to obesity: Phenotypes, food choices and activity. *British Journal of Nutrition*, *83*(S1), S33–S38. doi:10.1017/S0007114500000933 PMID:10889790

Brehm, B. J., & D'Alessio, D. A. (2014). Environmental factors influencing obesity. In Endotext. MD-Text. com, Inc.

Brown, P. J. (1991). Culture and the evolution of obesity. *Human Nature (Hawthorne, N.Y.)*, *2*(1), 31–57. doi:10.1007/BF02692180 PMID:24222189

Byard, R. W. (2017, February 6). *What risks do herbal products pose to the Australian community?* The Medical Journal of Australia. https://www.mja.com.au/journal/2017/206/2/what-risks-do-herbal-products-pose-australian-community

Cheng, T. O. (2006). Obesity is a global challenge. *The American Journal of Medicine*, *119*(6), e11. doi:10.1016/j.amjmed.2006.04.006 PMID:16750947

Csige, I., Ujvárosy, D., Szabó, Z., Lőrincz, I., Paragh, G., Harangi, M., & Somodi, S. (2018). The impact of obesity on the cardiovascular system. *Journal of Diabetes Research*, *2018*, 2018. doi:10.1155/2018/3407306 PMID:30525052

Darbre, P. D. (2017). Endocrine disruptors and obesity. *Current Obesity Reports*, *6*(1), 18–27. doi:10.100713679-017-0240-4 PMID:28205155

Dragomir, A., & Radulian, G. (2016). Eating habits in normal weight and obese people. *Romanian Journal of Diabetes, Nutrition, & Metabolic Diseases*, *23*(4), 387–395. doi:10.1515/rjdnmd-2016-0045

Epstein, L. H., Wing, R. R., Penner, B. C., & Kress, M. J. (1985). Effect of diet and controlled exercise on weight loss in obese children. *The Journal of Pediatrics*, *107*(3), 358–361. doi:10.1016/S0022-3476(85)80506-0 PMID:4032130

Field, A. E., Coakley, E. H., Must, A., Spadano, J. L., Laird, N., Dietz, W. H., Rimm, E., & Colditz, G. A. (2001). Impact of overweight on the risk of developing common chronic diseases during a 10-year period. *Archives of Internal Medicine*, *161*(13), 1581–1586. doi:10.1001/archinte.161.13.1581 PMID:11434789

Fried, M., Hainer, V., Basdevant, A., Buchwald, H., Deitel, M., Finer, N., ... Steffen, R. (2007). Interdisciplinary European guidelines for surgery for severe (morbid) obesity. *Obesity Surgery*, *17*(2), 260–270. doi:10.100711695-007-9025-2 PMID:17476884

Gupta, V., Winocour, J., Rodriguez-Feo, C., Bamba, R., Shack, R. B., Grotting, J. C., & Higdon, K. K. (2016). *Safety of aesthetic surgery*. Academic Press.

Harvey, J. R., & Ogden, D. E. (2014). Obesity treatment in disadvantaged population groups: Where do we stand and what can we do? *Prev Med (Baltim)*, *68*, 71–75. doi:10.1016/j.ypmed.2014.05.015 PMID:24878585

Health.gov. (2020). Available at: https://health.gov/sites/default/files/2019-09/paguide.pdf

Hollander, P., Maggs, D.G., Ruggles, J.A., Fineman, M., Shen, L., Koltetman, O.G., & Weyer, C. (2004). Effect of Pramlintide on weight in overweight an obese insulin-treated type2 diabetes patients. *Obese Res.*, *12*, 661-668.

Horne, B. D., Muhlestein, J. B., & Anderson, J. L. (2015). Health effects of intermittent fasting: Hormesis or harm? A systematic review. *The American Journal of Clinical Nutrition, 102*(2), 464–470. doi:10.3945/ajcn.115.109553 PMID:26135345

Jakicic, J. M., & Otto, A. D. (2005). Physical activity considerations for the treatment and prevention of obesity. *The American Journal of Clinical Nutrition, 82*(1), 226–229. doi:10.1093/ajcn/82.1.226S PMID:16002826

Kanter, R., & Caballero, B. (2012). Global gender disparities in obesity: A review. *Advances in Nutrition, 3*(4), 491–498. doi:10.3945/an.112.002063 PMID:22797984

Karri, S., Sharma, S., Hatware, K., & Patil, K. (2019). Natural anti-obesity agents and their therapeutic role in management of obesity: A future trend perspective. *Biomedicine and Pharmacotherapy, 110*, 224–238. doi:10.1016/j.biopha.2018.11.076 PMID:30481727

Kernan, W. N., Inzucchi, S. E., Sawan, C., Macko, R. F., & Furie, K. L. (2013). Obesity: A stubbornly obvious target for stroke prevention. *Stroke, 44*(1), 278–286. doi:10.1161/STROKEAHA.111.639922 PMID:23111440

Knutson, K. L. (2012). Does inadequate sleep play a role in vulnerability to obesity? *American Journal of Human Biology, 24*(3), 361–371. doi:10.1002/ajhb.22219 PMID:22275135

Landsberg, L., Aronne, L. J., Beilin, L. J., Burke, V., Igel, L. I., Lloyd-Jones, D., & Sowers, J. (2013). Obesity- related hypertension: Pathogenesis, cardiovascular risk, and treatment—a position paper of the obesity society and the American society of hypertension. *Obesity (Silver Spring, Md.), 21*(1), 8–24. doi:10.1002/oby.20181 PMID:23401272

Lavle, C. J., & Milani, R. V. (2005). Cardiac rehabilitation and exercise training pogrammes in metabolic syndrome and diabetes. *Journal of Cardiopulmonary Rehabilitation, 25*(2), 59–66. doi:10.1097/00008483-200503000-00001 PMID:15818190

Lazzer, S., Bedogni, G., Lafortuna, C. L., Marazzi, N., Busti, C., Galli, R., de Col, A., Agosti, F., & Sartorio, A. (2010). Relationship between basal metabolic rate, gender, age, and body composition in 8,780 white obese subjects. *Obesity (Silver Spring, Md.), 18*(1), 71–78. doi:10.1038/oby.2009.162 PMID:19478787

Leibel, R. L., Rosenbaum, M., & Hirsch, J. (1995). Changes in energy expenditure resulting from altered body weight. *The New England Journal of Medicine, 332*(10), 621–628. doi:10.1056/NEJM199503093321001 PMID:7632212

Little, T. J., Horowitz, M., & Feinle-Bisset, C. (2005). Role of cholecystokinin in appetite control and body weight regulation. *Obesity Reviews, 6*(4), 297–306. doi:10.1111/j.1467-789X.2005.00212.x PMID:16246215

Liu, Y., Sun, M., Yao, H., Liu, Y., & Gao, R. (2017). Herbal medicine for the treatment of obesity: An overview of scientific evidence from 2007 to 2017. *Evidence-Based Complementary and Alternative Medicine*. doi:10.1155/2017/8943059 PMID:29234439

Lv, L., Huang, W., Yu, X., Ren, H., & Sun, R. (2009). Comparative research of different Bupleurum chinense composition to influence of hepatotoxicity of rats and oxidative damage mechanism. *Zhongguo Zhongyao Zazhi*, *34*(18), 2364–2368. PMID:20030090

Makris, A., & Foster, G. D. (2011). Dietary approaches to the treatment of obesity. *Psychiatria Clinica*, *34*(4), 813–827. PMID:22098806

Mayo Clinic. (2020). *The Best Ways To Cut Calories From Your Diet*. Available at: https://www.mayoclinic.org/healthy-lifestyle/weight-loss/in-depth/calories/art-20048065

Mayoclinic.org. (2020a). *Blood Pressure Test - Mayo Clinic*. Available at: https://www.mayoclinic.org/tests-procedures/blood-pressure-test/about/pac-20393098

Mayoclinic.org. (2020b). *Cholesterol Test - Mayo Clinic*. Available at: https://www.mayoclinic.org/tests-procedures/cholesterol-test/about/pac-20384601

Mayoclinic.org. (2020c). *Liposuction - Mayo Clinic*. Available at: https://www.mayoclinic.org/tests-procedures/liposuction/about/pac-20384586

Mizutani, T., Suzuki, K., Kondo, N., & Yamagata, Z. (2007). Association of maternallife style including smoking during pregnancy with childhood obesity. *Obesity (Silver Spring, Md.)*, *15*(12), 33133–31399. doi:10.1038/oby.2007.373 PMID:18198324

Najafian, J., Abdar-Esfahani, M., Arab-Momeni, M., & Akhavan-Tabib, A. (2014). Safety of herbal medicine in treatment of weight loss. *ARYA Atherosclerosis*, *10*(1), 55. PMID:24963315

Nelson, J. C., & Papakostas, G. I. (2009). A Typical antipsychotic augmentation in major depressive disorder: A meta- analysis of placebo-controlled randomized trials. *The American Journal of Psychiatry*, *166*(9), 980–991. doi:10.1176/appi.ajp.2009.09030312 PMID:19687129

Ness-Abramof, R., & Apovian, C. M. (2006). Diet modification for treatment and prevention of obesity. *Endocrine*, *29*(1), 5–9. doi:10.1385/ENDO:29:1:5 PMID:16622287

Ng, M., Fleming, T., Robinson, M., Thomson, B., Graetz, N., Margono, C., Mullany, E. C., Biryukov, S., Abbafati, C., Abera, S. F., Abraham, J. P., Abu-Rmeileh, N. M. E., Achoki, T., AlBuhairan, F. S., Alemu, Z. A., Alfonso, R., Ali, M. K., Ali, R., Guzman, N. A., ... Gakidou, E. (2014). Global, regional, and national prevalence of overweight and obesity in children and adults during 1980- 2013: A systematic analysis for the Global Burden of Disease Study 2013. *Lancet*, *384*(9945), 766–781. doi:10.1016/S0140-6736(14)60460-8 PMID:24880830

Obata, S., Okauchi, S., Kimura, T., Hirukawa, H., Tanabe, A., Kinoshita, T., Kohara, K., Tatsumi, F., Shimoda, M., Kamei, S., Nakanishi, S., Mune, T., Kaku, K., & Kaneto, H. (2017). Advanced breast cancer in a relatively young man with severe obesity and type 2 diabetes mellitus. *Journal of Diabetes Investigation*, *8*(3), 395–396. doi:10.1111/jdi.12570 PMID:28470916

Padwal, R. S., & Majumdur, S. R. (2007). Drug treatments for obesity: Olistat, Sibutramine, rimonabant. *Lancet*, *369*(9555), 371–377. doi:10.1016/S0140-6736(07)60033-6 PMID:17208644

Parker, J., McCullough, K., Field, B., Minnion, J. S., Martin, N. M., Ghatei, M. A., & Bloom, S. R. (2013). Glucagon and GLP-1 inhibit food intake and increase c-fos expression in similar appetite regulating centres in the brainstem and amygdala. *International Journal of Obesity*, *37*(10), 1391–1398. doi:10.1038/ijo.2012.227 PMID:23337772

Poirier, P., Giles, T. D., Bray, G. A., Hong, Y., Stern, J. S., Pi-Sunyer, F. X., & Eckel, R. H. (2006). Obesity and cardiovascular diseases: Pathophysiology, evaluation, and effect of weight loss: an update of 1997 American Heart Association Scientific statement on obesity and heart disease from the obesity committee of the council on nutrition, physical activity, and metabolism. *Circulation*, *113*(6), 898–918. doi:10.1161/CIRCULATIONAHA.106.171016 PMID:16380542

Ranjbar, H. S., Jouyandeh, Z., & Abdollahi, M. (2013). *A Systematic Review Of Anti-Obesity Medicinal Plants - An Update*. J Diabetes Met Dis.

Ravi, R., & Krishnamurthy, V. (2019). Beneficial Effects of Medicinal Plants Used For the Management of Obesity-A Review. *International Journal of Health Sciences and Research*, *9*(12), 174–194.

Richette, P., & Bardin, T. (2010). Gout. *Lancet*, *375*(9711), 318–328. doi:10.1016/S0140-6736(09)60883-7 PMID:19692116

Serretti, A., & Mandelli, L. (2010). Antidepressants and body weight: A comprehensive review and meta-analysis. *The Journal of Clinical Psychiatry*, *71*(10), 1259–1272. doi:10.4088/JCP.09r05346blu PMID:21062615

Snow, V., Barry, P., Fitterman, N., Qaseem, A., & Weiss, K. (2005). Pharmacologic and surgical management of obesityin primary care: A clinical practice guideline from theAmerican College of Physicians. *Annals of Internal Medicine*, *142*(7), 525–531. doi:10.7326/0003-4819-142-7-200504050-00011 PMID:15809464

Sun, N.-N., Wu, T.-Y., & Chau, C.-F. (2016). Natural dietary and herbal products in anti- obesity treatment. *Molecules (Basel, Switzerland)*, *21*(10), 1351. doi:10.3390/molecules21101351 PMID:27727194

Thaker, V. V. (2017). Genetic and epigenetic causes of obesity. *Adolescent Medicine: State of the Art Reviews*, *28*(2), 379. PMID:30416642

Trollo, P. J., & Rogers, R. M. (1996). Obstructive sleep apnea. *The New England Journal of Medicine*, *334*(2), 99–104. doi:10.1056/NEJM199601113340207 PMID:8531966

Tzotzas, T., Papazisis, K., Perros, P., & Krassas, G. E. (2008). Use of somatostatin analogues in obesity. *Drugs*, *68*(14), 1963–1973. doi:10.2165/00003495-200868140-00003 PMID:18778119

Valizadeh, E., Ghalichi, F., & Ostadrahimi, A. (2016). Traditional herbal medicine for weight management: A review. *International Journal of Medical Research & Health Sciences*, *5*(11), 393–399.

Verhaegen, A. A., & Van Gaal, L. F. (2017). Drug-induced obesity and its metabolic consequences: A review with a focus on mechanisms and possible therapeutic options. *Journal of Endocrinological Investigation*, *40*(11), 1165–1174. doi:10.100740618-017-0719-6 PMID:28660606

Verma, R. K., & Paraidathathu, T. (2014). Herbal medicines used in the traditional indian medicinal system as a therapeutic treatment option for overweight and obesity management: A review. *International Journal of Pharmacy and Pharmaceutical Sciences*, *6*, 40–47.

Westerterp, K. R. (2004). Diet induced thermo- genesis. *Nutrition & Metabolism*, *1*(1), 5. doi:10.1186/1743-7075-1-5 PMID:15507147

Wiklund, P. (2016). The role of physical activity and exercise in obesity and weight management: Time for critical appraisal. *Journal of Sport and Health Science*, *5*(2), 151–154. doi:10.1016/j.jshs.2016.04.001 PMID:30356545

World Health Organization. (2011). *Global recommendations on physical activity for health*. WHO.

World Health Organization. (2000). *Obesity: Preventing and managing the global epidemic*. Technical report series No.894, Geneva: WHO.

Yannakoulia, M., Poulimeneas, D., Mamalaki, E., & Anastasiou, C. A. (2019). Dietary modifications for weight loss and weight loss maintenance. *Metabolism: Clinical and Experimental*, *92*, 153–162. doi:10.1016/j.metabol.2019.01.001 PMID:30625301

Zhang, J., Wider, B., Shang, H., Li, X., & Ernst, E. (2012). Quality of herbal medicines: Challenges and solutions. *Complementary Therapies in Medicine*, *20*(1-2), 100–106. doi:10.1016/j.ctim.2011.09.004 PMID:22305255

Section 2
Infertility Management

Chapter 6
An Insight on Polycystic Ovary Syndrome (PCOS) and Use of Herbal Medicines as Alternative Treatment

Sowmya Kiran Rao
Manipal Academy of Higher Education, UAE

ABSTRACT

One of the most common endocrine disorder in females during reproductive age which leads to infertility, metabolic derangements, and also psychological impairments is polycystic ovary syndrome (PCOS). This syndrome has been known to increases the risk of type 2 diabetes, obesity, hypertension, cardiovascular diseases, lipid disorders, and also autoimmune thyroiditis. Impending complication list includes malignancies like breast and endometrial cancer. The actual cause of this syndrome is unknown, and perhaps, it could be due to a combination of various unmodifiable genetic factors and modifiable environmental factors. Several research studies have been carried out on management of PCOS, and many medicinal plants have been used as an alternative therapy for oligo/amenorrhoea, hyperandrogenism, and PCOS in women. The chapter gives an insight on PCOS, its management, and elucidates the effects of medicinal plants on PCOS.

INTRODUCTION

In the developed world, one of the debatable heterogeneous endocrine disorder, known to affect females in reproductive age, causing health complications namely infertility, menstrual dysfunction, obesity, acne and metabolic syndrome is Polycystic ovary syndrome (PCOS) (Dargham etal,2017; Norman, 2007; Knochenhauer et al.,1998). About 12-24% have been known to be affected by PCOS leading to infertility (Nirav, 2017), characterized by imbalance of sex hormones (Khomami, 2015).

Infertility is known to affect three million couples in US and 17% of couples in industrialized countries are known to seek help for infertility. It is reported that 40% of cases are due to factors related to

DOI: 10.4018/978-1-7998-4808-0.ch006

females, 30% due to male, 20% are usually combination of both male and female factors and 10% are due to unknown cause. The cause for infertility may be due to endometriosis, tubal damage, ovary failure or low sperm count (Siladitya, 2010; Marcelle 2005). The problems in ovulation in females has been related to cause of infertility in PCOS women. Apart from PCOS, fertility is also affected by some of the other hormonal conditions like premature ovarian failure, diabetes, thyroid problems, and sometimes Cushing's syndrome. (Marcelle 2005).

The reproductive system is an integral part of the endocrine system, and this syndrome is characterized by endocrine, metabolic and genetic disorder (Zahra et al, 2018). The organs involved in PCOS are ovary, adrenal gland, pancreas and the pitutary gland (Shantaram, 2019). It is a condition with epigenetic origins influenced by uterine environment and also behavioral factors (Norman et al., 2007). Dietary pattern along with physical activity, stress and smoking are some of the environmental factors that have an important role to play in the manifestation of the syndrome (Xita &Tsatsoulis, 2006; Nardo et al, 2008; Abbott et al., 2002). The management depends on symptoms like ovulatory dysfunction, androgen-related symptoms or menstrual disorders (Ahmed & Abubaker, 2011). Traditional medicinal plants have found its use since thousands of years in the treatment of various ailments and research findings on herbal medicine and its effectiveness on PCOS treatment is available for some of the herbs.

The present chapter deals with PCOS prevalence, etiology, clinical manifestations, associated co-morbidities, conventional treatment and management along with its drawbacks, and an insight on alternative therapy for PCOS management with special reference to the beneficial effects of medicinal or herbal plants used in Ayurvedic practice in India, Tradition Arabic /Persian medicine, Traditional Chinese Medicine as well as Korean herbal medicine practice. Concerns related to herbal medicine supplements and strategies for safe use has also been dealt with in the chapter.

BACKGROUND

PCOS, also known as 'Stein-Leventhal Syndrome', is a persistent global health problem known to have an impact on multiple organ systems that exerts reproductive and metabolic manifestations (Nirav, 2017; Tracy et al., 2016). This complex (Tracy et al., 2016; March et al., 2010; El-Sharkawy et al., 2014; Richard et.al., 2013; Robert & David, 2016) trait results from the interaction of genetic and also environmental factors that manifests usually at puberty (Robert & David, 2016). The clinical characteristics and features of this syndrome first described in 1935 by Irving Stein and Michael Leventhal, develops when the ovaries are stimulated to produce excess androgens, particularly testosterone (Stein & Leventhal, 1935, Strauss, 2003). The resultant increase in male hormone leads to polycystic ovaries (Strauss, 2003).

Diagnostic criteria for PCOS have been set by National Institutes of Health (NIH) 1990, Rotterdam 2003, AE-PCOS Society 2006, NIH 2012/International PCOS Guidelines 2018. To determine the presence or absence of PCOS, each of these suggests criteria that have slightly different biological, clinical and image-based findings (Okoroh, 2012). An international evidence-based guideline for the assessment and management of PCOS released in 2018 recommends the use of the Rotterdam diagnostic criteria (Teede et al., 2018). Rotterdam criteria is accepted criteria in Asia, Australia and Europe (Stepto et al., 2013; Yildiz et al., 2012.). This criteria described presence of polycystic ovaries and hyperandrogenism in females with normal menstrual cycles, and also women with polycystic ovaries and ovulatory disturbance without hyperandrogenism (Broekmans et al., 2006). The diagnosis necessitates the presence of at least two of the three findings on ultrasound i.e., hyperandrogenism, ovulatory dysfunction, and polycystic ovarian morphology (Tracy, 2016).

PREVALENCE

Due to different sets of criteria's available, the inconsistencies and the high degree of variability, the determination of prevalence of his complex syndrome has become a challenge (Wendy,2018). It depends on the choice of diagnostic criteria being used to document the prevalence (Ahmed, 2016). An estimated 75% individuals are known to remain undiagnosed with PCOS when visiting their doctor. (Carmina, 2004; and Zahra et al, 2018) and many cases are not diagnosed even after consultation with many health care providers. (Wendy etal, 2018).

The prevalence rates are thought to be 3-10% but it is not known for sub-populations based on race or ethnicity and geographical location (Wendy et al, 2018). It has been reported to be between 6% and 9% documented across the United States, the United Kingdom, Spain, Greece, Australia, Asia, and Mexico (Ricardo et al., 2011).According to (Nirav, 2017) 12-24% have been known to be affected by PCOS.

Prevalence of PCOS by NIH guidelines in Qatari cohort is reported to be 12.1% which reflected 20% by Rotterdam criteria with a distinctly more metabolic phenotype than control Qatari population in the study. (Soha.R etal., 2017) Studies conducted in Palestine shows prevalence of 7.3% in 18–24 year old female subjects, and the prevalence was relatively high similar to other Mediterranean statistics and the study concluded by recommending further studies using wider age groups and more sample size to generalize the results (Samar.M etal., 2013).

Some of the available studies on PCOS consist of less sample sizes to arrive at any particular conclusion and studies generally conclude by recommending for a further study including a bigger, sample size. Notably there is a variation in PCOS prevalence rates with different diagnostic criteria used across ethnic groups. The prevalence rates have been stated to be 1.6% using all the three diagnostic criteria combination and 18% in similar Caucasian population when Rotterdam criteria is used projecting the fact that prevalence rates are affected due to changes in diagnostic criteria being used. (Azziz et al, 2004; Lim et al 2013; March et al 2010;Tao Ding et al, 2017). Hence, an ethnicity-specific guidelines may be needed in order to prevent under-or-over diagnosis of this complex syndrome (Tao Ding et al, 2017).

ETIOLOGY

The primary cause of the syndrome is unknown (Uche et al., 2013). This syndrome results in an increased ovarian androgens and also some degree of both adrenal and metabolic disorders in the females (Lankarani et al., 2005).

The histological features of this complex syndrome is known to include thickened capsule measuring >100 μ, Increased number of sub capsular follicle cysts, ovarian hypertrophy, paucity of corporea lutea or albicantia, premature luteinization of the theca cells and also hyperplasia and fibrosis of the ovarian stroma (Azziz et al, 2016).

Hypothalamus neurons in the reproductive axis referred to as Hypothalamic–pituitary–gonadal (HPG) or gonadotropic axis produces Gonadotropin-releasing hormone (GnRH) which stimulates the release of two gonadotropins namely Follicle-stimulating hormone (FSH) and Luteinizing hormone (LH). The function of FSH is to stimulates growth of small sacs in ovaries to a mature follicle containing egg and also produces additional hormones, and LH is to support FSH to stimulate the growth of the follicle and enables egg maturing and release (14th day of menstrual cycle), ready for fertilization by sperm; if not fertilized, shedding of endometrium after 14 days of ovulation (28 day normal cycle) takes place through menstrual flow in females. (Zahra et al, 2018; Bhagyashri et al, 2013; Dan Jiang, 2017)

In PCOS, there is hormonal imbalance and the follicular growth is affected during the ovarian cycle. This results in follicle release and the retained follicle forms a cyst. This process happens in all the ovarian cycle and new cysts are formed which shows up as multiple cysts when viewed with ultrasound scanning. The ultrasonic morphologic evidence of above or equal to 12 follicles which measure 2.9mm in diameter in single plane during quiescent phase of the ovary referring to 2.7 days of cycle is related with oligomenorrohea, anovulation, hyperandrogenism, obesity and hyperinsulinemia (Zahra et al, 2018; Bhagyashri et al, 2013; Dan Jiang, 2017).

Although the cause of this complex syndrome is unknown, it is reported that in increase in insulin secretion which is perhaps due to insulin resistance leads to increased frequency of GnRH pulses which is high coordination among GnRH neurons derived from neuro pulse generator known as GnRH pulse generator and this pulse mode is essential for normal functioning of gonadotropins and ability for normal reproduction. The slow GnRH pulse releases further FSH hormone and rapid pulses are compatible with increased LH hormone. The increase in LH levels compared to FSH, a hormonal change at the surfaces of theca and granulosa cells, leads to hike in the production of androgens and decrease in estradiol production which stops maturation of follicular cells disrupting ovulation. Increased insulin levels also reduces the serum sex hormone binding globin (SHBG) leading to higher free testosterone levels. Increased androgen levels causes anovulation. (Zahra et al, 2018; Bhagyashri et al, 2013; Dan Jiang, 2017)

Infertility in PCOS is caused due to problems in ovulation related to eggs produced in the ovaries, its movement from ovary to uterus and fertilized embryo being unable to attach to the lining of the uterus or to survive after attaching to the uterus lining. (Samiksha et al,2011). Due to increased androgen production and supressed maturation of the ovarian follicles, the ovum formation and release is affected leading to anovulation in PCOS. (Shantaram et al, 2019; Shubhashree et al,2012).Apart from imbalance in luteinizing hormone and follicle-stimulation hormone, increased or low body weight, pituitary tumors, injury to pituitary gland or hypothalamus are known to cause infertility (Rosencrantz et al., 2011; Balen et al., 2016).

Many studies have suggested that heredity has a role in the pathogenesis of PCOS (Roldan et al., 2004; Urbanek, 2007; Amato & Simpson, 2004; Crosignani & Nicolosi 2001). A family history of PCOS, premature pubarche, Caribbean, Hispanic or African American ancestry, and/ or obesity are more probable to develop the syndrome (Driscoll, 2000).

Clinical Manifestations

The symptoms of PCOS is related to reproductive and psychological problems in young female and metabolic symptoms in older women. (Teede et al., 2011). It is characterized by oligo/amenorrhea, polycystic ovaries and hyperandrogenism.

A menstrual interval of above 35 days is oligomenorrhea and absence of menstrual bleeding above 90 day is regarded as amenorrhea. Heavy menstrual bleeding is also a symptom along with other symptoms like gain in weight (Johanna,2011). Hyperandrogenism is caused due to increased ovarian and or increased adrenal androgen production in PCOS females (Johanna,2011). It is known to occur in approximately

60% of PCOS females, though this varies with the race and degree of obesity in PCOS females (Azziz et al. 2006). Hirsutism, acne are typical symptoms of hyperandrogenism .Acne has been reported in 38% of females with PCOS (Borgia 2004). Acanthosis nigricans, is a medical sign showing patches of thick dark and velvety hyperpigmentation of skin. (Lujan et al, 2013; Goodarzi et al,2011; March et al, 2010) Fatigue and fluid retention (Shantaram et al, 2019) are also symptoms observed in PCOS females.

ASSOCIATED CO-MORBIDITIES

Reproductive Consequences

Infertility and Pregnancy Related Complications

PCOS women have difficulty in conception and pregnancy. Approximately 90%–95% of anovulatory females visiting infertility clinics have PCOS (Sirmans and Pate, 2014). Oligo/anovulation and metabolic alterations causes three quarters of PCOS women sub fertile or infertile (Legro,1998; Diejomaoh et al, 2003). The rates of miscarriage is higher in PCOS females compared to normal females. These females are also overweight or obese and studies indicate higher prevalence of gestational diabetes and hypertension, premature birth and preeclampsia in PCOS females. (Boomsma et al,2006)

Cancer

The risk factors associated with PCOS for endometrial cancer are nulliparity, excessive weight, long time exposure to estrogens and hyper insulinemia. Females with PCOS are shown to be almost 3 times at higher risk of developing endometrial cancer compared to females without PCOS. (Chittenden et al,2009)

Metabolic Consequences

Metabolic Syndrome

Many features of PCOS is in common with the metabolic syndrome (Glueck et al, 2003) It has been reported that the metabolic syndrome is associated with an increased risk of cardio vascular diseases (CVD) and diabetes as well as all-cause mortality in general female population (Isomaa et al,2011; Trevisan et al, 1998) . Family history of diabetes, fasting insulin and obesity are the factors that have capacity to predict the metabolic syndrome in females with PCOS (Coviello et al, 2006; Ehrmann et al, 2006).

Insulin Resistance and Type 2 Diabetes Mellitus (T2DM)

In PCOS females, it has been found that, 50-70% are insulin-resistant and hyperinsulinemic. (Diamanti-Kandarakis et al,2008). According to a study (Legro et al, 1999) PCOS females have higher risk of impaired glucose tolerance (IGT) and T2DM at all body weights and at young ages. Another study on Mediterranean females with PCOS with a mean age of 28 years showed that approximately 16% had glucose intolerance and 2.5% were T2DM (Gambineri et al, 2004). One in five females with PCOS are known to develop T2DM. (Dunaif, 1999)

Obesity

Many studies have shown that female with PCOS in fertile age, compared to normal control population, have increased abdominal obesity and also increased visceral or abdominal fat status (Mannerås-Holm et al,2011; Douchi et al,2001). A meta-analysis study conducted on Iranian women to study the prevalence of PCOS and its associated complications revealed that the intensity of PCOS symptoms increased with age and was associated with accumulation of adipose tissue (Anahita et al., 2015).

Cardiovascular Consequences

Many studies have indicated increased CVD risk factors in PCOS females of fertile or premenopausal ages. The mothers of females with PCOS have a high risk of CVD events than control group (Cheang et al, 2008). Studies have indicated that, compared to controlled matched samples, PCOS females show significantly higher levels of circulating biomarkers of CVD which includes C-reactive protein and lipoprotein A. (61 cross- Bahceci et al., 2004; Meyer et al., 2005; (Yilmaz et al., 2005; Bahceci et al., 2007; Berneis et al., 2009; Rizzo et al., 2009). Hyperlipidemia- increased triglycerides (TG),low-density lipoproteins (LDL) levels and decreased high density lipo protein (HDL) levels has been common metabolic abnormality in PCOS females . (Diamanti-Kandarakis et al, 2007; Valkenburg et al,2008; Talbott EO et al, 2000; Talbott et al,1998).

Psychological Well-Being

Psychological stress and PCOS are shown to be related to each other bearing a consequence on the female with the syndrome. PCOS females are reported to be more prone to suffer from psychological disorders like depression and anxiety compared to normal healthy female controls. (Jedel et al., 2010; Veltman-Verhulst et al., 2012)

Apart from all the above mentioned consequences, cerebrovascular stroke, sleep apnea, fatty liver disease (non-alcoholic) and autoimmune thyroiditis have also been mentioned as prognosis of PCOS. (Ong KJ et al, 2006). Some of the complications of PCOS during different stages of a female life cycle is shown in Table 1.

Table 1. Complications of PCOS

Age group	Complications
Adolescent ages	Amenorrhea, oligo-menorrhea, hirsutism, obesity, acne
Fertility ages	Infertility, irregular ovulation, pregnancy complications
Pre-menopausal and post-menopausal ages	Insulin resistance, risk of Type 2 diabetes, hypertension, dyslipidemia, cardiovascular diseases, endometrial cancer, possibly breast cancer

(Adapted from Haji et al., 2007; Anahita et al., 2015)

Overall, the endocrine picture of PCOS women of fertile age is -normal to low FSH (Fauser et al,1991; Yen,1980), increased LH (van Santbrink,1997; Rebar et al,1976), normal to low Sex hormone binding globulin (SHBG) levels caused due to inhibitory effects of insulin on SHBG production in liver (Gerard C et al, 2014; Nestler et al 1991;, O`Malley & Strott, 1999), normal to increased estradiol levels (Franks et al, 1989; Polson et al, 1987) and increased androgens (Franks et al, 1989; Kumar, 2005). Thus, PCOS is a multifaceted disease caused due to genetic predisposition, raised insulin levels, strong stimulation in adrenals during childhood, hormonal imbalance, oxidative stress (Samer et al, 2016; Howkins & Bourne, 1999). With a multifactorial pathophysiology, the syndrome exhibits the effect of genetic, fetal, metabolic and environmental factors. The intensity of each factor decides the clinical and subclinical character with different therapeutic response (Elham, 2018). Careful physical examination and collection of history of the patient is required to ensure appropriate diagnosis, treatment (Tracy, 2016) and management of PCOS.

TREATMENT AND MANAGEMENT

As the primary cause of the syndrome is unknown, treatment is usually directed at the symptoms (Uche et al., 2013).The heterogeneity in PCOS phenotypes needs to be considered for therapeutic management and hence, careful individualized approach is essential to monitor females throughout their life (Gerard et al., 2014). It is suggested that the treatment for PCOS be individualized based on the patient's presentation and wish for pregnancy (Tracy et al., 2016). Table 2 illustrates the course of action generally performed when a case of PCOS is suspected in a female patient.

Table 2. Course of actions generally performed on PCOS patient

<table>
<tr><th colspan="3">Suspected PCOS Case</th></tr>
<tr><th>Perform</th><th>Reason</th><th>Rule out factors before confirming diagnosis</th></tr>
<tr><td>Complete medical history</td><td rowspan="2">To know about:
· Unexplained weight gain
· Menstrual cycle abnormalities
· hirsutism
· Skin changes
· Elevated blood pressure</td><td rowspan="4">· Adrenal hyperplasia
· Cushing's syndrome
· Hyperprolactinemia</td></tr>
<tr><td>Physical examination</td></tr>
<tr><td>Blood tests</td><td>To assess levels of:
· Hormones
· Glucose
· Lipid</td></tr>
<tr><td>Pelvic ultrasound</td><td>To scan ovarian cysts</td></tr>
</table>

(Adapted from NIH pub, 2008; Azziz et al., 2006; Lee & Rausch, 2012; Uche et al., 2013;Ahmed, 2016)

The management of androgen-related symptoms, menstruation related disorders, and infertility treatment is important (Susan & Kristen, 2014). The symptoms can be effectively managed with dietary modifications coupled with increase in physical activity (Patel, 2018).It is also noted that the effective-

Table 3. Treatment Approaches for PCOS

<table>
<tr><th>Pharmacological Approaches</th><th>Non-pharmacological Approaches</th></tr>
<tr><td>Anovulation
· Clomiphene
· Antidiabetic agents
· Gonadotropins
· Aromatase inhibitors</td><td rowspan="3">· Weight reduction for overweight patients
· Laparoscopic ovarian drilling</td></tr>
<tr><td>Androgenic Symptoms
· Antiandrogens
· Oral contraceptives</td></tr>
<tr><td>Other Therapies
· Medroxyprogesterone acetate
· Statins</td></tr>
</table>

(Adapted from Uche et al., 2013)

ness depends on the self-motivation of the patient to follow a diet and exercise pattern as routine. Table 3 depicts the approaches for treatment of the syndrome.

Overweight patients should be assessed for signs and symptoms of obstructive sleep apnea and also it is essential that patients should be screened for depression (Tracy et al., 2016). Currently, the treatment for PCOS ranges from lifestyle modification to pharmacological interventions (Harrison et al., 2011). Life style changes made to improve insulin sensitivity is essential in the management of PCOS (Norman et al., 2002). Studies have tried to establish the role of exercise in the treatment of obese PCOS patients (Bruner et al., 2006) and it has been observed that effective treatment in terms of lifestyle modification is weight reduction for overweight females (Harrison et al., 2011).

A Dietary pattern containing a carbohydrate diet that is rich in fibre sourced from healthy choices made from whole grains, legumes, vegetables and fruits is favorable for PCOS females (Zeinab et al., 2017). A diet therapy containing high carbohydrate of about 55% calories, low fat i.e. 30% of calories and an average protein of about 15% calories coupled with physical activity is recommended for PCOS females (Moran et al., 2008). Weight reduction in both overweight and obese PCOS females is known to cause ovulation. Thus, lifestyle changes with respect to increasing physical activity coupled with dietary modifications should be considered as a treatment choice for PCOS females (Moran et al., 2009; Thesssaloniki ESHRE/ASRM workshop, 2008). Table -4 illustrates management of PCOS.

DRAWBACKS OF CONVENTIONAL TREATMENT

Oral contraceptive pills, anti-androgens namely cyproterone acetate, spironolactone or flutamide, progestins like medroxyprogesterone acetate, insulin sensitizing drugs like metformin, clomiphene, are some of the medical treatment options for PCOS. These are known to have side effects of its own. oral contraceptive administered may have a negative effect on the metabolic aberrations of PCOS (Bargiota 2012); fluid retention, weight gain, as well as liver dysfunction and depression is associated with progestin used in the treatment (Romm, 2010); gastrointestinal disturbance and in rare incidence where complications of renal impairment as well as lactic acidosis has been identified with Insulin sensitizing drugs (Teede at al.2007); therapeutic intervention with statins in PCOS treatment to reduce hyperandrogenism as well as improve the lipid levels does have promising use however, more investigation is required to determine if

Table 4. Management of PCOS

Condition of Patient	Management	Purpose	Actions
Overweight & obese PCOS	-Diet regulation	Weight reduction -restore normal ovulation -menstruation Vitamin D -synthesize hormones of the adrenal cortex	Low-carbohydrate diet, Regular exercise Treating vitamin D deficiency
	-Medications	-Reduce insulin resistance -Improve insulin sensitivity	Metformin and Thiazolidinedione (Metformin – to women with PCOS and BMI above 25, when other therapy fails to produce results)
Infertility (due to PCOS)	-Diet -Medications -Procedures	Promote ovulation -Treat anovulation or infrequent ovulation -Aid in child bearing	Overweight anovulatory women with PCOS- weight loss and dietary modifications Clomiphene citrate and FSH-promote ovulation For non-responsive patients- Assisted reproductive technology procedures -controlled ovarian hyper-stimulation with FSH injections, In- vitro fertilization (IVF), laparoscopic procedure, ovarian drilling
Hirsutism and acne in PCOS	-Medications -Other treatments	Block action of androgens -reduce acne -reduce unwanted facial and body hair growth	Contraceptive pills- Cyproterone acetate Flutamide, Spironolactone, Metformin-reduce hirsutism Eflornithine cream-inhibit hair growth Bromocriptine -Acne Finasteride and Dutasteride (acne and control hair growth) Removal of facial, hair, electrolysis or laser treatments
Menstrual irregularity and endometrial hyperplasia in PCOS	Medications	-Convenience and sense of well-being -Conception in women who want to get pregnant	-Oral Progestogen -Progestin implant

(Adapted from Ahmed MK, 2016)

it can clinically impact PCOS females in long term especially young females and who may not require treatment with statin (Lisa et al, 2016).

In the treatment of PCOS, the short-term cosmetic and reproductive consequences is often focused while metabolic and psychological risks are usually not considered (Dinka et al., 2015). When viewed from the patient's perspective, the treatment possess psychological burden coupled with physical distress and side effect of drugs. The treatment for PCOS is usually associated with considerable cost and has been known to cause different side effects (Nowak et al, 2007). Available data estimates $4 billion annual cost for identification and management of this endocrinal disorder in USA (Azziz et al., 2005) and $400 million per year in Australia (Nirav, 2017). Due to the financial burden as well as physical and emotional distress of treatment regimens, patients are usually inclined to follow alternative therapies for treatment of PCOS.

HERBAL MEDICINE AS ALTERNATIVE THERAPY FOR PCOS

Complementary medicine has been used to improve health of females with PCOS (Arentz et al., 2014). Many medicinal plants studied are known to contain active compounds and have attracted much attention in the recent years to treat the syndrome as they have no major adverse effects (Zahra et al., 2018). Experimental studies on animals as well as human beings and many detailed review articles on these experimental works (Bhuvaneshwari et al.,2015; Ahmadi & Mostafavi, 2015; Hossein et al, 2015; Radha et al., 2016; Jelodar & Askari, 2012; Kashani and Akhondzadeh, 2016; Pachiappan et al., 2017; Nava et al, 2019) have shown beneficial effects of herbal medicine. No major adverse effects have been found in medicinal plants with active compounds hence, phytotherapy as an alternative treatment can be considered instead of chemical drugs which has several side effects (Ahmed, B & Abubaker, E, 2011).

Ayurveda, practiced in India, Traditional Arabic medicines, Traditional Chinese medicines and Korean Herbal medicines are all known to use herbal plants for treating various diseases and disorders including PCOS. Some of the published research articles on traditional herbal medicines and its effects on PCOS has been reviewed below

Although many of these herbs are known to have potential effects in reproductive endocrinology in PCOS, they do lack data on mechanism of effects for whole herbal extract. The information on herbs with known effects as well as some of the herbs with effects and mechanism of action are provided below. Some herbs finds its use traditionally in more than one country/region, in order to avoid repetition it has been included only once in the list.

Ayurveda

Originated in South Asia, Ayurveda means 'Knowledge of the life' and is being practiced for thousands of years in India. It has been recognized as a medical science equivalent to traditional Chinese medicine. (Witt et al, 2013; WHO Report, 2003; WHO Report, 2002; Kessler &Wirksamkeit,2017). Many herbs have been used for effective treatment of PCOS and they are known to have multi-potential effects on oligo/ amenorrhea treatment, hyperandrogenism, insulin resistance and also obesity (Pachiappan et al., 2017). Some of the available data on medicinal herbs used in Ayurveda for PCOS treatment is highlighted below.

Tribulus terrestris: (Puncture Vine), belongs to family Zygophyllaceae, is known to have beneficial effects in PCOS. Random control trials (RCT's) on effect of herb on rats with PCOS that were induced with oestradiol valerate showed improved ovulation rates compared to control.(Dehghan et al,2012; Esfandiari et al,2011). The ethanol extract of herb showed increased FSH levels in healthy women (Milanov et al,1981). Another study showed equivalence for ovulation induction for herb and Clomiphene for females with oligomenorrhea and anovulation caused infertility (Tabakova et al,1984). The aerial part and the fruit of *Tribulus terrestris* had been known to promote regular ovulation. This may reduce ovarian cyst in women with PCOS. (Amrin et al, 2016).

*Vitex agnus-castus: (*Chasetree), belongs to family Lamiaceae, an herb known to be in use since 2000yrs for the treatment of infertility and also menstrual irregularities. (Bergmann, et al, 2000; Shahnazi et al, 2016). It is known to be used in Ayurvedic treatment as well as in other traditional treatments around the world. A recent study on the herb extract on PCOS complications in experimental rat model revealed the potential ameliorative effects (Hamza et al,2019). Pre-clinical as well as clinical evidences was found for ethanol extracts of Vitex agnus-castus for infertility treatment, improving menstrual regularity as well as lowering prolactin levels (Arentz et al., 2014)). Results of a study has found similar effects of low dose estrogen and the herb on normalizing menstrual cycle in PCOS women (Shahnazi, et al, 2016). Therapeutically it is used for its dopamegic effects and in the treatment of latent hyperprolactinemia, corpus luteal insufficiency and pre-menstrual syndrome (Mills and Bone 2013). The herb is known to contain variety of compounds that bind receptors in brain (dopamine type 2 receptors), reduce cyclic adenosine mono phosphate and lower the secretion of prolactin (Arentz et al., 2014).

Withania somnifera: (Ashwagandha) also known as "Indian Ginseng" belongs to family Solanaceae. It is used for millennia in Ayurveda as a Rasayana- an herbal or metallic preparation that promotes physical and mental health. It is commonly available in powder form called churna, which is mixed with water, clarified butter or honey before consumption. It is known to promote reproductive health and maintain balance (Changhadi, 1938). Active compounds of herb includes alkaloids like anahygrine, cuseohygrine, isopelletierine etc, and saponins. Sitoindosides VII-X and Withaferin-A, these have significant anti-stress activity (Mishra, 2000 et al., 2000; Bhattacharya et al, 1987). The root of this herb is known to support overall functions of the endocrine system, It finds its use in the treatment of infertily in females. (Amrin et al, 2016).

Cinnamomum zeylanicum: (Cinnamon), of family Lauraceae, has been reported in both in vitro and in vivo studies to reduce the insulin resistance. In the insulin signaling pathway, it is known to increase the phosphatidylinositol 3-kinase activity thus potentiating insulin action. A human study on this herb shows improved insulin sensitivity in women with PCOS (Wang GJ etal,2007).

Ocimum tenuiflorum. L: (Holy Basil), commonly known as Tulsi in India belongs to family Lamiaceae. It is known to be an excellent antioxidant (Shantaram et al, 2019), has anti-androgenic properties and hence is effective in the management of PCOS. It also finds its use in treating multiple ailments and in management of obesity and related co-morbidities. (Shantaram et al, 2019; Pachiappan et al., 2017; Swayamjeet Satapathy et al, 2017).

Taraxacum officinale: (Dandelion Root), belong to family Asteraceae, has hepatoprotective properties, stimulates bile flow and detoxifies liver. In Ayurvedic treatment it is used in cleansing process of liver to get rid of build-up hormones and this clean up stimulates the production of Sex hormone binding globulin (SHBG) which reduces free testosterone levels (Cai L et al, 2017; Pachiappan et al., 2017)

Cimicifuga racemosa: known as Black Cohosh Root, belongs to family Ranunculaceae contains phytochemicals and suppresses the LH secretion. Black cohosh is known to be very effective for PMS, excessive menstrual cramps and hormone related symptoms (Dehghan et al, 2012). The herb was known to reduce LH in cell cultures from ovariectomised rats in laboratory studies (Düker et al 1991;Seidlova-Wuttke et al, 2003). Estrogen inhibition following selective binding of receptors of estrogen on the pitutary and hypothalamus is the known mechanism of action (Seidlova-Wuttke et al, 2003). Significant effects on reduced LH for PCOS women receiving the herb extract compared to clomiphene was observed in a randomized control study projecting the beneficial effect of the herb. (Kamel, 2013)

Trigonella foenumgraceum L: (Fenugreek), belongs to family Leguminosae, its seeds extract is successfully used in lowering blood glucose levels. In a study, PCOS women were given *Trigonella foenumgraceum* seed capsule along with metformin for eight weeks and the results showed improved insulin sensitivity as well as improved ultrasound results. Improvement in menstrual cycle and decrease in the polycystic ovaries in ultrasound scans was also reported (Bashtian, et al, 2013). However, there are no reports on fenugreek's effect on hormonal levels related to LH, FSH or free testosterone levels.

Asparagus Racemosus: (Shatavari), belongs to Asparagaceae, is known to have pharmacological effects, contains phytoestrogen which helps revitalize reproductive system, promote normal development of female ovarian follicles and regulate the menstrual cycle. (Pachiappan et al., 2017; Kumar et al, 2008)

Tinospora Cordifolia: (Guduchi), belongs to family Menispermaceae. It was used as one of the herb successfully used along with combination of herbs used in a study that was conducted to find out the clinical efficacy of Ayurveda treatment regimen on PCOS and subfertility (Siriwardene et al, 2010). It is known to exert hypoglycemic effect and has anti-inflammatory property. It revitalizes and boosts body's metabolism naturally (Chandrasekaran et al,2012; Pachiappan et al., 2017).

Lepidium meyenii: (Maca), belongs to Brassicaceae family, is known have fertility benefits and acts without any side effects. It is known to increase the serum levels of LH in female experimental rats (Fumiaki et al, 2013). Being a natural hormonal balancer, this herb stimulates the endocrine system (Gonzales etal, 2002).

Combination of Herbs: In a study on effect of combination of herbs namely *Tribulus terrestris Linn* and *Withania somnifera Dunalon* on letrozole induced PCOS rats were tested. Roots of Withania somnifera and fruits of Tribulus terrestris used as hydro alcoholic extract and results showed significant recovery of hormones LH and FSH along with testosterone and estradiole levels in serum. It also had anti androgenic effects as it was able to reduce the elevated testosterone levels and prevented the ovarian dysfunction. These observed properties of the test drugs may be due to the presence of phytoestrogens in the extract (Amrin et al, 2016)

Mohammed et al, 2019, tested a polyherbal formulation ("DXB-2030") consisting of combination of herbs namely, *Trigonella foenum-graecum* (used as insulin sensitizer in DM and in female reproductive disorders), *Aloe vera* (controls hyperglycemic conditions, modulates steroidogenesis), *Sphaeranthus indicus* (anticonvulsant activities, anxiolytic, central nervous system depressant), *Nardostachys jatamansi* (used in stress management), and *Symplocos racemosa* (used in menorrhagia and other female reproductive dysfunctions) and evaluated recently, for its effects on PCOS associated with hyperandrogenism in the experimental model of testosterone propionate induced PCOS female rats.. The active compounds in the formulations are known to be flavonoids, saponins, volatile oil, alkaloids, and polyphenols. The study findings revealed that the formulation reversed the pathophysiological changes due to administration of testosterone propionate in immature rats and the effect was related to synergistic effect of each individual herb used in the formulation. Herbs reversed the estrus cyclicity, reduced the volume of ovary and cyst size, decreased testosterone levels, showed anti androgenic effect and also restored the histology of ovarian tissue of female rats. The study concluded recommending further clinical studies to confirm the effects and mechanism of action of the formulation

Traditional Arabic Herbal Medicines

Despite the advances in modern medicine, traditional Arabic herbal medicine has always been practiced by people. There are many herbs which are known for their traditional medicinal use in Arab countries and available studies suggests effects and mechanism of actions for some as discussed below:

Traditional Persian Medicine

Traditional Persian medicine (TPM) uses different medicinal plants to treat oligomenorrhea and amenorrhea. In a recent study, five herbs namely *Foeniculum vulgare, Vitex agnus-castus,, Paeonia lactiflora, Mentha longifolia and, Sesamum indicum* L., were strongly suggested in TPM and also these herbs were proven effective in the conventional medicine references. (Arezoo et al, 2018).

1. *Foeniculum vulgare*: *(*Fennel), belongs to family Apiaceae, is an aromatic plant with medicinal value with estrogenic effect. Phenolic compounds extracted from *Foeniculum vulgare* are considered to have antioxidant activity. (Manzoor et al,2016). A study results reported that fennel and low-dose combined oral contraceptive can resolve depot medroxyprogesterone acetate induced amenorrhea (Mohebbi-Kian et al,2014). It is known as Shatapushpa and finds its use in Ayurvedic treatment also, for the management of PCOS. The seeds are known to be rich in phytoestrogens and helps in reducing insulin resistance and also known to reduce the cellular imbalance that leads to metabolic disturbances in PCOS. (Jungbauer etal, 2014).
2. *Paeonia lactiflora:* (Chinese peony), belongs to family Paeoniaceae, is known to be in use in Japan. China, Korea as well as in Iran for around 1200 years (Shirazi & Makhzan al-adviyah, 2019). In china, Korea and Japan, the dried root without the bark is used in the form of a decoction to treat dysmenorrhea, rheumatoid arthritis and many other conditions. The total glucosides of peony (TGP) which is the water/ ethanol extract of roots, contains more than 15 components which includes oxybenzoyl-paeoniflorin, galloylpaeoniflorin, paeonolide, paeonol, albiflorin, benzoylpaeoniflorin, paeoniflorin, oxypaeoniflorin, lactiflorin, paeonin and paeoniflorigenone (Dong-Yi & Sheng-Ming, 2011). It has been used in combination with *Glycyrrhiza glabra* for the treatment of PCOS details of which has been given under combination of herbs.
3. *Mentha longifolia: (*wild mint), member of family Lamiaceae, this herb is used in Iran and many other countries as traditional medicine is known to have many pharmacological and therapeutic effects (Peyman et al, 2013). The extract of *Mentha longifolia* is shown to regulate menstrual cycle (Mokaberinejad et al, 2012), and decrease FSH and induce menstruation in females with primary ovarian failure. (Mokaberinejad et al, 2014)
4. *Sesamum indicum L:* (Sesame), a flowering plant belonging to family Pedaliaceae, has been used in TPM as well as in Ayurveda to induce menstrual bleeding and to treat many other conditions (104-34). It is known to induce menstruation without any known side effects with females who have severe oligomenorrhea (Yavari et al, 2016; Yavari et al, 2014)

Herbal teas have been known to be beneficial in the management of PCOS and is used in many countries. Green tea, Marjoram tea, spearmint tea, and Mountain tea have been shown to have effects on PCOS.

*Origanum majorana: (*Marjoram), from family Lamiaceae, is known to have citrus flavor known for its traditional use in Iran and Jordon (Mitra K etal, 2017). It has antifungal and antibacterial activities, is an antioxidant, known to be cardio and hepato protective, and also anti-inflammatory, anticoagulant, antiulcer properties. Some of the active compounds found in herb are known to be flavonoids namely kaempferol, apigenin, quercetin hesperetin; phenolic glycosides – arbutin; monoterpene hydrocarbons like α-pinene, β-pinene,, γ-terpinene and camphene; as well as oxygenated monoterpenes namely terpineol, terpinene-4-ol, *cis*-sabinene hydrate (Fatemeh & Roja, 2017). A randomized clinical trial (RCT) on patients receiving sweet marjoram tea showed significant reduction in dehydroepiandrosterone-S

DHEA-S and fasting insulin levels. But the patients had side effects namely bloating, nausea, mild sedation (Haj-Husein et al, 2015). It is known to improve insulin sensitivity, in studies using Ethanol extracts of herb, it was found to activate the peroxisome proliferator-activated receptors (PPAR) (Rau et al,2006; Bhatia& Viswanathan, 2006).

Mentha spicata: (Mint), also known as spearmint belongs to family Lamiaceae, is commonly used in the Middle East to treat hirsutism. In the past years many biologically active compounds have been identified and two chemicals namely menthol and carvone are the major constituents in Mentha spicata along with 28 other compounds which includes limonene 1, 8-cineole, isomenthone and menthone (Bharat et al, 2009; Mitra et al,2017). Results of a RCT on spearmint tea has shown no side effects and the results revealed a significant decrease in total and free testosterone levels, rise in LH and FSH levels and also decrease hirsutism level (Grant P, 2010). A study finding on the essential oil of spearmint and its effect on PCOS in rats revealed that the essential oil increased Graafian follicles, reduced ovarian cysts aprt from reducing the weight of the body of PCOS rats and the levels of testosterone thus, showing potential on PCOS treatment (Mahmood et al, 2017).

Stachys lavandulifolia: (Mountain tea) belongs to family Lamiaceae, is known to have traditional use in Iran. It has anti-inflammatory effects and estrogenic properties (Mitra et al,2017). It is known to contain biologically active components like flavonoids, phenylethanoid and also terpenoid. (Mitra et al,2017). The herb is also regarded for its antimicrobial, antioxidant effects and finds it use in dysmenorrhea. (Pirbalouti &Mohammadi, 2013; Asadi & Bahrami,2010; Mitra et al,2017). RCT on the herb reveals that it may be used as an alternative for medroxy-progesterone acetate to manage the abnormal uterine bleeding in PCOS women.(Jalilian et al, 2013).

Camellia Sinensis: (Green Tea), belongs to family Theaceae, known to be traditionally used in India, China, Thailand and Japan (Chopade et al, 2008).It finds its use in Traditional Iranian medicine too. Green tea consumption resulted in decreased fasting insulin levels, weight loss and also showed decrease in free testosterone levels in PCOS women with overweight and obesity (Baker et al, 2013). It has positive affect on endocrine system as well as glucose and lipid metabolism as revealed through research study. In rats the herb was able to show reduced serum testesteron levels, weight, estradiol and leptin. Reduced LH, cholesterol and TG and also insulin and glucose levels. (Basu et al, 2011) . Anti-androgenic effects of green tea has been associated with Epigallocatechin-3-gallate (EGCG), the component of green tea, and 5α-reductase inhibitor. (Grant & Ramasamy, 2012)

Combination of Herbs: *Glycyrrhiza uralensis* and *Paeonia lactiflora*: combination of these herbs has shown significant reductions in the free and total testosterone levels in animals and clinical trials in PCOS females. (Takeuchi et al, 1989; Takahashi& Kitao,1994). Paeonia lactiflora in combination with Glycyrrhiza spp in aqueous extract (TJ-68) had been shown to reduce LH (Takeuchi et al, 1989), LH:FSH ratio (Takahashi& Kitao,1994) and showed improvement in ovulation in females with PCOS (Yaginuma et al, 1982).

Paeonia lactiflora and Cinnamomum cassia: herbal combination in aqueous extract Unkei-to investigated for steroid hormonal effects on cultured human granulosa cells from IVF treatment women, showed increased granulosa production of progesterone and oestradiol (Sun et al,2004). Clinical trial of these two herbs on females with oligo/amenorrhoea resulted in decreased LH and also improved ovulation rates (Ushiroyama et al, 2001)

A current study on herbal remedies for infertility in males and females has furnished information on herbal medicines obtained from 51 traditional healers from areas of nine regions of West Bank/ Palestine. Information on names of plants, and its parts used as well as modes (powders, infusion, paste, decoctions) and methods of preparation has been furnished (Nidal& Abdel, 2019). According to the study, the most common herbal medicine used for female infertility were:

*Ceratonia siliqua: (*Carob), belongs to Fabaceae, known to have phytoestrogens (Abdullatif et al, 2017). Its pollen grains (powder) is known to find its use in female infertility (Nidal& Abdel, 2019). A study on the effect of Carob male flower showed significant effect on ovulation in mice (Abdullatif et al, 2017).

*Anastatica hierochuntica: (*Mary's flower*)* belongs to family Brassicaceae. Its fruits infusion is known to have an effect on female infertility (Nidal& Abdel, 2019). Aqueous extract on female mice *showed* significant effect on levels of Luetinizing harmone, FSH compared to control (Baker et al, 2013).

Parietaria Judaica: (spreading pellitory), belongs to family Urticaceae. The decoction of leaves are known to have beneficial effect on female infertility (Nidal& Abdel, 2019).

More scientific evidences and studies are required to establish facts on effects and mechanism of action of these herbs.

Traditional Chinese Medicine

According to results of a recently published study, 89.22% PCOS patients had a relatively high tendency to consult Traditional Chinese Medicine (TCM) practitioners in Taiwan. TCM is known for treating gynecological problems in women and also for infertility ((Wan-Ting ey al, 2018).). Chinese herbal medicine has been studied and identified to improve ovulation rates as well as menstrual health of females (Ried, 2015). Acupuncture in TCM is confirmed to restore balance between Yin and Yang which according to western Medicine is to restore the equilibrium between parasympathetic and sympathetic activity [Takahashi, 2011]. Animal study on combination treatment with Chinese medicinal herbs and acupuncture on PCOS revealed the beneficial effects of herbs on the treatment and also projected the positive effect of acupuncture on the absorption of herbal extracts used for treatment (Ma R.J et al, 2011).

In TCM, single herbs as well as combinations of different herbs have been known to be effective in the treatment of PCOS. Both of these have been included here.

The most commonly used single herbs for the PCOS treatment are found to be:

1. *Cyperi Rhizoma (Xiang Fu):* most commonly prescribed herb for PCOS treatment (Wan-Ting et al, 2018). The pharmacological effects known for this herb are anti-androgenic, anti-diabetic, anti-lipidemic, anti-obesity, and weight-control effects in obese patients which may help its use in the treatment of PCOS. (Pirzada et al, 2015; Lemaure et al, 2007). According to reports available, it is known to exhibit antidepressant activity in the forced swimming test in experimental animal models (Kim et al, 2015).
2. *Radix Salvia Miltiorrhiza (Dan-Shen*): It is an herb obtained from dried roots of Salvia miltiorrhiza Bunge, known to regulate menstruation. (Yen-Nung et al, 2018), Tannshinone is identified as the main ingredient of Salvia miltiorrhiza Bunge. (Xia Y et al, 2017). Salvia miltiorrhiza Bunge used widely in china and other Asian countries to treat cardio vascular diseases.(Wang et al, 2017), and this may have beneficial effects in decreasing level of androgen, lowering total cholesterol and triglycerides and also increasing the levels of HDL in PCOS females.(Zhang et al, 2015)
3. *Coptidis Rhizoma (Huang Lian):* it originates from dried roots of *Coptis chinensis Franch.* Its known effects on the body according to principles of TCM is clearing heat, eliminating dampness and induce detoxification. (Yen-Nung et al, 2018). Berberine, are derived from this herb (Ong et al, 2017). Studies have shown that berberine is a potent oral hypoglycemic agent with modest ef-

fect on lipid metabolism. It regulates glucose and lipid metabolism both in vitro and in vivo (Jun Yin et al, 2008). Berberine when compared with metformin, has shown to increase live birth rate with less gastrointestinal adverse effects in PCOS patients undergoing IVF treatments (An Y et al, 2014).

4. *Leonurus (Yi-Mu-Cao):* known as Chinese Motherwort, promotes blood flow and can be used to regulate menstrual disorders. Reports on treatment with motherwort extract SCM-198 (4-guanidino-n-butyl syringate) has shown to cause a decrease in fasting blood glucose (FBS) levels and plasma triacylglycerol levels (TG) and also an increase in High density lipoprotein (HDL) levels and plasma insulin concentrations. It is known to exhibit anti-inflammatory activity and have an ameliorating effect on symptoms of diabetes through inhibition of the nuclear factor-kB /IkB kinase pathway [Huang et al,2012].

Other herbs namely, Corydalis yanhusuo W. T. Wang known as,Yan-Hu-Suo in Chinese is known for treating dysmenorrhea and is known to have analgesic effects in humans. (Yuan et al, 2004; Chen et al, 2014). *Rheum officinale* Baill (Chinese rhubarb) Da-Huang, in Chinese is a common traditional medicine known for its pharmacological activities. It contains Emodin, which is proposed as a possible treatment for Type2 DM and other metabolic disorders (Wan-Ting et al, 2018).

Some of the other common single Chinese herbs known to be popularly used TCM for treatment of PCOS are Gan-Cao (Glycyrrhiza uralensis Fisch.), Tu-Si-Zi (Cuscuta chinensis Lam.), Huang-Qin (Scutellaria baicalensis Georgi), Bei-Mu (Fritillaria thunbergii Miq.) and, Du-Zhong (Eucommia ulmoides Oliv) (Wan-Ting et al, 2018).

Herbal formulations used are: Gui-Zhi-Fu-Ling-Wan, known to rejuvenate blood, transform blood stasis, improve glucose tolerance (Scheidt et al, 2009; Nakagawa et al, 2008) and Dang-Gui-Shao-Yao-San used in treating dysmenorrhea and abdominal pain,(Wan-Ting et al, 2018). Table.5 shows some of the common Chinese herbal formulations and its effects on PCOS.

Korean Herbal Medicine Therapy

Korean medicine clinics have treated PCOS with herbal remedies and lifestyle management using Korean herbal medicine therapy (KHM). A case report published on an obese –type woman with PCOS revealed effectiveness of KHM (Ji Hyeon & Junyoung, 2017). According to the study, the patient received two courses of therapy, of five and two months duration, respectively with a daily dose and KHM, a decoction made out of *Coicis Semen* (coix seed), *Rehmanniae Radix, Citri Unshius Pericarpium, Poria, Dioscoreae Rhizoma, Radix Angelicae, Ephedrae Herba, Cnidii Rhizoma, Astragali Radix, Acanthopanacis Cortex, Glycyrrhizae Radix et Rhizoma, Foeniculi Fruct, Magnoliae Cortex, Coptidis Rhizoma, Cyperi Rhizoma* and *Gardeniae Fructus*, administered three times a day before each meal with no other conventional treatment. The results revealed that KHM coupled with lifestyle management was able to normalize both reproductive hormone and menstrual cycle of the patient.

Panax ginseng and *Glycyrrhizae radix et rhizome* have been used in the treatment of PCOS. *Panax ginseng*: (Korean ginseng) known as "the king of herbs", belongs to family Araliaceae. It has been in use in oriental countries since more than two thousand years. It has been known to have various pharmacological properties (Cho, 2012; Kim et al, 2018). The herb can significantly increase serum estradiol and reduced FSH as well as LH levels (Xu Y et al, 2014).Used as a natural estrogen replacement therapy, its extracts are known to activate growth of estrogen receptor positive cells in vitro. Ginsenoside Rb1 and

Table 5. Some Chinese herbal formulations used in the treatment of PCOS

Herbal formulations	Herb combination	Effects	Ref
Jia-Wei-Xiao-Yao-San/Dan-Zhi-Xiao-Yao-San	· *Moutan Radicis Cortex* · *Radix Paeoniae Rubra* · *Bupleuri Radix,* · *Angelicae Sinensis Radix* · *Poria, Glycyrrhizae Radix* · *Atractylodes Ovatae Rhizoma* · *Zingiberis Rhizoma Recens* · *Menthae Herba*	-Disperses stagnated liver qi -Suppresses heat, nourishes blood. -Danzhi xiaoyao pill In anovulation infertility: -improved ovulation and pregnancy rates	Yen-Nung et al, 2018; Liu, 2013; Chen,2015.
Wen-Jing-Tang	· *Cinnamomi Ramulus* · *Evodiae Fructus* · *Ligustici Rhizoma* · *Angelicae sinensis Radix* · *Paeoniae Radix* · *Ginseng Radix* · *Glycyrrhizae Radix* · *Zingiberis Rhizoma Recens* · *Moutan Radicis Cortex Ophiopogonis Tuber* · *Pinelliae Tuber* · *Asini Corii Gelatinum*	-Promote blood circulation -Regulating endocrine conditions	Yen-Nung et al, 2018; Ushiroyama et al, 2006; Tang et al, 2006.
Cang-Fu-Dao-Tan-Wan	· *Atractylodes Lanceae Rhizoma* · *Cyperi Rhizoma, Pinelliae Rhizoma* · *Citri Reticulata Pericarpium* · *Poria* · *Citrus aurantium L* · *Glycyrrhiza Radix* · *Arisaema heterophyllum Bl.*	-Improve PCOS symptoms -Increase ovarian artery blood flow -Lower FSH and LH	Yen-Nung et al, 2018; Hong & Sun, 2016.

Rg1 is reported to stimulate ERs with estrogen-like activity (Ding et al, 2015; Cho et al, 2004; Wu et al, 2012). A Current research on potential of KRG extract in water (Korea Ginseng Corporation, Daejeon, Korea) using dehydroepiandrosterone (DHEA)- mediated rat model showed that the extract could prevent DHEA induced PCOS through its antioxidant and anti-inflammatory activities (Choi JH et al, 2019).

Glycyrrhizae radix et rhizome (Licorice), in Korean medicinal formula is used for its potential effects in metabolic and reproductive diseases. Recent study on rat model of PCOS suggested that the ethanol extract of Licorice was successful in regulating imbalances in hormonal levels and was able to control levels of FSH, LH/FSH ratio in serum, and irregular ovarian follicular phase as well as abnormal changes in the rat's administered with sustained release letrozole pellets (*Hyun et al, 2018*)

Some Herbs and its Side Effects in PCOS Treatment

Herbs namely *Urtica Dioica, Cimicifuga racemosa, Trifolium pretense* are known to have beneficial effects in the treatment of PCOS however, they are also known to have side effects as mentioned below:

Urtica Dioica: (Stinging Nettle), belongs to family Urticaceae, and the root of this herb is known to produce SHBG and help in normalizing the hormone level. However, long term use can result in lowering the blood pressure and if a patient is on hypertensive medicine or on diuretics, it can lead to further complications (Shantaram et al, 2019).

Cimicifuga racemosa: (Black Cohosh Root), member of family Ranunculaceae, has an effect on endocrine system, and is known to contain phytochemicals that can suppress LH secretion. But it has been associated with liver disease/complications, gastro intestinal issues, weight gain, vaginal spotting etc., to name a few (Shantaram et al, 2019).

Trifolium pretense: (Red Clover),belongs to family Fabaceae, contains phytoestrogens and finds its use in purifying blood and treating acne in PCOS females. Side effects of this herb includes vaginal bleeding, headache, rashes, muscle ache, nausea. This herb usage is to be avoided by pregnant and lactating women, patients with breast or ovarian cancer, endometriosis and in patients with conditions of bleeding disorders. (Shantaram et al, 2019)

Concerns about Herbal Medicine Usage

Practice of traditional herbal medicine is based on beliefs and knowledge about herbs and not scientific evidences (Davyson et al, 2014).The quality issue categories are external issues, which are contamination of herbal medicine, adulteration and misidentification; while the ingredient non-uniformity and complexity in herbal medicine are regarded as internal issues (Dilip, 2018). Herbal medicines contain active pharmacological components as well as minerals and trace metals (Rania et al, 2015). Lack of proper standardization of herbal preparation results in inferior quality. This is turn leads to side effects and complications. The metal content present and toxicity associated with it is a public health problem. A study result on 252 herbal Ayurveda samples revealed that 65% had lead, 38% had mercury and 32% arsenic. The study also found that mercury, lead and arsenic exceeded the pharmaceutical impurities' recommended daily intake value by up to several thousand times in some of the herbal samples (Marek et al, 2017).

Another aspect in complementary medicines to be noted is that the benefit-risk assessment is difficult due to lack of information. (Joanne, 2003). Data for mechanism of action of many herbs is unavailable The data are generally lacking on various other information related to pharmacokinetics, pharmacology, toxicology, active constituents, metabolites, adverse effects, drug-herb interactions and also interaction with food and alcohol, safety of its use in specific disease group, elderly, pregnancy and lactating women (Joanne, 2003).

The herbal medicines are introduced without any mandatory safety or toxicological evaluation in many countries and the products are also available to consumers without prescription (Bandaranayake, 2006).) There is also a lack of consistent terminology for describing the herb (Rivera et al, 2013). Increasing popularity in over-the-counter herbal medications have increased the concern on safety and quality aspects of herbs and its use. Presence of heavy metals, microbial contaminants and banned pesticides as well as chemical toxins are a cause of concern (Chan, 2003). Short-term toxic effects of some herbal drugs are related to gastrointestinal disturbances and dermatological effects but some have also been associated with hepatotoxicity, nephrotoxicity and tumors with long –term use (Davyson et al, 2014).

STRATEGIES FOR SAFE USE

The plethora of problems associated with use of herbal medicine can be handled by strategies mentioned below:

1. Applying evidence-based herbal medicine knowledge into conventional health care practice, Good clinical practice (GCP)
2. Quality determined by modern science-based public monographs
3. Controlling environmental related factors by:
    - Implementing standard operating procedures (SOP)
    - Good agricultural and collection practices (GACP)
    - Good Laboratory practice (GLP) and safety determined by Hazard Analysis Critical Control Point (HACCP)
    - Good manufacturing practice (GMP), and regulations for the same.
    - Good supply practice (GSP)
4. Awareness and education on benefits as well as associated possible risks of herbs to both providers as well as patients
5. Understanding of claims made on herbal products
6. Purchasing herbs only from a reputed practitioner or provider /company.

(Rivera et al, 2013; Chan, 2003; Arnold et al, 2009; Luisa, 2005; Dilip, 2018; Marek et al, 2017).

CONCLUSION AND FUTURE IMPLICATIONS

PCOS is a multifaceted disease which involves, uncontrolled ovarian steroidogenesis, abnormal insulin signaling, coupled with oxidative stress, and genetic and or environmental factors (Samer et al, 2016). Herbal medicine have been used in treating many human ailments since thousands of years. They do contain constituents that have an effect on the female endocrinology (Ren et al., 2001; Grant & Ramasamy, 2012; Whitten & Naftolin, 1998) and many researchers have worked on beneficial effects of medicinal plants in the treatment of PCOS (Ainehchi et al., 2019; Grant P, 2010; Kort & Lobo, 2014; Hajimonfarednejad et al, 2018; Borzoei et al, 2018). Meta –analysis and studies on herbal medicines reveal that herbal medicine not just regularizes the reproductive function, but some also have an effect on decreasing the insulin resistance and abnormal lipid levels of patients thereby, assisting in the management of PCOS. (Nava et al, 2019 ; Susan et al., 2014).

Traditional herbal medicines used in India, Arab countries, China and Korea have shown promising use of herbs in the treatment of PCOS as discussed in the chapter. Although many herbs are available for treatment, there is a dearth of scientific evidences to prove mechanism of action for many. Controlled, randomized, double-blind, clinical studies along with case studies are required to understand the reproductive endocrinological effects, mechanism of actions of various herbs (Dilip, 2018; Susan et al, 2014). Herbal medicine's quality, efficacy and safety are of at most importance and this can be achieved provided there is a strong association and support between the drug regulatory authorities, industries that manufacture the herbal products and scientist who provide evidences (Kuruvilla, 2002).

Given the paramount importance of health of women in any country, effective management of PCOS becomes essential. This might become easier if future research focuses on the complexities of this endocrinal disorder for better understanding and management. Awareness about this multifaceted syndrome among young girls and women is important. Approaching a health care provider at the start of the symptoms of PCOS might help in the better management. Many herbal medicines have been used as an alternative medicine for their prominent positive effect on female reproductive system and available animal as well as human studies do show the potential use of herbal medicines in the treatment. There is a lot of scope for in depth research in this area to establish facts. Further research on the beneficial effects of herbal medicine might add on to the existing evidences and help herbal medicine establish a niche of its own in the successful treatment of the syndrome.

REFERENCES

Abbott, D. H., Dumesic, D. A., & Franks, S. (2002). Developmental origin of polycystic ovary syndrome - a hypothesis. *The Journal of Endocrinology*, *174*(1), 1–5. doi:10.1677/joe.0.1740001 PMID:12098657

Aggarwal & Kunnumakkara. (2009). Molecular Targets and Therapeutic Uses of Spices: Modern Uses for Ancient Medicine. World Scientific Publishing Co. Pte. Ltd.

Ahmadi, A., & Mostafavi, M. (2015). Study on the effects of licorice root hydroalcoholiclicorice extract on mice uterus histological structure and level of testosterone improvement with hyperandrogenism following experimental polycystic ovary syndrome. *Majallah-i Pizishki-i Urumiyyah*, *26*, 571–581.

Ahmed, B., & Abubaker, E. (2011). Treatment options for polycystic ovary syndrome. *International Journal of Women's Health*, *3*, 25–35. PMID:21339935

Ahmed, M. K. (2016). Polycystic Ovarian Syndrome: Insights into Pathogenesis, Diagnosis, Prognosis, Pharmacological and Non-Pharmacological Treatment. *Journal of Pharma Research*, *1*, 1.

Ainehchi, N., Khaki, A., Farshbaf-Khalili, A., Hammadeh, M., & Ouladsahebmadarek, E. (2019). The Effectiveness of Herbal Mixture Supplements with and without Clomiphene Citrate in Comparison to Clomiphene Citrate on Serum Antioxidants and Glycemic Biomarkers in Women with Polycystic Ovary Syndrome Willing to be Pregnant: A Randomized Clinical Trial. *Biomolecules*, *9*(6), E215. doi:10.3390/biom9060215 PMID:31163689

Amato, P., & Simpson, J. L. (2004). The genetics of polycystic ovary syndrome. *Best Practice & Research. Clinical Obstetrics & Gynaecology*, *18*(5), 707–718. doi:10.1016/j.bpobgyn.2004.05.002 PMID:15380142

An, Y., Sun, Z., Zhang, Y., Liu, B., Guan, Y., & Lu, M. (2014). The use of berberine for women with polycystic ovary syndrome undergoing IVF treatment. *Horumon To Rinsho*, *80*(3), 425–431. doi:10.1111/cen.12294 PMID:23869585

Anahita, J., Faezeh, K., Fatemeh, S., Kourosh, S., Zahra, K., & Malihe, A. (2015). Prevalence of polycystic ovary syndrome and its associated complications in Iranian women: A meta-analysis. *Iranian Journal of Reproductive Medicine*, *13*(10), 591–604. PMID:26644787

Arentz, S., Abbott, J. A., Smith, C. A., & Bensoussan, A. (2014). A survey of the use of complementary medicine by a self- selected community group of Australian women with polycystic ovary syndrome. *BMC Complementary and Alternative Medicine*, *14*(1), 472. doi:10.1186/1472-6882-14-472 PMID:25481654

Asadi, M., & Bahrami, S. (2010). The effect of stachys lavandulifolia Vahl. and mespilus germanica L. leaves hydroalcoholic extracts on leishmania major (MRHO/IR/75/ER) in vitro. *Jundishapur Journal of Natural Pharmaceutical Products*, *5*(1), 39–43.

Ataabadi, Alaee, Bagheri, & Bahmanpoor. (2017). Role of Essential Oil of Mentha Spicata (Spearmint) in Addressing Reverse Hormonal and Folliculogenesis Disturbances in a Polycystic Ovarian Syndrome in a Rat Model. *Adv Pharm Bull, 7*(4), 651-654.

Azab, A. (2017). Carob (Ceratonia siliqua): Health, Medicine And Chemistry. *European Chemical Bulletin, 6*(10), 456–469. doi:10.17628/ecb.2017.6.456-469

Azeemuddin, Anturlikar, Onkaramurthy, Baig, Ashok, Rao, Rafiq, & Rangesh. (2019). Effect of "DXB-2030," a Polyherbal Formulation, on Experimental Polycystic Ovary Syndrome Associated with Hyperandrogenism. *Advances in Pharmacological Sciences*. . doi:10.1155/2019/8272850

Azziz, R., Carmina, E., Dewailly, D., Diamanti-Kandarakis, E., Escobar-Morreale, H. F., Futterweit, W., Janssen, O. E., Legro, R. S., Norman, R. J., Taylor, A. E., & Witchel, S. F. (2006). Position statement: Criteria for defining polycystic ovary syndrome as a predominantly hyperandrogenic syndrome. An Androgen Excess Society guideline. *The Journal of Clinical Endocrinology and Metabolism, 91*(11), 4237–4245. doi:10.1210/jc.2006-0178 PMID:16940456

Azziz, R., Marin, C., Hoq, L., Badamgarav, E., & Song, P. (2005). Health care-related economic burden of the polycystic ovary syndrome during the reproductive life span. *The Journal of Clinical Endocrinology and Metabolism, 90*(8), 4650–4658. doi:10.1210/jc.2005-0628 PMID:15944216

Azziz, R., Nestler, J. E., & Dewailly, D. (2006). *Androgen excessdisorders in women: polycystic ovary syndrome and otherdisorders*. Humana Press.

Azziz, R., Woods, K. S., Reyna, R., Key, T. J., Knochenhauer, E. S., & Yildiz, B. O. (2004). The prevalence and features of the polycystic ovary syndrome in an unselected population. *The Journal of Clinical Endocrinology and Metabolism, 89*(6), 2745–2749. doi:10.1210/jc.2003-032046 PMID:15181052

Bahceci, M., Aydemir, M., & Tuzcu, A. (2007). Effects of oral fat and glucose Tolerance test on serum lipid profile, apolipoprotein, and CRP concentration, and insulin resistance in patients with polycystic ovary syndrome. *Fertility and Sterility, 87*(6), 1363–1368. doi:10.1016/j.fertnstert.2006.11.031 PMID:17362944

Balen, A. H., Morley, L. C., Misso, M., Franks, S., Legro, R. S., Wijeyaratne, C. N., Stener-Victorin, E., Fauser, B. C. J. M., Norman, R. J., & Teede, H. (2016). The management of anovulatory infertility in women with polycystic ovary syndrome: An analysis of the evidence to support the development of global WHO guidance. *Human Reproduction Update, 22*(6), 687–708. doi:10.1093/humupd/dmw025 PMID:27511809

Bandaranayake, W. M. (2006). Qualitycontrol, screening, toxicity, and regulation of herbal drugs. Modern Phyto medicine Turning Medicinal Plants into Drugs, 25–57.

Bargiota. (2012). The effects of old, new and emerging medicines on metabolic aberrations in PCOS. Therapeutic Advances in Endocrinology and Metabolism, 3(1), 27–47. PubMed

Barnes, J. (2003). Quality, efficacy and safety of complementary medicines: fashions, facts and the future. Part II: Efficacy and safety. 2003 Blackwell Publishing Ltd. *British Journal of Clinical Pharmacology, 55*(4), 331–340. doi:10.1046/j.1365-2125.2003.01811.x PMID:12680880

Bashtian, H. M., Emami, A. S., & Mousavifar, N. (2013). Evaluation of fenugreek (Trigonella Foenum-graceum L.), effects seeds extract on insulin resistance in women with polycystic ovarian syndrome. *Iranian J. Pharm. Res.: IJPR*, *12*, 475. PMID:24250624

Basu, A., Du, M., Sanchez, K., Leyva, M. J., Betts, N. M., Blevins, S., Wu, M., Aston, C. E., & Lyons, T. J. (2011). Green tea minimally affects biomarkers of inflammation obese subjects with metabolic syndrome. *Nutrition (Burbank, Los Angeles County, Calif.)*, *27*(2), 206–213. doi:10.1016/j.nut.2010.01.015 PMID:20605696

Bergmann, J., Luft, B., Boehmann, S., Runnebaum, B., & Gerhard, I. (2000). Phyto-Hypophyson_ L for female infertility. Randomized, placebo-controlled, clinical double-blind study. *Forschende Komplementarmedizin und Klassische Naturheilkunde*, *7*(4), 190–199. PMID:11025394

Berneis, K., Rizzo, M., Hersberger, M., Rini, G. B., DiFede, G., Pepe, I., Spinas, G. A., & Carmina, E. (2009). Atherogenic forms of dyslipidaemia in women with polycystic ovary syndrome. *International Journal of Clinical Practice*, *63*(1), 56–62. doi:10.1111/j.1742-1241.2008.01897.x PMID:19125993

Bhatia, V., & Viswanathan, P. (2006). Insulin resistance and PPAR insulin sensitizers. *Current Opinion in Investigational Drugs (London, England)*, *7*(10), 891–897. PMID:17086933

Bhattacharya, Johnson, Tijani, Hart, Pandey, & Gibreel. (2010). Female Infertility. *BMJ Clin Evid, 819.*

Bhattacharya, S. K., Goel, R. K., Kaur, R., & Ghosal, S. (1987). Anti - stress activity of Sitoindosides VII and VIII. New Acylsterylglucosides from *Withania somnifera. Phytotherapy Research*, *1*(1), 32–37. doi:10.1002/ptr.2650010108

Bhuvaneshwari, S., Poornima, R., & Averal, H. (2015). Management of obesity in polycystic ovary syndrome induced albino rats with Pergularia daemia. *Int. J. Appl. Res*, *1*, 779–783.

Bina, F., & Rahimi, R. (2017). Sweet Marjoram, A Review of Ethnopharmacology, Phytochemistry, and Biological Activities. *Journal of Evidence-Based Complementary & Alternative Medicine*, *22*(1), 175–185. doi:10.1177/2156587216650793 PMID:27231340

Boomsma, C. M., Eijkemans, M. J., Hughes, E. G., Visser, G. H., Fauser, B. C., & Macklon, N. S. (2006, November-December). A meta-analysis of pregnancy outcomes in women with polycystic ovary syndrome. *Human Reproduction Update*, *12*(6), 673–683. doi:10.1093/humupd/dml036 PMID:16891296

Borgia, F., Cannavo, S., Guarneri, Cannavo, S.P., Vaccaro, M., & Guarneri, B(2004Correlation between endocrinological parameters and acne severity in adult women. *Acta Derm Venereol., 84*(3), 201–204.

Borzoei, A., Rafraf, M., Niromanesh, S., Farzadi, L., Narimani, F., & Doostan, F. (2018). Effects of cinnamon supplementation on antioxidant status and serum lipids in women with polycystic ovary syndrome. *Journal of Traditional and Complementary Medicine*, *8*(1), 128–133. doi:10.1016/j.jtcme.2017.04.008 PMID:29322000

Broekmans, F., Knauff, E., Valkenburg, O., Laven, J., Eijkemans, M., & Fauser, B. (2006). PCOS according to the Rotterdam consensus criteria: Change in prevalence among WHO-II anovulation and association with metabolic factors. *BJOG*, *13*(10), 1210–1217. doi:10.1111/j.1471-0528.2006.01008.x PMID:16972863

Bruner, B., Chad, K., & Chizen, D. (2006). Effects of exercise and nutritional counseling in women with polycystic ovary syndrome. *Applied Physiology, Nutrition, and Metabolism*, *31*(4), 384–391. doi:10.1139/h06-007 PMID:16900227

Cai, L., Wan, D., & Yi, F. (2017). Purification, preliminary characterisation and hepatoprotective effects of polysaccharides from dandelion root. *Molecules (Basel, Switzerland)*, *22*(9), 1409. doi:10.3390/molecules22091409 PMID:28841174

Carmina, E. (2004). Diagnosis of polycystic ovary syndrome: From NIH criteria to ESHRE-ASRM guidelines. *Minerva Ginecologica*, *56*, 1–6. PMID:14973405

Cassidy-Vu, Joe, & Kirk. (2016). Role of Statin Drugs for Polycystic Ovary Syndrome. *Journal of Family & Reproductive Health*, *10*(4), 165–175. PMID:28546815

Cedars, M., & Jaffe, R. B. (2005). Infertility and women. *The Journal of Clinical Endocrinology and Metabolism*, *90*(4), E2. doi:10.1210/jcem.90.4.9997

Chan, K. (2003). Some aspects of toxic contaminants in herbal medicines. *Chemosphere*, *52*(9), 1361–1371. doi:10.1016/S0045-6535(03)00471-5 PMID:12867165

Chandrasekaran, C. V., Vijayalakshmi, M. A., Prakash, K., Bansal, V. S., Meenakshi, J., & Amit, A. (2012). Herbal Approach for Obesity Management Review Article. *American Journal of Plant Sciences*, *3*(No.7A), 1003–1014. doi:10.4236/ajps.2012.327119

Cheang, K. I., Nestler, J. E., & Futterweit, W. (2008). Risk of cardiovascular events in mothers of women with polycystic ovary syndrome. *Endocrine Practice*, *14*(9), 1084–1094. doi:10.4158/EP.14.9.1084 PMID:19158047

Chen, H. W., Chiang, W. J., & Chen, C. L. (2015). Characteristics and Prescription Patterns of Traditional Chinese Medicine in Polycystic Ovary Syndrome. *Journal of Chengdu University of TCM.*, *38*, 120–123.

Chen, H. Y., Lin, Y. H., Su, I. H., Chen, Y. C., Yang, S. H., & Chen, J. L. (2014). Investigation on Chinese herbal medicine for primary dysmenorrhea: Implication from a nationwide prescription database in Taiwan. *Complementary Therapies in Medicine*, *22*(1), 116–125. doi:10.1016/j.ctim.2013.11.012 PMID:24559826

Chen, J.-T., Tominaga, K., Sato, Y., Anzai, H., & Matsuoka, R. (2010). Maitake mushroom (Grifola frondosa) extract induces ovulation in patients with polycystic ovary syndrome: A possible monotherapy and a combination therapy after failure with first-line clomiphene citrate. *Journal of Alternative and Complementary Medicine (New York, N.Y.)*, *16*(12), 1295–1299. doi:10.1089/acm.2009.0696 PMID:21034160

Chittenden, B. G., Fullerton, G., Maheshwari, A., & Bhattacharya, S. (2009). Polycystic ovary syndrome and the risk of gynaecological cancer: A systematic review. *Reproductive Biomedicine Online*, *19*(3), 398–405. doi:10.1016/S1472-6483(10)60175-7 PMID:19778486

Cho, I. (2012). Effects of Panax ginseng in neurodegenerative diseases. *Journal of Ginseng Research*, *36*(4), 342–353. doi:10.5142/jgr.2012.36.4.342 PMID:23717136

Cho, J., Park, W., Lee, S., Ahn, W., & Lee, Y. (2004). Ginsenoside-Rb1 from Panax ginseng C.A. Meyer activates estrogen receptor-alpha and -beta, independent of ligand binding. *The Journal of Clinical Endocrinology and Metabolism*, *89*(7), 3510–3515. doi:10.1210/jc.2003-031823 PMID:15240639

Choi, J. H., Jang, M., Kim, E.-J., Lee, M. J., Park, K. S., Kim, S.-H., In, J.-G., Kwak, Y.-S., Park, D.-H., Cho, S.-S., Nah, S.-Y., Cho, I.-H., & Bae, C.-S. (2019). Korean Red Ginseng alleviates dehydroepiandrosterone-induced polycystic ovarian syndrome in rats via its antiinflammatory and antioxidant activities. *Journal of Ginseng Research*. Advance online publication. doi:10.1016/j.jgr.2019.08.007

Chopade, V., Phatak, A., Upaganlawar, A., & Tankar, A. (2008). Green tea (Camellia sinensis): Chemistry, traditional, medicinal uses and its pharmacological activities - A review. *Phcog Rev.*, *2*, 157–162.

Coviello, A. D., Legro, R. S., & Dunaif, A. (2006). Adolescent girls with polycystic ovary syndrome have an increased risk of the metabolic syndrome associated with increasing androgen levels independent of obesity and insulin resistance. *The Journal of Clinical Endocrinology and Metabolism*, *91*(2), 492–497. doi:10.1210/jc.2005-1666 PMID:16249280

Crosignani, P. (2001). A. Polycystic ovarian disease: Heritability and heterogeneity. *Human Reproduction Update*, *7*(1), 3–7. doi:10.1093/humupd/7.1.3 PMID:11212071

Dargham, S. R., Ahmed, L., Kilpatrick, E. S., & Atkin, S. L. (2017). The prevalence and metabolic characteristics of polycystic ovary syndrome in the Qatari population. *PLoS One*, *12*(7), e0181467. doi:10.1371/journal.pone.0181467 PMID:28723965

Dargham, Ahmed, Kilpatrick, & Atkin. (2017). *The prevalence and metabolic characteristics of polycystic ovary syndrome in the Qatari population*. doi:10.1371/journal.pone.0181467

Dayani Siriwardene, S. A., Karunathilaka, L. P. A., Kodituwakku, N. D., & Karunarathne, Y. A. U. D. (2010). Clinical efficacy of Ayurveda treatment regimen on Subfertility with Poly Cystic Ovarian Syndrome (PCOS). *Ayu*, *31*(1), 24–27. doi:10.4103/0974-8520.68203 PMID:22131680

Dehghan, A., Esfandiari, A., & Bigdeli, S. M. (2012). Alternative Treatment of Ovarian Cysts with Tribulus terrestris Extract: A Rat Model. *Reproduction in Domestic Animals*, *47*(1), 12–15. doi:10.1111/j.1439-0531.2011.01877.x PMID:21883512

Dghaim, R., Al Khatib, S., Rasool, H., & Khan, M. A. (2015). Determination of Heavy Metals Concentration in Traditional. Herbs Commonly Consumed in the United Arab Emirates. Journal of Environmental and Public Health. Hindawi Publishing Corporation.

Diamanti-Kandarakis, E., Argyrakopoulou, G., Economou, F., Kandaraki, E., & Koutsilieris, M. (2008). Defects in insulin signaling pathways in ovarian steroidogenesis and other tissues in polycystic ovary syndrome (PCOS). *The Journal of Steroid Biochemistry and Molecular Biology*, *109*(3-5), 242–246. doi:10.1016/j.jsbmb.2008.03.014 PMID:18440223

Diamanti-Kandarakis, E., Papavassiliou, A. G., Kandarakis, S. A., & Chrousos, G. P. (2007). Pathophysiology and types of dyslipidemia in PCOS. *Trends in Endocrinology and Metabolism*, *18*(7), 280–285. doi:10.1016/j.tem.2007.07.004 PMID:17692530

Diejomaoh, M., Jirous, J., Al-Azemi, M., Baig, S., Gupta, M., & Tallat, A. (2003). The relationship of recurrent spontaneous miscarriage with reproductive failure. *Medical Principles and Practice*, *12*(2), 107–111. doi:10.1159/000069122 PMID:12634466

Ding, H., & Petersen, W. Qu, & Baio. (2017). The prevalence of polycystic ovary syndrome in reproductive aged women of different ethnicity: a systematic review and meta-analysis. Oncotarget, 8(56), 96351–96358. PubMed

Ding, J., Xu, Y., Ma, X., An, J., Yang, X., Liu, Z., & Lin, N. (2015). Estrogenic effect of the extract of Renshen (Radix Ginseng) on reproductive tissues in immature mice. *Journal of Traditional Chinese Medicine*, *35*(4), 460–467. doi:10.1016/S0254-6272(15)30125-4 PMID:26427118

Dinka, P. B., Lana, S., & Roya, O. (2015). Polycystic Ovary Syndrome: Important Underrecognized Cardiometabolic Risk Factor in Reproductive-Age Women. *International Journal of Endocrinology*, 1–17.

Douchi, T., Oki, T., Yamasaki, H., Kuwahata, R., Nakae, M., & Nagata, Y. (2001). Relationship of androgens to muscle size and bone mineral density in women with polycystic ovary syndrome. *Obstetrics and Gynecology*, *98*(3), 445–449. PubMed

Driscoll, D. A. (2000). Polycystic ovary syndrome in adolescence. *Seminars in Reproductive Medicine*, *21*(3), 301–307. PMID:14593553

Düker, E. M., Kopanski, L., Jarry, H., & Wuttke, W. (1991). Effects of extracts from Cimicifuga racemosa on gonadotropin release in menopausal women and ovariectomized rats. *Planta Medica*, *57*(5), 420–424. doi:10.1055-2006-960139 PMID:1798794

Dunaif, A. (1999). Insulin action in the poly cystic ovary syndrome. *Endocrinology and Metabolism Clinics of North America*, *28*(2), 341–359. doi:10.1016/S0889-8529(05)70073-6 PMID:10352922

Ehrmann, D. A., Liljenquist, D. R., Kasza, K., Azziz, R., Legro, R. S., & Ghazzi, M. N. (2006). Prevalence and predictors of the metabolic syndrome in women with polycystic ovary syndrome. *The Journal of Clinical Endocrinology and Metabolism*, *91*(1), 48–53. doi:10.1210/jc.2005-1329 PMID:16249284

El Hayek, Bitar, Hamdar, Mirza, & Daoud. (2016). Poly Cystic Ovarian Syndrome: An Updated Overview. *Frontiers in Physiology, 7.*

El-Sharkawy, A. A., Abdelmotaleb, G. S., Aly, M. K., & Kabel, A. M. (2014). Effect of metformin on sleep disorders in adolescent girls with polycystic ovarian syndrome. *Journal of Pediatric and Adolescent Gynecology*, *27*(6), 347–352. doi:10.1016/j.jpag.2014.01.004 PMID:25256878

Elham, P. (2018). Lean Women with Polycystic Ovary Syndrome. In Debatable Topics in PCOS Patients. Intech Publishers.

Esfandiari, A., Dehghan, A., Sharifi, S., Najafi, B., & Vesali, E. (2011). Effect of Tribulus terrestris extract on ovarian activity in immature Wistar rat: A histological evaluation. *Journal of Animal and Veterinary Advances*, *10*(7), 883–886. doi:10.3923/javaa.2011.883.886

Fauser, B. C., Pache, T. D., Lamberts, S. W., Hop, W. C., de Jong, F. H., & Dahl, K. D. (1991). Serum bioactive and immunoreactive luteinizing hormone and follicle-stimulating hormone levels in women with cycle abnormalities, with or without polycystic ovarian disease. *The Journal of Clinical Endocrinology and Metabolism*, *73*(4), 811–817. doi:10.1210/jcem-73-4-811 PMID:1909705

Franks, S. (1989). Polycystic ovary syndrome: A changing perspective. *Horumon To Rinsho*, *31*(1), 87–120. doi:10.1111/j.1365-2265.1989.tb00457.x PMID:2513151

Futterweit, W. (1999). Polycystic ovary syndrome: Clinical perspectives and management. *Obstetrical & Gynecological Survey*, *54*(6), 403–413. doi:10.1097/00006254-199906000-00024 PMID:10358853

Gambineri, A., Pelusi, C., Manicardi, E., Vicennati, V., Cacciari, M., Morselli-Labate, A. M., Pagotto, U., & Pasquali, R. (2004). Glucose intolerance in a large cohort of mediterranean women with polycystic ovary syndrome: Phenotype and associated factors. *Diabetes*, *53*(9), 2353–2358. doi:10.2337/diabetes.53.9.2353 PMID:15331545

Gerard, C., Didier, D., & Evanthia, D. (2014). The polycystic ovary syndrome: A position statement from the European Society of Endocrinology. *European Journal of Endocrinology*, *171*(4), 1–29. doi:10.1530/EJE-14-0253 PMID:24849517

Ghafurniyan, H., Azarnia, M., Nabiuni, M., & Karimzadeh, L. (2015). The effect of green tea extract on reproductive improvement in estradiol valerate-induced polycystic ovarian syndrome in rat, Iran. *J. Pharm. Res: IJPR*, *14*, 1215. PMID:26664389

Ghosh, D. (2018). Quality issues of herbal medicines: Internal and external factors. *Internationa Journal of Complementary & Alternative Medicine*, *11*(1), 67–69. doi:10.15406/ijcam.2018.11.00350

Glueck, C. J., Papanna, R., Wang, P., Goldenberg, N., & Sieve-Smith, L. (2003). Incidence and treatment of metabolic syndrome in newly referred women with confirmed polycystic ovarian syndrome. *Metabolism: Clinical and Experimental*, *52*(7), 908–915. doi:10.1016/S0026-0495(03)00104-5 PMID:12870169

Gonzales, G.F., Cordova, A., Vega, K., Chung, A., Villena, A., & Gonez, C. (2002). *Effect of Lepidium meyenii (MACA) on sexual desire and its absent relationship with serum testosterone levels in adult healthy men*. Academic Press.

Goodarzi, M. O., Dumesic, D. A., Chazenbalk, G., & Azziz, R. (2011). Polycystic ovary syndrome:etiology, pathogenesis and diagnosis. *Nature Reviews. Endocrinology*, *7*(4), 219–231. doi:10.1038/nrendo.2010.217 PMID:21263450

Goodarzi, M. O., Dumesic, D. A., Chazenbalk, G., & Azziz, R. (2011). Polycystic ovary syndrome: Etiology, pathogenesis and diagnosis. *National Review*, *7*(4), 219–231. doi:10.1038/nrendo.2010.217 PMID:21263450

Grant, P. (2010). Spearmint herbal tea has significant anti-androgen effects in polycystic ovarian syndrome. a randomized controlled trial. *Phytotherapy Research*, *24*(2), 186–188. doi:10.1002/ptr.2900 PMID:19585478

Grant, P., & Ramasamy, S. (2012). An Update on Plant Derived Anti-Androgens. *International Journal of Endocrinology and Metabolism*, *2*(2), 497–502. doi:10.5812/ijem.3644 PMID:23843810

Haj-Husein, I. S., Tukan, S., & Alkazaleh, F. (2016). The effect of marjoram (Origanum majorana) tea on the hormonal profile of women with polycystic ovary syndrome: A randomised controlled pilot study. *Journal of Human Nutrition and Dietetics*, *29*(1), 105–111. doi:10.1111/jhn.12290 PMID:25662759

Haji Shafiha, M., Zabiri, T., & Salari Lak, S. H. (2007). Investigating validity criteria of vaginal ultrasound (ovarian volume, the ovarian stroma and the stromal surface of the ovary) in the diagnosis of polycystic ovary syndrome. *Majallah-i Pizishki-i Urumiyyah*, *3*, 538–543.

Hajimonfarednejad, M., Nimrouzi, M., Heydari, M., Zarshenas, M. M., Raee, M. J., & Jahromi, B. N. (2018). Insulin resistance improvement by cinnamon powder in polycystic ovary syndrome: A randomized double-blind placebo controlled clinical trial. *Phytotherapy Research*, *32*(2), 276–283. doi:10.1002/ptr.5970 PMID:29250843

Hamza, A. H., AlBishri, W. M., & Alfaris, M. H. (2019). Effect of Vitex agnus-castus plant extract on polycystic ovary syndrome complications in experimental rat model. *Asian Pacific Journal of Reproduction*, *8*, 63–69.

Harrison, C. L., Lombard, C. B., Moran, L. J., & Teede, H. J. (2011). Exercise therapy in polycystic ovary syndrome: A systematic review. *Human Reproduction Update*, *17*(2), 171–183. doi:10.1093/humupd/dmq045 PMID:20833639

He, D.-Y., & Dai, S.-M. (2011). Anti-Inflammatory and Immunomodulatory Effects of Paeonia Lactiflora Pall, a Traditional Chinese Herbal Medicine. *Frontiers in Pharmacology*, *2*, 10. doi:10.3389/fphar.2011.00010 PMID:21687505

Hong, Y., & Sun, B. (2016). Curative Estimation of Using Modified Cangfu Daotan Pill and Clomiphene in the Treatment of Polycystic Ovarian Syndrome Complicated with Infertility. *Journal of Sichuan of Traditional Chinese Medicine*, *34*, 90–93.

Hossein, K. J., Leila, K. J., Ebrahim, T., Nazanin, S., Farzad, P., Elham, R., Mohammad, P., & Zahra, H. (2015). The effect of pomegranate juice extract on hormonal changes of female wistar rats caused by polycystic ovarian syndrome. *Biomedical & Pharmacology Journal*, *8*(2), 971–977. doi:10.13005/bpj/849

Howkins & Shaw. (1999). *Textbook of Gynaecology* (12th ed.). B.I. Churchill Livingstone Pvt. Ltd.

Huang, H., Xin, H., Liu, X., Xu, Y., Wen, D., Zhang, Y., & Zhu, Y. Z. (2012). Novel anti-diabetic effect of SCM-198 via inhibiting the hepatic NF-kappaB pathway in db/db mice. *Bioscience Reports*, *32*(2), 185–195. doi:10.1042/BSR20110017 PMID:21859425

Isomaa, B., Almgren, P., Tuomi, T., Forsen, B., Lahti, K., Nissen, M., Taskinen, M.-R., & Groop, L. (2001). Cardiovascular morbidity and mortality associated with the metabolic syndrome. *Diabetes Care*, *24*(4), 683–689. doi:10.2337/diacare.24.4.683 PMID:11315831

Jalilian, N., Modarresi, M., Rezaie, M., Ghaderi, L., & Bozorgmanesh, M. (2013). Phytotherapeutic management of polycystic ovary syndrome: Role of aerial parts of wood betony (Stachys lavandulifolia). *Phytotherapy Research*, *27*(11), 1708–1713. doi:10.1002/ptr.4921 PMID:23307315

Jaradat, N., & Zaid, A. N. (2019). Herbal remedies used for the treatment of infertility in males and females by traditional healers in the rural areas of the West Bank/Palestine. *BMC Complementary and Alternative Medicine*, *19*(1), 194. doi:10.118612906-019-2617-2 PMID:31366346

Jazani, Hamdi, Tansaz, Nazemiyeh, Bazargani, Fazljou, & Azgomi. (2018). *Herbal Medicine for Oligomenorrhea and Amenorrhea: A Systematic Review of Ancient and Conventional Medicine*. Hindawi BioMed Research International. doi:10.1155/2018/3052768

Jedel, E., Waern, M., Gustafson, D., Landén, M., Eriksson, E., Holm, G., Nilsson, L., Lind, A.-K., Janson, P. O., & Stener-Victorin, E. (2010). Anxiety and depression symptoms in women with polycystic ovary Syndrome compared with controls matched for body mass index. *Human Reproduction (Oxford, England)*, *25*(2), 450–456. doi:10.1093/humrep/dep384 PMID:19933236

Jelodar, K. A. (2012). Effect of Vitex agnus-castus fruits hydroalcoholic extract on sex hormones in rat with induced polycystic ovary syndrome (PCOS). *Physiol. Pharmacol.*, *16*, 62–69.

Jiang, D. (2017). TCM Treatment of Polycystic Ovary and PCOS. *J Complement Med Alt Healthcare J*, *2*(1), 1–5. doi:10.19080/JCMAH.2017.02.555578

Jungbauer, A., & Medjakovic, S. (2014). Phytoestrogens and the metabolic syndrome. *The Journal of Steroid Biochemistry and Molecular Biology*, *139*, 277–289. doi:10.1016/j.jsbmb.2012.12.009 PMID:23318879

Kamel, H. H. (2013). Role of phyto-oestrogens in ovulation induction in women with polycystic ovarian syndrome. *European Journal of Obstetrics, Gynecology, and Reproductive Biology*, *168*(1), 60–63. doi:10.1016/j.ejogrb.2012.12.025 PMID:23347605

Kashani,, L., & Akhondzadeh, S. (2016). Herbal Medicine in the Treatment of Polycystic Ovary Syndrome. *Faslnamah-i Giyahan-i Daruyi*, *15*, 59.

Khanage, S. G., Subhash, T. Y., & Bhaiyyasaheb, I. R. (2019). Herbal drugs for the treatment of Polycystic ovary syndrome (PCOS) and its complications. *Pharmaceutical Research*, *2*(1), 5–13. PMID:31823112

Khomami, M. B., Tehrani, F. R., Hashemi, S., Farahmand, M., & Azizi, F. (2015). Of PCOS symptoms, hirsutism has the most significant impact on the quality of life of Iranian women. *PLoS One*, *10*(4), e0123608. doi:10.1371/journal.pone.0123608 PMID:25874409

Khot, Lad, Patil, & Kakad. (2013). Clinical Efficacy Of Ayurveda Treatment On Polycystic Ovarian Syndrome. *IOSR Journal of Pharmacy*, *3*(4), 21-25.

Kim, K. H., Lee, D., Lee, H. L., Kim, C. E., Jung, K., & Kang, K. S. (2018). Beneficial effects of Panax ginseng for the treatment and prevention of neurodegenerative diseases: Past findings and future directions. *Journal of Ginseng Research*, *42*(3), 239–247. doi:10.1016/j.jgr.2017.03.011 PMID:29989012

Kim, S. H., Han, J., Seog, D. H., Chung, J. Y., Kim, N., Hong Park, Y., & Lee, S. K. (2015). Antidepressant effect of Chaihu-Shugan-San extract and its constituents in rat models of depression. *Life Sciences*, *76*(11), 1297–1306. doi:10.1016/j.lfs.2004.10.022 PMID:15642599

Knochenhauer, E. S., Key, T. J., Kahsar-Miller, M., Waggoner, W., Boots, L. R., & Azziz, R. (1998). Prevalence of the polycystic ovary syndrome in unselected black and white women of the Southeastern United States: A prospective study. *The Journal of Clinical Endocrinology and Metabolism*, *83*(9), 3078–3082. doi:10.1210/jc.83.9.3078 PMID:9745406

Kort, D. H., & Lobo, R. A. (2014). Preliminary evidence that cinnamon improves menstrual cyclicity in women with polycystic ovary syndrome: A randomized controlled trial. *American Journal of Obstetrics and Gynecology*, *211*(5), 487.e481–487.e486. doi:10.1016/j.ajog.2014.05.009 PMID:24813595

Kumar, A., Woods, K. S., Bartolucci, A. A., & Azziz, R. (2005). Prevalence of adrenal androgen excess in patients with the polycystic ovary syndrome (PCOS). *Horumon To Rinsho*, *62*(6), 644–649. doi:10.1111/j.1365-2265.2005.02256.x PMID:15943823

Kuruvilla, A. (2002). Herbal Formulations as Pharmacotherapeutic Agents. *Indian Journal of Experimental Biology*, *40*, 7–11. PMID:12561961

Lankarani, M., Valizadeh, N., Heshmat, R., Shafaee, A.R., Amini, M.R., & Ardeshir Larijani, M.B. (2005). Evaluation of dyslipidemia in polycystic ovary syndrome. *J Diabetes Metab Disord*, *4*, E11+E11i-E11x.

Lee, T. T., & Rausch, M. E. (2012). Polycystic ovarian syndrome: Role of imaging in diagnosis. *Radiographics*, *32*(6), 1643–1657. doi:10.1148/rg.326125503 PMID:23065162

Leea, J. H., & Jo, J. (2017). Successful treatment with Korean herbal medicine and lifestyle management in an obese woman with polycystic ovarian syndrome. *Integrative Medicine Research*, *6*(3), 325–328. doi:10.1016/j.imr.2017.06.002 PMID:28951847

Legro, R. S. (1998). Polycystic ovary syndrome: Current and future treatment paradigms. *American Journal of Obstetrics and Gynecology*, *179*(6 Pt 2), S101–S8. doi:10.1016/S0002-9378(98)70240-6 PMID:9855616

Legro, R. S., Kunselman, A. R., Dodson, W. C., & Dunaif, A. (1999). Prevalence and predictors of risk for type 2 diabetes mellitus and impaired glucose tolerance in polycystic ovary syndrome: A prospective, controlled study in 254 affected women. *The Journal of Clinical Endocrinology and Metabolism*, *84*(1), 165–169. PMID:9920077

Lemaure, B., Touché, A., Zbinden, I., Moulin, J., Courtois, D., Macé, K., & Darimont, C. (2007). Administration of Cyperus rotundus tubers extract prevents weight gain in obese Zucker rats. *Phytotherapy Research*, *21*(8), 724–730. doi:10.1002/ptr.2147 PMID:17444573

Liao, Hu, & Hung. (2018). *Complementary Therapy with Traditional Chinese Medicine for Polycystic Ovarian Syndrome*. Intech Open Science. doi:10.5772/intechopen.71654

Liao, W.-T., Chiang, J.-H., Li, C.-J., Lee, M.-T., Su, C.-C., & Yen, H.-R. (2018). Investigation on the Use of Traditional Chinese Medicine for Polycystic Ovary Syndrome in a Nationwide Prescription Database in Taiwan. *Journal of Clinical Medicine*, *7*(7), 179. doi:10.3390/jcm7070179 PMID:30037150

Lim, S. S., Norman, R. J., Davies, M. J., & Moran, L. J. (2013). The effect of obesity on polycystic ovary syndrome: A systematic review and meta-analysis. *Obesity Reviews*, *14*(2), 95–109. doi:10.1111/j.1467-789X.2012.01053.x PMID:23114091

Liu, Y., & Mao, L. H. (2013). Effect of danzhi xiaoyao pill on ovulation induction of polycystic ovarian syndrome patients of pathogenic fire derived from stagnation of gan-qi. Zhongguo. *Zhong Xi Yi Jie He Za Zhi.*, *33*, 1191–1195. PMID:24273971

Lujan, M. E., Jarrett, B. Y., Brooks, E. D., Reines, J. K., Peppin, A. K., Muhn, N., Haider, E., Pierson, R. A., & Chizen, D. R. (2013). Updated ultrasound criteria for polycystic ovary syndrome: Reliable thresholds for elevated follicle population and ovarian volume. *Human Reproduction (Oxford, England)*, *28*(5), 1361–1368. doi:10.1093/humrep/det062 PMID:23503943

Ma, R. J., Zhou, J., Fang, J. Q., Yang, D. H., & Qu, F. (2011). Combination of acupuncture and chinese medicinal herbs in treating model rats with polycystic ovary syndrome. *Afr. J. Tradit. Complement. Altern. Med. AJTCAM.*, *8*(4), 353–361. doi:10.4314/ajtcam.v8i4.3 PMID:22654211

Manneräs-Holm, L., Baghaei, F., Holm, G., Janson, P. O., Ohlsson, C., Lonn, M., & Stener-Victorin, E. (2011). Coagulation and fibrinolytic disturbances in women with polycystic ovary syndrome. *The Journal of Clinical Endocrinology and Metabolism*, *96*(4), 1068–1076. doi:10.1210/jc.2010-2279 PMID:21252248

March, W. A., Moore, V. M., Willson, K. J., Phillips, D. I., Norman, R. J., & Davies, M. J. (2010). The prevalence of polycystic ovary syndrome in a community sample assessed under contrasting diagnostic criteria. *Human Reproduction (Oxford, England)*, *25*(2), 544–551. doi:10.1093/humrep/dep399 PMID:19910321

March, W. A., Moore, V. M., Willson, K. J., Phillips, D. I., Norman, R. J., & Davies, M. J. (2010). The prevalence of polycystic ovary syndrome in a community sample assessed under contrasting diagnostic criteria. *Human Reproduction (Oxford, England)*, *25*(2), 544–555. doi:10.1093/humrep/dep399 PMID:19910321

Mikaili, Mojaverrostami, & Moloudizargari, & Aghajanshakeri. (2013). Pharmacological and therapeutic effects of Mentha Longifolia L. and its main constituent, menthol. *Ancient Science of Life*, *33*(2), 131–138. PMID:25284948

Mikulskia, M. A., Wichmanb, M. D., Simmonsc, D. L., Phama, A. N., Clotteya, V., & Fuortesa, L. J. (2017). Toxic metals in ayurvedic preparations from a public health lead poisoning cluster investigation. *International Journal of Occupational and Environmental Health*, *23*(3), 187–192. doi:10.1080/10773525.2018.1447880 PMID:29528276

Milanov, S., Maleeva, A., & Tashkov, M. T. (1981). Effect on the concentration of some hormones in the serum of healthy subjects. Sofia, Bulgaria: Company Documentation, Chemical Pharmaceutical Research Institute.

Mills & Bone. (2013). *The Principles and Practices of Phytotherapy*. Churchill.

Mishra, L. C., Singh, B. B., & Dagenais, S. (2000). Scientific basis for the therapeutic use of Withania somnifera (ashwagandha): A Review. *Alternative Medicine Review*, *5*(4), 334–346. PMID:10956379

Mitra, K., Afsaneh, K., & Ahmad, K. (2017). The Effect of Herbal Teas on Management of Polycystic Ovary Syndrome: A Systematic Review. *Journal of Midwifery and Reproductive Health*, *5*(4), 1098–1106.

Mohebbi-Kian, E., Mohammad-Alizadeh-Charandabi, S., & Bekhradi, R. (2014). Efficacy of fennel and combined oral contraceptive on depot medroxyprogesterone acetate-induced amenorrhea: A randomized placebo-controlled trial. *Contraception*, *90*(4), 440–446. doi:10.1016/j.contraception.2014.05.001 PMID:24981150

Mokaberinejad, R., Akhtari, E., Tansaz, M., Bioos, S., Kamalinejad, M., Zafarghandi, N., Ghobadi, A., Sohrabvand, F., & Akhbari, A. (2014). Effect of Mentha longifolia on FSH Serum Level in Premature Ovarian Failure. *Open Journal of Obstetrics and Gynecology*, *4*(7), 356–360. doi:10.4236/ojog.2014.47053

Mokaberinejad, R., Zafarghandi, N., Bioos, S., Dabaghian, F. H., Naseri, M., Kamalinejad, M., Amin, G., Ghobadi, A., Tansaz, M., Akhbari, A., & Hamiditabar, M. (2012). Mentha longifolia syrup in secondary amenorrhea: A double-blind, placebo-controlled, randomized trials. *Daru: Journal of Faculty of Pharmacy, Tehran University of Medical Sciences*, *20*(1), 97. doi:10.1186/2008-2231-20-97 PMID:23351184

Moran, L. J., Brinkworth, G. D., & Norman, R. J. (2008). Dietary therapy in polycystic ovary syndrome. *Seminars in Reproductive Medicine*, *26*(1), 85–92. doi:10.1055-2007-992928 PMID:18181086

Moran, L. J., Pasquali, R., Teede, H. J., Hoeger, K. M., & Norman, R. J. (2009). Treatment of obesity in polycystic ovary syndrome: A position statement of the Androgen Excess and Polycystic Ovary Syndrome Society. *Fertility and Sterility*, *92*(6), 1966–1982. doi:10.1016/j.fertnstert.2008.09.018 PMID:19062007

Moreira, D. L., Teixeira, S. S., Monteiro, M. H. D., De-Oliveira, A. C. A. X., & Paumgartten, F. J. R. (2014). Traditional use and safety of herbal medicines. *Revista Brasileira de Farmacognosia*, *24*(2), 248–257. doi:10.1016/j.bjp.2014.03.006

Musmar, S., Afaneh, A., & Mo'alla, H. (2013). Epidemiology of polycystic ovary syndrome: A cross sectional study of university students at An-Najah national university-Palestine. *Reproductive Biology and Endocrinology*, *11*(1), 47. doi:10.1186/1477-7827-11-47 PMID:23688000

Nakagawa, T., Goto, H., Hussein, G., Hikiami, H., Shibahara, N., & Shimada, Y. (2008). Keishibukuryogan ameliorates glucose intolerance and hyperlipidemia in Otsuka Long-Evans Tokushima Fatty (OLETF) rats. *Diabetes Research (Edinburgh, Lothian)*, *80*(1), 40–47. doi:10.1016/j.diabres.2007.11.019 PMID:18242756

Nardo, L. G., Patchava, S., & Laing, I. (2008). Polycystic ovary syndrome: Pathophysiology, molecular aspects and clinical implications. *Panminerva Medica*, *50*(4), 267–278. PMID:19078868

National Institutes of Health, Department of Health and Human Services. (2008). *Beyond Infertility: Polycystic Ovary Syndrome (PCOS)*. NIH Pub, No. 08-5863.

Nava, A., Azizeh, F. K., Aliyeh, G., Kobra, H., Arash, K., Elaheh, O., Abbas, D., Fahimeh, B., & Masoumeh, M. (2019). The Effect of Herbal Medicine Supplementation on Clinical and Para-clinical Outcomes in Women With PCOS: A Systematic Review and Meta-analysis. *International Journal of Women's Health and Reproduction Sciences*, *7*(4), 423–433. doi:10.15296/ijwhr.2019.72

Nestler, J. E., Powers, L. P., Matt, D. W., Steingold, K. A., Plymate, S. R., Rittmaster, R. S., Clore, J. N., & Blackard, W. G. (1991). A direct effect of hyperinsulinemia on serum sex hormone-binding globulin levels in obese women with the polycystic ovary syndrome. *The Journal of Clinical Endocrinology and Metabolism*, *72*(1), 83–89. doi:10.1210/jcem-72-1-83 PMID:1898744

Nirav, R. S. (2017). Current Management on PCOS (Polycystic Ovary Syndrome)/Stein-Leventhal Syndrome. *Invest Gynecol Res Women's Health*, *1*(3), 46–48.

Norman, R. J., Davies, M. J., Lord, J., & Moran, L. J. (2002). The role of lifestyle modification in polycystic ovary syndrome. *Trends in Endocrinology and Metabolism*, *13*(6), 251–257. doi:10.1016/S1043-2760(02)00612-4 PMID:12128286

Norman, R. J., Dewailly, D., Legro, R. S., & Hickey, T. E. (2007). Polycystic ovary syndrome. *Lancet*, *370*(9588), 685–697. doi:10.1016/S0140-6736(07)61345-2 PMID:17720020

Nowak, D. A., Snyder, D. C., Brown, A. J., & Wahnefried, W. D. (2007). The Effect of Flaxseed Supplementation on Hormonal Levels Associated with Polycystic Ovarian Syndrome: A Case Study. *Current Topics in Nutraceutical Research*, *5*(4), 177–181. PMID:19789727

O'Malley, B., & Strott, C. (1999). Steroid hormones: Metabolism and mechanism of action. In Reproductive Endocrinology- Physiology, pathophysiology and clinical management. Philadelphia: WB Saunders Company.

Oelker, L. (2005). Quality control in herbal supplements. *Annali dell'Istituto Superiore di Sanita*, *41*(1), 43–48. PMID:16037649

Okoroh, E. M., Hooper, W. C., Atrash, H. K., Yusuf, H. R., & Boulet, S. L. (2012). Prevalence of polycystic ovary syndrome among the privately insured, United States, 2003–2008. *Obstetrics and Gynecology*, *207*, 299.e1–299.e7. PMID:22921097

Ong, K. J., Theodoru, E., & Ledger, W. (2006). Long-term consequence of polycystic ovarian syndrome. *Current Obstetrics & Gynaecology*, *16*(6), 333–336. doi:10.1016/j.curobgyn.2006.09.002

Ong, M., Peng, J., Jin, X., & Qu, X. (2017). Chinese Herbal Medicine for the Optimal Management of Polycystic Ovary Syndrome. *The American Journal of Chinese Medicine*, *45*(03), 405–422. doi:10.1142/S0192415X17500252 PMID:28359195

Pachiappan, Matheswaran, Pushkalai, Saravanan, & Muthusamy. (2017). Medicinal plants for polycystic ovary syndrome: A review of phytomedicine research. *International Journal of Herbal Medicine, 5*(2), 78-80.

Patel, S. (2018). Polycystic ovary syndrome, an inflammatory, systemic, lifestyle endocrinopathy. *The Journal of Steroid Biochemistry and Molecular Biology*, *182*, 27–36. doi:10.1016/j.jsbmb.2018.04.008 PMID:29678491

Pirbalouti, A. G., & Mohammadi, M. (2013). Phytochemical composition of the essential oil of different populations of Stachys lavandulifolia Vahl. *Asian Pacific Journal of Tropical Biomedicine*, *3*(2), 123–128. doi:10.1016/S2221-1691(13)60036-2 PMID:23593591

Pirzada, A. M., Ali, H. H., Naeem, M., Latif, M., Bukhari, A. H., & Tanveer, A. (2015). Traditional uses, phytochemistry, and pharmacological activities. *Journal of Ethnopharmacology*, *174*, 540–560. doi:10.1016/j.jep.2015.08.012 PMID:26297840

Polson, D. W., Franks, S., Reed, M. J., Cheng, R. W., Adams, J., & James, V. H. (1987). The distribution of oestradiol in plasma in relation to uterine cross-sectional area in women with polycystic or multifollicular ovaries. *Horumon To Rinsho*, *26*(5), 581–588. doi:10.1111/j.1365-2265.1987.tb00813.x PMID:3665120

Radha, M., & Laxmipriya, N. (2016). Efficacy of non-polar extract (NPE) of aloe barbadensis mill. In polycystic ovarian syndrome (PCOS) rodent model-an 'in vivo' study. *International Journal of Pharmaceutical Sciences and Research*, *7*, 4933.

Rajaa, K. (2013). The Effect Of Aqueous Extract Of Anastatica Hierochuntica On Some Hormones In Mouse Females. *Ibn Al-Haitham Jour. for Pure & Appl. Sci.*

Rathera, M. A., Dara, B. A., Sofia, S. N., Bhata, B. A., & Qurishi, M. A. (2016). Foeniculum vulgare: A comprehensive review of its traditional use, phytochemistry, pharmacology, and safety. *Arabian Journal of Chemistry*, *9*(2), S1574–S1583. doi:10.1016/j.arabjc.2012.04.011

Rau, O., Wurglics, M., Dingermann, T., Abdel-Tawab, M., & Schubert-Zsilavecz, M. (2006). Screening of herbal extracts for activation of the human peroxisome proliferator-activated receptor. *Die Pharmazie-An International Journal of Pharmaceutical Sciences.*, *61*(11), 952–956. PMID:17152989

Rebar, R., Judd, H. L., Yen, S. S., Rakoff, J., Vandenberg, G., & Naftolin, F. (1976). Characterization of the inappropriate gonadotropin secretion in polycystic ovary syndrome. *The Journal of Clinical Investigation*, *7*(5), 1320–1329. doi:10.1172/JCI108400 PMID:770505

Ren, M. Q., Kuhn, G., Wegner, J., & Chen, J. (2001). Isoflavones, substances with multibiological and clinical properties. *European Journal of Nutrition*, *40*(4), 135–146. doi:10.1007/PL00007388 PMID:11905954

Ricardo Azziz, M. P. H., & Daniel, A. (2011). Polycystic ovary syndrome: An ancient disorder? *Fertility and Sterility*, *95*(5), 1544–1548. doi:10.1016/j.fertnstert.2010.09.032 PMID:20979996

Richard, S. L., Silva, A. A., David, A. E., & Kathleen, M. H. (2013). Diagnosis and Treatment of Polycystic Ovary Syndrome: An Endocrine Society Clinical Practice Guideline. *The Journal of Clinical Endocrinology and Metabolism*, *98*(12), 4565–4592. doi:10.1210/jc.2013-2350 PMID:24151290

Ried, K. (2015). Chinese herbal medicine for female infertility: An updated meta-analysis. *Complementary Therapies in Medicine*, *23*(1), 116–128. doi:10.1016/j.ctim.2014.12.004 PMID:25637159

Rivera, Loya, & Ceballo. (2013). Use of Herbal Medicines and Implications for Conventional Drug Therapy Medical Sciences. *Altern Integ, 2*(6).

Rizzo, M., Berneis, K., Hersberger, M., Pepe, I., DiFede, G., Rini, G. B., Spinas, G. A., & Carmina, E. (2009). Milder forms of atherogenic dyslipidemia inovulatory versus anovulatory Polycystic ovary syndrome phenotype. *Human Reproduction (Oxford, England)*, *24*(9), 2286–2292. doi:10.1093/humrep/dep121 PMID:19454589

Robert, L. R., & David, A. E. (2016). The Pathogenesis of Polycystic Ovary Syndrome (PCOS): The Hypothesis of PCOS as Functional Ovarian Hyperandrogenism Revisited. *Endocrine Reviews*, *37*(5), 467–520. doi:10.1210/er.2015-1104 PMID:27459230

Roldan, B., San Millan, J. L., & Escobar-Morreale, H. F. (2004). Genetic basis of metabolic abnormalities in polycystic ovary syndrome: Implications for therapy. *American Journal of Pharmacogenomics, 4*(2), 93–107. doi:10.2165/00129785-200404020-00004 PMID:15059032

Romm, A. (2010). *Botanical Medicine for Women's Health*. Churchill Livingstone.

Rosencrantz, M. A., Coffler, M. S., Haggan, A., Duke, K. B., Donohue, M. C., Shayya, R. F., Su, H. I., & Chang, R. J. (2011). Clinical evidence for predominance of delta-5 steroid production in women with polycystic ovary syndrome. *The Journal of Clinical Endocrinology and Metabolism, 96*(4), 1106–1113. doi:10.1210/jc.2010-2200 PMID:21270326

Saiyed, Jahan, Makbul, Ansari, Bano, & Habib. (2016). Effect of combination of Withania somnifera Dunal and Tribulus terrestris Linn on letrozole induced polycystic ovarian syndrome in rats. *Integr Med Res, 5*, 293–300.

Santosh, K. (2008). Mehla RK, Dang AK. (2008). Use of shatavari (Asparagus Racemosus) as a galactopoietic and therapeutic herb-A review. *Agricultural Reviews (Karnal), 29*(2), 132–138.

Satapathy, S., Das, N., Bandyopadhyay, D., Mahapatra, S. C., Sundar Sahu, D., & Meda, M. (2017). Effect of Tulsi (Ocimum sanctum Linn.) Supplementation on Metabolic Parameters and Liver Enzymes in Young Overweight and Obese Subjects. *Indian Journal of Clinical Biochemistry, 32*(3), 357–363. doi:10.100712291-016-0615-4 PMID:28811698

Scheidt, P., Dellarco, M., & Dearry, A. A. (2009). Major milestone for the National Children's Study. *Environmental Health Perspectives, 117*(1), A13. doi:10.1289/ehp.12416 PMID:19165365

Schmidt, J. (2011). *Polycystic ovary syndrome Ovarian pathophysiology and consequences after the menopause* (Thesis). Geson Hylte Tryck.

Seidlova-Wuttke, D., Hesse, O., Jarry, H., Christoffel, V., Spengler, B., Becker, T., & Wuttke, W. (2003). Evidence for selective estrogen receptor modulator activity in a Black Cohosh (Cimicifuga racemosa) extract: Comparison with estradiol-17beta. *European Journal of Endocrinology, 149*(4), 351–362. doi:10.1530/eje.0.1490351 PMID:14514351

Shahnazi, M., Khalili, A. F., Hamdi, K., & Ghahremaninasab, P. (2016). The effects of combined low-dose oral contraceptives and Vitex agnus on the improvement of clinical and paraclinical parameters of polycystic ovarian syndrome: A triple-blind, randomized, controlled clinical trial. *Iranian Red Crescent Medical Journal, 18*(12). doi:10.5812/ircmj.37510

Sharma. (1938). *Ashwagandharishta - Rastantra Sar Evam Sidhyaprayog Sangrah-Krishna-Gopal Ayurveda Bhawan*. Dharmarth Trust.

Sharma, S., Khinchi, M. P., Sharma, N., Agrawal, D., & Gupta, M. K. (2011). Female Infertility: An Overview. *IJPSR, 2*(1). https://ijpsr.com/bft-article/female-infertility-an-overview/?view=fulltext

Shirazi, A. (2009). The Storehouse of Medicaments. Tehran University of Medical Sciences: Institute for Islamic and Complementary Medicine, Tehran, Iran.

Shubhashree, M. N. (2012). Female Infertility: An Overview (12th ed.). Academic Press.

Sirmans, S., & Pate, K. (2014). Epidemiology, diagnosis, and management of polycystic ovary syndrome. *Clinical Epidemiology*, *6*, 1–13. PubMed

Soumya, V., Muzib, Y. I., Venkatesh, P., & Hariprasath, K. (2014). GC-MS analysis of Cocus nucifera flower extract and its effects on heterogeneous symptoms of polycystic ovarian disease in female Wistar rats. *Chinese Journal of Natural Medicines*, *12*(9), 677–684. doi:10.1016/S1875-5364(14)60103-5 PMID:25263979

Stein, I., & Leventhal, M. (1935). Amenorrhea associated with bilateral polycystic ovaries. *American Journal of Obstetrics and Gynecology*, *29*(2), 181–191. doi:10.1016/S0002-9378(15)30642-6

Stepto, N. K., Cassar, S., Joham, A. E., Hutchison, S. K., Harrison, C. L., Goldstein, R. F., & Teede, H. J. (2013). Women with polycystic ovary syndrome have intrinsic insulin resistance on euglycaemic-hyperinsulaemic clamp. *Human Reproduction (Oxford, England)*, *28*(3), 777–784. doi:10.1093/humrep/des463 PMID:23315061

Strauss, J.F. (2003). Some new thoughts on the pathophysiology and genetics of polycystic ovary syndrome. *Ann 1N Y Acad Sci, 997*, 42-48.

Sun, W. S., Imai, A., Tagami, K., Sugiyama, M., Furui, T., & Tamaya, T. (2004). In vitro stimulation of granulosa cells by a combination of different active ingredients of unkei-to. *The American Journal of Chinese Medicine*, *32*(4), 569–578. doi:10.1142/S0192415X0400220X PMID:15481646

Susan, A., Jason, A. A., Caroline, A. S., & Alan, B. (2014). Herbal medicine for the management of polycystic ovary syndrome (PCOS) and associated oligo/amenorrhoea and hyperandrogenism; a review of the laboratory evidence for effects with corroborative clinical findings. *BMC Complementary and Alternative Medicine*, *14*(1), 511. doi:10.1186/1472-6882-14-511 PMID:25524718

Susan, M. S., & Kristen, A. P. (2014). Epidemiology, diagnosis, and management of polycystic ovary syndrome. *Clinical Epidemiology*, *6*, 1–13. PMID:24379699

Tabakova, P., Dimitrov, M., & Tashkov, B. (1984). *Clinical studies on the preparation Tribestan in women with endocrine infertility or menopausal syndrome*. Sofia, Bulgaria: 1st Obstetrical and Gynecological Hospital.

Takahashi, K., & Kitao, M. (1994). Effect of TJ-68 (shakuyaku-kanzo-to) on polycystic ovarian disease. *International Journal of Fertility and Menopausal Studies*, *39*(2), 69. PMID:8012442

Takahashi, T. (2011). Mechanism of acupuncture on neuromodulation in the gut—A review. *Neuromodulation*, *14*(1), 8–12. doi:10.1111/j.1525-1403.2010.00295.x PMID:21992155

Takeuchi, T., Nishii, O., Okamura, T., & Yaginuma, T. (1989). Effect of traditional herbal medicine, shakuyaku-kanzo-to on total and free serum testosterone levels. *The American Journal of Chinese Medicine*, *17*(1-2), 35–44. doi:10.1142/S0192415X89000073 PMID:2511749

Talbott, E., Clerici, A., Berga, S. L., Kuller, L., Guzick, D., Detre, K., Daniels, T., & Engberg, R. A. (1998). Adverse lipid and coronary heart disease risk profiles in young women with polycystic ovary syndrome: Results of a case-control study. *Journal of Clinical Epidemiology*, *51*(5), 415–422. doi:10.1016/S0895-4356(98)00010-9 PMID:9619969

Talbott, E. O., Guzick, D. S., Sutton-Tyrrell, K., McHugh-Pemu, K. P., Zborowski, J. V., Remsberg, K. E., & Kuller, L. H. (2000). Evidence for association between polycystic ovary syndrome and premature carotid atherosclerosis in middle-aged women. *Arteriosclerosis, Thrombosis, and Vascular Biology*, *20*(11), 2414–2421. doi:10.1161/01.ATV.20.11.2414 PMID:11073846

Tang, T., Glanville, J., Hayden, C. J., White, D., Barth, J. H., & Balen, A. H. (2006). Combined lifestyle modification and metformin in obese patients with polycystic ovary syndrome. A randomized, placebo-controlled, double-blind multicentre study. *Human Reproduction (Oxford, England)*, *21*(1), 80–89. doi:10.1093/humrep/dei311 PMID:16199429

Teede, H., Hutchinson, S.K., & Zoungas, S. (2007). The management of insulin in polycystic ovary syndrome. *Trends in Endocrinology and Metabolism*(18273-279.

Teede, H. J., Misso, M. L., Costello, M. F., Dokras, A., Laven, J., Moran, L., Piltonen, T., & Norman, R. J. (2018). The International PCOS Network. Recommendations from the international evidence-based guideline for the assessment and management of polycystic ovary syndrome. *Horumon To Rinsho*, *89*(3), 251–268. doi:10.1111/cen.13795 PMID:30024653

Teede, H. J., Misso, M. L., Deeks, A. A., Moran, L. J., Stuckey, B. G., Wong, J. L., Norman, R. J., & Costello, M. F. (2011). Assessmentandmanagementofpolycysticovarysyndrome: Summary of an evidence-based guideline. *The Medical Journal of Australia*, *195*(S6), S65–S112. doi:10.5694/mja11.10915 PMID:21929505

Thessaloniki ESHRE/ASRM-Sponsored PCOS Consensus Workshop Group. (2008). Consensus on infertility treatment related to polycystic ovary syndrome. *Human Reproduction, 23*, 462–477.

Tracy, W., Rami, M., & Samuel, P. (2016). Diagnosis and Treatment of Polycystic Ovary Syndrome. *American Family Physician*, *94*(2), 106–113. PMID:27419327

Trevisan, M., Liu, J., Bahsas, F.B., & Menotti, A. (1998). Syndrome X and mortality: a population based study. Risk Factor and Life Expectancy Research Group. *Am J Epidemiol, 148*(10), 958-66.

Uche, A. N., Angie, E., & Monica, R. G. (2013). Polycystic Ovary Syndrome A Review of Treatment Options With a Focus on Pharmacological Approaches. *P&T*, *38*(6), 336–355. PMID:23946629

Uchiyama, Jikyo, Takeda, & Ogata. (2013). Lepidium Meyenii (Maca) Enhances the Serum Levels of Luteinising Hormone in Female Rats. *J Ethnopharmacol., 151*(2), 897-902.

Urbanek, M. (2007). The genetics of the polycystic ovary syndrome. *Nature Clinical Practice. Endocrinology & Metabolism*, *3*(2), 103–111. doi:10.1038/ncpendmet0400 PMID:17237837

Ushiroyama, T., Hosotani, T., Mori, K., Yamashita, Y., Ikeda, A., & Ueki, M. (2006). Effects of switching to wen-jing-tang (unkei-to) from preceding herbal preparations selected by eight-principle pattern identification on endocrinological status and ovulatory induction in women with polycystic ovary syndrome. *The American Journal of Chinese Medicine*, *34*(02), 177–187. doi:10.1142/S0192415X06003746 PMID:16552830

Ushiroyama, T., Ikeda, A., Sakai, M., Hosotani, T., Suzuki, Y., Tsubokura, S., & Ueki, M. (2001). Effects of unkei-to, an herbal medicine, on endocrine function and ovulation in women with high basal levels of luteinizing hormone secretion. *The Journal of Reproductive Medicine*, *46*(5), 451–456. PMID:11396371

Valkenburg, O., Steegers-Theunissen, R. P., Smedts, H. P., Dallinga-Thie, G. M., Fauser, B. C., Westerveld, E. H., & Laven, J. S. E. (2008). A more atherogenic serum lipoprotein profile is present in women with polycystic ovary syndrome: A case-control study. *The Journal of Clinical Endocrinology and Metabolism*, *93*(2), 470–476. doi:10.1210/jc.2007-1756 PMID:18056772

van Santbrink, E. J., Hop, W. C., & Fauser, B. C. (1997). Classification of normogonadotropic infertility: Polycystic ovaries diagnosed by ultrasound versus endocrine characteristics of polycystic ovary syndrome. *Fertility and Sterility*, *67*(3), 452–458. doi:10.1016/S0015-0282(97)80068-4 PMID:9091329

Veltman-Verhulst, S. M., Boivin, J., Eijkemans, M. J., & Fauser, B. J. (2012). Emotional distress is a common risk in women with polycystic ovary syndrome: A systematic review and meta-analysis of 28 studies. *Human Reproduction Update*, *18*(6), 638–651. doi:10.1093/humupd/dms029 PMID:22824735

Vlietinck, A., Pieters, L., & Apers, S. (2009). Legal Requirements for the Quality of Herbal Substances and Herbal Preparations for the Manufacturing of Herbal Medicinal Products in the European Union. *Planta Medica*, *75*(7), 683–688. doi:10.1055-0029-1185307 PMID:19204891

Wang, G. J., Anderson, A. R., Graham, M. G. III, Chu, M. C., Sauer, M. V., Guarnaccia, M. M., & Lobo, R. A. (2007). The effect of cinnamon extract on insulin resistance parameters in polycystic ovary syndrome: A pilot study. *Fertility and Sterility*, *88*(1), 240–243. doi:10.1016/j.fertnstert.2006.11.082 PMID:17296187

Wang, L., Ma, R., Liu, C., Liu, H., Zhu, R., Guo, S., Tang, M., Li, Y., Niu, J., Fu, M., Gao, S., & Zhang, D. (2017). Salvia miltiorrhiza: A Potential Red Light to the Development of Cardiovascular Diseases. *Current Pharmaceutical Design*, *23*(7), 1077–1097. doi:10.2174/1381612822666161010105242 PMID:27748194

Whitten, P. L., & Naftolin, F. (1998). Reproductive actions of phytoestrogens. *Bailliere's Clinical Endocrinology and Metabolism*, *12*(4), 667–690. doi:10.1016/S0950-351X(98)80010-4 PMID:10384819

Wirksamkeit. (2007). *Ayurveda bei chronischen Erkrankungen. Systematische Analysen klinischer Ayurveda-Studien*. Essen: KVC.

Witt, C. M., Michalsen, A., Roll, S., Morandi, A., Gupta, S., Rosenberg, M., Kronpass, L., Stapelfeldt, E., Hissar, S., Muller, M., & Kessler, C. (2013). Comparative effectiveness of a complex Ayurvedic treatment and conventional standard care in osteoarthritis of the knee – study protocol for a randomized controlled trial. *Trials*, *14*(1), 149. doi:10.1186/1745-6215-14-149 PMID:23701973

Wolf, W. M., Wattick, R. A., Kinkade, O. N., & Olfert, M. D. (2018). Geographical Prevalence of Polycystic Ovary Syndrome as Determined by Region and Race/Ethnicity. *International Journal of Environmental Research and Public Health*, *15*(11), 2589. doi:10.3390/ijerph15112589 PMID:30463276

World Health Organization. (2002). *Traditional Medicine in Asia*. WHO Regional Publications.

World Health Organization (WHO). (2003). *Traditional Medicine*. Report by the Secretariat. A 56/18. https://extranet.who.int/iris/restricted/handle/10665/78244

Wu, J., Pan, Z., Wang, Z., Zhu, W., Shen, Y., Cui, R., Lin, J., Yu, H., Wang, Q., Qian, J., Yu, Y., Zhu, D., & Lou, Y. (2012). Ginsenoside Rg1 protection against beta-amyloid peptide-induced neuronal apoptosis via estrogen receptor alpha and glucocorticoid receptor-dependent anti-protein nitration pathway. *Neuropharmacology*, *63*(3), 349–361. doi:10.1016/j.neuropharm.2012.04.005 PMID:22534050

Xia, Y., Zhao, P., Huang, H., Xie, Y., Lu, R., & Dong, L. (2017). Cryptotanshinone reverses reproductive disturbances in rats with dehydroepiandrosterone-induced polycystic ovary syndrome. *American Journal of Translational Research*, *15*(9), 2447–2456. PMID:28559995

Xita, N., & Tsatsoulis, A. (2006). Review: fetal programming of polycystic ovary syndrome by androgen excess: evidence from experimental, clinical, and genetic association studies. *The Journal of Clinical Endocrinology and Metabolism*, *91*(5), 1660–1666. doi:10.1210/jc.2005-2757 PMID:16522691

Xu, Y., Ding, J., Ma, X.P., Ma, Y.H., Liu, Z.Q., & Lin, N. (2014). Treatment with Panax ginseng antagonizes the estrogen decline in ovariectomized mice. *Int J Mol Sci, 15*, 7827-40.

Yaginuma, T. I., Yasui, R., Arai, H., & Kawabata, T. (1982). Effect of traditional herbal medicine on serum testosterone levels and its induction of regular ovulation in hyperandrogenic and oligomenorrheic women. *Nippon Sanka Fujinka Gakkai Zasshi*, *34*(7), 939. PubMed

Yang, K. Pyun, & Lee. (2018). Licorice ethanol extract improves symptoms of polycytic ovary syndrome in Letrozole-induced female rats. Integrative Medicine Research, 7, 264–270. PubMed

Yavari, M., Rouholamin, S., Tansaz, M., Bioos, S., & Esmaeili, S. (2014). Sesame a treatment of menstrual bleeding cessation in iranian traditional medicine: Results from a pilot study. *Shiraz E Medical Journal*, *15*(3). Advance online publication. doi:10.17795emj21893

Yavari, M., Rouholamin, S., Tansaz, M., Bioos, S., & Esmaeili, S. (2016). Sesame a Treatment of Menstrual Bleeding Cessation in Iranian Traditional Medicine: Results From a Pilot Study. *Shiraz E Medical Journal*, *5*(3), 114–121.

Yen, S. S. (1980). The polycystic ovary syndrome. *Horumon To Rinsho*, *12*(2), 177–207. doi:10.1111/j.1365-2265.1980.tb02132.x PMID:6772357

Yildiz, B. O., Bozdag, G., Yapici, Z., Esinler, I., & Yarali, H. (2012). Prevalence, phenotype and cardiometabolic risk of polycystic ovary syndrome under different diagnostic criteria. *Human Reproduction (Oxford, England)*, *27*(10), 3067–3073. doi:10.1093/humrep/des232 PMID:22777527

Yilmaz, M., Bukan, N., Ayvaz, G., Karakoç, A., Törüner, F., Cakir, N., & Arslan, M. (2005). The effects of rosiglitazone and metformin on oxidative stress and Homocysteine levels in lean patients with polycystic ovary syndrome. *Human Reproduction (Oxford, England)*, *20*(12), 3333–3340. doi:10.1093/humrep/dei258 PMID:16123091

Yin, J., Xing, H., & Ye, J. (2008). Efficacy of Berberine in Patients with Type 2. *Diabetes & Metabolism*, *57*(5), 712–717. PMID:18442638

Yuan, C. S., Mehendale, S. R., Wang, C. Z., Aung, H. H., Jiang, T., Guan, X., & Shoyama, Y. (2004). Effects of Corydalis yanhusuo and Angelicae dahuricae on cold pressor-induced pain in humans: A controlled trial. *Journal of Clinical Pharmacology*, *44*(11), 1323–1327. doi:10.1177/0091270004267809 PMID:15496650

Zahra, A., Ayoob, R., Mohsen, M., Masih, H., & Mahmoud, R. (2018). A review on role of medicinal plants in polycystic ovarian syndrome: Pathophysiology, neuroendocrine signaling, therapeutic status and future prospects. *Middle East Fertility Society Journal*, *23*(4), 255–262. doi:10.1016/j.mefs.2018.04.005

Zeinab, F., Siavash, F., Mahdi, S., & Reza, G. (2017). Nutritional management in women with polycystic ovary syndrome: A review study. *Diab Met Syndr: Clin Res Rev*, *11*(S1).

Zhang, J. Y., Xue, H. Y., Su, J., Zuo, Y. H., Fan, X. Q., & Cheng, Y. Q. (2015). Clinical effects of tanshinone on polycystic ovary syndrome patients with hyperandrogenism. *Guangxi Medical Journal*, *37*, 767–769.

KEY TERMS AND DEFINITIONS

Alternative Medicine: Any healing or treatment regimen of diseases generally not included in the traditional medical curricula of the U.S. and Britain.

Diet: Food and drink regularly included for consumption as part of a meal pattern.

Herbal Medicine: Plants and their parts used as medicine due to their beneficially effects in maintaining health as well as to prevent or cure diseases.

Ovarian Cysts: Sacs of fluid or slimy fluid called mucus within the ovaries.

Chapter 7
Male Infertility Management With Alternative Medicine:
Promises, Practice, and Perspectives – Treatment of Male Infertility Using Plant-Based Alternative Medicine

Sreepoorna Pramodh
College of Natural and Health Sciences, Zayed University, UAE

ABSTRACT

In this chapter, the main causes of male factor infertility, specifically endocrine abnormalities and effect of endocrine disrupters, will be outlined. For many patients, conventional therapy presents considerable financial strain and moral dilemma. In this context, many patients are preferring complementary medicine (CAM). Hence, the promises offered by herbal medicine including Ayurveda, Arab, and Chinese medicine will be explored in this chapter. Many naturopathic medicaments such as Withania somnifera, Asparagus racemosus, Curculigo orchioides, Zingiber officinale, etc. are being routinely used as part of traditional medicine practice in Ayurveda and Arab medicine and gaining wider acceptance in other countries. Common herbs, targeted infertility condition, and results thereafter shall be discussed. In the concluding part of the chapter, the potential deleterious contraindications of alternate medicine such as lead toxicity from Ayurvedic medications shall be briefly discussed.

INTRODUCTION

Infertility is a major health concern that affects nearly 15% of sexually active couples. Male infertility contributes to approximately 50% of these cases (Pasqualotto, 2004). While there are many causes for male infertility, endocrinological reasons are relatively easier to treat. Infertility results due to impaired spermatogenesis and is affected by Hypothalamus-Pituitary-Gonadal Axis (HPG). Hormonal imbalance due to disruptions of HPG, inevitably result in poor sperm production. Exposure to endocrine disruptors can also cause infertility (Anawalt, 2013). This chapter discusses in depth the process of

DOI: 10.4018/978-1-7998-4808-0.ch007

spermatogenesis, impact of HPG axis and influence of endocrine disruptors to understand etiology of infertility. Conventional treatment strategy involves treatment with hormones and health supplements such as vitamins and antioxidants. Due to various disadvantages associate with this option, many couples worldwide are resorting to complementary alternative medication (CAM) involving plant based herbal medicines. Three popular herbal treatment practices are- Ayurveda, Arab Traditional Medicine (ATM) and Chinese herbal medicine. Important herbs recommended by each of these regimens is discussed in detail. Certain limitations associated with herbal treatment such as toxicity concerns, lack of sufficient data and absence of information regarding mode of action are reviewed and finally recommendations for overcoming these issues are suggested in the concluding part of the chapter.

BACKGROUND

Infertility is classically defined as the inability for a couple to conceive after 12 months of frequent vaginal intercourse without the use of contraception (Gnoth, 2005). The most common cause of male subfertility is primary testicular dysfunction and a defect in spermatogenesis that is generally due to irrever ible damage, and these men typically require treatment with Assisted Reproductive Technology (ART) (Jungwirth, 2012).

Infertility can occur when there is a low sperm count, or problems with the motility (movement) or morphology (appearance or shape) of the sperm. The World Health Organization (WHO) estimates that approximately 50-80 million people suffer from infertility. Causes of male infertility can be divided into three main categories:

A) Sperm production disorders affecting the quality and/or the quantity of sperm (Non Obstructive Azoospermia, NOA). NOA may be manifested as Sertoli cell-only pattern (SCO), maturation arrest (MA), or hypospermatogenesis.
B) Anatomical obstructions (Obstructive Azoospermia)
C) Other factors such immunological disorders.

Approximately a third of all cases of male infertility can be attributed to immune or endocrine problems, as well as to a failure of the testes to respond to the hormonal stimulation triggering sperm production. However, in a great number of cases of male infertility due to inadequate spermatogenesis (sperm production) or sperm defects, the origin of the problem still remains unexplained. The etiology of male infertility is either congenital or acquired due to environmental toxins or disease processes (Anawalt, 2013). In order to evaluate factors that may cause infertility, it is crucial to understand the process by which sperm are produced in male testis, namely Spermatogenesis and mechanisms of its regulation.

Spermatogenesis

The sequence of cytological events that result in the formation of the mature spermatozoa from precursor cells is known as spermatogenesis. Spermatogenesis is largely orchestrated, by complex endocrine and auto/paracrine regulation as well as by direct cell to cell interactions (Sharpe, 1986). Defects in the process or regulation of spermatogenesis result in infertility.

Spermatogenesis takes place within the seminiferous tubules of the testis. The major cell types within the testis are-

1. Germ cells

Germ cells are cells that ultimately give rise to sperm. Primitive germ cells- the PGCs colonize the genital ridge in the embryo and after a series of cell divisions form the precursor to the germ cell – i.e. the goncocyte. The gonocytes on receiving appropriate environmental cues from the surrounding milieu, at the predicted developmental stage, give rise to spermatogonia. Spermatogonia undergo proliferation and differentiation to give rise to other differentiated cells, the spermatocytes. Spermatocytes enter into meiosis and transform into haploid spermatids (Skinner, 1991). Spermatids eventually develop into sperm and post spermiation, are released into the rete testis and epididymis (Fig. 1).

2. Sertoli Cells

Sertoli cells are the somatic cells of the testis that are essential for testis formation and spermatogenesis. They facilitate the progression of germ cells to spermatozoa via direct contact and by controlling the environment milieu within the seminiferous tubules. Sertoli cells provide critical factors in the form of physical support, junctional complexes, or biochemical stimulation in the form of growth factors necessary for the successful progression of germ cells into spermatozoa (Figure. 1). These cells play an undisputed role in nurturing the germ cells by being the site of hormonal action (FSH) and secreting numerous regulatory molecules like Inhibin, transferrin, SCF, GDNF, lactate etc. They also harbour receptors for many ligands such as EGF and FSH (Spiteri-Grech, 1993). Sertoli cells undergo series of mitotic division and proliferation post birth. On attaining puberty, in response to the changing hormonal milieu, the cells stop dividing and undergo maturation.

3. Leydig Cells

Leydig cells or interstitial cells of leydig are present in lumen of seminiferous tubule (Figure. 1). Leydig cells are major site of steroidogenesis in testis. The principal function of the Leydig cell is production of steroid hormones namely testosterone (Sharpe, 1994).

Spermatogenesis can be divided into three main stages: 1) mitotic proliferation of spermatogonial stem cells and premeiotic differentiation of spermatogonia cells to diploid primary spermatocytes; 2) meiotic differentiation of primary spermatocytes to haploid early round spermatids via two successive divisions — the reductional division, in which homologous chromosomes are separated into two haploid secondary spermatocytes (each chromosome consists of two chromatids), and an equational division in which the two chromatids of each chromosome are separated into two haploid round spermatids; and 3) spermiogenesis, a cellular and nuclear reorganization process that turns spermatids into spermatozoa. The development of the germ cells begins with the spermatogonia at the periphery of the seminiferous tubule and advances towards the lumen over spermatocytes I (primary spermatocytes), spermatocytes II (secondary spermatocytes), spermatids and finally to mature sperm cells (Sharpe, 1994). While the basic phenomenon of spermatogenesis is conserved among species, subtle differences exist in the number and type of spermatogonia, the number of mitotic divisions, the number and arrangement of cellular associations/stages and the time duration of each cycle of the seminiferous epithelium.

Figure 1. Histological section of adult human testis depicting different cell types within testis

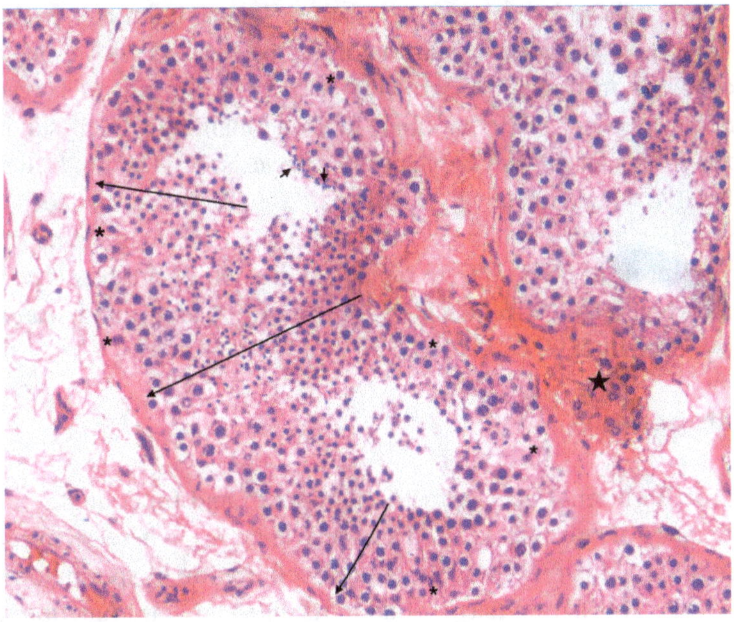

Figure 1. Histological section of adult human testis depicting different cell types within testis.

Black arrows indicate germ cells, arranged from the basement towards lumen of each tubule. Cells near the basement membrane with large spherical nuclei are spermatogonia, followed by spermatocytes. Smaller cells at the lumen are haploid spermatids. Mature sperm are indicated by black arrowheads. Somatic Sertoli cells are dispersed throughout the tubule, a few Sertoli oval nuclei have been labelled with *. Leydig cells responsible for producing Testosterone are present outside the tubule and have been indicated by a star.

Endocrine control of spermatogenesis

Spermatogenesis is influenced by many hormones which act directly or indirectly. Two important hormones that regulate spermatogenesis are FSH and Testosterone. The production of these hormones is in turn regulated by the hypothalamus and pituitary glands in the brain. Hence, commonly these glands along with testis are referred to as a single entity- The Hypothalamus- Pituitary- Gonadal Axis (HPG) (Ramaswamy, 2015).

The Hypothalamus synthesizes and releases a hormone known as Gonadotropin Releasing hormone (GnRH) in a pulsatile manner, which is delivered to the anterior region of Pituitary. In response to this, Pituitary releases two hormones Luteinizing Hormone (LH) in a robust pulsatile manner and Follicle Stimulating Hormone (FSH) in a sluggish pulsatile manner, into the blood stream. These hormones travel to the testis and act on different targets within and outside the seminiferous tubules of the testis. Both hormones mediate their effects by binding to transmembrane receptors LH-R and FSH-R respectively. While LH binds to LH-R on interstitial cells called Leydig Cells, outside the seminiferous tubules, FSH acts on FSH-R present on Sertoli cells that are somatic cells present within tubules. Importantly, both these hormones bind to non-germ cells and appear to exert their influence indirectly on them. LH upon binding to LH receptors on Leydig cells, causes synthesis of Testosterone. Testosterone receptors are present on Sertoli cells, hence effects mediated by T are via Sertoli cells. Sertoli cells on stimulation by FSH, produce Androgen Binding Protein (ABP) that binds to T and maintains increased intratesticular levels of T that may be important for specific stages of spermatogenesis. FSH action also results in production of Inhibin by Sertoli cells, which selectively regulates FSH (Ramaswamy, 2015). Inhibin and Testosterone together are the major feedback signals that control the HPC axis via negative feedback inhibition (Figure.2). Abnormal levels of FSH or T are typically associated with issues in spermatogenesis, resulting in azoospermia. Hence faulty feedback inhibition of gonadotrophins can also result in severe testicular abnormalities (Sigman, 1997).

Role of FSH in spermatogenesis

FSH plays a very important role in normal development, maturation and functioning of Sertoli cells. FSH is also needed for maintenance of cell cytoskeleton and cell junctions, where germ cells attach and develop. During spermatogenesis, FSH is reported to regulate proliferation of spermatogonia and their differentiation into spermatocytes. This action may be due to its anti-apoptotic function rather than as a mitogen (McLachlan, 2000).

Role of Testosterone in spermatogenesis

Testosterone in addition to regulating spermatogenesis, is also essential for development of secondary sexual characteristics, maintenance of accessory sexual organs. T has been reported to be indispensable for spermatid adhesion to Sertoli junctions and its absence can impact spermatid production. The rapid fall in human sperm count (within 4 weeks) seen with recent contraceptive regimens suggests an effect of gonadotrophin withdrawal at a late stage in spermatogenesis.

In summary, both FSH and testosterone are essential for meiosis, support spermatocytes and round spermatids, and help in spermatid maturation and spermiation. Therefore, both LH/testosterone and FSH are necessary for quantitatively normal spermatogenesis (McLachlan, 2000).

In addition to hormonal imbalance, stress, increasing age, smoking and alcohol, exposure to toxic chemicals such as endocrine disruptors and drugs, and nutritional deficiencies can all negatively affect fertility.

Endocrine disruptors and infertility

Endocrine disruptors (ED) are chemicals that can disrupt endocrine function, cause hormonal imbalance and hence result in infertility. They are found in environment and used in agriculture, pharmacology etc. They act on HPG axis and impact hormone synthesis, storage, release, transport or clearance. They may also affect hormone receptor binding, post binding activation as well as induce oxidative stress in testis. Common ED include agricultural and industrial chemicals such as Dibromochloropropane (DBCP), dichlorodiphenyl-trichloroethane (DDT), polychlorinated biphenyls (PCBs), Dioxins, and Methyl chloride. These are reported to decrease fertility, reduce semen quality and also cause fetal loss and birth defects. Heavy metals such as Lead, Mercury, Cadmium, Cobalt and Chromium may also act

Figure 2. Hypothalamus Pituitary Gonadal Axis

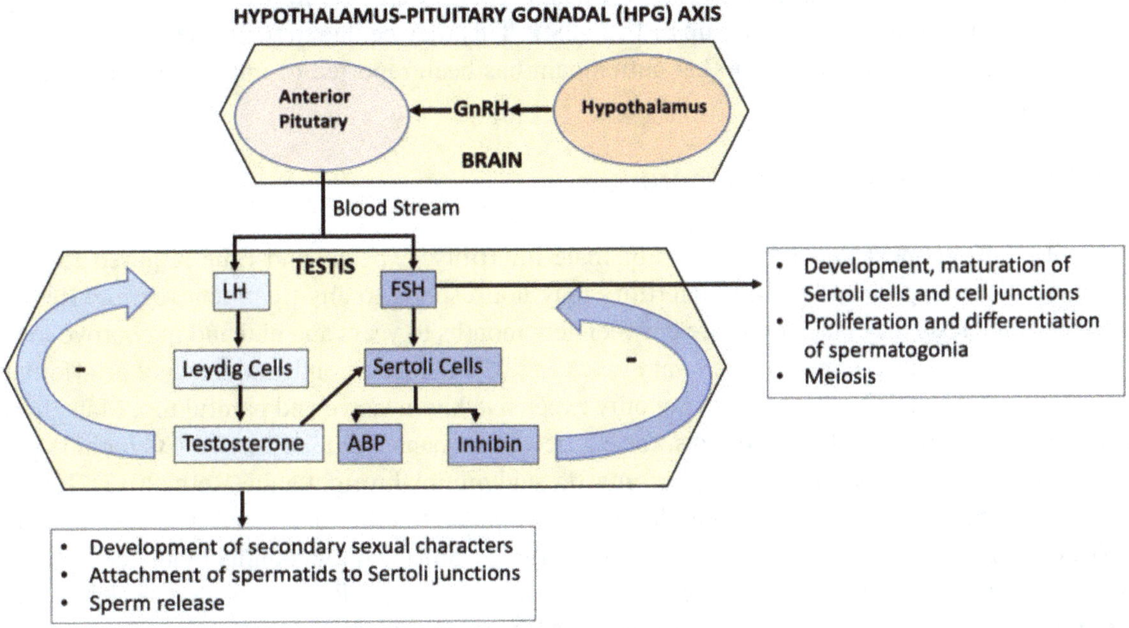

Figure 2. Hypothalamus Pituitary Gonadal Axis

as ED by causing testicular damage and lowering spermatogenesis.Pharmacological agents such X-rays, γ-rays GnRH-analogs, Narcotics, Anabolic steroids and Ethanol, cause endocrine disruption by causing germ cell and Leydig cell damage, decreasing sperm count and lowering steroidogenesis (Sikka, 2008).

Conventional treatment for infertility

The two main strategies being used in infertility management are hormonal treatment and antioxidant supplementation. Hormonal treatment includes use of gonadotropins, androgens, oestrogen receptor blockers and aromatase inhibitors. Gonadotropins are traditionally used in treating infertility due to congenital or acquired hypogonadotropism. Human chorionic gonadotropin (hCG) is an LH analog that is commonly used for Replacement therapy. hCG thus increases intratesticular and serum testosterone levels to improve spermatogenesis. hCG alone has shown to be able to maintain spermatogenesis only for short periods of time (Depenbusch, 2002).

Estrogen receptor modulators/blockers such as Clomiphene Citrate (CC) have been recommended for use in patients with low T levels or low Testosterone/Estrogen ratio. It blocks negative feedback of HPG and enhances LH and FSH excretion, thereby increasing T secretion and spermatogenesis. This treatment may not be effective in patients with high FSH levels.

Aromatase, is a cytochrome p450 enzyme present in many tissues such as testes, prostate, brain, bone, and adipose tissue. It converts testosterone and androstenedione to estradiol that negatively feeds back on HPG, reduces gonadotropic secretions and affects spermatogenesis. Aromatase inhibitors (AI) such as Letrozole and Anastrazole, decrease estrogen production by inhibiting cytochrome p450 isoenzymes. AIs increase FSH and T production and improve sperm parameters (Ring, 2016).

Antioxidants such as vitamins, zinc, carnitines, coenzyme Q-10 have been studied for their role in improving fertility. The most effective antioxidants reported are Vitamin E and Zinc, that improved live birth rate from sub-fertile males up to 11%–28%. This may be due to their effect on lowering DNA fragmentation. Coenzyme Q10, another antioxidant has been reported to improved semen parameters (Ring, 2016).

Limitations of conventional therapy

Conventional treatment depends on type of male infertility, expense and time required for effective treatment. Some types of idiopathic infertility may not respond to any treatment regime. Resumption of spermatogenesis may take anywhere between few months to years and end and may prove to be very expensive for patients. Treatment costs vary between 60-500 per month and may not be affordable for all (Gumus, 2012). hCG injections are not only expensive but invasive and painful too. Many hormonal treatments have undesirable side-effects, for e.g. few documented side effects of CC include gastrointestinal distress, dizziness, hair loss, gynecomastia, and minimal weight gain (Roth, 2013). Hence, they are only recommended for patients who have not responded to other hormonal treatments or for those who are willing to bear expenses. Large heterogeneity in results and low-quality evidence from many of these treatment studies warrant more placebo-controlled trails to validate their results (Ring, 2016). In addition to treatment regimens described earlier, ART may be needed in conjunction with medication. ART is emotionally and financially draining. It may not be accepted by many conserved communities. Hence, due to all these limitations, many patients across the globe have been considering complementary alternative medicine (CAM).

MAIN FOCUS OF THE CHAPTER

Complementary Alternative Medicine- does it hold promise for cure from infertility?

Uncertainty surrounding infertility treatment regimens and their associated high failure rates are compelling many patients to seek CAM. Centers for Disease Control (CDC), defines CAM as *group of diverse medical and health care systems, practices, and products that are not presently considered to be part of conventional medicine*. This broad definition includes many practices such as herbal and traditional medicines, acupuncture, mind-body techniques, energy healing etc. The focus of this chapter is use of herbal and traditional medicine in alleviating male infertility. CAM allows incorporation of cultural traditions and is reported to relieve stress and anxiety (Miner, 2018). Three types of plant-based medications have been discussed in this chapter, namely- Ayurveda (practiced in India), Iranian traditional medicine (practiced in Middle East) and Chinese herbal medicine (originated in China). It is interesting to note that these treatments have originated centuries ago in countries that are far apart and yet many common herbs are being shared by them. This is strikingly apparent in Ayurveda and Iranian medicine, which may lead to the conclusion that many of these herbal medicines may have strong role in infertility management, since they have been in use since a long period of time in multiple locations. Main herbs used in each of these three treatment modalities, targeted condition and treatment outcomes are discussed in detail in the following paragraphs.

1. Treatment of male infertility in Ayurveda

Ayurveda is the ancient Indian traditional medicine practice that has been extensively studied, described and practiced in India. This form of medicine has gained wide acceptance and is being practiced in many countries besides India. Ayurveda is based on balancing key elements in the body using diet and plant-based medication. The branch of Ayurveda dealing with psychological and physical sexual issues such as impotence, poor libido, semen quality etc. is known as Vajikarana Chikitsa (Vyas, 2018). Different plant derived aphrodisiacs have been described for various issues such as poor/late production of semen, improving semen quality, delaying ejaculation etc. Few examples pertaining to improving spermatogenesis and semen quality are described here (Chauhan, 2014) and summarized in Table 1.

Table 1. Summary of important herbs recommended in Ayurveda

	Herb	Form	Effects	Mode of Action	Reference
1	**Curculigo orchiodes**	Ethanolic and/or aqueous extracts of rhizomes	1. Improvement in the sexual behavior (penile erection, mating performance and vigor, mount frequency and ejaculation) 2. Spermatogenic potential and has anabolic effects 3. Overcoming testicular damage	The presence of the steroidal saponins in the extracts may be cause of testosterone and nitric oxide-mediated effects and also improved gonadotropic activity.	Chauhan, 2007; Thakur, 2008, 2009.
2	**Tribulus terrestris**	Granules	1. Stimulatory effect on spermatogenesis by increasing plasma T levels and other T derivatives 2. Enhanced relaxant effect 3. Improved seminal count and motility in oligospermic men	Increase in LH production that leads to increased testosterone levels	Gauthaman & Ganesan, 2008; Adaikan, 2000; Georgiev, 1988; Balanathan, 2001; Koumanov, 1997.
3	**Mucuna pruriens**	Seeds:Aqueous, alcohol extract	1. Reduced levels of stress markers (SOD, GSH, catalase etc.) 2. Aphrodisiac properties and stimulatory effects on spermatogenesis 3. Stimulates sexual function 4. In infertile men it improved T, LH, dopamine, adrenaline, and noradrenaline levels and reduced levels of FSH and PRL 5. Improved sperm count and motility of infertile men and reactivates their antioxidant defense system	Reduction in the ROS level, restoration of mitochondrial membrane potential and regulation of apoptosis.	Shukla, 2010; Tripathi & Upadhyay, 2002; Singh, 2013; Saksena, 1987; Amin, 1996; Ahmad, 2008; KK shukla, 2008, 2009.
4	**Withania somnifera**	Roots, dry leaves: Aqueous extracts, root powder	Improves spermatogenesis by-1. Improving semen parameters 2. Increasing serum hormone levels (increased serum T and LH and reduced levels of FSH and PRL) 3. Improves the level of antioxidants 4. Inhibits lipid peroxidation	1. By reducing serum cortisol levels and ROS.2. Increased LH and testosterone-like effects as well as the induction of nitric oxide synthase	Iuvone, 2003; Ambiye, 2013; Ahmad, 2010; Mahdi, 2011; Abdel-Magied, 2012.
5	**Chlorophytum borivilianum**	Roots: aqueous extract	1. Potent aphrodisiac 2. Enhanced sexual behavior 3. Used in treatment of decreased libido, premature ejaculation, erectile dysfunction and oligospermic conditions 4. Anabolic and spermatogenic effect 5. Increases sperm count	Enhanced sexual behavior may be due to testosterone like effects of extract, role in penile erection suggests role of NO.	Thakur, 2009; Kenjale, 2008; Thakur and V. K. Dixit 2006.
6	**Asparagus racemosus**	Roots: Hydro-alcoholic and aqueous extracts	1. Strong aphrodisiac 2. Increased sexual behavior (Penile Erection Index, latency in mount, intromission and ejaculation and hesitation time, mount frequency)	Not sufficiently described	Wani, 2011; Mishra, 2010; Thakur, 2009.

a. *Curculigo orchiodes*

This plant is commonly known as Kali musli and is considered to be a strong aphrodisiac. Various studies on rats have indicated that treatment with ethanolic or aqueous extract of this rhizome improves sexual behavior such as penile erection, mating performance and vigour, mount frequency and ejaculation (Chauhan, 2008). In addition, an anabolic effect indicated by gain in body weight as well as reproductive organs was observed (Chauhan, 2007). The plant extract has also been reported to play a role in overcoming sexual dysfunction due to testicular damage (Thakur, 2008). The presence of steroidal saponins in plant extracts suggests that these could be involved in gonadotropic activity and observed results could be due to testosterone or Nitrous Oxide mediated effects of saponins (Thakur, 2009)

b. *Tribulus terrestris*

Tribulus terrestris is a creeping herb, also known as Chhota Gokhru in India. In addition to treatment for sexual dysfunction, it has also been used in treatment for urinary infections, leucorrhoea and inflammations (Chopra, 2006). It is reported to have a stimulatory effect on spermatogenesis (Brown, 2001), probably due to its ability to increase LH production, serum testosterone and other T derivatives such as Dihydrotestosterone, dehydroepiandrosterone in rats (Gauthaman & Ganesan, 2008). Similar effects were observed in treated male rams and lambs (Georgiev, 1988). Oral treatment of this extract on New Zealand white rabbits showed an enhanced relaxant effect, substantiating its aphrodisiac effect (Adaikan, 2000). In oligospermic males, treatment with the extract led to improvement of sperm count (Sellandi, 2012). High levels of LH and T along with improved seminal quality was also reported in patients with erectile dysfunction (Balanathan, 2001).

c. *Mucuna pruriens*

Seeds of the plant *Mucuna pruriens* have been used in Ayurveda since a long time. The plant is referred to as atmagupta in traditional texts. The seeds are reported to contain neurotransmitter L- DOPA that stimulates spermatogenesis (Molloy, 2006). Seed extracts have been known to inhibit lipid peroxidation, improve sperm concentration and motility and recover levels of antioxidant vitamins and fructose in oligospermic patients (Misra & Wagner, 2007; Prakash, 2001). Use of the extract has resulted in reduced stress marker levels such as SOD, GSH, catalase, thereby helping in stress management in infertility (Shukla, 2010). In rats, treatment with extract has resulted in weight gain of reproductive organs (Saksena & Dixit, 1987) and improving sexual function (in mounting frequency, intromission frequency and ejaculation latency) (Amin, 1996). It is postulated that this recovery of spermatogenesis may be mediated by reduction in the ROS level, restoration of mitochondrial membrane potential and regulation of apoptosis (Singh, 2013). In clinical studies on humans, treatment with seed extract resulted in increased sperm concentration and motility and recovery of antioxidants, vitamins and fructose similar to rodent studies (Ahmad, 2008). *Mucuna pruriens* improved T, LH, dopamine, adrenaline, and noradrenaline levels and reduced levels of FSH and PRL in infertile men and improved semen quality, by its action on HPG axis in infertile men (Shukla, 2010).

d. *Withania somnifera.*

Withania somnifera is also known as Ashwagandha or Indian ginseng and is commonly used in Ayurvedic medicine as a aphrodisiac. Aqueous extracts of its leaves, as well as root powder have been used in improving spermatogenesis and sexual function. The extract has been reported to contain many flavonoids, neurotransmitters, steroids and alkaloids that are used in treating several ailments in addition to infertility (Dhuley, 1998). Aqueous extract treatment in rats led to changes in pituitary gonadotropins and high epididymal sperm pattern (Al-Qarwi, 2000). Other rodent studies have reported testicular development, improved serum testosterone levels and elevated sperm production (Abdel-Magied, 2001; Mishra, 2012). Administration of extract for 90 days to oligospermic patients resulted in elevated serum hormone levels and improvement of sperm parameters (Ambiye, 2013). Similar to *Mucuna pruriens,* this extract has also been implicated in inhibiting lipid peroxidationand improving levels of antioxidants, vitamins A, C, and E and corrected fructose, as well as increasing serum levels of hormones T and LH and reducing levels of FSH and PRL (Ahmad, 2010).

It is proposed that these effects of *Withania somnifera could be* due to increased interstitial cell stimulating hormone and testosterone-like effects as well as the induction of nitric oxide synthase and by reducing serum cortisol levels and ROS (Iuvone, 2003).

e. *Chlorophytum borivilianum*

Root extracts of *Chlorophytum borivilianum* have been used to treat reproductive health issues. It is commonly known as safed musli in India and is considered to be a powerful aphrodisiac (Mayank et al in 2009) and an equivalent to Viagra (Pratap & Rajender, 2012). In animals, treatment with this extract was helpful for oligospermia, erectile dysfunction and low libido. These effects could be attributed to testosterone lie effects of the extract and also a possible role of NO (Kenjale, 2008; Thakur, 2009). Sexual arousal, vigor, and libido improved in treated Wistar rats and their sperm count increased significantly. Similar effect on sexual behavior and an increase in body and reproductive organ weights was reported by Thakur and Dixit (2006).

f. *Asparagus racemosus*

Asparagus racemosus, is a climbing plant commonly known as Shatavari. It is regarded as a potent aphrodisiac (Lohiya, 2016). Aqueous and hydro alcoholic extract of its roots have been found to markedly elevate sexual behavior such as Penile Erection Index, latency in mount, intromission and ejaculation and hesitation time, mount frequency etc. in rodents (Wani, 2011). When used in combination with Chlorophytum borivilianum and Curculigo orchiodes, Chlorophytum borivilianum and Curculigo orchiodes, Asparagaus racemosus demonstrated anabolic effects, evidenced by weight gain in reproductive organs. Improved sexual performance was observed as expected. The saponins in the extract are assumed to be responsible for steroidogenesis and cause these effects (Thakur, 2009).

From these and other documented studies it is apparent that plant-based medications prescribed by Ayurvedic practice appear to have stimulatory effects on spermatogenesis. The extracts either function by influencing HPG axis or as antioxidants protecting sperm DNA from damage. While clinical trials have been carried out to validate few herbs, such data is not available for many of the recommended herbs. Problems related to toxicity have also been reported, which need to be considered. These issues are discussed ahead.

2. Treatment of male infertility in Arab Traditional Medicine (ATM)

Similar to Ayurveda, Arab Traditional Medicine (ATM) has been widely utilized by people in Middle East, since ancient time for maintenance of good health and treatment of ailments (Saad, 2008). 2600 known plant species have been reported in the Middle east, of which at least 200-250 are still being used for treatment and prevention of diseases (Said, 2002; Azaizeh, 2006). In Iranian medicine, sexual dysfunction is caused by imbalance of heat/cold, moisture/dryness in the body which may be associated with specific organ failure, neurological issues, drug abuse and other psychological issues (Nejatbakhsh, 2016). Hence while specific medicaments for sexual issues have been indicated, majority of treatments target the systemic disorder and recommend lifestyle changes, herbal medications and other therapies such as massage, aromatherapy etc. (Nejatbakhsh, 2012). In this chapter, only herbal medications related to alleviation of infertility is discussed.

Both Ayurveda and ATM recommend many common herbs as aphrodisiacs such as *Tribulus terrestris, Chlorophytum borivilianum, Mucuna pruriens* and *Withania somnifera*. Since these have been discussed before, additional herbs used in ATM are described in this section.

a. Crocus sativus

Crocus sativus is a plant cultivated in Iran, Europe, Turkey, Central Asia, India, China and Algeria. It is commonly referred to as saffron. Treatment with aqueous extract of saffron show increased sexual behavior such as increased mounting, intromission and erection frequencies) in rodents (Hosseinzadeh, 2008). Asadi et al. (2014) reported improvement in semen parameters in rats treated with aqueous extract. Similarly, in men with idiopathic infertility, oral intake of saffron milk improved number and motility of sperm. These observations could be due to increased testosterone levels induced by saffron (Heidary, 2008). Saffron is also reported to show a protective effect against DNA damage and chromosomal aberrations in sperm (Mardani, 2014). This was confirmed by another study which reported that Saffron reduced cytological and testicular alterations induced by sodium valproate (Sakr et al., 2014). These effects may be due to antioxidant properties of many water-soluble carotenoids such as safranal crocin and its derivatives crocetin and dimethyl crocetin found in saffron extract (Asadi, 2014; Heidary, 2008; Mardani, 2014).

b. Nigella sativa

Nigella sativa, also known as Kalijiri or black cumin, has been used in the Middle East as a traditional medicine for a wide range of illnesses. Seed oil as well as aqueous extract have been used in various studies and have been implicated in stimulating spermatogenesis by increasing weight of reproductive organs, improving sperm motility (Al-Sa'aidi, 2009) and viability (Tawfeek, 2006). In a trial on infertile men, administration of seed oil led to improvement of all sperm parameters (Kolahdooz, 2014). It is proposed that these effects may be due to various constituents such as thymoquinone, carvacrol, unsaturated fatty acids present in seed extract that enhance activity of enzymes involved in testosterone synthesis pathway (Kolahdooz, 2014).

c. Zingiber officinale

Whole ginger, is widely used in Arabic and Indian cuisine. It is known to have anti-inflammatory and antioxidant properties (Rahmani, 2014). Many constituents of ginger such as Gingerdiol, Zingibrene, gingerols and shogaols have antioxidant properties which may be responsible for its effects on spermatogenesis. Khaki et al., 2009 reported improvement of sperm parameters in rats post treatment with the rhizome. Similar effect on diabetic reports was also reported (Hafez, 2010). Other studies reveal that Ginger can reduce toxic effects of chemical like cyclophosphamide, gentamicin, deltamethrin etc. on epididymal sperm parameters (Bordbar, 2013; Hafez, 2010).

d. Sesamum indicum

Sesamum indicum, commonly known as sesame, is an integral part of Arab diet. Sesame seed oil is known to improve sperm parameters such as count, motility, viability etc. in male rats (Abbasi, 2013; Amini, 2013). Sesame seed oil contains sesamin and sesamolin, which are strong antioxidants, and these may be responsible for improvement in sperm parameters (Abbasi, 2013). In infertile men, treatment with

Table 2. Summary of important herbs recommended in Arab Traditional Medicine

	Herb	Form	Effects	Mode of Action	References
1	**Crocus sativus**	Stigma-aqueous extract	1. Enhanced sexual behavior (increased mounting, intromission and erection frequencies) in rodents 2. Improvement in sperm parameters 3. Protective role against DNA damage, chromatin anomalies and sperm membrane integrity 4. Increased number and motility of sperm in men with idiopathic infertility	1. The antioxidant effect of carotenoids including safranal, crocin and its derivatives crocetin and dimethyl crocetin may be responsible for beneficial effects on sperm parameters 2. Increasing blood testosterone level may improve sperm parameters	Asadi, 2014; Modaresi, 2008; Hosseinzadeh, 2008; Sakr, 2014; Heidary, 2008; Safarinejad, 2011; Bakhtiary, 2014.
2	**Nigella sativa**	seed-oil, aqueous extract	1. Increase in weight of reproductive organs in rodents 2. Improved sperm motility and viability 3. Significant increase in spermatogenesis activity in seminiferous tubule of rats 4. Reduced reproductive toxicity induced by various compounds 5. Increased percentage of live/ dead spermatozoa 6. Improvement of all semen parameters in treated infertile men	Antioxidant effects of constituents like thymoquinone and carvacrol, unsaturated fatty acids which enhance the activity of enzymes involved in testosterone synthesize pathway	Al-Sa'aidi, 2009; Abdul Rahman, 2013; Elshama, 2013; Tawfeek, 2006; Bashandy, 2007; Kolahdooz, 2014);
3	**Zingiber officinale**	Rhizome-methanolic extract	1.Antioxidative and androgenic activity 2. Improvement in sperm parameters in rats 3. Compensates harmful effect of toxic substances	Phenolic compounds including zingerone, gingerdiol, zingiberene, gingerols and shogaols have potent antioxidant properties which improve sperm parameters	Khaki, 2008; Khaki, 2009; Hafez, 2010; Bordbar, 2013; Zahedi, 2010;
4	**Sesamum indicum**	Seed-oil	Improvement in sperm parameters (sperm count, sperm motility, sperm viability) in rodents and men	Sesame seed oil contains sesamin and sesamolin, which are strong antioxidants, and these may be responsible for improvement in sperm parameters	Abbasi, 2013; Amini, 2013; Khani, 2013.

sesame led to improvement in sperm count and motility without improvement of sperm morphology (Khani, 2013).

In addition to these common herbs that directly impact spermatogenesis, several other plants have been described to improve sexual function by influencing various other targets and have been listed in Table 3. From this overview it is apparent that Ayurveda and Arab traditional medicine share many features, such as treatment modality and types of common herbs used. Also considering that both practices are ancient, these medications have stood the test of time and if they had not been proven efficient, they would have been discontinued.

Table 3. Herbs targeting different aspects of infertility described in ART

Function	Target	Herbs	References
Optimizing testicular function	Connective tissue repair	*Trachyspermum ammi, Alhagi persarum manna, Alyssum alyssoides, and Zingiber zerumbet*	Hosein Farzaei, 2014
	Hypogonadotropic hypogonadism	*A. hir- tifolium, Z. zerumbet, F. assa-foetida, A. europaeum, F. persica, C. rotun- dus, A. calamus, P. nigrum, Lepidium sativum, L. usitatissimum, N. sativa, Urtica, L. officinale*	Tansaz, 2016
	Autoantibodies against spermatozoa	*L. sativum, M. chamomilla, P. emblica, W. somnifera, F. persica, C. sativus, C. mukul, B. carteri, L. officinale, Urtica and Zingiber officinalis*	Amirghofran, 2010
Optimizing ejaculation	Peripheral neurological defects	*A. alyssoides, A. officinarum and E. sativa*	Nejatbakhsh, 2016
Optimizing libido	Neurological. Psychological effects	*P. emblica, Z. officinalis, L. officinale, P. nigrum, A. calamus, F. persica and B. niger*	Shahabi, 2008

3. Traditional Chinese medicine (TCM)

TCM is an ancient practice dating back to thousands of years and enormous volume of research has been carried out in this area. On similar lines with Ayurveda and ATM, TCM follows a holistic approach for treating disorders such as infertility. TCM focusses on different targets of spermatogenesis, such as HPG axis, boosting function of accessory cells such as Sertoli and Leydig cells, reducing oxidative stress and improving seminal quality (Zhou, 2019). A brief overview of studies in these areas and Chinese herbs recommended for the same are discussed in this section.

a. Effect on HPG

According to TCM, the kidney is the most vital organ in the body and plays an important role in growth and reproduction. Hence problems related to fertility, trace their origins in kidney. Alterations in HPG can cause both kidney and spermatogenic dysfunction and hence herbs targeting HPG axis can ameliorate issues pertaining to both. Different medications have been studied for impacting HPG axis by increasing or decreasing FSH and LH levels, by increasing Testosterone levels or by bidirectionally regulating FSH and LH. *Lycium barbarum* could significantly raise FSH and LH levels in rat model (Luo, 2006), while *liuwei dihuang* pill could do the same in infertile men (Ye Z, 2013). High FSH or LH levels are usually indicative of impaired spermatogenesis, hence medications that could lower these could help recover spermatogenesis. 2 medications- *Schizandra chinensis* polysaccharide, and *jingui shenqi* pill were capable of achieving this endpoint by decreasing FSH and LH levels (Zhang, 2013, Ma, 2011). Bidirectional regulation of increasing LH and simultaneously lowering FSH could be accomplished by *bushen shengjing* pill in a controlled trial of infertile men (Yue, 1996). Testosterone the other key regulator of HPG axis, could be elevated by *Cistanche tubulosa* and *Cistanche tubulosa,* which enhanced the steroid biosynthesis pathways (Jiang, 2016).

b. Stimulating accessory cells

The importance of Sertoli cells and Leydig cells in regulation of spermatogenesis has already been discussed. Stimulating these cells can thus impact spermatogenesis. WYP and *liuwei dihuang* pill extract were capable of stimulating Sertoli cells by enhancing cytochrome c oxidase, increasing vimentin expression, thereby increasing proliferation of these cells (Yang, 2010; Wang QZ, 2013). Two other extracts- *yangjing* capsule (YC) and icariin treatment were reported to influence Leydig cells by upregulating testosterone synthesis, reducing apoptosis and promoting their proliferation (Gu Y, 2015).

c. Reducing free radicle action

Reactive oxygen species (ROS) are known to cause oxidative stress by damaging sperm membrane and fragmenting its DNA. Studies have revealed that several TCM could reduce oxidative stress by scavenging ROS, increasing superoxide dismutase (SOD) levels and reducing malondialdehyde (MDA) content (Zhou, 2019). These include *Wuzi yanzong* (Yin, 2013), *jinkui shenqi* pill (Li, 2007) and *Morinda officinalis (*Wu, 2015).

d. Improving semen quality

TCM could improve seminal concentrations of metabolites, as well as sperm motility. *Jiawei wuziyanzong* decoction treatment (Chen, 2013) and *shengjing* prescription (Sun, 2012) could increase fructose levels, which are the main energy source for sperm. *Jiawei wuzi yanzong* decoction, *liuwei dihuang* pill treatments, *qilin* pill and the WYP could improve sperm motility and vitality (Shang, 2011).

The mechanism of action of most TCM appears to be similar to Ayurveda and ATM, i.e., by targeting hormones, reducing oxidative stress and improving blood circulation. Limitations associated with this area are also analogous to the other fields and include issues such as small sample size, lack of description of adverse effects and poor-quality data.

Issues, Controversies, Problems

The practice of using plant-based medications for treatment of ailments was a personalized form of treatment during ancient times. The knowledge regarding diagnosis, selection, preparation and dosage of herb extracts would be traditionally handed down generations in the physician's family. Ideally the practitioner would hand pick herbs or grown them in his own facility and personally formulate the medication according to the patients need. However, with changing time and increasing demand this entire process has been compromised, much to the patient's dilemma. Low professionalism of practitioners and mass production of medication has let to many issues such as adulteration, contamination and sub-standard quality of formulations. Lack of regulation by many international health administrators has aggravated this issue. This is evident by the rise in cases related to adverse effects and toxicity, post consumption of herbal medicines from various ethnic groups (Elvin- Lewis, 2001; Chan, 2003).

Many Ayurvedic medications consist of herbs, intentionally mixed with metals such as lead, mercury, iron, zinc etc., under the belief that these are therapeutic and that their toxicity is reduced during processing and preparation of the formulation (Breeher, 2013). Some of these medications are under regulation, however many are not. The absence of detailed ingredient list in many non-branded medications makes them an unrecognized source of toxicity. The alarming increase in lead toxicity cases after taking Ayurvedic medicines has become a public health concern. The presence of lead in various unbranded herbal and traditional medicines used in India to treat various ailments has been reported (Auyeng, 2002; Roche, 2005). During 2000-2003, a total of 12 cases of lead poisoning among adults was reported to CDC in US (CDC, 2004). Many case studies of lead toxicity have since been reported (Breeher, 2013; Geraldine, 2007). Other causes of herbal toxicity could be due to contamination with pesticides and microbes, contamination of cultivated soils and surroundings with heavy metals and poor harvest and storage practice (Saad, 2008).

Another major problem associated with CAM related to herbal medications is lack of standardization of study protocols. Low evidence, poor quality of generated data and small sample sizes makes comparison across studies difficult (Miner, 2018). Blinded randomized controlled trials have been very rare, and details of methodology, adverse reactions of drugs tested is scarce. One of the major obstacles in using herbal medications for treating infertility is that the mechanism of action of many of these treatments is largely unknown. While improvements in condition are monitored, mechanism of how this improvement occurred is not investigated. Hence evidence-based trials to validate these studies and to understand the molecular mechanism involved is essential (Zhou, 2019).

The absence of standards for evaluation of efficacy of treatment is also troublesome, as most studies focus on improvement of sperm parameters and not on restoration of spermatogenesis (Lohiya, 2016). Another neglected area in complementary medicine is assessment of mental health and quality of life (QoL) of patients. Although traditional medicine is considered holistic in approach, there are no reports about evaluating mental issues related to infertility. Hence largescale multicenter trails are the need of the hour to validate efficacy of herbal medications in treating male infertility.

SOLUTIONS AND RECOMMENDATIONS

Herbal medicines have stood the test of time and have been widely accepted by ethnic communities across the globe. This is because they are considered generally safe, effective and economic (Saad, 2008). Various studies have reported promising results, where sperm parameters and sexual function have improved significantly post treatment. Although adverse reactions and side effects of herbal medications are rare compared to allopathy, rigorous testing of formulations for safety should be mandatory. Good manufacturing practice by manufacturers and good agricultural practice by farmers to ensure appropriate soil quality, harvest and storage conditions, avoiding pesticide and microbial contamination is recommended.

In depth evidence-based studies, preferably multicentric and with large sample sizes should be conducted to validate efficacy of herbs that have been reported to be beneficial, negative results if any, should also be reported. Studies with valid research designs and higher level of evidence should be implemented. Research towards unravelling cellular and molecular mechanisms behind drug action need to be undertaken. Educating and creating awareness about adverse effects, toxicity issues and uncertainty in improvement of condition, post treatment is vital among potential users of herbal medications. Strong regulation by health administration is also necessary to prevent fake practitioners and adulterations in formulations.

CONCLUSION

Male infertility is a serious disorder that can affect the quality of life of young couples. While infertility can manifest due to different conditions, those related to endocrinological issues may be addressed and lead to alleviation of the condition. Conventional therapy for male infertility poses many disadvantages such as it is time consuming, expensive and may have numerous side effects due to hormonal treatments. Complementary alternative medicine (CAM), specifically involving herbal medications have become popular as they provide a more personalized treatment regimen, are inexpensive and may not have as many adverse effects. These medications have persisted since ancient times and are also more acceptable for many conserved communities. Many herbs find common mention in Ayurvedic and Arab literature (E.g. *Tribulus terrestris, Chlorophytum borivilianum, Mucuna pruriens, Withania somnifera* etc.) indicating their therapeutic nature and effectiveness. Chinese medicine has survived the test of time and many studies show improvement of spermatogenesis. Herbs used in Indian, Arab and Chinese practice, that have been documented to be efficient in treating male infertility have been discussed in this chapter. Their common mode of action appears to be reduction of oxidative stress, improving serum hormone concentration (increasing LH and Testosterone, reducing FSH levels) by effecting HPG axis or by influencing NO synthesis. Few human based studies have been described, where improvement of sperm parameters have been reported. Considering the advantages of plant-based herb medications in treating male infertility, this treatment modality should be revived, however the dearth of high-quality evidence, lack of information about mechanism of action and reports of toxicity and adverse effects precludes them from clinical acceptance.

It is very important to preserve the traditional knowledge about medicinal plants. This can be possible only if their benefits are validated and alternative plant-based therapy is encouraged. Therefore, well designed, multicentric randomized trials must be conducted to provide irrefutable proof of safety and efficacy of herbal medications in treating infertility. Molecular studies to decipher mode of action of these agents should be carried out. Strict regulations for production and formulation of these agents by certified practitioners should be enforced. Finally, all such research pertaining to herbal agents should be well funded, to encourage young researchers to take up this promising area of research.

REFERENCES

Abbasi, Z., Tabatabaei, S. R. F., Mazaheri, Y., Barati, F., & Morovvati, H. (2013). Effects of Sesame Oil on the Reproductive Parameters of Diabetes Mellitus-Induced Male Rats. *The World Journal of Men's Health*, *31*(2), 141. doi:10.5534/wjmh.2013.31.2.141 PMID:24044109

Abdel-Magied, E. M., Abdel-Rahman, H. A., & Harraz, F. M. (2001). The effect of aqueous extracts of *Cynomorium coccineum* and *Withania somnifera* on testicular development in immature Wistar rats. *Journal of Ethnopharmacology*, *75*(1), 1–4. doi:10.1016/S0378-8741(00)00348-2 PMID:11282435

Adaikan, P. G., Gauthaman, K., Prasad, R. N. V., & Ng, S. C. (2000). Proerectile pharmacological effects of *Tribulus terrestris* extract on the rabbit corpus cavernosum. *Annals of the Academy of Medicine, Singapore*, *29*(1), 22–26. PMID:10748960

Ahmad, M., Mahdi, A., Shukla, K., Islam, N., Jaiswar, S., & Ahmad, S. (2008). Effect of Mucuna pruriens on semen profile and biochemical parameters in seminal plasma of infertile men. *Fertility and Sterility*, *90*(3), 627–635. doi:10.1016/j.fertnstert.2007.07.1314 PMID:18001713

Ahmad, M. K., Mahdi, A. A., Shukla, K. K., Islam, N., Rajender, S., Madhukar, D., Shankhwar, S. N., & Ahmad, S. (2010). Withania somnifera improves semen quality by regulating reproductive hormone levels and oxidative stress in seminal plasma of infertile males. *Fertility and Sterility*, *94*(3), 989–996. doi:10.1016/j.fertnstert.2009.04.046 PMID:19501822

Al-Qarwi, A. A., Abdel-Rehman, H. A., El-Badry, A. A., Harraz, F., Razig, N. A., & Abdel-Magied, E. M. (2000). The effect of extracts of *Cynomorium coccineum* and *Withania somnifera* on gonadotrophins and ovarian follicles of immature Wistar rats. *Phytotherapy Research*, *14*(4), 288–290. doi:10.1002/1099-1573(200006)14:4<288::AID-PTR603>3.0.CO;2-9 PMID:10861976

Al-Sa'aidi, J. A. A., Al-Khuzai, A. L. D., & Al-Zobaydi, N. F. H. (2009). Effect of alcoholic extract of Nigella sativa on fertility in male rats. *Iraqi Journal of Veterinary Sciences*, *23*, 123–128.

Ambiye, V. R., Langade, D., Dongre, S., Aptikar, P., Kulkarni, M., & Dongre, A. (2013). Clinical Evaluation of the Spermatogenic Activity of the Root Extract of Ashwagandha (Withania somnifera) in Oligospermic Males: A Pilot Study. *Evidence-Based Complementary and Alternative Medicine*, *2013*, 1–6. doi:10.1155/2013/571420 PMID:24371462

Amin, Y. M. N., Rehman, Z. S., & Khan, N. A. (1996). Sexual function improving effect of *M. pruriens* in sexually normal male rats. *Fitoterapial*, *67*, 53–58.

Anawalt, B. D. (2013). Approach to Male Infertility and Induction of Spermatogenesis. *The Journal of Clinical Endocrinology and Metabolism*, *98*(9), 3532–3542. doi:10.1210/jc.2012-2400 PMID:24014811

Asadi, M. H., Zafari, F., Sarveazad, A., Abbasi, M., Safa, M., Koruji, M., ... Miran, R. A. (2013). Saffron Improves Epididymal Sperm Parameters in Rats Exposed to Cadmium. *Nephro-Urology Monthly*, *6*(1). Advance online publication. doi:10.5812/numonthly.12125 PMID:24719804

Auyeng, T. W., Chang, K. K. F., To, C. H., Mak, A., & Szeto, M. L. (2002). Three patients with lead poisoning following use of a Chinese herbal pill. *Hong Kong Medical Journal*, *8*, 60–62. PMID:11861997

Azaizeh, H., Saad, B., Khaleel, Kh., & Said, O. (2006) The state of the art of traditional Arab herbal medicine in the eastern region of the Mediterranean: a review. *eCAM*, *3*, 229–235.

Balanathan, K., Omar, M. H., Zainul Rashid, M. R., Ong, F. B., Nurshaireen, A., & Jamil, M. A. (2001). A clinical study on the effect of *Tribulus terrestris* (Tribestan) on the semen profile in males with low sperm count and low motility. *Malayasian Journal of Obstetrics Gynecology*, *7*, 69–78.

Bordbar, H., Esmaeilpour, T., Dehghani, F., & Panjehshahin, M. R. (2013). Stereological study of the effect of ginger's alcoholic extract on the testis in busulfan-induced infertility in rats. *Iranian Journal of Reproductive Medicine*, *11*, 467–472. PMID:24639780

Breeher, L., Gerr, F., & Fuortes, L. (2013). A case report of adult lead toxicity following use of Ayurvedic herbal medication. *Journal of Occupational Medicine and Toxicology (London, England)*, *8*(1), 26. doi:10.1186/1745-6673-8-26 PMID:24083830

Brown, G. A., Vukovich, M. D., Martini, E. R., Kohut, M. L., Franke, W. D., Jackson, D. A., & King, D. S. (2001). Endocrine and lipid responses to chronic androstenediol-herbal supplementation in 30 to 58 year old men. *Journal of the American College of Nutrition*, *20*(5), 520–528. doi:10.1080/07315724.2001.10719061 PMID:11601567

CDC. (2004). Lead poisoning associated with Ayurvedic medications – five states, 2000–2003. *MMWR. Morbidity and Mortality Weekly Report*, *53*, 582–584. PMID:15241300

Chan, K. (2003). Some aspects of toxic contaminants in herbal medicines. *J Chemosphere*, *52*(9), 1361–1371. doi:10.1016/S0045-6535(03)00471-5 PMID:12867165

Chauhan, N. S., & Dixit, V. K. (2008). Spermatogenic activity of rhi-zomes of *Curculigo orchioides* gaertn in male rats. *International Journal of Applied Research in Natural Products*, *1*(2), 26–31.

Chauhan, N. S., Rao, C. V., & Dixit, V. K. (2007). Effect of Curculigo orchioides rhizomes on sexual behaviour of male rats. *Fitoterapia*, *78*(7-8), 530–534. doi:10.1016/j.fitote.2007.06.005 PMID:17643866

Chauhan, N. S., Sharma, V., Dixit, V. K., & Thakur, M. (2014). A Review on Plants Used for Improvement of Sexual Performance and Virility. *BioMed Research International*, *2014*, 1–19. doi:10.1155/2014/868062 PMID:25215296

Chen, D., Zhong, J., Chen, S., Zhang, Y., Zhang, W., & Wang, G. (2013). Effect of supplemented Wuzi Yanzong decoction on the quality of sperm and secretion of seminal fructose. *Journal of Traditional Chinese Medicine*, *54*, 401–404.

Chopra, R. N. (2006). *Chopras indigenous drugs of India*. Academic Publishers.

Depenbusch, M., Eckardstein, S. V., Simoni, M., & Nieschlag, E. (2002). Maintenance of spermatogenesis in hypogonadotropic hypogonadal men with human chorionic gonadotropin alone. *European Journal of Endocrinology*, *147*(5), 617–624. doi:10.1530/eje.0.1470617 PMID:12444893

Dhuley, J. N. (1998). Effect of ashwagandha on lipid peroxidation in stress induced animals. *Journal of Ethnopharmacology*, *60*(2), 173–178. doi:10.1016/S0378-8741(97)00151-7 PMID:9582008

Elvin-Lewis, M. (2001). Should we be concerned about herbal remedies. *Journal of Ethnopharmacology*, *75*(2-3), 141–164. doi:10.1016/S0378-8741(00)00394-9 PMID:11297844

Gauthaman, K., & Ganesan, A. P. (2008). The hormonal effects of *Tribulus terrestris* and its role in the management of male erectile dysfunction – an evaluation using primates, rabbit and rat. *Phytomedicine*, *15*(1-2), 44–54. doi:10.1016/j.phymed.2007.11.011 PMID:18068966

Georgiev, P., Dimitrov, M., & Vitanov, S. (1988). Effect of Tribestan (from *Tribulus terrestris*) on plasma testosterone and spermatogenesis in male lambs and rams. *Veterinarna Sbirka*, *86*(3), 20–22.

Geraldine, M., Herman, D. S. S., & Venkatesh, T. (2006). Lead poisoning as a result of infertility treatment using herbal remedies. *Archives of Gynecology and Obstetrics*, *275*(4), 279–281. doi:10.100700404-006-0227-y PMID:16947057

Gnoth, C., Godehardt, E., Frank-Herrmann, P., Friol, K., Tigges, J., & Freundl, G. (2005). Definition and prevalence of subfertility and infertility. *Human Reproduction (Oxford, England)*, *20*(5), 1144–1147. doi:10.1093/humrep/deh870 PMID:15802321

Gu, Y., Zhang, X., Sun, D., Zhao, H., Cai, B., & Gao, C. (2015). The Stimulative Effect of Yangjing Capsule on Testosterone Synthesis through Nur77 Pathway in Leydig Cells. *Evidence-Based Complementary and Alternative Medicine*, 1–8. doi:10.1155/2015/408686 PMID:26413123

Gumus, G., & Lee, J. (2011). Alternative Paths To Parenthood: Ivf Or Child Adoption? *Economic Inquiry*, *50*(3), 802–820. doi:10.1111/j.1465-7295.2011.00401.x

Hafez, D. A. (2010). Effect of extracts of ginger goots and cinnamon bark on fertility of male diabetic rats. *The Journal of American Science*, *6*, 940–947.

Heidary, M., Vahhabi, S., Reza Nejadi, J., Delfan, B., Birjandi, M., Kaviani, H., & Givrad, S. (2008). Effect of saffron on semen parameters of infertile men. *Urology Journal*, *5*, 255–259. PMID:19101900

Hosseinzadeh, H., Ziaee, T., & Sadeghi, A. (2008). The effect of saffron, Crocus sativus stigma, extract and its constituents, safranal and crocin on sexual behaviors in normal male rats. *Phytomedicine*, *15*(6-7), 491–495. doi:10.1016/j.phymed.2007.09.020 PMID:17962007

Iuvone, T., Esposito, G., Capasso, F., & Izzo, A. A. (2003). Induction of nitric oxide synthase expression by Withania somnifera in macrophages. *Life Sciences*, *72*(14), 1617–1625. doi:10.1016/S0024-3205(02)02472-4 PMID:12551750

Jiang, Z., Wang, J., Li, X., & Zhang, X. (2016). Echinacoside and Cistanche tubulosa (Schenk) R. wight ameliorate bisphenol A-induced testicular and sperm damage in rats through gonad axis regulated steroidogenic enzymes. *Journal of Ethnopharmacology*, *193*, 321–328. doi:10.1016/j.jep.2016.07.033 PMID:27422164

Jungwirth, A., Giwercman, A., Tournaye, H., Diemer, T., Kopa, Z., Dohle, G., & Krausz, C. (2012). European Association of Urology Guidelines on Male Infertility: The 2012 update. *European Urology*, *62*(2), 324–332. doi:10.1016/j.eururo.2012.04.048 PMID:22591628

Kenjale, R., Shah, R., & Sathaye, S. (2008). Effects of *Chlorophytum borivil- ianum* on sexual behaviour and sperm count in male rats. *Phytotherapy Research*, *22*(6), 796–801. doi:10.1002/ptr.2369 PMID:18412148

Khaki, A. A. (2012). Pp-1 The Effects Of Ginger On Spermatogenesis And Sperm Parameters Of Rat. *Reproductive Biomedicine Online*, *24*, S5. Advance online publication. doi:10.1016/S1472-6483(12)60133-3

Khani, B., Rabbani Bidgoli, S., Moattar, F., & Hassani, H. (2013). Effect of sesame on sperm quality of infertile men. *Journal of Research in Medical Sciences*, *18*(3), 184–187. PMID:23930112

Kolahdooz, M., Nasri, S., Modarres, S. Z., Kianbakht, S., & Huseini, H. F. (2014). Effects of Nigella sativa L. seed oil on abnormal semen quality in infertile men: A randomized, double-blind, placebo-controlled clinical trial. *Phytomedicine*, *21*(6), 901–905. doi:10.1016/j.phymed.2014.02.006 PMID:24680621

Li, W. L., Dai, Y., Xu, D., & Ji, Y. B. (2007). Effects of different polar fractions from Jinkuishenqiwan on testosterone and oxidative stress in rats with kidney-yang deficiency induced by hydrocortisone. *Zhongguo Xin Yao Zazhi*, *16*, 1944–1946.

Lohiya, N. K., Balasubramanian, K., & Ansari, A. S. (2016). Indian folklore medicine in managing mens health and wellness. *Andrologia*, *48*(8), 894–907. doi:10.1111/and.12680 PMID:27681646

Luo, Q., Li, Z., Huang, X., Yan, J., Zhang, S., & Cai, Y.-Z. (2006). Lycium barbarum polysaccharides: Protective effects against heat-induced damage of rat testes and H2O2-induced DNA damage in mouse testicular cells and beneficial effect on sexual behavior and reproductive function of hemicastrated rats. *Life Sciences*, *79*(7), 613–621. doi:10.1016/j.lfs.2006.02.012 PMID:16563441

Ma, L., Jia, M., Nan, Y. Y., Liu, M. L., Wang, Z. R., & Ma, J. (2011). Effects of Jin- gui Shenqi pills on sperm quality and contents of hormones in adenine-induced infertility rats. *J Shandong Univ Tradit Chin Med*, *35*, 431–433.

Mahabadi, J. A., Bafrani, H. H., Nikzad, H., Taherian, A., & Salehi, M. (2013). Effect of Diet Contains Sesame Seed on Adult Wistar Rat Testis. *International Journal of Morphology*, *31*(1), 197–202. doi:10.4067/S0717-95022013000100033

Mardani, M., Vaez, A., & Razavi, S. (2014). Effect of saffron on rat sperm chromatin integrity. *Iranian Journal of Reproductive Medicine*, *12*, 343–350. PMID:25031579

Mclachlan, R. I. (2000). The endocrine control of spermatogenesis. *Best Practice & Research. Clinical Endocrinology & Metabolism*, *14*(3), 345–362. doi:10.1053/beem.2000.0084 PMID:11097780

Miner, S. A., Robins, S., Zhu, Y. J., Keeren, K., Gu, V., Read, S. C., & Zelkowitz, P. (2018). Evidence for the use of complementary and alternative medicines during fertility treatment: A scoping review. *BMC Complementary and Alternative Medicine*, *18*(1), 158. Advance online publication. doi:10.118612906-018-2224-7 PMID:29764413

Mishra, R. K., Verma, H. P., Singh, N., & Singh, S. K. (2012). Male infertility: Lifestyle and oriental remedies. *Journal of Science Research*, *56*, 93–101.

Misra, L., & Wagner, H. (2007). Extraction of bioactive principle from *Mucuna pruriens* seeds. *Indian Journal of Biochemistry & Biophysics*, *44*, 56–60. PMID:17385342

Molloy, S. A., Rowan, E. N., Brien, J. T. O., McKeith, I. G., Wesnes, K., & Burn, D. J. (2006). Effect of levodopa on cognitive function in Parkinson's disease with and without dementia with Lewy bodies. *Journal of Neurology, Neurosurgery, and Psychiatry*, *77*(12), 1323–1328. doi:10.1136/jnnp.2006.098079 PMID:16952917

Nejatbakhsh, F., Nazem, E., Goushegir, A., & Isfahani, M. M., Nikbakht Nasrabadi, A., & Baygom Siahpoosh, M. (2012). Recommended foods for male infertility in Iranian traditional medicine. *Iranian Journal of Reproductive Medicine*, *10*, 511–516. PMID:25246919

Nejatbakhsh, F., Shirbeigi, L., Rahimi, R., & Abolhassani, H. (2016). Review of local herbal compounds found in the Iranian traditional medicine known to optimise male fertility. *Andrologia*, *48*(8), 850–859. doi:10.1111/and.12675 PMID:27681643

Pasqualotto, F. F., Lucon, A. M., Sobreiro, B. P., Pasqualotto, E. B., & Arap, S. (2004). Effects of medicaltherapy, alcohol, smoking, and endocrine disruptors on male infertility. *Revista do Hospital das Clínicas*, *59*(6), 375–382. doi:10.1590/S0041-87812004000600011 PMID:15654492

Prakash, D., Niranjan, A., & Tewari, S. K. (2001). Some nutritional properties of the seeds of three *Mucuna species*. *International Journal of Food Sciences and Nutrition*, *52*, 79–82. doi:10.1080/09637480020027264 PMID:11225181

Pratap, S. A., & Rajender, S. (2012). Potent natural aphrodisiacs for the management of erectile dysfunction and male sexual debilities. *Frontiers in Bioscience (Scholar Edition)*, *4*(1), 167–180. doi:10.2741259 PMID:22202051

Rahmani, A.H., Al shabrmi, F.M., Aly, S.M. (2014). Active ingredients of ginger as potential candidates in the prevention and treatment of diseases via modulation of biological activities. *International Journal of Physiology, Pathophysiology and Pharmacology*, *6*, 125–136. PMID:25057339

Ramaswamy, S., & Weinbauer, G. F. (2014). Endocrine control of spermatogenesis: Role of FSH and LH/ testosterone. *Spermatogenesis*, *4*(2), e996025. Advance online publication. doi:10.1080/21565562.2014.996025 PMID:26413400

Ring, J., Lwin, A., & Köhler, T. (2016). Current medical management of endocrine-related male infertility. *Asian Journal of Andrology*, *18*(3), 357. doi:10.4103/1008-682X.179252 PMID:27098657

Roche, A., Florkowski, C., & Walmsley, T. (2005). Lead poisoning due to ingestion of Indian herbal remedies. *The New Zealand Medical Journal*, *118*(1219), U1589. PMID:16059407

Roth, L. W., Ryan, A. R., & Meacham, R. B. (2013). Clomiphene citrate in the management of male infertility. *Seminars in Reproductive Medicine*, *31*(04), 245–250. doi:10.1055-0033-1345271 PMID:23775379

Saad, B., Azaizeh, H., & Said, O. (2008). Arab herbal medicines. In Botanical Medicine in Clinical Practice (pp.31–39). CABI. doi:10.1079/9781845934132.0031

Said, O., Khalil, K., Fulder, S., & Azaizeh, H. (2002). Ethnopharmacological survey of medicinal herbs in Israel, the Golan Heights and the West Bank region. *Journal of Ethnopharmacology*, *83*(3), 251–265. doi:10.1016/S0378-8741(02)00253-2 PMID:12426094

Sakr, S. A., Zowail, M. E., & Marzouk, A. M. (2014). Effect of saffron (Crocus sativusL.) on sodium valporate induced cytogenetic and testicular alterations in albino rats. *Anatomy & Cell Biology*, *47*(3), 171. doi:10.5115/acb.2014.47.3.171 PMID:25276476

Saksena, S., & Dixit, V. K. (1987). Role of total alkaloids of *Mucuna pruriens* Baker in spermatogenesis in Albino rats. *Indian Journal of Natural Products*, *3*, 3–7.

Sellandi, T. M., Thakar, A. B., & Baghel, M. S. (2012). Clinical study of *Trib- ulus terrestris* Linn. in Oligozoospermia: A double blind study. *Ayu*, *33*(3), 356–364. doi:10.4103/0974-8520.108822 PMID:23723641

Shang, X. J., Guo, J., Chen, L., Deng, C. H., Sun, X. Z., & Geng, Q. (2011). Qilin pills for oligoasthenospermia: A multi-centered clinical trial. *Natl J Androl*, *17*, 1139–1142. PMID:22235686

Sharpe, R. M. (1986). Paracrine control of the testis. *Clinics in Endocrinology and Metabolism, 15*(1), 185–207. doi:10.1016/S0300-595X(86)80049-4 PMID:3514003

Shukla, K. K., Mahdi, A. A., Ahmad, M. K., Jaiswar, S. P., Shankwar, S. N., & Tiwari, S. C. (2010). *Mucuna pruriens* reduces stress and improves the quality of semen in infertile men. *Evidence-Based Complementary and Alternative Medicine: eCAM, 7*, 137–144.

Sigman, M., & Jarow, J. P. (1997). Endocrine evaluation of infertile men. *Urology, 50*(5), 659–664. doi:10.1016/S0090-4295(97)00340-3 PMID:9372871

Sikka, S. C., Kendirci, M., & Naz, R. (2004). Endocrine Disruptors and Male Infertility. *Endocrine Disruptors (Austin, Tex.)*, 291–312. doi:10.1201/9781420038866-9

Singh, A. P., Sarkar, S., Tripathi, M., & Rajender, S. (2013). *Mucuna pruriens* and its major constituent L-DOPA recover spermatogenic loss by com- bating ROS, loss of mitochondrial membrane potential and apoptosis. *PLoS One, 8*(1), e54655. doi:10.1371/journal.pone.0054655 PMID:23349947

Skinner, M. K. (1991). Cell-cell interaction in the testis. *Endocrine Reviews, 12*(1), 45–77. doi:10.1210/edrv-12-1-45 PMID:2026122

Spiteri-Grech, J., & Nieschlag, E. (1993). Paracrine factors relevant to the regulation of spermatogenesis-a review. *Journal of Reproduction and Fertility, 98*(1), 1–14. doi:10.1530/jrf.0.0980001 PMID:8345452

Sun, Z. G., Lian, F., Jiang, K. P., Zhang, J. W., Ma, F. M., & Zhang, N. (2012). Shengjing prescription improves semen parameters of oligo-asthenozoospermia patients: Efficacy and mechanism. *Natl J Androl, 18*, 764–767. PMID:22934526

Tawfeek, F. K. (2006). Effect of nigella sativa oil treatment on the sex organs and sperm characters in rats exposed to hydrogen peroxide. *Mesopotamia Journal of Agriculture, 34*(1), 2–8. doi:10.33899/magrj.2006.38488

Thakur, M., Chauhan, N. S., Bhargava, S., & Dixit, V. K. (2009). A Comparative Study on Aphrodisiac Activity of Some Ayurvedic Herbs in Male Albino Rats. *Archives of Sexual Behavior, 38*(6), 1009–1015. doi:10.100710508-008-9444-8 PMID:19139984

Thakur, M., Loeppert, R., Praznik, W., & Dixit, V. K. (2008). Effect of Some Ayurvedic Vajikaran Rasayana Herbs on Heat Induced Testicular Damage in Male Albino Rats. *Journal of Complementary & Integrative Medicine, 5*(1). Advance online publication. doi:10.2202/1553-3840.1112

Vyas, N., Gamit, K., & Raval, M. (2018). Male infertility: A major problem worldwide and its management in Ayurveda. *Pharma Science Monitor, 9*, 1.

Wang, Q. Z., Wang, D. F., Liu, H. L., Feng, D. J., Wang, H. H., & Guo, Z. B. (2013). Effects of extracts from Liuwei dihuang Pill on the proliferation of mouse Sertoli cells. *Lishizhen Med Mat Medica Res, 24*, 1363–1365.

Wani, J. A., Achur, R. N., & Nema, R. K. (2011). Phytochemical screening and aphrodisiac property of *Asparagus racemosus. International Journal of Pharmaceutical Sciences and Drug Research, 3*, 112–115.

Wu, Z.-Q., Chen, D.-L., Lin, F.-H., Lin, L., Shuai, O., Wang, J.-Y., Qi, L.-K., & Zhang, P. (2015). Effect of bajijiasu isolated from Morinda officinalis F. C. how on sexual function in male mice and its antioxidant protection of human sperm. *Journal of Ethnopharmacology*, *164*, 283–292. doi:10.1016/j.jep.2015.02.016 PMID:25686781

Yang, A., Liu, B., Zhang, S., Xie, C., Li, L., & Zhou, Q. (2010). Mechanism of Wuziyanzong Pills in improvement of function of Sertoli cells in rats with insufficiency of kidney essence. *J Beijing Univ Tradit Chin Med*, *33*, 378–380.

Ye, Z., Chen, D., Zhong, J., Zhang, Y., Zhang, W., & Wang, G. (2013). Effect of Jiawei Wuzi Yanzong decoction on sperm quality and hormone level. *World Chin Med*, *8*, 626–629.

Yin, J. L., Xu, Y., & Wu, B. (2013). Wuziyanzong compound relieves oxidative stress injury and inhibits the apoptosis of Sertoli cells. *J Natl Androl*, *19*, 257–261. PMID:23700734

Yue, G. P., Chen, Q., & Dai, N. (1996). Eighty-seven cases of male infertility treated by bushen shengjing pill in clinical observation and evaluation on its curative effect. *Chin J Integr Tradit West Med*, *16*, 463–466. PMID:9387745

Zhang, Y., Shen, N., Qi, L., Chen, W., Dong, Z., & Zhao, D. H. (2013). Efficacy of Schizandra chinesis polysaccharide on cyclophosphamide induced dyszoospermia of rats and its effects on reproductive hormones. *Chin J Integr Tradit West Med*, *33*, 361–364. PMID:23713251

Zhou, S. H., Deng, Y. F., Weng, Z. W., Weng, H. W., & Liu, Z. D. (2019). Traditional Chinese medicine as a remedy for male infertility: A review. *The World Journal of Men's Health*, *37*(2), 175–185. doi:10.5534/wjmh.180069 PMID:30644235

KEY TERMS AND DEFINITIONS

HPG Axis: The hypothalamus-pituitary-testis are often referred to as one single entity. Hypothalamus and Pituitary secrete hormones that control spermatogenesis in testis.

Infertility: Infertility is the failure of conception after at least 12 months of unprotected intercourse.

Spermatogenesis: The sequence of cytological events that occur within the testis, that result in the formation of the mature spermatozoa from precursor cells- spermatogoniais known as spermatogenesis.

Section 3

Cancer Treatment and Prevention

Chapter 8
Combinational Therapy Using Chemotherapeutic Agents and Dietary Bioactive Compounds:
A Pragmatic Approach to Cancer Treatment

Madhumitha Kedhari Sundaram
Manipal Academy of Higher Education, UAE

Shefina Silas
Manipal Academy of Higher Education, UAE

Arif Hussain
Manipal Academy of Higher Education, UAE

ABSTRACT

Diet-derived phytochemicals find prominent use in traditional medicine and have been credited with lowering cancer risk significantly. Dietary agents demonstrate anticancer activity by modulating various molecular targets and cell signaling pathways. Several studies have focused on combinations of dietary bioactive compounds and conventional chemotherapeutic agents to augment their therapeutic response and mitigate the side effects of conventional chemotherapy. The observed synergistic response heralds promise for successful future chemopreventive and chemotherapeutic strategies in cancer management. Animal models and pre-clinical trials of the effective combinations must be undertaken to clearly understand the mechanism of action. This chapter catalogues recent studies that have used dietary bioactive compounds (sulforaphane, EGCG, curcumin, genistein, resveratrol, eugenol) in combination with conventional chemopreventive agents and with other phytochemicals.

DOI: 10.4018/978-1-7998-4808-0.ch008

INTRODUCTION

Cancer is a multi-step, multi-factorial disorder that continues to claim numerous lives across the world each year. A cancer cell is characterized by its ability to achieve replicative immortality, unrestricted proliferation, capacity to invade, migrate, form new blood vessels, alter their energetics and promote inflammation (Hanahan & Weinberg, 2000, 2011). Inflammation and genomic instability are pertinent enablers of carcinogenesis, while altered energetics and immune response are being considered as emerging hallmarks of cancer. These capabilities are dependent on their ability to alter several growth-signaling pathways, death inducing pathways and cell regulatory pathways. The molecular biology that underlies these competencies are represented by two main classes of genes; the oncogenes and the tumour suppressor genes (TSGs) including those involved in DNA repair (Burstein & Schwartz, 2008; Herceg et al., 2018). While epigenetic mechanisms are at the centrestage of normal development, any abnormality alters cellular function by disturbing the balance between various proteins and regulators in the cells. Changes in the key regulators, leads to modifications in the epigenetic patterns impacting gene expression and results in development of malignancies (Soto, Song, & McLaughlin-Drubin, 2017). Alteration in epigenetic mechanisms including DNA methylation and histone modifications fuel widespread changes in expression of TSGs and oncogenes (Sharma S, Kelly TK, 2010). An ideal therapeutic strategy would be to target one or more of these cancer hallmarks and induce cell death.

Significant understanding of the biology of cancer has been achieved and several treatment avenues have been developed. Despite the huge advancements in diagnosis and treatment, cancer is responsible for a significant number of human mortality with more than 9.6 million people succumbing to it in 2018 alone (Bray et al., 2018). The number of new cancer incidences is set to increase to 22 million and a major proportion of them are expected in the developing countries of Africa, Asia, and Central and South America (Jacques Ferlay et al., 2015). In India, it is expected that more females (712,758) than males (679,421) will be affected in 2020, with 98.7 per 100,000 population affected (Mathur et al., 2020). It is estimated that if the risk factors such as tobacco, infection are modified then nearly 70% of cancers incidence across India can be prevented (Gandhi, Kumar, Bhandari, Devnani, & Rath, 2017). This highlights the need for comprehensive health care guidelines and the importance of healthy diet and lifestyle practices. In terms of both cancer incidence and mortality, cancers of the breast, lung and cervix are the top three respectively, amongst women across the globe (J. Ferlay et al., 2019). While for men, cancers of the lung, prostate and stomach have the highest incidence and cancers of the lung, liver and stomach have the highest mortality (J. Ferlay et al., 2019). Therefore, considerable attention needs to be given to the development of effective cancer treatments.

Chemotherapeutics And Its Limitations

For almost 60 years now, chemotherapeutic drugs have endured as the keystone of cancer treatment (DeVita & Chu, 2008). Despite, being the gold standard of treatment, high level of success has been elusive. Chemotherapeutic agents are capable of disrupting the cell cycle and reduce cell proliferation (Tao, Visvanathan, & Wolff, 2016). Further, they promote the onset of apoptosis, leading to cancer cell death. A similar mechanism of action is displayed by the majority of chemotherapeutic agents. Unfortunately, conventional cancer therapies and existing epigenetic modifiers are characterized by low specificity with non-specific action towards all rapidly dividing cells, resulting in substantial cellular and clinical toxicity and/or poor quality of life for the patient (Aslam et al., 2014; Beaver & Magnan, 2016; Chan &

Ismail, 2014; Savard, Ivers, Savard, & Morin, 2015; Tao et al., 2016). Several toxic effects have been documented such as headache, nausea, hairloss, ailments of blood cells and reduced immunity (Beaver & Magnan, 2016). For instance, the FDA-approved epigenetic agent, 5-aza- 2-deoxycytidine (5-Aza-dC) was found to bring about inhibition of DNA methylation by suppressing the action of DNA methyltransferases and ensuring anti-cancer effect by restoring the expression of TSGs (Derissen, Beijnen, & Schellens, 2013; Kaminskas, Farrell, Wang, Sridhara, & Pazdur, 2005; Stresemann & Lyko, 2008). However, the intercalation of 5-Aza-dC into the DNA makes it toxic for normal cells and hence, safer non-nucleoside compounds are being sought (Compagni et al., 2008). Another popular agent, cisplatin belongs to a class of platinum-containing chemotherapeutic compounds and is administered for treating solid malignancies. Cisplatin is associated with nausea, anaemia, loss of hearing and electrolyte imbalance (Florea & Büsselberg, 2011). Cisplatin-resistance is also observed in many patients (Chou & Talalay, 1984). 5-fluorouracil has broad spectrum activity against solid tumors and is used alone or in combination with other chemotherapy regimens. It interferes with nucleoside metabolism to bring about cell death and produces side effects similar to cisplatin (Longley, Harkin, & Johnston, 2003).

In order to avoid these debilitating side effects, drug doses may be reduced rendering the chemotherapeutic agents ineffective against cancer. Further, side effects also contribute to the patient's non-adherence to the treatment regimen and results in poor therapeutic outcome (Barthélémy et al., 2015; Huang, Chen, Lin, & Chang, 2016; Torresan et al., 2015). The inadequate efficacy of available treatment options by itself accounts for the high incidence of mortality (Mokhtari et al., 2017). Moreover, the complexity and multi factorial nature of cancer precludes the use of a single agent for optimum efficacy. Another reason for the recurrence of cancer and associated increase in mortality is the development of resistance to chemotherapeutic drugs (Cornelison, Llaneza, & Landen, 2017; Pan, Li, He, Qiu, & Zhou, 2016).

The toxicity associated with existing agents clearly indicates the need to identify safe chemopreventive and chemotherapeutic agents that can effectively cancer cells with a high degree of specificity.

Dietary Bioactive Compounds A Treasure Trove Of Anti—Carcinogenic Agents

In epidemiological studies, people with high dietary consumption of phytochemicals evidence reduced risk of mortality from cancer (Bal, Foerster, Backman, & Lyman, 2001). Further, it is estimated that increasing the dietary proportion of vegetables and fruits may reduce global cancer incidence by 7-31% (Bal et al., 2001). Several *in vitro* and clinical studies have shown that dietary bioactive compounds could be successfully used to inhibit or delay various stages of cancer (van Berleere & Dauchet, 2017; Q.-J. Wu et al., 2016). Phytochemicals effectively suppress various stages of carcinogenesis by modulating inflammation, immune system, oxidative stress, apoptosis and cell signaling pathways (Afroze, Pramodh, Hussain, Waleed, & Vakharia, 2020; M. A. Khan et al., 2015; Raina, Hussain, & Sharma, 2020; M. K. Sundaram et al., 2018, 2017; M. Sundaram et al., 2019). Further, several studies have documented that dietary bioactive compounds modulate the epigenetic machinery and thereby target the expression of multiple molecular targets (Kedhari Sundaram, Hussain, Haque, Raina, & Afroze, 2019; Sundaram, Unni, Somvanshi, & Bhardwaj, 2019). Figure 1 presents the consolidated effect of phytochemicals on various molecular targets and establishes their potential as chemotherapeutic and chemopreventive agents. Dietary bioactive compounds such as curcumin, epigallocatechin-3-gallate, sulforaphane, quercetin, genistein and eugenol display anti-proliferative, anti-inflammatory, anti-oxidant and pro-apoptotic properties and their combinations form the basis of this review (Hussain et al., 2012; C Sharma et al., 2012; M. K. Sundaram et al., 2018; M. Sundaram et al., 2019; Sur & Panda, 2017).

Figure 1. Dietary bioactive compounds impact various hallmarks of cancer through different signaling pathways.

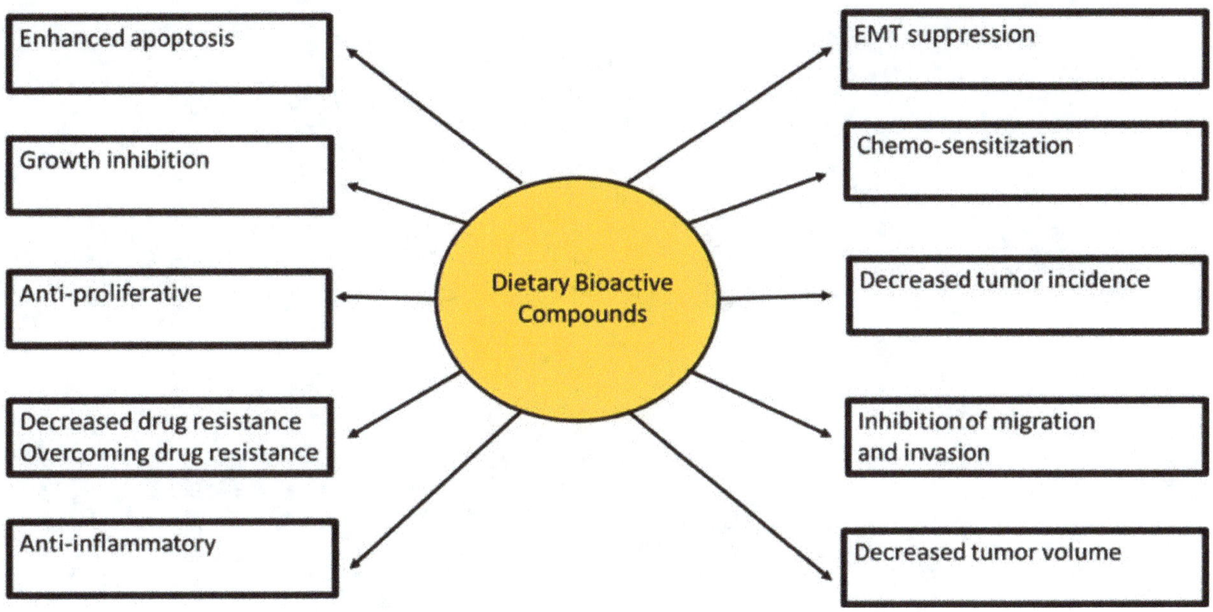

Rationale For Combination Treatments Using Phytochemicals As Adjuncts To Chemotherapeutic Agents

Combination treatments employ different compounds or agents concurrently which may interact in various ways such as additive (no advantage is conferred), synergistic (enhanced therapeutic outcome), or antagonistic (reduced therapeutic benefit) (Chou & Talalay, 1984). A multi-dimensional therapeutic strategy employing synergistic agents in combination may augment their effectiveness at a lesser dosage (Kerr, Adhikary, Grun, George, & Eckert, 2018b; Toden et al., 2015). This may have the added benefit of reducing toxicity in non-cancerous cells, relieving unfavorable side effects and delaying or blocking chemoresistance (Ben-Arye, Schiff, Steiner, & Silbermann, 2011; Fantini et al., 2015; Gopal et al., 2012; Mukherjea & Rybak, 2011; Rejhová, Opattová, Čumová, Slíva, & Vodička, 2018). The increase in therapeutic index can be attributed to the modulation of different signaling pathways by the individual agents (Asati, Mahapatra, & Bharti, 2016; X. Li et al., 2018). Further, it could greatly aid in patient adherence to treatment schedules and enhance the quality and quantity of life after cancer diagnosis.

Several studies indicate that dietary bioactive compounds can positively impact the response to chemotherapy. Given these advantages, augmentation of therapeutic efficacy with the use of safer dietary bioactive compounds as adjuncts to chemotherapeutic agents seems a viable and attractive strategy. This review summarizes the recent advances in synergistic combinatorial therapies involving the interaction of dietary bioactive compounds with conventional, clinically used chemotherapeutic drugs (Figure 2 and Tables 1-6).

Figure 2. Combination of dietary bioactive compounds and chemotherapeutic agents impact various hallmarks of cancer through different molecular targets.

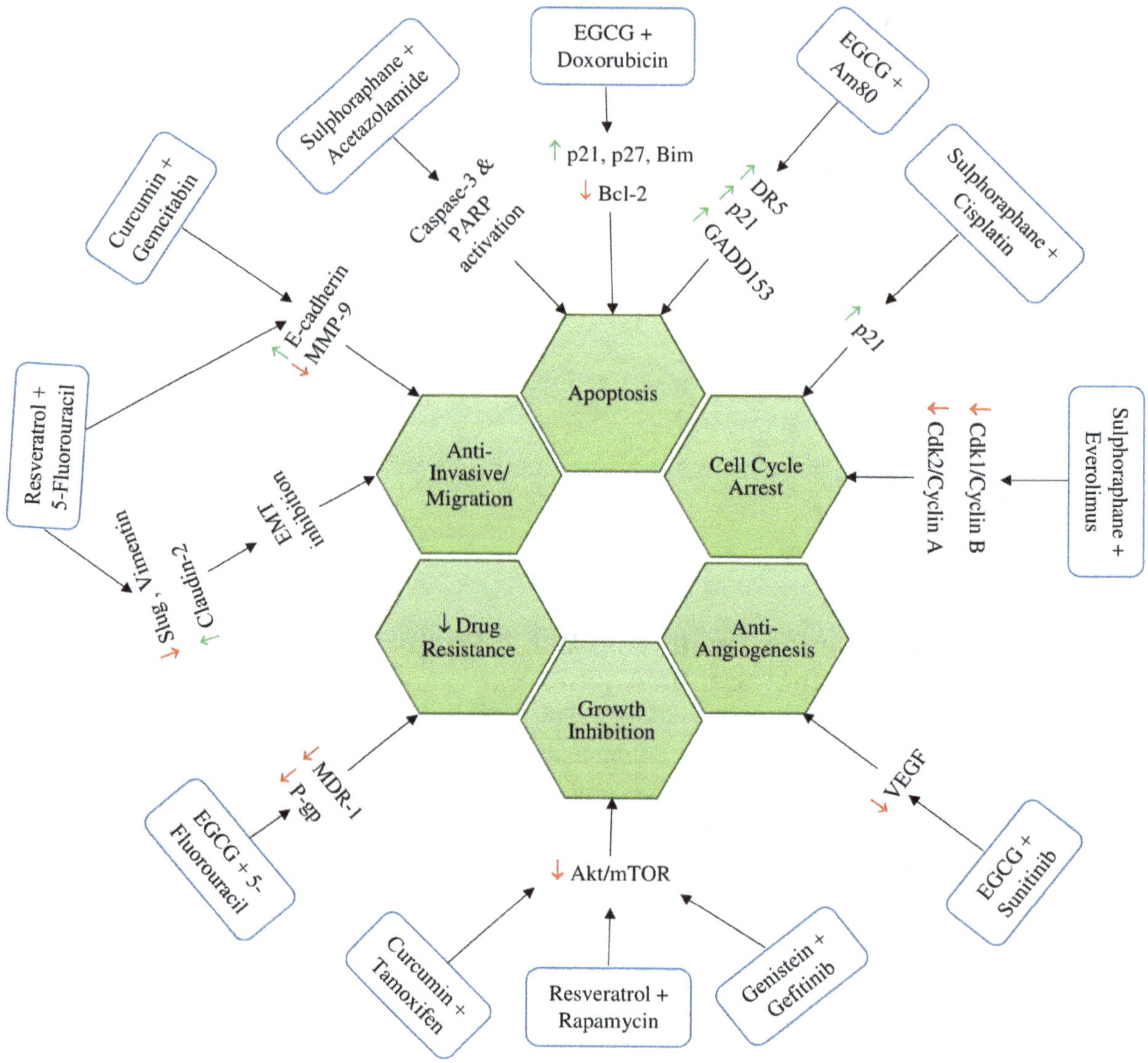

COMBINATIONAL THERAPY INVOLVING DIETARY BIOACTIVE COMPOUNDS AND CHEMOTHERAPEUTIC AGENTS

1. Synergistic Effect Of Sulforaphane In Combination With Chemotherapeutic Agents

A key member of the isothiocynate family, sulforaphane (SFN), can be sourced from cruciferous vegetables such as cabbage, cauliflower and broccoli. SFN individually has been observed to mediate cell cycle arrest, induce apoptosis and inhibit migration and angiogenesis in several cancer cell lines (Hussain et

Table 1. Studies that show synergistic effect of sulforaphane in combination with chemotherapeutic agents

Chemotherapeutic Agent	Cell line/animal model	Enhanced effect observed	Genes modulated	Reference
Doxorubicin	Rat breast cancer model	Apoptosis	Reduced IL-6 and TNFα	(Bose, Awasthi, Sharma, Benes, et al., 2018)
5-Fluorouracil	breast cancer cells MDA-MB-231	Autophagic cell death	Reduced thymidylate synthetase	(Malgorzata Milczarek et al., 2018)
Acetazolamide	bladder tumor cell lines HTB-9 and RT112(H)	Apoptosis, anti-metastatic	Caspase-3 and PARP activation	(S. S. Islam et al., 2016)
Everolimus	renal cell carcinoma cells A498, Caki-1, KTCTL-26	Growth and proliferation inhibition, cell cycle arrest	Reduced cdk1-cyclin B and cdk2-cyclin A	(Juengel et al., 2017)
Clofarabin	breast cancer cells MCF-7 and MDA-MB-231	Tumor growth inhibition	Upregulation of PTEN and RARbeta2	(Lubecka-Pietruszewska et al., 2015)
Cisplatin	skin keratinocytes, SCC-13 and HaCaT cells	Anti-proliferative, anti-invasive, anti-migratory	Increased p21 Cip1 level	(Kerr et al., 2018b)
Bicalutamide and enzalutamide	prostate cancer cells LNCaP and C4-2B	Anti-proliferative	Decreased PSA, androgen receptor expression	(Chandra, 2017)

al., 2013; Park, Kim, Bae, Yoo, & Choi, 2007; Chhavi Sharma et al., 2011). Its anti-cancer property has been attributed to its ability to modulate multiple signal transduction pathways including the epigenetic pathways (Ali Khan et al., 2015). SFN targets the Keap1-Nrf2 pathway that plays a role in regulating the stress response system. This increases Nrf2 and enhances transcription of Nrf2 target genes (Leone et al., 2017). SFN was shown to exhibit anti-cancer activity in the T4 human bladder cancer cells through the ROS-mediated intrinsic apoptotic pathway by activating ER stress and the Nrf2 signaling pathway (Jo, Kim, Kim, Park, & Choi, 2014). SFN inhibited proliferation of human thyroid cancer cell lines by repressing phosphorylation of Akt, upregulating p21 expression via the Erk and p38 signaling cascade and promoting mitochondrial-mediated apoptosis via ROS-dependent pathway (L. Wang et al., 2015). ERK 1/2-dependent signaling was also implicated along with upregulation of Bax and downregulation of Bim in SFN-mediated apoptosis of non-small cell lung cancer cells (Geng et al., 2017). Interestingly, SFN specifically targets precancerous and cancerous cells while non-transformed normal cells remain unaffected (Clarke, Hsu, Yu, Dashwood, & Ho, 2011).

Various studies have shown that SFN potentiates the action of chemotherapeutic agents in various cancers including cervical cancer and pancreatic cancer (Ahmad Ganai, Rashid, Abdullah, & Altaf, 2017; M. K. Sundaram, Raina, et al., 2019). SFN has been shown to potentiate the action of cisplatin and reduce the proliferation of HeLa cells and induce apoptosis. The study also showed that combination of SFN with another phytochemical, quercetin was also equally effective; highlighting the use of a cocktail of phytochemicals in lieu of chemotherapeutic agents (M. K. Sundaram, Raina, et al., 2019). SFN and cisplatin have also been shown to synergistically reduce proliferation, and migration of skin keratinocytes (HaCaT and SCC-13 cells) (Kerr, Adhikary, Grun, George, & Eckert, 2018a). Enhanced suppression of tumor formation was also observed in SCC-13 cell xenograft model treated with cisplatin and SFN (Kerr et al., 2018b). Similarly, SFN along with Everolimus prevented the development of

Table 2. Studies that show synergistic effect of EGCG in combination with chemotherapeutic agents

Chemotherapeutic Agent	Cell line/animal model	Enhanced effect observed	Genes modulated	Reference
Doxorubicin	Hep3B cells xenograft tumor model	Increased apoptosis and reduction in tumor growth, suppression of autophagy	Reduced LC3 protein, Atg5 and Beclin1 expression	(L. Chen et al., 2014)
Cisplatin	non-small cell lung cancer cells A549, H460 and H1299; mouse xenograft	Enhanced cisplatin sensitivity, growth inhibition	CTR1 upregulation	(P. Jiang et al., 2016)
Am80	Lung cancer cell line PC-9	Growth arrest, apoptosis	Upregulation of GADD153, death receptor 5, and p21^{waf1} gene	(Oya, Mondal, Rawangkan, Umsumarng, Iida, Watanabe, Kanno, Suzuki, Li, Kagechika, et al., 2017)
Erlotinib	SCCHN cells	Enhanced apoptosis	Increased Bim, p21, p27 and reduced Bcl-2	(Haque et al., 2015)
Actinomycin D/ Methotrexate	human placenta choriocarcinoma JAR cell line	Reduced cell proliferation & metastasis	Increased caspase-3 and Bax, decreased HER2	(Telli et al. 2018)
Sunitinib	Breast cancer cells MCF-7, H460, and H1975 cell lines; MCF-7 and H460 xenograft tumors	Anti-proliferative, anti-angiogenesis, tumor-shrinkage	VEGF reduction; suppression of IRS/ MAPK/p-S6K1	(Y. Zhou et al., 2016)
Temozolomide	Glioma stem- like cells (GSLCs)	Apoptosis, anti-migratory, inhibited cell viability	Down-regulation of cyclin D1, p-Akt and Bcl-2; overexpression of Bax, CD133, ALDH1, ABCB1	(Yong Zhang et al., 2014)
Cisplatin	Ovarian cancer cells (SKOV3 and OVCAR3); xenograft mice	Increased cisplatin sensitivity	CTR1 upregulation	(Xuemin Wang, Jiang, Wang, Yang, & Wang, 2015)
quercetin+ Doc	LAPC-4-AI and PC-3 cells	Cell cycle arrest, increased apoptosis	Decreased MRP1expression	(P. Wang et al., 2016)
5-Flourouracil	SGC7901/FU xenograft	Anti-proliferative, reversal of 5-FU resistance	Reduced MDR-1 and P-gp, VEGF, TFAP2A	(Tang et al., 2017)
IIF	SK-Ch-A1 cholangiocarcinoma cell line and colon carcinoma cell lines (LoVo and LoVoMDR)	Growth-inhibition, apoptosis, anti-invasive	Increased Forkhead boxO3	(Papi et al., 2016)
5-aza 2' dC	Breast cancer cells MCF-7, MDA-MB 231	Growth-inhibition, apoptosis	Increased RSG and pro-apoptotic proteins; decreased CCNE2 and CCNA1 CCND1, BCL2, survivin, wnt, DNMT3B, DNMT3A	(Angeles & Abbvie, 2015)

Table 3. Studies that show synergistic effect of genistein in combination with chemotherapeutic agents

Chemotherapeutic Agent	Cell line/animal model	Enhanced effect observed	Genes modulated	Reference
5- Fluorouracil	pancreatic cancer cell MIA PaCa-2	Apoptosis and autophagy	Decreased Bcl-2 and increased LC-3 and Beclin-1.	(Suzuki et al., 2014)
5- Fluorouracil	Murine xenograft of the PaCa-2 cell	Reduction in tumor volume	Increased LC-3B expression	(Suzuki et al., 2014)
Cisplatin	Non-small lung cancer, A549 cell line; xenograft of A549	Tumor growth suppression	Increased activity of caspase-3, -8 and -10; reduction in p-AKT and PI3K	(LIU et al., 2014)
Cisplatin	H446 small-cell lung cancer cell	Anti-proliferative	Downregulation of Cdc25, cyclin B1 and survivin	(Tian et al., 2014)
Gefitinib	H1975, NSCLC cell	Enhanced apoptosis, anti-proliferative	Reduced p-EGFR, p-Akt, and p-mTOR expressions	(Zhu et al., 2012)
Cisplatin	Cervical cancer cells, HeLa	Inhibition of NF-κB and Akt/mTOR pathways	Reduced expressions of NF-κB, p-mTOR, p-p70S6K1, p-4E-BP1, and p-Akt	(Sahin et al., 2012)
Topotecan	prostate cancer cells LNCaP	Enhanced apoptosis	Caspase-3 and -9 activation	(Hormann, Kumi-Diaka, Durity, & Rathinavelu, 2012)
Trichostan A	ERα-negative MDA-MB-231 breast cancer cells	Enhances hormonal therapy sensitivity	Increased ERα and decreased HDACs and DNMT expression	(Y. Li et al., 2013)
Tamoxifen	ERα-negative MDA-MB-231 xenograft mouse model	Enhances hormonal therapy sensitivity	Increased ERα	(Y. Li et al., 2013)
Trastuzumab	ERα/β-positive BT-474 breast cancer cells	Growth inhibitory	Increased expression of the tumor suppressor ERβ variant, cx	(Lattrich et al., 2011)
Cisplatin	hepatocellular carcinomaHCCLM3 xenograft in nude mice	Inhibition of tumor recurrence and metastasis	Decreased MMP-2 expression	(P. Chen et al., 2013)
Gemcitabine	Osteosarcoma MNNG/HOS tumor model	Tumour growth inhibition	Down-regulation of NF-κB and Akt	(Liang et al., 2012)

resistance in renal cell carcinoma cell lines (A498, Caki-1, KTCTL-26) and modulated the cdk2-cyclin A and cdk1-cyclin B axis to reduce proliferation (Juengel et al., 2017).

SFN potentiated the effect of doxorubicin requiring a lower concentration to bring about tumour regression in rats with breast cancer (Bose, Awasthi, Sharma, Beneš, et al., 2018). This combination could also induce apoptosis in cells harboring mutations in the crucial TSG, p53 (Fimognari, Lenzi, Sciuscio, Cantelli-Forti, & Hrelia, 2007). Further, SFN treatment helped overcome development of resistance to doxorubicin (Fimognari et al., 2007). SFN and 5-fluorouracil have been shown to synergistically induce premature senescence and autophagic cell death in MDA-MB-231, breast cancer cells (Małgorzata Milczarek et al., 2018). Similar results have also been obtained with salivary gland adenoid cystic carcinoma high metastatic cell line (ACC-M) and low metastasis cell line (ACC-2 cells) via inhibition of

Table 4. Studies that show synergistic effect of curcumin in combination with chemotherapeutic agents

Chemo-therapeutic Agent	Cell line/animal model	Enhanced effect observed	Genes modulated	Reference
Paclitaxel	Cervical cancer cells HeLa, CaSki	Enhanced apoptosis	Increased p53 and caspase-3	(Dang et al., 2015)
Paclitaxel	Xenograft of cervical cancer cells HeLa cells	Decreased tumor incidence and tumor volume	Downregulation of NF-κB, Akt and MAP kinases	(Sreekanth et al., 2011)
Bortezomib	Multiple myeloma MM1.R cells	Anti-proliferative, enhanced apoptosis	Increased caspase-3 and -9, decreased NF-κB and HSP-90	(Zheng et al., 2016)
Paclitaxel	ovarian cancer cell A2780	Decreased drug resistance	Reduced P-glycoprotein (P-gp)	(Z. Liu et al., 2016)
Gemcitabine	Gemcitabine-resistant PDAC cell lines, xenograft mouse model	Chemo-sensitization	Decreased PRC2 subunit EZH2 and the lncRNA, PVT1	(Yoshida et al., 2017)
5- Fluorouracil	colorectal cancer cells HCT116 and SW480	Enhanced apoptosis, Anti-proliferative, EMT suppression	Downregulation of BMI1, SUZ12 and EZH2	(Toden et al., 2015)
5- Fluorouracil	colorectal cancer cells HCT116	Apoptosis, anti-proliferative	Increased caspase-8, -9, -3, PARP and Bax; decreased Bcl-xL and cyclin D1	(Shakibaei et al., 2013)
FOLFOX	Patient-derived explants of colorectal liver metastases	Anti-proliferative and pro-apoptotic	Reduction in stem cell-associated markers such as ALDH and CD133	(James et al., 2015)
Tamoxifen	breast cancer cell lines MCF-7/LCC2 and MCF-7/LCC9	Growth inhibition, apoptosis	Inactivation of NF-κB, Src and Akt/mTOR pathways; reduced EZH2	(M. Jiang et al., 2013)
Bicalutamide	Prostate cancer cell lines PC3, and DU145	Growth inhibition	Reduced NF-κB subunit p65; increased phosphorylation of ERK1/2 and SAPK/JNK	(J. Li et al., 2015)
Carboplatin	Non- small lung cancer cells A549	Inhibition of tumor cell growth, migration, and invasion	Increased p53, caspase-3 and caspase-9; decreased Bcl-2, MMP-2 and MMP-9	(Kang et al., 2015)
Cisplatin	Non- small lung cancer cells A549 and H2170	Cell growth arrest, apoptosis, migratory inhibition	Increased p21, Apaf1, caspase-9; reduced cyclin D1	(Baharuddin et al., 2016)
Mitomycin C	MCF-7 breast cancer cells	Apoptosis	Increased Bax, Bak, Bad, Bik, and Bim; reduced Bcl-2 and Bcl-w	(Q.-M. Zhou et al., 2017b)
Gemcitabine	MiaPaCa-2 cells	Apoptosis, anti-proliferative, decreased cell migration/invasion	Increased E-cadherin, reduced MMP-9	(Avan et al., 2016b)

the NFkB pathway (Xiao-Feng Wang, Wu, Li, Lu, & Yang, 2009). The carbonic anhydrase inhibitor acetazolamide is potentiated by SFN in the bladder tumor cells (HTB-9 and RT112(H)) and induces apoptosis via inhibition of AKT pathway and activation of PARP and caspase cascade (S. S. Islam et

Table 5. Studies that show synergistic effect of resveratrol in combination with chemotherapeutic agents

Chemotherapeutic Agent	Cell line/animal model	Enhanced effect observed	Genes modulated	Reference
5- Fluorouracil	HCT116, SW480	Anti-invasive, EMT inhibition	Decreased vimentin and slug; increased claudin-2, E-cadherin, MMP-9, caspase-3	(Buhrmann et al., 2015)
Cisplatin	Lung cancer (A549) cells	Apoptosis and autophagy	Reduced P-AKT expression, increased LC3	(Hu et al., 2016)
5- Fluorouracil	B16 murine melanoma model	Cell growth and angiogenesis suppression	Reduced levels of AMPK, VASP, VEGF and COX2	(Lee et al., 2015)
Raamycin	TSC1$^{-/-}$ MEF cells	Apoptosis	Inhibition of mTOR and PI3K signaling	(Alayev et al., 2017)
Paclitaxel	MCF-7/Adr xenografts	Drug resistance reversal; tumor growth inhibition	-	(Meng et al., 2016)
Paclitaxel	HepG2 cells	Apoptosis, anti-proliferative, anti-angiogenesis, anti-migratory	Up-regulation of caspase-3, caspase-8, caspase-9, Bax, p53, p21, IκB-α, Fas, FasL, TIMP-1 & TIMP-2; down-regulation of Bcl-2, Bcl-xL, HIAP-1, HIAP-2, NF-κB, COX-2, iNOS, MMP-2, MMP-9, EGF, EGFR, VEGF, Fit-1	(Q. Jiang et al., 2017)
Vemurafenib	Vemurafenib-resistant (BRAF V600E mutation) melanoma cells	Anti-proliferative	Increased -pAKT	(Luo et al., 2016)

al., 2016). This combination also reduced the metastatic potential of the tumor cells via downregulation of pro-metastasis genes (S. S. Islam et al., 2016).

SFN reactivates epigenetically-silenced TSGs in breast cancer cells (MCF-7 and MDA-MB-231) on its own and enhances the efficacy of clofarabine (Lubecka-Pietruszewska et al., 2015). This com-

Table 6. Studies that show synergistic effect of resveratrol in combination with chemotherapeutic agents

Chemotherapeutic Agent	Cell line/animal model	Enhanced effect observed	Genes modulated	Reference
Cisplatin	Triple-negative breast cancer cells	Growth and EMT inhibition	Inhibition of NF-κB pathway, downregulation of IL-6 and IL-8	(S. Islam et al., 2017)
2-Methoxyestradiol	Prostate cancer cells	Enhanced apoptosis and growth inhibition	Decreased Bcl-2 and increased Bax expression	(Ghosh et al., 2009)
Gemcitabine	HeLa cervical cancer cells	Anti-inflammatory and anti-apoptotic effects	Down-regulation of Bcl-2, COX-2 and IL-1β	(Hussain et al., 2011)
Cisplatin	HeLa cervical cancer cells	Enhanced apoptosis and cell cycle arrest	Increased caspase-3 activity	(Yi et al., 2015)
5- Fluorouracil	HeLa cervical cancer cells	Cell cycle arrest	-	(Hemaiswarya & Doble, 2013)

bination also restored the expression of the TSG, CDKN2A and retarded tumour growth (Lubecka, Kaufman-Szymczyk, & Fabianowska-Majewska, 2018). SFN is also considered as a promising adjunct to increase the efficacy of anti-androgens for the treatment of aggressive prostate cancer cells (Chandra, 2017). Across various cell types, sulforaphane was found to be effective and contributed to synergistic anti-cancer effect; the studies and their outcome are listed in table 1.

2. Synergistic Effect Of EGCG In Combination With Chemotherapeutics

EGCG or (-)-epigallocatechin- 3-gallate, a catechin present abundantly in green tea, has anti-oxidant and anti-inflammatory properties (Fujiki, Sueoka, Watanabe, & Suganuma, 2015; Papi et al., 2016; Shen et al., 2014). EGCG also exhibits anti-proliferative, anti-angiogenic and anti-metastatic capability (Fujiki, Sueoka, et al., 2015; Papi et al., 2016; Shen et al., 2014). Epidemiological study suggests that 10 cups of EGCG a day brings about a signification reduction in cancer risk (Fujiki, Imai, et al., 2015). It is able to mediate cell cycle arrest and reduce telomerase activity in cervical cancer cells and gastric carcinoma cells (Gonzalez, 2014; C Sharma et al., 2012). By inhibiting the Wnt/β-catenin pathway, it suppresses carcinogenic potential of colorectal cancer cells (Y. Chen et al., 2017). Another study showed that the inhibition of p38MAPK, Akt or ERK1/2 led to partial blocking of EGCG-induced tumor cell death, thereby suggesting that these pathways play a role in the anti-cancer activities of EGCG (Cerezo-Guisado et al., 2015). EGCG is also able to modulate the epigenetic pathways in cervical cancer cells (M. Khan et al., 2015). It also demonstrates the capability to potentiate other therapeutic agents.

Synergistic decline in proliferation, angiogenesis resulting in tumor shrinkage was noted in MCF-7, H460, and H1975 cell lines as well as MCF-7 and H460 xenograft tumors treated with EGCG and sunitinib (Y. Zhou, Tang, Du, Ding, & Liu, 2016). The effectiveness of this combination against a wide array of cell lines is significant. Zhou *et al* reported that the combination worked by suppressing the IRS/MAPK/p-S6K1 signaling cascade and regulating the PI3K/AKT and MEK/ERK signaling, leading to a reduction in VEGF. Treatment of xenograft tumor model of Hep3B cells with a combination of EGCG and doxorubicin synergistically increased apoptosis and reduced tumor growth (L. Chen et al., 2014). EGCG was also able to enhance cisplatin-induced growth inhibition in non-small cell lung cancer cells such as A549, H460 and H1299, and in a mouse xenograft model (P. Jiang, Wu, Wang, Huang, & Feng, 2016). Further, it sensitised ovarian cancer cells (SKOV3 and OVCAR3) and xenograft mice to cisplatin via increase in expression of CTR1 (Wang et al. 2015).

The human lung cancer cell line PC-9 when subjected to Am80, a synthetic retinoid, in combination with EGCG showed increased apoptosis and up-regulation of p21, WAF1, Death Receptor 5 and GADD153 genes (Oya, Mondal, Rawangkan, Umsumarng, Iida, Watanabe, Kanno, Suzuki, Li, & Kagechika, 2017). In head and neck cancers cells, a combination of erlotinib and EGCG, exhibited synergistic anti-cancer effects by inhibiting Bcl-2 expression, phosphorylation of AKT, ERK and upregulating p21, p27 and Bim (Haque et al., 2015). Methotrexate (MTX) and actinomycin-D (ACD), which are usually used to treat gestational trophoblastic neoplasia, showed better survival outcomes in JAR (human placenta choriocarcinoma) cell line when used in combination with EGCG, as evidenced by increased caspase-3 activation and Bax expression (Telli et al. 2018).

Temozolomide, a DNA-methylating agent which is utilized as the first line of chemotherapy for glioma, when used in combination with EGCG was shown to synergistically inhibit the stem cell characteristics, cell viability and migration of glioma stem-like cells (GSLCs) (Yong Zhang, Ma, & Xie, 2014). This was an outcome of a decrease in the expression of p-Akt, cyclin D1 and Bcl-2, as well as an increase in the expression of ALDH1, CD133, Bax and the drug-resistance gene, ABCB1 (Yong Zhang et al., 2014). The combination of EGCG, quercetin and docetaxel was shown to synergistically inhibit proliferation in LAPC-4-AI cells when compared to docetaxel treatment alone (P. Wang, Henning, Heber, Vadgama, & Angeles, 2016). This was accomplished through an increased inhibition of the STAT3 and PI3K/Akt signaling pathways. In addition, this combination treatment showed a greater inhibition of tumor cell invasion and colony formation as well as a reduction in the levels of CD44+/CD24− stem-like LAPC-4-AI cells and multi drug resistance-related protein (MRP1) (P. Wang et al., 2016).

EGCG in combination with 5-fluorouracil in gastric cancer cells suppressed tumor growth and proliferation and reduced angiogenesis via down-regulation of VEGF (Tang, Zeng, Wang, Zhang, & Ruan, 2017). This combination also suppressed the development of drug resistance by downregulating MDR-1 and P-gp in gastric cancer cells and in SGC7901/FU xenograft (Tang et al., 2017).

The capacity of EGCG to bring about epigenetic changes in combination is well documented. Breast cancer cell lines (MCF-7, MDA-MB 231) treated with a combination of EGCG and the DNA methylation inhibitor, 5-aza-2¢-deoxycytidine, showed enhanced apoptosis and tumor inhibition (Angeles & Abbvie, 2015). Crucially, normal breast epithelial cells remained unaffected. Significant downregulation of DNA methyltransferases DNMT3B, DNMT3A and genes involved in cell cycle and apoptosis such as CCNE2, CCNA1, CCND1, BCL2, survivin and WNT1 with simultaneous upregulation of pro-apoptotic proteins was observed.

EGCG was also found to exert synergistic interaction in combination with other therapeutic ligands under development. The combined treatment of EGCG and RXRg ligand, 6-OH-11-Ohydroxyphenantrene in cholangiocarcinoma (SK-Ch-A1) and colon carcinoma cell lines (LoVo and LoVoMDR) showed synergistic growth inhibition and apoptosis, accompanied by the upregulation of Forkhead box O3 expression (Papi et al., 2016). Moreover, tumor cell invasion was inhibited through the suppression of activity of metalloproteinase and its inducer (EMMPRIN), following combination treatment in the SK-Ch-A1 cell line (Papi et al., 2016). Another report supports the use EGCG in combination with a PDE5 inhibitor for treating early stage CLL with overexpression of PDE5 and 67LR (Weinkauf & Dreyling, 2015). These studies and their outcome are listed in table 2.

3. Synergistic Effect Of Curcumin In Combination With Chemotherapeutics

Curcumin is a polyphenol obtained from the roots of the turmeric plant (*Curcuma longa*), which is widely used in Ayurvedic medicine. Curcumin has been studied extensively to understand its anticancer properties and mechanism of action. In addition to its anticancer properties, it is well-known for its wound healing, anti-inflammatory and anti-microbial activity. Curcumin is known to elicit chemo-preventive action by activating the Nrf2 signaling, inducing phase II antioxidant enzymes; modulating pro-inflammatory proteins such as TGF-β and COX2 and restoring p53 expression (Das & Vinayak, 2015). Curcumin inhibits proliferation of breast cancer cells by down-regulating NF-κBp65, and by inhibiting the JAK2/STAT3 pathway in H460 lung cancer cells (D. Liu & Chen, 2013; L. Wu et al., 2015).

Several studies have shown the ability of curcumin to enhance the anti-tumor effects of various chemotherapeutic drugs (Table 3). For instance, the combination of curcumin with mitomycin c (MMC) synergistically enhanced apoptosis in MCF-7 breast cancer-like stem cells; and the combination of bortezomib with curcumin could inhibit proliferation and enhance apoptosis in human multiple myeloma MM1R cells while decreasing NF-κB and HSP-90 expressions (Zheng, Fan, Wu, Cai, & Shi, 2016; Q.-M. Zhou et al., 2017a).

The combination of paclitaxel and curcumin induced apoptosis in MCF-7 cells, with repression of paclitaxel-induced EGFR signaling (Zhan, Chen, Liu, Zhang, & Zhang, 2014). In cervical cancer cells, the same combination synergistically increased apoptosis via NFκB-p53-caspase3 pathway, which increased p53 and cleaved caspase 3 while reducing the phosphorylation of IκBα and the p65NFκB subunit levels (Dang, Yuan, Tian, Li, & Liu, 2015). Downregulation of the activity of NF-κB, AKT and MAP kinases was also supported by another study (Z. Liu, Zhu, Li, & Ning, 2016). In A2780, ovarian cancer cell line also reduction of P-glycoprotein expression and elevation of paclitaxel concentration in the tumor cells was found (Z. Liu et al., 2016). These outcomes were validated *in vivo*, by decline in tumor incidence and volume in xenograft model of HeLa cells in NOD-SCID mice (Sreekanth, Bava, Sreekumar, & Anto, 2011).

Good synergy was also evident with the chemotherapeutic agent, gemcitabine in several cancers. In pancreatic ductal adenocarcinoma (PDAC) cells, synergistic enhancement of pro-apoptotic and anti-proliferative properties was observed, alongside decline in cell migration/invasion, evidenced by the increased E-cadherin and reduced MMP9 expressions (Avan et al., 2016a). Curcumin was also able to sensitize gemcitabine-resistant PDAC cells by inhibiting EZH2 expression, and its related long, non-coding RNA, PVT1 that are involved in mediating cancer stemness and epithelial-to-mesenchymal transition, linked to drug resistance (Yoshida, Toden, Ravindranathan, Han, & Goel, 2017). They also documented a similar observation in a xenograft mouse model. The ability of curcumin to modulate EZH2 and restore expression of tumour suppressor genes further supports its effect on the epigenetic pathways (M. Jiang et al., 2013).

The combination of curcumin and 5-fluorouracil was able to elicit anti-proliferative and pro-apoptosis effects in chemo-resistant colorectal cancer through miRNA-mediated suppression of EMT(Toden et al., 2015). By inhibiting IκBα phosphorylation curcumin reduced 5-fluorouracil-induced drug resistance in colorectal cells (Shakibaei et al., 2013). The combination therapy of curcumin with oxaliplatin/5-flourouracil (FOLFOX) in patient-derived explants of colorectal liver metastases resulted in enhanced apoptosis as well as a reduction in stem cell-associated markers such as CD133 and ALDH (James et al., 2015). Treatment of antiestrogen-resistant breast cancer cell lines (MCF-7/LCC2 and MCF-7/LCC9), with tamoxifen and curcumin combination resulted in synergistic growth inhibition. This was accomplished through the inactivation of AKT/mTOR, Src and NF-κB pathways and downregulation of EZH2, which ultimately led to reduced expression of anti-apoptotic and pro-growth molecules (M. Jiang et al., 2013).

Androgen-independent prostate cancer cells showed synergistic inhibition of growth when treated with curcumin and the androgen receptor antagonist, bicalutamide via increased SAPK/JNK, ERK1/2 phosphorylation and reduction in NF-κB subunit p65 (J. Li et al., 2015). Curcumin enhanced the anti-tumor activity of carboplatin in the A549 NSCLC cell line by suppressing NF-κB (Kang et al., 2015). This was mediated by inhibition of the Akt/IKKα pathway, and supported by increase in p53 expression and ERK1/2 activity (Kang et al., 2015).

Curcumin was also found to enhance cisplatin-induced anti-migratory effects in NSCLC cell lines by inhibiting the highly migratory CD166+/EpCAM+ cancer stem-like cell (CSC) subpopulation (Baharuddin et al., 2016). This combined treatment also promoted growth arrest and intrinsic apoptosis as evidenced by the down-regulation of cyclin D1, increased p21 expression and activation of Apaf1 and caspase-9 in the CSC subpopulation (Baharuddin et al., 2016).

4. Synergistic Effect Of Genistein In Combination With Chemotherapeutics

Genistein (4'5, 7-trihydroxyisoflavone), a glycoside found in soyabean, is popular in Chinese and Japanese medicine and has for long found favor with researchers. This is further supported by epidemiological data which links consumption of soy with lowered risk of cancer (Yukun Zhang & Chen, 2011). Genistein's reputation as a strong anti-cancer agent has been built through various reports of its inhibitory effect on cancers affecting the various organs (He & Chen, 2013; Shanmugam, Kannaiyan, & Sethi, 2011). It regulates various aspects of cell growth by functioning as a tyrosine kinase inhibitor, angiogenesis inhibitor and anti-oxidant (He & Chen, 2013). Through these roles its effect is evident on the proliferation signal cascades (Shanmugam et al., 2011). Recently, studies have also connected genistein to epigenetic modulation via reactivation of TSGs (M. K. Sundaram et al., 2018). TSG re-expression following genistein treatment has been shown in cervical and prostate cancer cells (Majid et al., 2008; M. K. Sundaram et al., 2018). Further, it suppresses tumor cell propagation via inactivation of the IGF-1R-PI3 K/Akt pathway and induces apoptosis by downregulating the Bcl-2/Bax protein ratio in breast cancer cells (J. Chen et al., 2015). Similarly, genistein-mediated suppression of proliferation in human endometrial hyperplastic cells was accomplished by inhibiting EGFR and downstream signaling molecules such as NF-κB and PI3K/Akt,; alongside of inducing apoptosis through the intrinsic pathway (Shukla et al., 2015). Further, GEN-27, derived from genistein, showed anti-tumor activities in colorectal cancer cells through various means such as inhibition of NF-κB/p65 nuclear localization, inhibition of β-catenin activity and increased APC and AXIN2 expressions (Qianming Du et al., 2016).

Genistein is known to augment the anti-tumor effects of various conventional chemotherapeutic drugs in different types of cancers (Table 4). Genistein enhances the anti-tumor action of cisplatin in cervical cancer cells (HeLa) via inhibition of the Akt/mTOR and NF-κB pathways, as seen by the reduced expressions of p-Akt, p-mTOR, p-4E-BP1, p-p70S6K1 and NF-κB (Sahin et al., 2012). This combination also inhibited tumor recurrence and metastasis in nude mice bearing human hepatocellular carcinoma (HCCLM3) xenograft by abolishing MMP-2 expression (P. Chen, Hu, Deng, & Li, 2013). Similar synergistic effects were also seen in A549 NSCLC cells and xenograft of A549 cells (Liu et al., 2014). This combination was also shown to synergistically induce anti-proliferative effects in H466, a small-cell lung cancer cell line, by attenuating FoxM1 and downregulating its target such as Cdc25, cyclin B1 and survivin, which play a role in cell cycle regulation (Tian et al., 2014).

The combination of genistein and topotecan was more efficacious in inducing apoptosis in LNCaP prostate cancer cells through the intrinsic pathway via the activation of caspase-3 and -9 (Hörmann, Kumi-Diaka, Durity, & Rathinavelu, 2012).

In human pancreatic cell line, PaCa-2, genistein and 5-fluorouracil induced apoptosis and autophagy, by reducing Bcl-2 and the increasing beclin-1 protein levels (Suzuki et al., 2014). This study also showed reduction in tumor volume in a murine xenograft of the PaCa-2 cell line. Genistein can act as an agonist to the estrogen receptor, ERβ which is often found to be co-expressed with HER2 in breast cancer. Treatment of ERα/β-positive, BT-474 breast cancer cells overexpressing HER2, with a combination of genistein and trastuzumab (a monoclonal antibody against HER2/neu), significantly enhanced growth inhibition (Lattrich et al., 2011). Genistein and gemcitabine co-treatment of human osteosarcoma tumor model inhibited growth by down-regulating NF-κB and Akt pathways (Liang et al., 2012). Genistein when administered with gefitinib enhanced anti-tumor effects in a gefitinib resistant NSCLC cell line, H1975 by downregulating p-Akt, p-mTOR and p-EGFR (Zhu et al., 2012). This is in accordance with genistein's capability to impede tyrosine kinases including EGFR.

The combination of genistein with trichostatin A, a HDAC inhibitor was shown to synergistically restore the expression of ERα in MDA-MB-231 (ERα-negative breast cancer cells). Genistein accomplishes this by reducing gene expression of HDACs and DNMTs and their binding to ERα promoter (Y. Li et al., 2013). This highlights ability of genistein to modulate epigenetic pathways in combination treatments as well. Reports also suggest that a combination of epigenetic drugs and known chemotherapeutic agents may allow re- sensitization of drug-resistant tumors. Genistein enhanced the anti-tumor activity of tamoxifen in ERα-negative MDA-MB-231 xenograft mouse model by re-sensitizing them to anti-hormone therapy (Y. Li et al., 2013). Synergistic studies involving genistein are listed in table 4.

5. Synergistic Effects Of Resveratrol In Combination With Chemotherapeutics

Resveratrol, is a phytoalexin that can be isolated from the skin of red grapes, protects the cardiovascular system and demonstrates anti-carcinogenic effects by interacting with multiple molecular targets involved in cancer development. It is particularly known to suppress angiogenesis and metastasis. For instance, resveratrol suppresses migration and invasion by inhibiting the PI-3K/Akt/NF-κB signaling pathway in pancreatic cancer cells. This was demonstrated by a reduction in the phosphorylation of Akt and NF-κB, decrease in the expression of N-cadherin, vimentin and increased E-cadherin (W. Li et al., 2013). Resveratrol also suppresses the NF-κB pathway; by reducing the transcriptional activity of p65, and blocking ubiquitination of both NEMO and IκB kinase (Ren et al., 2013). Autophagy in prostate cancer cell lines (DU145 and PC3) has been reported by targeting STIM1 and downregulating the mTOR pathway, resulting in the depletion of Ca^{2+} in ER and subsequent ER stress (Selvaraj, Sun, Sukumaran, & Singh, 2016). Tumour growth and metastasis was suppressed in colorectal cells (HCT116 and SW48) by targeting Sirt1 and suppressing NF-κB activation (Buhrmann, Shayan, Popper, Goel, & Shakibaei, 2016). Another similar study demonstrated G1-S-phase cell cycle arrest in response to resveratrol, as evidenced by the reduction in the expression of cell-cycle regulatory genes (CDK2, CDK4, p21, cyclin D1 and PCNA) (B. Liu et al., 2014).

Several studies have shown that resveratrol in combination with chemotherapeutic agents can augment their anti-cancer activities. For instance, resveratrol was shown to improve the anticancer effects of paclitaxel in HepG2 cells by upregulating IκB-α and downregulating iNOS, COX-2 and NF-κB expression. In addition, this combination showed increased apoptosis and upregulation of Bax, a pro-apoptotic protein and down-regulation of Bcl2, Bcl-xL and other anti-apoptotic proteins (Q. Jiang, Yang, Qu, Zhou, & Zhang, 2017). Treatment of resveratrol with 5-fluorouracil reduces tumor growth and angiogenesis via downregulation of AMPK, VEGF and COX-2 in B16 murine melanoma cells (Lee, Koo, Park, & Kim, 2015). In human colorectal cancer cells, this combination up-regulated intercellular junctions and down-regulated the NF-κB pathway, resulting in chemosensitzation and inhibition of EMT phenotype (Buhrmann et al., 2015).

Resveratrol and cisplatin synergistically induces the autophagic cell death pathway apoptosis in lung cancer (A549) cells with downregulation of pAKT and Bcl2 family of proteins (Hu et al., 2016). Inhibition of the mTOR pathway and Akt, resulting in apoptosis was the outcome in breast cancer cells treated with resveratrol and rapamycin (Alayev, Berger, Kramer, Schwartz, & Holz, 2015). The same combination evoked a similar mechanism of cell death in human bladder cancer cell lines (Alayey et al., 2017). Gu *et al* review highlights resveratrol's ability to prevent doxorubicin induced cardiac toxicity while exerting a synergistic therapeutic effect in tumour cells (Gu, 2015).

Resveratrol not only potentiates the cytotoxic effects of various drugs but also reverses drug-resistance in tumor cells. For instance, resveratrol in combination with vemurafenib repressed cell proliferation and AKT phosphorylation in vemurafenib-resistant (BRAF V600E mutation) melanoma cells. (Luo, Umebayashi, Doi, & Morisaki, 2016). Synergistic combination studies using resveratrol are listed in table 5.

6. Synergistic Effects Of Eugenol In Combination With Chemotherapeutics

Eugenol is a phenolic compound that is abundantly present in cloves and has been shown to be effective for several medical applications including anticancer properties. Eugenol showed a dose-dependent cytotoxic response as well as downregulation of MMP-1, 3, 7, 9 and 11 in MDA-MB-231 cells. Eugenol was therefore, able to significantly inhibit cell migration and suppress metastasis (Rajoriya et al., 2019). Eugenol significantly induced apoptosis in MCF-7 cells by increasing N-terminal phosphorylation of β-catenin, thereby enhancing its degradation. Furthermore, eugenol was found to downregulate CSC markers in spheroid cultures, as demonstrated by reduction in CD44+/CD24-/low cell population (Choudhury et al., 2020). Eugenol encapsulated in a chitosan polymer was able to induce autophagy and anti-cancer effects in rat C6 glioma cells (Z. Li et al., 2020). In cervical cancer cells (HeLa), eugenol was seen to reverse the hypermethylation of RASSF1A gene, which is involved in suppressing Ras-dependent oncogenesis, highlighting its ability to mediate epigenetic effects (Saloni, Sharma, Mathur, & Jha, 2019).

Eugenol potentiates the action of some chemotherapeutic agents (Table 6). When used in conjunction with cisplatin, it inhibited the growth of triple- negative breast cancer cells by suppressing the NF-κB signaling pathway and down-regulation of IL-6, IL-8 (S. Islam et al., 2017). Moreover, this combination was able to inhibit ALDH-positive tumor infiltrating cells and ALDH enzyme activity, which are significantly increased in cancer cells (S. Islam et al., 2017). Similarly, methyl eugenol with cisplatin inhibited proliferation and induced apoptosis in HeLa cells (Yi et al., 2015).

The combination of eugenol and methoxyestradiol enhanced apoptosis in prostate cancer cells by up-regulating the pro-apoptotic protein, Bax and down-regulating the anti-apoptotic protein, Bcl-2. The combination could induce apoptosis and inhibit growth at concentrations much lower than either agent alone (Ghosh, Ganapathy, Alworth, Chan, & Kumar, 2009). Eugenol potentiated gemcitabine induced apoptosis and growth inhibition in cervical cancer cells (HeLa) while normal cells remained unaffected (Hussain et al., 2011). Eugenol and 5-fluorouracil also brought about cell cycle arrest and limited proliferation synergistically in HeLa cells (Hemaiswarya & Doble, 2013). Studies highlighting synergistic combinations with eugenol are listed in table 6.

7. Synergistic Effect Of Combination Of Phytochemicals

It is interesting that not only combinations of phytochemicals with established chemotherapeutic agents are effective, but combinations of the phytochemicals themselves are very promising. Curcumin and resveratrol in combination was shown to contribute to chemoprevention against lung cancer in mice by modulating p53 hyperphosphorylation and showing improved activity of apoptotic enzymes including caspase-3 and -9 (Malhotra, Nair, & Dhawan, 2014). The combination of curcumin and resveratrol also showed increased anti-proliferative effects on hepatocellular carcinoma, Hepa1-6 cells. This was accompanied by upregulation of ROS levels, activation of caspase-3, -8 and -9, and downregulation of XIAP and survivin (Qin Du et al., 2013). Co-treatment of EGCG and curcumin suppress breast cancer stem cells by inhibiting the phosphorylation of STAT3 and its interaction with NF-κB (Chung & Vadgama,

2015). Curcumin improved the anti-proliferative effect of EGCG on prostate cancer cells, PC3, with synergistic up-regulation of p21 (Eom et al., 2015). Genistein and curcumin synergistically improved the anti-angiogenic effects on PC3 cells through downregulation of ARNT, HIF-1α and lowered VEGF production (Aditya, Shim, Yang, Lee, & Ko, 2014). Sulforaphane and quercetin limited proliferation and migration in HeLa cells at higher levels when low doses were administered together in comparison to individually (M. K. Sundaram, Raina, et al., 2019). These studies highlight the potential of a cocktail of phytochemicals in lieu of chemotherapeutic agents for therapeutic efficacy.

8. Clinical Studies Studying Effect Of Combination Of Phytochemicals

Over the past few years, several combination therapies have been studied as part of clinical trials. These have validated the claims of synergy and established the success of combinational therapy. Some of the clinical studies have been elaborated below.

A randomized, placebo-controlled, double-blind clinical trial on Norwegian patients who received 30 mg genistein or placebo capsules daily for 3-6 weeks before prostatectomy showed an overall reduction in Myc activity and increased PTEN activity (Bilir et al., 2017). A phase I trial involving sixteen pancreatic cancer patients treated with 400 mg to 1600 mg of AXP107-11 (a novel, multi-component crystalline form of the naturally occurring compound genistein) in combination with gemcitabine found no hematological and non-hematological toxicity. The median overall survival time was found to be 4.9 months and 19% were alive at the one-year follow-up (Löhr et al., 2016). A phase I dose escalation trial employing gemicitabine with AXP107-11, a multi-component crystalline form of genistein, to treat pancreatic cancer patients showed a favorable pharmacokinetic-profile (Lohr et al., 2016).

Twenty patients (10 per dose) with histologically confirmed colorectal cancer were given either 0.5 g or 1.0 g of resveratrol for eight days prior to surgical resection. The patients showed no adverse reactions in response to resveratrol and both doses were tolerated well. Tumor cell proliferation reduced by 5% as evidenced by Ki-67 staining in post-intervention surgical tissue (Patel et al., 2010). In a pilot study of nine patients with colorectal cancer and hepatic metastases, six were given 5 g of SRT501 (micronized resveratrol) for 14 days. Malignant hepatic tissue showed a significant increase in cleaved caspase-3 when compared with tissue from the placebo-treated patients (Howells et al., 2011). A phase 2 clinical trial of SRT501 (resveratrol) with or without bortezomib in relapsed multiple myeloma however, demonstrated an unacceptable safety profile and minimal efficacy in this category of patients (Popat et al., 2013).

In a phase I study, EGCG was sprayed on the chest wall of breast cancer patients after post- mastectomy radiotherapy for 2 weeks. Patients were observed to have reduced levels of dermatitis (Zhao et al., 2014).

A phase I study was conducted on 24 surgically unresectable stage III non-small-cell lung cancer patients using a combination of EGCG, standard chemoradiation and either cisplatin or etoposide. EGCG was found to reduce the development of esophagitis (Zhao et al., 2016). A phase II randomized, three-arm trial involving unresectable stage III NSCLC or limited SCLC patients showed that acute radiation-induced esophagitis in patients treated with EGCG was significantly lower than for those given conventional therapy (Zhao et al., 2019).

In phase I/II study of gemcitabine-resistant pancreatic cancer patients, a combination of gemcitabine and curcumin was found to be safe and effective (Kanai et al., 2011). The phase I dose-escalation study of curcumin in combination with FOLFOX chemotherapy for the treatment of colorectal liver metastases patients also highlighted its safety profile (James et al., 2015).

FUTURE RESEARCH DIRECTIONS

Several studies consistently show that phytochemicals have immense potential as chemotherapeutic and chemopreventive agents. Reports on anticancer properties have been followed by detailed constructions of the mechanism of action and their impact on various molecular targets and signaling pathways (Figure 1). A more detailed understanding of the metabolism and stability of these phytochemicals is required. Interactions of these phytochemicals with various targets and off-target proteins including the CYP enzymes are warranted. If these interactions are not clearly elucidated, combination of such phytochemicals may result in harmful side effects (Mohan, Narayanan, Sethuraman, & Maheswari Krishnan, 2013; Ulbricht & Chao, 2010). Enhanced understanding of the pathways targeted by combination of therapeutic agents. The targeting of multiple pathways while beneficial may also result in increased toxicity due to potentiation of off-target activity. Delbaldo *et al*, report in their meta-analysis that there could be unwanted side-effects from combinations and that addition of three agents, while reducing dosage and increasing response may not necessarily result in good quality of life for the patient. Hence, it is imperative that future studies focus on all aspects of a patient response from tumour regression, side-effects and quality of life (Catherine Delbaldo, Stefan Michiels, Nathalie Syz, Jean-Charles Soria, Thierry Le Chevalier, 2017).

Noting that cancer stem cells may contribute to relapse of cancer in patients, future efforts must be targeted at addressing the effect of these stem cell population to combination therapy. The efficacy of some dietary compounds against cancer are negatively impacted due to their low bioavailability. Nanotechnology based formulations may help offset this and increase the bioavailability of these phytochemicals. Several *in vitro* studies demonstrate increased availability and enhanced anti-carcinogenic effect when nanoparticle encapsulation was utilized (Tabrez et al., 2013). In order to assess the effect of combination therapy it is necessary to undertake a more comprehensive approach to their mechanism of action. This process may be hastened or made more feasible by undertaking *in silico* studies. Prior to testing the combinations *in vitro* for synergy, an *in silico* assessment of their individual mechanism of action may be undertaken. *In silico* studies will help in screening a wider array of possible combinations and ensure a more wide-ranging approach. The development of tools such as CytoScape will further aid in this regard (Paul Shannon et al., 1971). Network-biology based assessment of drug discovery methods will ensure a more targeted approach while understanding the breadth of possible off-target responses.

Given that several of these agents impact epigenetic pathways which are the early precancer changes their candidature as potential chemopreventive agents is also very high. However, the success seen in these *in vitro* studies needs to be replicated at clinical trials in order to harness their properties for clinical use. There are as yet only a limited number of clinical studies that have assessed combinatorial therapies for cancer treatment and there is a need to increase clinical studies focusing on assessing the risks and benefits of combination treatments. Further effort also needs to be directed towards understanding the various genetic, proteomic and environmental influences on therapeutics. Development and updation of databases of therapeutic targets will ensure that a wider net is cast while looking for potential therapeutic interactions.

Various genotypic, pharmacokinetic differences exist between different cancers and different patients, so it continues to be important to explore the anticancer properties of different phytochemicals and build an array of drug candidates.

CONCLUSION

Combination therapy involving dietary agents and chemotherapeutic agents appear to be a promising therapeutic strategy for the treatment of cancer (Figure 3). There have been several *in vitro* studies and a few *in vivo* studies documenting the immense scope of this strategy as detailed in this chapter. However, there are some gaps which need to be overcome so that it can become a viable therapeutic solution. Identification of novel bioactive agents with chemopreventive potential can be viewed as an important goal of cancer research as well as public health initiative to ensure population-wide chemoprevention strategies. There is an urgent need to assess the effect of combination of these phytochemicals with chemotherapeutic agents, so that pharmacologically safe and effective compositions that can act on all the stages of carcinogenesis can be reliably identified.

Figure 3. Dietary bioactive compounds can potentiate the action of chemotherapeutic agents.

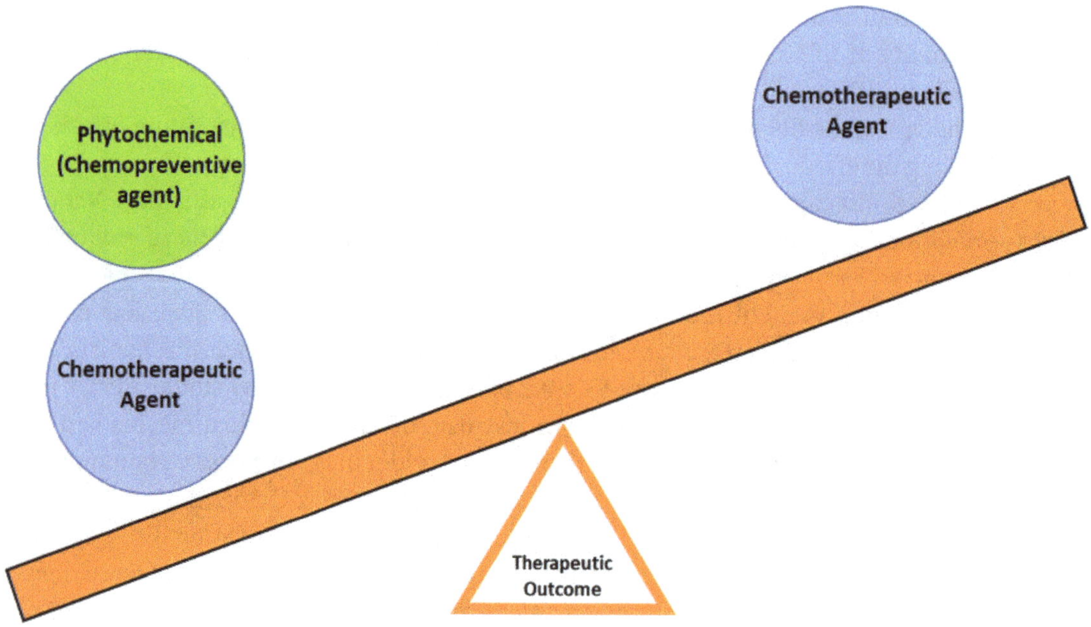

ACKNOWLEDGMENT

The authors are grateful to Dr. Kota Reddy, Academic President, Manipal Academy of Higher Education, Dubai, for his constant support and encouragement.

REFERENCES

Aditya, N. P., Shim, M., Yang, H., Lee, Y. J., & Ko, S. (2014). Antiangiogenic effect of combined treatment with curcumin and genistein on human prostate cancer cell line. *Journal of Functional Foods*, *8*, 204–213. doi:10.1016/j.jff.2014.03.014

Ahmad Ganai, S. (2017). Plant derived inhibitor Sulforaphane in combinatorial therapy against therapeutically challenging Pancreatic Cancer. *Anti-Cancer Agents in Medicinal Chemistry (Formerly Current Medicinal Chemistry-Anti-Cancer Agents)*, *17*(3), 365–373.

Ali Khan, M., Kedhari Sundaram, M., Hamza, A., Quraishi, U., Gunasekera, D., Ramesh, L., Goala, P., Al Alami, U., Ansari, M. Z., Rizvi, T. A., Sharma, C., & Hussain, A. (2015). Sulforaphane Reverses the Expression of Various Tumor Suppressor Genes by Targeting DNMT3B and HDAC1 in Human Cervical Cancer Cells. *Evidence-Based Complementary and Alternative Medicine*, *2015*, 2015. doi:10.1155/2015/412149 PMID:26161119

Amararathna, M., Johnston, M. R., & Vasantha Rupasinghe, H. P. (2016). Plant polyphenols as chemopreventive agents for lung cancer. *International Journal of Molecular Sciences*, *17*(8), 1352. doi:10.3390/ijms17081352 PMID:27548149

Angeles, L. & Abbvie, P.M. (2015). *Potentiation of growth inhibition and epigenetic modulation by combination of green tea polyphenol and 5-aza-2 ¢ -deoxycytidine i*. Academic Press.

Aslam, M. S., Naveed, S., Ahmed, A., Abbas, Z., Gull, I., & Athar, M. A. (2014). Side Effects of Chemotherapy in Cancer Patients and Evaluation of Patients Opinion about Starvation Based Differential Chemotherapy. *Journal of Cancer Therapy*, *5*(8), 817–822. doi:10.4236/jct.2014.58089

Avan, A. (2016). 257P Molecular mechanisms involved in the synergistic interaction of novel formulated curcumin with gemcitabine in pancreatic cancer cells. *Annals of Oncology*, 27(suppl_9), p.mdw582.038-mdw582.038. Available at: . doi:10.1093/annonc/mdw582.038

Baharuddin, P., Satar, N., Fakiruddin, K. S., Zakaria, N., Lim, M. N., Yusoff, N. M., Zakaria, Z., & Yahaya, B. H. (2016). Curcumin improves the efficacy of cisplatin by targeting cancer stem-like cells through p21 and cyclin D1-mediated tumour cell inhibition in non-small cell lung cancer cell lines. *Oncology Reports*, *35*(1), 13–25. doi:10.3892/or.2015.4371 PMID:26531053

Bal, D. G., Foerster, S. B., Backman, D. R., & Lyman, D. O. (2001). Dietary change and cancer: Challenges and future direction. *The Journal of Nutrition*, *131*(1), 181S–185S. doi:10.1093/jn/131.1.181S PMID:11208961

Barthélémy, P., Asmane-De la Porte, I., Meyer, N., Duclos, B., Serra, S., Dourthe, L.-M., Amé, S., Litique, V., Giron, C., Goldbarg, V., Fornecker, L., Quoix, E., & Kurtz, J.-E. (2015). Adherence and Patients' Attitudes to Oral Anticancer Drugs: A Prospective Series of 201 Patients Focusing on Targeted Therapies. *Oncology*, *88*(1), 1–8. doi:10.1159/000366226 PMID:25247774

van Berleere, M., & Dauchet, L. (2017). Fruits, Vegetables, and Health: Evidence From Meta-analyses of Prospective Epidemiological Studies. In *Vegetarian and Plant-Based Diets in Health and Disease Prevention* (pp. 215–248). Elsevier. doi:10.1016/B978-0-12-803968-7.00013-7

Cellular, V., Biology, D. & Gen, H. (2018). *In vitro evaluation of combination of EGCG and Erlotinib with classical chemotherapeutics on JAR cells*. Academic Press.

Chan, H.-K., & Ismail, S. (2014). Side Effects of Chemotherapy among Cancer Patients in a Malaysian General Hospital: Experiences, Perceptions and Informational Needs from Clinical Pharmacists. *Asian Pacific Journal of Cancer Prevention, 15*(13), 5305–5309. doi:10.7314/APJCP.2014.15.13.5305 PMID:25040993

Chandra, P. (2017). *Sulforaphane increases the efficacy of anti- androgens by rapidly decreasing androgen receptor levels in prostate cancer cells Sulforaphane increases the efficacy of anti-androgens by rapidly decreasing androgen receptor levels in prostate cancer cells*. Academic Press.

Chen, J., Duan, Y., Zhang, X., Ye, Y., Ge, B., & Chen, J. (2015). Genistein induces apoptosis by the inactivation of the IGF-1R/p-Akt signaling pathway in MCF-7 human breast cancer cells. *Food & Function, 6*(3), 995–1000. doi:10.1039/C4FO01141D PMID:25675448

Chen, P. (2013). Genistein reinforces the inhibitory effect of Cisplatin on liver cancer recurrence and metastasis after curative hepatectomy. *Asian Pacific journal of cancer prevention, 14*(2), 759–764. PMID:23621233

Chou, T.-C., & Talalay, P. (1984). Quantitative analysis of dose-effect relationships: The combined effects of multiple drugs or enzyme inhibitors. *Advances in Enzyme Regulation, 22*, 27–55. doi:10.1016/0065-2571(84)90007-4 PMID:6382953

Chung, S. S., & Vadgama, J. V. (2015). Curcumin and epigallocatechin gallate inhibit the cancer stem cell phenotype via down-regulation of STAT3-NFkappaB signaling. *Anticancer Research, 35*(1), 39–46. PMID:25550533

Cornelison, R., Llaneza, D. C., & Landen, C. N. (2017). Emerging therapeutics to overcome chemoresistance in epithelial ovarian cancer: A mini-review. *International Journal of Molecular Sciences, 18*(10), 1–20. doi:10.3390/ijms18102171 PMID:29057791

Dang, Y.-P., Yuan, X.-Y., Tian, R., Li, D.-G., & Liu, W. (2015). Curcumin improves the paclitaxel-induced apoptosis of HPV-positive human cervical cancer cells via the NF-kappaB-p53-caspase-3 pathway. *Experimental and Therapeutic Medicine, 9*(4), 1470–1476. doi:10.3892/etm.2015.2240 PMID:25780454

Das, L., & Vinayak, M. (2015). Long Term Effect of Curcumin in Restoration of Tumour Suppressor p53 and Phase-II Antioxidant Enzymes via Activation of Nrf2 Signalling and Modulation of Inflammation in Prevention of Cancer. *PLoS One, 10*(4), e0124000. doi:10.1371/journal.pone.0124000 PMID:25860911

Du, Q., Wang, Y., Liu, C., Wang, H., Fan, H., Li, Y., Wang, J., Zhang, X., Lu, J., Ji, H., & Hu, R. (2016). Chemopreventive activity of GEN-27, a genistein derivative, in colitis-associated cancer is mediated by p65-CDX2-beta-catenin axis. *Oncotarget, 7*(14), 17870–17884. doi:10.18632/oncotarget.7554 PMID:26910375

Du, Q., Hu, B., an, H.-M., Shen, K.-P., Xu, L., Deng, S., & Wei, M.-M. (2013). Synergistic anticancer effects of curcumin and resveratrol in Hepa1-6 hepatocellular carcinoma cells. *Oncology Reports, 29*(5), 1851–1858. doi:10.3892/or.2013.2310 PMID:23446753

Eom, D.-W., Lee, J. H., Kim, Y.-J., Hwang, G. S., Kim, S.-N., Kwak, J. H., Cheon, G. J., Kim, K. H., Jang, H.-J., Ham, J., Kang, K. S., & Yamabe, N. (2015). Synergistic effect of curcumin on epigallocatechin gallate-induced anticancer action in PC3 prostate cancer cells. *BMB Reports*, *48*(8), 461–466. doi:10.5483/BMBRep.2015.48.8.216 PMID:25441423

Farvid, M. S., Chen, W. Y., Michels, K. B., Cho, E., Willett, W. C., & Eliassen, A. H. (2016). Fruit and vegetable consumption in adolescence and early adulthood and risk of breast cancer: Population based cohort study. *BMJ (Clinical Research Ed.)*, i2343. doi:10.1136/bmj.i2343 PMID:27170029

Fujiki, H., & Imai, K. (2015). Innovative strategy of cancer treatment with the combination of green tea catechins and anticancer compounds. Academic Press.

Fujiki, H., Sueoka, E., Watanabe, T., & Suganuma, M. (2015). Primary cancer prevention by green tea, and tertiary cancer prevention by the combination of green tea catechins and anticancer compounds. *Journal of Cancer Prevention*, *20*(1), 1–4. doi:10.15430/JCP.2015.20.1.1 PMID:25853098

Ghosh, R., Ganapathy, M., Alworth, W. L., Chan, D. C., & Kumar, A. P. (2009). Combination of 2-methoxyestradiol (2-ME2) and eugenol for apoptosis induction synergistically in androgen independent prostate cancer cells. *The Journal of Steroid Biochemistry and Molecular Biology*, *113*(1–2), 25–35. doi:10.1016/j.jsbmb.2008.11.002 PMID:19084597

Gu, J. (2015). *Protects against doxorubicin-induced cardiotoxicity Resveratrol alleviates cardiomyocytes oxidative stress induced by doxorubicin Resveratrol modulates doxorubicin- induced cardiocyomytes autophagy Resveratrol mitigates cardiomyocytes apoptosis induced by*. Academic Press.

Hemaiswarya, S., & Doble, M. (2013). Combination of phenylpropanoids with 5-fluorouracil as anti-cancer agents against human cervical cancer (HeLa) cell line. *Phytomedicine*, *20*(2), 151–158. doi:10.1016/j.phymed.2012.10.009 PMID:23207250

Hormann, V., Kumi-Diaka, J., Durity, M., & Rathinavelu, A. (2012). Anticancer activities of genistein-topotecan combination in prostate cancer cells. *Journal of Cellular and Molecular Medicine*, *16*(11), 2631–2636. doi:10.1111/j.1582-4934.2012.01576.x PMID:22452992

Hu, S. (2016). *The synergistic effect of resveratrol in combination with cisplatin on apoptosis via modulating autophagy in A549 cells*. Academic Press.

Huang, W.-C., Chen, C.-Y., Lin, S.-J., & Chang, C.-S. (2016). Medication adherence to oral anticancer drugs: Systematic review. *Expert Review of Anticancer Therapy*, *16*(4), 423–432. doi:10.1586/14737140.2016.1159515 PMID:26935964

Hussain, A., Brahmbhatt, K., Priyani, A., Ahmed, M., Rizvi, T. A., & Sharma, C. (2011). Eugenol enhances the chemotherapeutic potential of gemcitabine and induces anticarcinogenic and anti-inflammatory activity in human cervical cancer cells. *Cancer Biotherapy & Radiopharmaceuticals*, *26*(5), 519–527. doi:10.1089/cbr.2010.0925 PMID:21939359

Hussain, A., Harish, G., Prabhu, S. A., Mohsin, J., Khan, M. A., Rizvi, T. A., & Sharma, C. (2012). Inhibitory effect of genistein on the invasive potential of human cervical cancer cells via modulation of matrix metalloproteinase-9 and tissue inhibitiors of matrix metalloproteinase-1 expression. *Cancer Epidemiology*, *36*(6), e387–e393. doi:10.1016/j.canep.2012.07.005 PMID:22884883

Hussain, A., Mohsin, J., Prabhu, S. A., Begum, S., Nusri, Q. E.-A., Harish, G., Javed, E., Khan, M. A., & Sharma, C. (2013). Sulforaphane inhibits growth of human breast cancer cells and augments the therapeutic index of the chemotherapeutic drug, gemcitabine. *Asian Pacific Journal of Cancer Prevention, 14*(10), 5855–5860. doi:10.7314/APJCP.2013.14.10.5855 PMID:24289589

Islam, S., Mokhtari, R. B., Akbari, P., Hatina, J., Yeger, H., & Farhat, W. A. (2017). Simultaneous Targeting of Bladder Tumor Growth, Survival, and Epithelial-to-Mesenchymal Transition with a Novel Therapeutic Combination of Acetazolamide (AZ) and Sulforaphane (SFN). *Targeted Oncology, 11*(2), 209–227. doi:10.100711523-015-0386-5 PMID:26453055

James, M. I., Iwuji, C., Irving, G., Karmokar, A., Higgins, J. A., Griffin-Teal, N., Thomas, A., Greaves, P., Cai, H., Patel, S. R., Morgan, B., Dennison, A., Metcalfe, M., Garcea, G., Lloyd, D. M., Berry, D. P., Steward, W. P., Howells, L. M., & Brown, K. (2015). Curcumin inhibits cancer stem cell phenotypes in <em>ex vivo</em> models of colorectal liver metastases, and is clinically safe and tolerable in combination with FOLFOX chemotherapy. *Cancer Letters, 364*(2), 135–141. doi:10.1016/j.canlet.2015.05.005 PMID:25979230

Jiang, M., Huang, O., Zhang, X., Xie, Z., Shen, A., Liu, H., Geng, M., & Shen, K. (2013). Curcumin Induces Cell Death and Restores Tamoxifen Sensitivity in the Antiestrogen-Resistant Breast Cancer Cell Lines MCF-7/LCC2 and MCF-7/LCC9. *Molecules (Basel, Switzerland), 18*(1), 701–720. doi:10.3390/molecules18010701 PMID:23299550

Juengel, E., Euler, S., Maxeiner, S., Rutz, J., Justin, S., Roos, F., Khoder, W., Nelson, K., Bechstein, W. O., & Blaheta, R. A. (2017). Sulforaphane as an adjunctive to everolimus counteracts everolimus resistance in renal cancer cell lines. *Phytomedicine, 27*, 1–7. doi:10.1016/j.phymed.2017.01.016 PMID:28314474

Kalsi, T., Babic-Illman, G., Ross, P. J., Maisey, N. R., Hughes, S., Fields, P., Martin, F. C., Wang, Y., & Harari, D. (2015). The impact of comprehensive geriatric assessment interventions on tolerance to chemotherapy in older people. *British Journal of Cancer, 112*(9), 1435–1444. doi:10.1038/bjc.2015.120 PMID:25871332

Kanai, M., Yoshimura, K., Asada, M., Imaizumi, A., Suzuki, C., Matsumoto, S., Nishimura, T., Mori, Y., Masui, T., Kawaguchi, Y., Yanagihara, K., Yazumi, S., Chiba, T., Guha, S., & Aggarwal, B. B. (2011). A phase I/II study of gemcitabine-based chemotherapy plus curcumin for patients with gemcitabine-resistant pancreatic cancer. *Cancer Chemotherapy and Pharmacology, 68*(1), 157–164. doi:10.100700280-010-1470-2 PMID:20859741

Kang, J. H., Kang, H. S., Kim, I. K., Lee, H. Y., Ha, J. H., Yeo, C. D., Kang, H. H., Moon, H. S., & Lee, S. H. (2015). Curcumin sensitizes human lung cancer cells to apoptosis and metastasis synergistically combined with carboplatin. *Experimental Biology and Medicine, 240*(11), 1416–1425. doi:10.1177/1535370215571881 PMID:25716014

Kerr, C. (2018). Combination cisplatin and sulforaphane treatment reduces proliferation, invasion, and tumor formation in epidermal squamous cell carcinoma. Academic Press.

Khan, M., Hussain, A., Sundaram, M. K., Alalami, U., Gunasekera, D., Ramesh, L., Hamza, A., & Quraishi, U. (2015). (-)-Epigallocatechin-3-gallate reverses the expression of various tumor-suppressor genes by inhibiting DNA methyltransferases and histone deacetylases in human cervical cancer cells. *Oncology Reports*, *33*(4), 1–9. doi:10.3892/or.2015.3802 PMID:25682960

Lattrich, C., Lubig, J., Springwald, A., Goerse, R., Ortmann, O., & Treeck, O. (2011). Additive effects of trastuzumab and genistein on human breast cancer cells. *Anti-Cancer Drugs*, *22*(3), 253–261. doi:10.1097/CAD.0b013e3283427bb5 PMID:21160418

Lee, S. O. L. H. W. A. (2015). Anti - angiogenic effects of resveratrol in combination with 5 - fluorouracil on B16 murine melanoma cells. Academic Press.

Li, J., Xiang, S. T., Zhang, Q. H., Wu, J. J., Tang, Q., Zhou, J. F., Yang, L. J., Chen, Z. Q., & Hann, S. S. (2015). Combination of curcumin and bicalutamide enhanced the growth inhibition of androgen-independent prostate cancer cells through SAPK/JNK and MEK/ERK1/2-mediated targeting NF-κB/p65 and MUC1-C. *Journal of Experimental & Clinical Cancer Research*, *34*(1), 46. doi:10.118613046-015-0168-z PMID:25971429

Li, Y., Meeran, S. M., Patel, S. N., Chen, H., Hardy, T. M., & Tollefsbol, T. O. (2013). Epigenetic reactivation of estrogen receptor-α (ERα) by genistein enhances hormonal therapy sensitivity in ERα-negative breast cancer. *Molecular Cancer*, *12*(1), 9. doi:10.1186/1476-4598-12-9 PMID:24063558

Liang, C., Li, H., Shen, C., Lai, J., Shi, Z., Liu, B., & Tao, H. (2012). Genistein potentiates the anti-cancer effects of gemcitabine in human osteosarcoma via the downregulation of Akt and nuclear factor-kappaB pathway. *Anti-cancer Agents in Medicinal Chemistry*, *12*(5), 554–563. doi:10.2174/187152012800617867 PMID:22263786

Liu, D. (2014). Genistein enhances the effect of cisplatin on the inhibition of non-small cell lung cancer A549 cell growth in vitro and in vivo. *Oncology Letters*, *8*(6), 2806–2810. Available at: https://www.ncbi.nlm.nih.gov/pmc/articles/PMC4214458/

Liu, D., & Chen, Z. (2013). The effect of curcumin on breast cancer cells. *Journal of Breast Cancer*, *16*(2), 133–137. doi:10.4048/jbc.2013.16.2.133 PMID:23843843

Liu, Z., Zhu, Y.-Y., Li, Z.-Y., & Ning, S.-Q. (2016). Evaluation of the efficacy of paclitaxel with curcumin combination in ovarian cancer cells. *Oncology Letters*, *12*(5), 3944–3948. doi:10.3892/ol.2016.5192 PMID:27895754

Lohr, J.-M. (2016). A phase I dose escalation trial of AXP107-11, a novel multi-component crystalline form of genistein, in combination with gemcitabine in chemotherapy-naive patients with unresectable pancreatic cancer. *Pancreatology*, *16*(4), 640–645.

Lubecka-Pietruszewska, K. (2015). Sulforaphane Alone and in Combination with Clofarabine Epigenetically Regulates the Expression of DNA Methylation-Silenced Tumour Suppressor Genes in Human Breast Cancer Cells. *Lifestyle Genomics*, *8*(2), 91–101. https://www.karger.com/DOI/10.1159/000439111 PMID:26372775

Lubecka, K., Kaufman-Szymczyk, A., & Fabianowska-Majewska, K. (2018). Inhibition of breast cancer cell growth by the combination of clofarabine and sulforaphane involves epigenetically mediated CDKN2A upregulation. *Nucleosides, Nucleotides & Nucleic Acids*, *37*(5), 1–10. doi:10.1080/15257770.2018.1453075 PMID:29634384

Luo, H.A.O. (2016). *Resveratrol Overcomes Cellular Resistance to Vemurafenib Through Dephosphorylation of AKT in BRAF -mutated Melanoma Cells*. Academic Press.

Malhotra, A., Nair, P., & Dhawan, D. K. (2014). Study to evaluate molecular mechanics behind synergistic chemo-preventive effects of curcumin and resveratrol during lung carcinogenesis. *PLoS One*, *9*(4), e93820. doi:10.1371/journal.pone.0093820 PMID:24705375

Pan, S. T., Li, Z.-L., He, Z.-X., Qiu, J.-X., & Zhou, S.-F. (2016). Molecular mechanisms for tumour resistance to chemotherapy. *Clinical and Experimental Pharmacology & Physiology*, *43*(8), 723–737. doi:10.1111/1440-1681.12581 PMID:27097837

Panda, A. K., Chakraborty, D., Sarkar, I., Khan, T., & Sa, G. (2017). New insights into therapeutic activity and anticancer properties of curcumin. *Journal of Experimental Pharmacology*, *9*, 31–45. doi:10.2147/JEP.S70568 PMID:28435333

Papi, A., Govoni, M., Ciavarella, C., Spisni, E., Orlandi, M., & Farabegoli, F. (2016). Epigallocatechin-3-gallate increases RXRγ-mediated pro-apoptotic and anti-invasive effects in gastrointestinal cancer cell lines. *Current Cancer Drug Targets*, *16*(4), 373–385. doi:10.2174/15680096156661508171209 31 PMID:26278714

Park, S. Y., Kim, G., Bae, S.-J., Yoo, Y., & Choi, Y. (2007). Induction of apoptosis by isothiocyanate sulforaphane in human cervical carcinoma HeLa and hepatocarcinoma HepG2 cells through activation of caspase-3. *Oncology Reports*, *18*(1), 181–187. doi:10.3892/or.18.1.181 PMID:17549366

Rodriguez-Casado, A. (2016). The Health Potential of Fruits and Vegetables Phytochemicals: Notable Examples. *Critical Reviews in Food Science and Nutrition*, *56*(7), 1097–1107. doi:10.1080/10408398.2012.755149 PMID:25225771

Shakibaei, M., Mobasheri, A., Lueders, C., Busch, F., Shayan, P., & Goel, A. (2013). Curcumin Enhances the Effect of Chemotherapy against Colorectal Cancer Cells by Inhibition of NF-κB and Src Protein Kinase Signaling Pathways. *PLoS One*, *8*(2), e57218. doi:10.1371/journal.pone.0057218 PMID:23451189

Sharma, C., Nusri, Q. E.-A., Begum, S., Javed, E., Rizvi, T. A., & Hussain, A. (2012). (-)-Epigallocatechin-3-gallate induces apoptosis and inhibits invasion and migration of human cervical cancer cells. *Asian Pacific Journal of Cancer Prevention*, *13*(9), 4815–4822. doi:10.7314/APJCP.2012.13.9.4815 PMID:23167425

Sharma, C., Sadrieh, L., Priyani, A., Ahmed, M., Hassan, A. H., & Hussain, A. (2011). Anti-carcinogenic effects of sulforaphane in association with its apoptosis-inducing and anti-inflammatory properties in human cervical cancer cells. *Cancer Epidemiology*, *35*(3), 272–278. doi:10.1016/j.canep.2010.09.008 PMID:20956097

Shukla, V., Chandra, V., Sankhwar, P., Popli, P., Kaushal, J. B., Sirohi, V. K., & Dwivedi, A. (2015). Phytoestrogen genistein inhibits EGFR/PI3K/NF-kB activation and induces apoptosis in human endometrial hyperplasial cells. *RSC Advances*, *5*(69), 56075–56085. doi:10.1039/C5RA06167A

Sreekanth, C. N., Bava, S. V., Sreekumar, E., & Anto, R. J. (2011). Molecular evidences for the chemosensitizing efficacy of liposomal curcumin in paclitaxel chemotherapy in mouse models of cervical cancer. *Oncogene*, *30*(28), 3139–3152. doi:10.1038/onc.2011.23 PMID:21317920

Suzuki, R. (2014). Genistein potentiates the antitumor effect of 5-fluorouracil by inducing apoptosis and autophagy in human pancreatic cancer cells. *Anticancer Research*, *34*(9), 4685–4692. https://www.ncbi.nlm.nih.gov/pmc/articles/PMC4240628/ PMID:25202045

Tang, H. (2017). *Reversal of 5-fluorouracil resistance by EGCG is mediate by inactivation of TFAP2A / VEGF signaling pathway and down- regulation of MDR-1 and P-gp expression in gastric cancer.* Academic Press.

Tao, J. J., Visvanathan, K., & Wolff, A. C. (2016). Long term side effects of adjuvant chemotherapy in patients with early breast cancer. *The Breast*, *24*(2), 1–12. PMID:26299406

Taylor, P. (2014). *Digestive System Effects of Dietary Components on Cancer of the Digestive System.* Academic Press.

Tian, T., Li, J., Li, B., Wang, Y., Li, M., Ma, D., & Wang, X. (2014). Genistein exhibits anti-cancer effects via down-regulating FoxM1 in H446 small-cell lung cancer cells. *Tumour Biology*, *35*(5), 4137–4145. doi:10.100713277-013-1542-0 PMID:24379139

Toden, S., Okugawa, Y., Jascur, T., Wodarz, D., Komarova, N. L., Buhrmann, C., Shakibaei, M., Boland, C. R., & Goel, A. (2015). Curcumin mediates chemosensitization to 5-fluorouracil through miRNA-induced suppression of epithelial-to-mesenchymal transition in chemoresistant colorectal cancer. *Carcinogenesis*, *36*(3), 355–367. doi:10.1093/carcin/bgv006 PMID:25653233

Torresan, M. M., Garrino, L., Borraccino, A., Macchi, G., De Luca, A., & Dimonte, V. (2015). Adherence to treatment in patient with severe cancer pain: A qualitative enquiry through illness narratives. *European Journal of Oncology Nursing*, *19*(4), 397–404. doi:10.1016/j.ejon.2015.01.001 PMID:25691299

Turati, F., Rossi, M., Pelucchi, C., Levi, F., & La Vecchia, C. (2015). Fruit and vegetables and cancer risk: A review of southern European studies. *British Journal of Nutrition*, *113*(S2), S102–S110. doi:10.1017/S0007114515000148 PMID:26148912

Wang, P., Henning, S. M., Heber, D., & Vadgama, J. V. (2016). Sensitization to docetaxel in prostate cancer cells by green tea and quercetin. *The Journal of Nutritional Biochemistry*, *26*(4), 408–415. doi:10.1016/j.jnutbio.2014.11.017 PMID:25655047

Wang, X. (2015). EGCG Enhances Cisplatin Sensitivity by Regulating Expression of the Copper and Cisplatin Influx Transporter CTR1 in Ovary Cancer. Academic Press.

Wang, X. (2014). Fruit and vegetable consumption and mortality from all causes, cardiovascular disease, and cancer: systematic review and dose-response meta-analysis of prospective cohort studies. *BMJ*, *349*(3), g4490–g4490. Available at: https://www.bmj.com/cgi/doi/10.1136/bmj.g4490

Weinkauf, M. & Dreyling, M. (2015). *Vardenafil, a clinically available phosphodiesterase inhibitor, potentiates the killing effect of EGCG on CLL cells*. Academic Press.

Wu, L., Guo, L., Liang, Y., Liu, X., Jiang, L., & Wang, L. (2015). Curcumin suppresses stem-like traits of lung cancer cells via inhibiting the JAK2/STAT3 signaling pathway. *Oncology Reports*, *34*(6), 3311–3317. doi:10.3892/or.2015.4279 PMID:26397387

Wu, Q.-J., Wu, L., Zheng, L.-Q., Xu, X., Ji, C., & Gong, T.-T. (2016). Consumption of fruit and vegetables reduces risk of pancreatic cancer: Evidence from epidemiological studies. *European Journal of Cancer Prevention*, *25*(3), 196–205. doi:10.1097/CEJ.0000000000000171 PMID:26075658

Yang, J. (2015). Effect of curcumin on Bcl-2 and Bax expression in nude mice prostate cancer. *International Journal of Clinical and Experimental Pathology*, *8*(8), 9272–9278. PMID:26464676

Yi, J.-L. (2015). Myricetin and methyl eugenol combination enhances the anticancer activity, cell cycle arrest and apoptosis induction of cis-platin against HeLa cervical cancer cell lines. *International Journal of Clinical and Experimental Pathology*, *8*(2), 1116–1127. https://www.ncbi.nlm.nih.gov/pmc/articles/PMC4396221/ PMID:25972998

Yi, J. L. (2015). Myricetin and methyl eugenol combination enhances the anticancer activity, cell cycle arrest and apoptosis induction of cis-platin against HeLa cervical cancer cell lines. *International Journal of Clinical and Experimental Pathology*, *8*(2), 1116–1127. PMID:25972998

Zhan, Y., Chen, Y., Liu, R., Zhang, H., & Zhang, Y. (2014). Potentiation of paclitaxel activity by curcumin in human breast cancer cell by modulating apoptosis and inhibiting EGFR signaling. *Archives of Pharmacal Research*, *37*(8), 1086–1095. doi:10.100712272-013-0311-3 PMID:24318305

Zhang, Y., Ma, S.W.J. & Xie, H.L.J.Y.S. (2014). *Laboratory investigation EGCG inhibits properties of glioma stem-like cells and synergizes with temozolomide through downregulation of P-glycoprotein inhibition*. Academic Press.

Zheng, C. (2016). Synergistic effects of curcumin and bortezomib on multiple myeloma cells. *International Journal of Clinical and Experimental Medicine*, *9*(11), 21787–21793.

Zhou, Q.-M., Sun, Y., Lu, Y.-Y., Zhang, H., Chen, Q.-L., & Su, S.-B. (2017). Curcumin reduces mitomycin C resistance in breast cancer stem cells by regulating Bcl-2 family-mediated apoptosis. *Cancer Cell International*, *17*(1), 84. doi:10.118612935-017-0453-3 PMID:28959140

Zhou, Y., Tang, J., Du, Y., Ding, J., & Liu, J.-Y. (2016). The green tea polyphenol EGCG potentiates the antiproliferative activity of sunitinib in human cancer cells. *Tumour Biology*, *37*(7), 8555–8566. doi:10.100713277-015-4719-x PMID:26733173

Zhu, H., Cheng, H., Ren, Y., Liu, Z. G., Zhang, Y. F., & De Luo, B. (2012). Synergistic inhibitory effects by the combination of gefitinib and genistein on NSCLC with acquired drug-resistance in vitro and in vivo. *Molecular Biology Reports*, *39*(4), 4971–4979. doi:10.100711033-011-1293-1 PMID:22160570

Chapter 9
Role of Herbal Medicine/ Phyto-Therapy in Cancer Prevention by Inhibiting Epithelial-Mesenchymal Transition (EMT) Pathways

Rekha Gahtori
Department of Biotechnology, Bhimtal Campus, Kumaun University, India

Ashutosh Paliwal
Department of Biotechnology, Bhimtal Campus, Kumaun University, Nainital, India

ABSTRACT

Human life is surrounded and dependent on its environment. Human civilization is nurtured by nature as it provides raw materials that are used in the manufacturing of various essential products like medicine, food items, etc. Not only developing countries but developed countries also depend on herbal-based medications. Cancer is a global health burden. Epithelial-mesenchymal-transition (EMT) plays a key role in cancer progression and is also stimulated by different extracellular signals and could be regulated at different levels. Conventional therapies exhibit a cytotoxic effect, which encourages the development of a new approach that could be used with synthetic drugs. Phytotherapy emerged as an effective weapon against cancer. Herbal drugs directly target different signaling pathways that promote EMT and eventually lead to cancer.

DOI: 10.4018/978-1-7998-4808-0.ch009

INTRODUCTION

The human population have been in close contact with the environment since the beginning of human civilization and also dependent on nature for their food and medicinal need. Nature could be referred to as the best friend of the human since development of human civilization, as human population totally dependent on nature for their basic daily requirements. Various products required in daily life are manufactured by raw materials collected from different parts of plants. Plants provide different products which are the basis for treating different chronic diseases (Firenzuoli *et al.*, 2007). Use and adequacy of plants with medicinal values increasing day by day. The interest of researchers and pharmaceutical industries in medicinal plants also increased. Without plants and plant-derived compounds human survival could be quite difficult. Plants are not only important for the ecosystem but also important for the survival of humans. Plants produce a number of secondary metabolites that exhibited a wide spectrum of bioactivities which also support its acceptability. Different ancient civilizations have a history of usage of medicinal plants such as China, Egypt, Greece, and India. Hamilton, (2004) documented different role and application of plants such as drugs, disinfectant and aromatic agents in ancient Persia. Additionally, medicinal plants have a long history of using as a disease control agent against different diseases for mankind (Halberstein, 2005). Only the tenth part of explored medicinal plants are used by pharmaceutical industries and only collected from the wildlife population. Indeed, the demand for wildlife sources has increased by 8-15% per year in Europe, North America and Asia in recent decades (Verma and Singh, 2008). Plant species that possess medicinal properties are called medicinal plants and these plants have the ability to produce compounds, from which drugs can be synthesized (Rasool, 2012). Sometimes the whole plant is considered as medicinal plant whereas sometimes some part of plants *viz.* seeds, root, leaf, fruit, skin and the flower used for medication purposes. These plants have different substances and stored compounds which showed physiological effect on the living organisms (Phillipson, 2001). Raw materials obtained from medicinal plants used by humans to maintain health and for treatment or cure of diseases (Shakya, 2016). Synergistic properties of medicinal plants make it an appropriate candidate for treating diseases. Plant-derived compounds have the potential to improve chronic diseases such as cancer. The cytotoxic and adverse effect of conventional drugs could prevent by the use of plant-based drugs and this property is behind its high demand in the medical industry (Rasool, 2012).

A phenomenon in which uncontrolled growth of cells occurs called cancer. In a report, the World Health Organization (WHO) estimated that approximately 14 million people are suffering from different type of cancers worldwide and 8 million people died from cancer in 2012. Cancer exhibited high mortality and morbidity rate which makes it a global health and economic burden which requires immediate prevention measures. Currently, radiotherapy, chemotherapy and immunotherapy are available treatments against cancer progression. But these treatments have their limitations and showed adverse effects on healthy cells which encouraged an urgent need for new and safe alternative approaches against cancer prevention. Interestingly, herbal therapy or use of herbs in the treatment of cancer could be an alternative, better and safe approach (Saini et al., 2012).

EPITHELIAL TO MESENCHYMAL TRANSITION (EMT)

A cellular process where epithelial cell represses their cellular characteristics *i.e.* cellular morphology, controlled cell growth, cell-cell adhesion and developed invasive and migratory properties during wound healing and inflammation. This transitional phase is called an Epithelial-to-Mesenchymal transition (EMT) (Savagner, 2015). Apart from simple definition, EMT is a complex and diverse phenomenon that is stimulated by various pathological conditions such as organ fibrosis and cancer (Lamouille *et al.*, 2014). EMT is regarded as a critical event during embryonic development, tumor metastasis and organ fibrosis (Thompson and Newgreen, 2005; Yang and Weinberg, 2008; Thiery *et al.*, 2009). Study of Brabletz, (2012); De Craene and Berx, (2016); Nieto *et al.*, (2016) suggested the association of EMT with tumor initiation, malignant progression, tumor stemness, tumor cell migration, blood intravasation and metastasis. On the basis of different extracellular environment conditions and state of the tissue, different modes of EMT exhibited by cells which give rise to vastly different phenotype readouts, including behaviors in cancer progression and metastasis. Loss of apical-basal polarity and the disassembly of the epithelial cell-cell contacts including tight junctions (TJs), adherens junctions (AJs) and desmosomes, the actin cytoskeletal architecture in the cells undergoing EMT are the common hallmarks of EMT. Additionally, EMT is also characterized by degradation and invasion of their basal extracellular matrix. Different Matrix-Metallo Proteins (MMPs) are expressed during this phenomenon. EMT has long been considered as a binary process with two distinct cell populations, epithelial and mesenchymal (Puisieux *et al.*, 2014; Nieto *et al.*, 2016) and also characterized by the loss of epithelial markers and the gain of mesenchymal markers. Epithelial markers such as E-cadherin (endothelial cadherin), plakoglobin and desmoplakin were repressed and up-regulation of mesenchymal markers such as Vimentin, fibronectin and N-cadherin reported during epithelial-mesenchymal transition (Thompson and Newgreen, 2005; Yang and Weinberg, 2008; Yang and Wu, 2008; Thiery *et al.*, 2009). Additionally, EMT also associated with various cellular states in which epithelial and mesenchymal markers expressed at different levels and showing intermediate morphological, transcriptional and epigenetic features, between epithelial and mesenchymal cells (Jordan *et al.*, 2011; Huang *et al.*, 2013; Zhang *et al.*, 2014; Jolly *et al.*, 2016; Pastushenko *et al.*, 2018). Partial, incomplete, or hybrid EMT states are intermediate states between epithelial and fully mesenchymal states. Different transcriptional factors *i.e.*Twist1, Snail, Slug, Zeb1 (also known as T-cell Factor 8, TCF8 & δEF1), SIP1 (also known as ZEB2) and E47 (also known as TCF3) induce EMT by repressing CDH1 which encode E-cadherin (Remacle *et al.*, 1999; Cano *et al.*, 2000; Comijn *et al.*, 2001; Perez-Moreno *et al.*, 2001; Hajra *et al.*, 2002; Yang *et al.*, 2004). EMT facilitates gastrulation, neural crest delamination and the generation of diverse cell and tissue types during embryonic development (Nieto *et al.*, 2016).

EMT AND CANCER PROGRESSION

EMT, an essential and crucial phenomenon that plays an important role during the developmental process which finally leads to the formation of different tissues and organ formation. These cells supposed to have migration ability and they migrate individually or collectively in a coordinated manner. Single-cell migration commonly requires a more complete EMT with reduced cell adhesion, loss of apical-basal polarity, the gain of front-rear polarity, and increased individual motility (Figure 1) (Friedl and Mayor, 2017). The expression pattern of different inducers of EMT differs among various cancer types. Various scientific reports established a correlation between EMT and cancer progression. Study of Yang *et al.*, (2004); Tran *et al.*, (2014) and Xu *et al.*, (2017) claimed that metastasis was stimulated by transcriptional factors Snail and Twist1 in the breast cancer patients. In Pancreatic cancer, Zeb1 strongly stimulates metastasis (Krebs *et al.*, 2017). Initially, EMT promotes metastasis in the lungs by decreasing the expression of Twist1 in breast cancer cell lines (Yang *et al.*, 2004). On the contrary, it was proposed that EMT was dispensable for metastasis as the presence of metastasis in a mouse model of pancreatic tumors in which either Twist1 or Snai1 were deleted (Zheng *et al.*, 2015), or in a mouse mammary tumor model with overexpression of mir200, a microRNA that targets Zeb1 and Zeb2 and inhibits EMT (Fischer *et al.*, 2015). Moreover, these assumptions are made without any experimental data in which depicted that the deletion of Twist1 or Snai1 or overexpression of mir200 is completely responsible for EMT inhibition in the mouse models (Aiello *et al.*, 2017; Ye *et al.*, 2017). Another study in the same mouse model claimed that depletion of invasive property in highly aggressive tumor cells reported due to the deletion of Zeb1 which resulted in inhibition of metastasis. The outcome of this study suggests that EMT could not only suppressed by the deletion of Twist1 and Snai1 whereas deletion of Zeb1 exhibited a much greater impact on tumor phenotype and metastasis formation (Krebs *et al.*, 2017). The study of Ocana *et al.*, (2012) revealed the effect of transcriptional factors on EMT. During this study, it was shown that EMT was up-regulated in kidney epithelial cells due to overexpression of Prrx1 which also enhances the invasive potential of cells in human cancer cell lines. The cells in which Prrx1 was overexpressed resulted in failure to give rise to lung metastasis after intravenous injection, lung colonization was enhanced while Prrx1 expression was silenced. This depicted the importance of EMT suppression for the colonization of lungs (Ocana *et al.*, 2012). On the other side, effect of overexpression of Prrx1 was discussed, tumor cells could lock in late EMT state due to overexpression of Prrx1 and also reduce the potential of tumor cells to undergo mesenchymal to epithelial transition (MET), thereby limiting the capacity to give rise to lung colonization and the growth of metastasis. The study of Takano *et al.*, (2016) documented the opposite role of two Prrx1 isoforms *i.e.* Prrx1a and Prrx1b on EMT. Both isoforms work in an antagonistic manner. Increase in E-cadherin and decrease invasion potential was associated with overexpression of Prrx1a while overexpression of Prrx1b resulted in a reduction in E-cadherin, increased invasive potential and also associated with a poorly differentiated phenotype (Takano *et al.*, 2016). In addition increase in blood dissemination of tumor cells was associated with Prrx1b while Prrx1a also stimulates metastatic outgrowth after lung colonization and knockdown of both Prrx1a and Prrx1b isoforms suppresses blood dissemination and metastasis in this model (Takano *et al.*, 2016). Twist1 overexpression in mouse skin SCC encourages tumor invasion and intravasation of tumor cells into blood circulation, and these CTCs display an EMT phenotype. However, the down-regulation of Twist1 is required for efficient lung metastasis formation (Tsai *et al.*, 2012). Altogether, these studies suggest that EMT is important for initiating the metastatic cascade in some tumors, its down-regulation is required for metastatic outgrowth. Interestingly, cancer cells often undergo a partial or transient EMT, whereas different markers of EMT reported co-expressed in various combinations. Various recent reports acknowledged multiple subpopulations of cells associated with different EMT stages from primary skin and mammary tumors that display distinct chromatin landscapes and gene expression signatures (Pastushenko *et al.*, 2018). Breast cancer patients reported with related hybrid states of EMT were epithelial and mesenchymal characteristics co-expressed in circulating tumor cells (Yu *et al.*, 2013). These findings are also supported by a series of *in vitro* studies confirming the co-expression of epithelial and mesenchymal markers and stepwise transition in breast, ovarian, and lung cancer cell lines (Huang *et al.*, 2013; Zhang *et al.*, 2014 and Bierie *et al.*, 2017). Collectively we can say EMT exhibited vast diversity in cancer progression and also stimulated by different extracellular signals and could be regulated at different levels (Figure 2). Different hybrid or intermediate EMT status may also have distinct connections with increased tumor stemness, metastatic ability, and resistance to therapy (Nieto *et al.*, 2016).

PHYTOTHERAPY

Figure 1. Different changes occurs during Epithelial-Mesenchymal-Transition

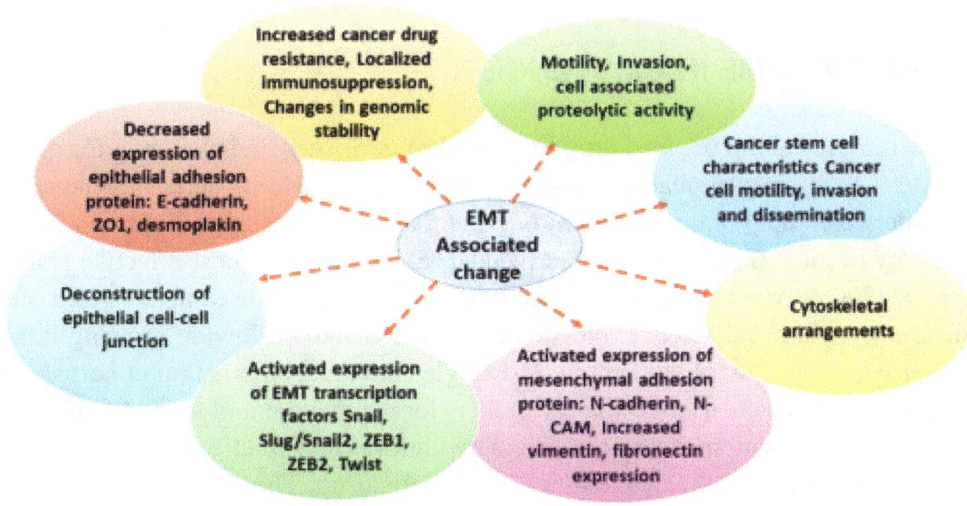

Figure 2. An overview: Link between EMT and Cancer progression

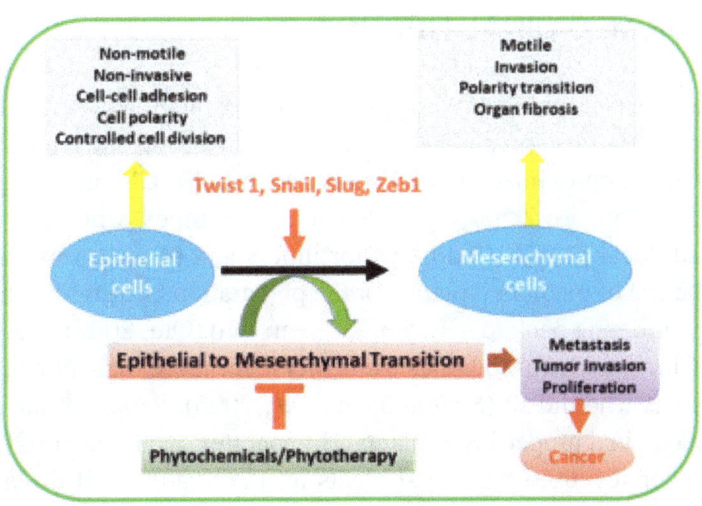

The study of natural heritages as medicine for the treatment of any disease or as human health-promoting agents and a science deals with the study of herbal medical practices, known as phytotherapy. The plants with biological properties such as antimicrobial, anticancerous, antioxidant, antiinflammation, antidiabetic, and antibiotic, etc. take part in the development of the phytotherapy. Due to these properties, nowadays, phytotherapy is becoming the leading interest among the scientific community.

WHY PHYTOTHERAPY CAME IN EXISTENCE

Phytotherapy is a new resource and processed drug used *in vitro* or *in vivo*, and clinically for the treatment of many diseases. According to pharmaceutical companies, the sale of herbal medicines also increased in last decade which help in the treatment of wide range of diseases (Capasso *et al.*, 2000). Nowadays, phytotherapy become therapeutic alternative and safe choice, less cost-effective and treatable also (Dattner *et al.*, 2003). Apart from this, in recent time, phytotherapy used in advanced science fields such as nanoscience, chemical science, biochemical science and worldwide growing different techniques of bioscience also used for phytotherapy. The single herb and combination of herbal decoction and with minerals, vitamins were used by the researchers for the treatment of several fatal diseases (Falzon *et al.*, 2017). The combination of phyto-medicine with known synthetic drugs also increased the potential of that drug by reducing the cytotoxicity of synthetic drug. The pharmaceutical industry is also demanding and producing more and more phytomedicines because herbal plants are considered as treasures of phyto-compounds.

Therefore, phytotherapy is an alternative therapeutic approach and urgent need in the field of drug discovery. Numerous studies have shown that isolated single compounds from the extract of medicinal plants which play an important role in the inhibition of many targeted pathways of some common diseases. Some factors such as less effective potential of synthetic drugs, occurring drug resistance due to long term use, expensive, and cost-effective, etc. are responsible for taking phytotherapy in existence.

HISTORIC OVERVIEW OF MEDICINAL HERBS

It is quite difficult to estimate the exact timing of using plants as drugs but Solecki and Shanidar, (1975) reported that approximately 60,000 years ago plants used as a drug first time. Various scientific reports claimed that plants used as a drug approximately 5000 years ago in India, China and Egypt and on the other hand history of the herbal drug are 2,500 years old. In ancient times, when the pharmaceutical industry is not well developed, local people used herbs for illness and treating various diseases. The earliest written evidence of the use of medicinal plants for the preparation of drugs has been found on a Sumerian clay slab from Nagpur dating back to nearly 5,000 years ago (Qiu, 2007). According to some inscriptions, Egyptians, and Chinese who used plants as medicine for more than 27 centuries BC were among the earliest human beings who did so (Schippmann *et al.*, 2006). People of ancient Greek was also familiar with the use of medicinal properties of plants. Hippocrates, the founder of Greek medicine and Aristotle, a pupil of Hippocrates, used medicinal plants for the treatment of diseases. After that, Theophrastus, a Greek scientist, founded the School of Medicinal Plants. Then, Pedanius Dioscorides, lived in the first century A.D., a physician and surgeon in the years 75-45 BC, wrote an encyclopedia, called De Materia Medica, to describe 600 therapeutic medicinal plants in the form of a series of scientific studies on medicinal plants (Madsen and Bertelsen, 1995; Rios and Recio, 2005).

The use of natural plant materials or plant-based drugs without industrial modifications which are used by the local population for treatment and control of disease is called Traditional Medicines by World Health Organization (WHO) (Tilburt and Kaptchuk, 2008). Plants have been a strong base for traditional medicines since long back and also provide different medications to mankind for several years. Traditional herbal medicines have been used in developed and developing countries for a thousand years as they exhibited fewer cytotoxic effects (Wichtl, 2004). The first book written about medicine were the first book written about plants, including the texts of the Ebers Papyrus, written 1500 BC, in which the name of many plants have been appeared (Ackerknecht, 1973). In the world various traditional medicine system was in use but Traditional Chinese Medicine system is most popular among all of them, and among all medicine system, plants are very frequently used or we can say that plant is the base for all traditional medicine systems (Liu, 2011).

In a study, WHO claimed that approximately 80% of the world population relies on herbal traditional system or plant-based medication which accounts a major source of health care (Farnsworth *et al.*, 1985). Today, approximately 70–95% of the population of developing countries use traditional medicines (Fridlender *et al.*, 2015). These statics not only give an account of India, China and developing countries but also for all developed countries (Ganesan, 2008). Scientific reports estimated that 50% of all manufactured drugs are based on plant-derived formulations now (Yarnell and Abascal, 2002; Harvey, 2008). An alternative herbal therapy, namely Phytotherapy, in which plant-derived compounds are used in the treatment of numerous diseases, most accepted and used worldwide.

There are 35,000 plants classified by National Cancer Institute (NCI) which have anticancer potential (Desai *et al.*, 2008). Plant kingdom is blessed with diversity which facilitates a prospect for the development of novel anticancer drugs. In drug discovery, isolation and characterization of a particular compound with anticancer potential continues to expand in research. Phytochemicals/phyto-compounds could sensitize the synthetic drugs as well as could enhance the efficacy of available conventional drugs. Phyto-compounds are natural and also minimize the risk of resistance over constant use. In combination with conventional drugs, phyto-compounds reduce the side effect of synthetic drugs and also sensitize the efficacy of drugs.

INHIBITION OF EMT PATHWAYS BY HERBAL MEDICINE

Epithelial to mesenchymal transition (EMT) is a complex process in which different signaling pathways are involved. Presently EMT becoming the primary interest of cancer biologists because in cancer, for encouraging drug resistance and metastasis, it plays a major role. In drug resistance and metastasis many EMT related factors, genes and pathways are involved. To increase the movement of epithelial to mesenchymal transition increasing the cancer rate. In recent years, phytotherapy is taking credit for the medication of it. According to many shreds of evidence, the phyto-compounds alone or either in combination revealed a significant role in the inhibition of the EMT (Aarthi *et al.*, 2019). Brusatol, a diterpenoid reported as a strong enemy of cancer. It also reverses the EMT pathways in pancreatic cancer (Lee *et al.*, 2019). The Oroxylin A, a natural compound isolated from *Scutellariae radix* well known for its medicinal values like anticoagulation, anticancer, antiinflammation, etc. Oroxylin A showed the inhibitory effect against breast cancer by inhibiting cell migration, invasion, proliferation and EMT pathways. It suppressed the protein and mRNA expression of mesenchymal markers N-cadherin and Vimentin however shown the reverse effect for epithelial markers E-cadherin. Oroxylin A also decreased the inflammation by suppressing the expression of inflammatory markers such as TNF-α, COX-2 and NF-κB. These inflammatory markers also are known as an EMT inducing agent (Sun et *al.*, 2019).

In the study of Zhu and Wen Astragaloside IV, a natural compound is a lanolin alcohol-shaped tetracyclic triterpenoid saponin, extracted from the A*stragalus membranaceus.* Astragaloside IV has been reported as an anticancer and antimetastasis agent by inhibiting the EMT pathways. Similarly, as above Astragaloside IV also suppresses the expression of markers and also inhibiting the PI3K/Akt/NF-κB by which prevents the TGF-β1-induced EMT in gastric cancer cells (Zhu e*t al.*, 2018). The A*rtemisia annua* medicinal plant reported as a strong potential of the antimalarial activity. According to the study of Y. S. Ko e*t al., (*2016) the polyphenols of A*rtemisia annua* demonstrated as a therapeutic agent against cancer metastasis on MDA-MB-231 cells of breast cancer. It inhibited the cell viability, cell adhesion, matrix metalloproteinase-2 and matrix metalloproteinase-9 and phosphorylation of Akt pathways. Salehi e*t al.,* also reviewed the involvement of phytochemicals such as Curcumin, Honokiol, Emodin, Gallic acid, Licochalcone A, Quercetin, Fisetin, Luteolin, Chrysin, Cyanidin, Oxymatrine, Berberine, Paeoniflori, Oleanolic acid, Vincristine, Vinflunine, Communic acid, Istanbulin A, Resveratrol, Garcinol, etc in the EMT. They reported many signaling pathways regulated by phytochemicals which includes NF-κB, WNT/β-catenin, JAK/STAT3, HIF-1α, FAK/Src and TGF-β1 pathways (Salehi e*t al.,* 2019). Similarly, Ginsenoside Rb2 is also a phyto-compound isolated from the P*anax ginseng* medicinal herb well-known for its antioxidant and anticancer potential. In one study, Ginsenoside Rb2 reported as an inhibitor of epithelial to mesenchymal transition by suppressing the TGF-β/Smad signaling pathways in colorectal cancer. Both i*n vitro* and i*n vivo* studies in xenograft mice proved the Ginsenoside Rb2 as an anti-EMT agent (Dai e*t al.,* 2019). Shao-Cheng Liu e*t al.,* (2019) also studied the Ovatodiolide macrocyclic diterpenoid phyto-compound isolated from A*nisomeles indica.* It is highly bioactive compound reported as an anticancer agent. It inhibited the viability of nasopharyngeal carcinoma (NPC) cells and induced the apoptosis by increasing the Bax/Bcl-xL ratio and also regulate the EMT markers (Liu e*t al.*, 2019). According to the study of Ming Wang e*t al.,* (2017). Poricoic acid tetracyclic triterpenoid compound isolated from P*oria cocos,* it is a medicinal mushroom also known as Indian bread and also well known for an anti-diuretic agent and renoprotective agent. This study demonstrated that Poricoic acid inhibits the Ras pathway and TGFβ1/Smad pathway by phosphorylation (Wang e*t al.,* 2017). Sulforaphane is also another natural compound abundantly present in cruciferous plants. It is known for its medicinal values such as antioxidants and the strong potential of anticancer effect. It suppressed the EGFR signaling pathway in lung cancer (non-small cell lung cancer- NSCLC) and another one is, miR-616-5p directly targeted GSK3β whereas Sulforaphane decreased the miR-616-5p level which suppresses the GSK3β/β-catenin signaling pathway and inhibition of EMT (Wang e*t al.*, 2017). In phytotherapy, not only single isolated phyto-compounds, but rather direct medicinal plant extracts also used as an EMT inhibitor. Study of Yung-Chien Hsu reported the Licorice (G*lycyrrhiza spp.*) root extract as inhibitors of renal tubular EMT by suppressing the Notch2 Signaling pathway.

Several studies demonstrated the effective role of phytochemicals on cancer cells. Alena Liskova *et al.,* (2019) reported the dietary phytochemicals targeting cancer stem cells. Some seaweeds extractions also showed anticancer properties. *Padina tetrastromatica*, *Hormophysa triquerta* and *Spatoglossum asperum* were studied for the pancreatic cancer and also have ability to target the signaling pathways which regulate the EMT pathways (Liskova *et al*., 2019). *Gynura divaricata* showed the anticancer potential on liver cancer stem cells by regulation of Wntβ/-catenin pathway (Yen *et al*., 2018). Similarly,

Green algae *Capsosiphon fluvescens* down-regulate the Wnt-1 signaling pathway and inhibited the gastric cancer cell migration. *Punica granatum* also a rich source of phytochemicals and reported as strong anticancer agent. *Trianthema portulacastrum* also exhibited the various pharmacological activities such as antioxidant, antibacterial, antifungal, antiinflammatory and it was also found to prevent breast carcinogenesis by inhibiting the NF-kβ and Nrf signaling pathways (Aravindan *et al.*, 2015). Other than this *Geissospermum vellosii, Rauwolfia vomitoria* and *Myrica rubra* also a rich sources of phytochemicals and have potential of targeting cancer Wntβ-catenin signaling pathways. Some other phytochemicals such as Pterostilbene, Genistein, Curcumin, Sulforaphane, Phenethyl isothiocyanate and Diallyl trisulfide reported as an anticancer compound by inhibiting the different mechanisms of signaling pathways (Liskova *et al.*, 2019). Zubair (2017), listed some phytochemicals such as Curcumin which targeted the COX2, iNOS, TLR/IL-1R, Keap1/Nrf2 and NF-kβ signaling pathways, whereas, Resveratrol target IL-1β, IL-6, IL-8, Keap1/Nrf2, and NF-kβ pathways. Moreover Honokiol, Plumbagin phytochemicals also targeted numerous signaling pathways and showed the antiinflammatory activity which further inhibit the EMT pathways (Zubair *et al.*, 2017). Kim *et al.*, (2016) reviewed the role of the phytochemicals that inhibit the EMT in cancer metastasis. They listed numerous phenolic compounds such as curcumin, Licochalcone A, Emodin (1, 3, 8-trihydroxy-6-methylanthraquinone) and flavonoid compound such as flavone luteolin and quercetin exhibited inhibitory effects on various cancers (Kim *et al.*, 2016). Fisetin, natural flavonoid suppress the EMT by targeting MAPK and NF-kβ signaling pathways (Pal *et al.*, 2014). Similarly, Procyanidin C1, supress the TGF-β-induced EMT in the lung cancer cell line (Kin *et al.*, 2013). Furthermore, Chrysin, Diosmetin flavonoid compounds also down-regulated the TGF-β1-induced the cell migration and refracted the expression of EMT markers like N-cadherin, E-cadherin (Kim *et al.*, 2016). Monophenols such as Shogaol component of ginger, similarly Eugenol, Capsaicin, Vanillin, Carvacrol and Thymol all are reported as an anticancer agents. Some polyphenols such as Garcinol, Honokiol, Kaemferol, Luteolin, Fisetin, Rhamnetin and crisiliol also revealed as a suppresser of EMT (Das *et al.*, 2019). Same study also showed other phytochemicals alkaloids including tetrandrine, restrain, berberine, matrine, sanguinarine, piperine and evodiamine serve as an anticancer drug (Lu *et al.*, 2012). Apart from these other phytochemicals Withaferin A isolated from *Withania somnifera*, Shikonin isolated from *Lithospermum erythrorhizon*, strongly targeted the NF-κB signaling pathway and other oncogenic signaling pathways (Lee *et al.*, 2016).

The study of Xu *et al.*, (2017), reported that resveratrol prevent the resistance of the doxorubicin by inhibiting EMT via targeting PTEN/Akt signaling pathway in gastric cancer (Xu *et al.*, 2017). In the same way, Da-xuan Wang *et al.*, (2017) used the Sulforaphane bioactive compound for the study. In this study Sulforaphane suppressed the EMT and metastasis in lung cancer by regulating GSK3β/β-catenin signaling pathways. It also inhibited the migration and invasion of lung cancer cell lines (Wang *et al.*, 2017). The prostate cancer is the most common with high mortality rate disease. Epidermal growth factors play an important role in metastasis in prostate cancer. Quercetin play a significant role against prostate cancer. According to this study quercetin down-regulate the EGF induced EMT pathways by targeting EGFR/PI3K/Akt signaling pathway (Bhat *et al.*, 2017). According to the study of Zuo *et al.*, (2015), pristimerin, a triterpenoid showed inhibitory potential of EMT and metastasis in prostate cancer cells (Zuo *et al.*, 2015). In another study it was revealed that the Diosgenin suppresses EMT by down-regulation of the vimentin and Madm2 in DU145 prostate cancer cell lines (Chang *et al.*, 2011). Silibinin, a bioactive flavonoid compound showed as strong potential of anticancer by modulating the cell proliferation, migration and invasion of cancer cells and suppressed the IR-induced EMT (Nambiar *et al.*, 2015).

Paclitaxel is a most common plant alkaloid used for the treatment of cancer. It used by researcher in combinatorial setting with some known cancer drugs or with other phyto-compounds where it enhanced the anticancer potential of that combined drug. Schmid *et al.,* (2018), demonstrated the role of paclitaxel in triple-negative breast cancer with Atezolizumab. Result showed that paclitaxel enhanced the anticancer activity of Atezolizumab (Schmid *et al.*, 2018). The additive and synergistic effect of plant compounds against cancer also published by the various researches. Di Zhang *et al.,* (2017), aimed the combinatorial therapeutic effect of Schisandrin B and Glycyrrhizic acid in bleomycin-induced pulmonary

Table 1. Role of Phyto-compounds on inhibition of epithelial to mesenchymal transition by targeting different signaling pathways.

Phytocompound	Sources	Research study	Reference(s)
Calycosin	*Astragalus membranaceus*	Inhibition of EMT in Pancreatic cancer	**Zhang *et al.*, 2020**
β-E lemene	*Curcuma wenyujin*	Inhibit metastasis on MDR gastric cancer cells and inhibit EMT	**Deng *et al.*, 2020**
Rosmarinic acid	*Labiatae, Boraginaceae,* and *Umbelliferae*	Anticancer effect on osteosarcoma cells by suppressing the PTEN-PI3K-Akt signaling pathway and inhibit the EMT	**Ma *et al.*, 2020**
Piperine	*Piper nigrum*	Inhibit EMT by inhibiting the TGF-Signaling Pathways in Human Lung Adenocarcinoma Cells	**Marques da Fonseca *et al.*, 2020**
Dulcitol	*Euonymus alatus*	Inhibit Proliferation and Migration of Hepatocellular Carcinoma by regulating SIRT1/p53 pathway	**Lin *et al.*, 2020**
Evodiamine	*Euodiae fructus*	Inhibited NSCLC cells metastasis and EMT in lung cancer	**Yang *et al.*, 2019**
Baicalein	*Scutellaria baicalensis*	Inhibit metastasis and EMT by regulating ERK signaling pathway in osteosarcoma	**Hang Lin *et al.*, 2020**
6α-hydroxy-4[14], 10[15]-guainadien-8β, 12-olide (SRCP1)	*Cyathocline purpurea*	Inhibit EMT and Wnt/ β -catenin pathway in breast cancer cells	**Javir *et al.*, 2020**
Hydroxygenkwanin	*Daphne genkwa*	Suppression of Hepatocellular Carcinoma (liver cancer) by inhibiting EMT	**Chou *et al.*, 2020**
Quercetin	Many fruits, vegetables, leaves, and grains	Inhibit metastasis by targeting EMT pathways in Oral Squamous Cell Carcinoma	**Kim *et al.*, 2020**
Silibinin	Milk thistle seeds	Inhibition of TGF-β1 signaling pathway	**Liu *et al.*, 2020**
Calebin A	*Curcuma longa*	Target the p65-NF-kB signaling pathways in Human colorectal cancer	**Buhrmann *et al.*, 2020**
Polyphyllin	*Paris polyphylla*	Induce apoptosis and regulate EMT markers in lung cancer	**Feng *et al.*, 2019**
Celastrol	*Tripterygium wilfordii*	Target TGF-β1/Smad signaling in colorectal cancer which induces EMT	**Jiang *et al.*, 2019**

fibrosis. Both compound showed synergistic effect and suppress the expression of the TGF-β and Smad2 signaling pathways (Zhang *et al.*, 2017). Apart from this, there are many natural compounds studied by the researchers for targeting EMT pathways for cancer are listed below:

FUTURE DIRECTIONS

Still, the discovery of cancer drug remains a huge challenge. Presently, the phytotherapy provides a new opportunity for new drug discovery from biologically active natural compounds. Medicinal compounds alone and in combination reported as a chemotherapeutic agent. In a combinatorial study, phyto-compounds also demonstrate the additive and synergistic effect. The combination of phytomedicine which targeted different EMT pathways also provides the new direction of research in this field. Apart from this phytotherapy in combination with other therapies also might be the hopeful therapeutic approach for treatment of cancer (Zhang *et al.*, 2018). In Phytotherapy, clinical trials of isolated phyto-compound after *in vitro* and *in vivo* studies, play a vital role in new drug discovery. Rather than new drug discovery, it is also very important to have a drug target system. For this, nanotechnology coming ahead as advanced scientific tool. Green synthesis is an important part of it. Here docking of nanoparticles with standardized herbal drug could provide a new way to target the particular pathways in EMT. Thus phytotherapy will become the popular in developed countries for treatment of cancer via targeting EMT pathways.

CONCLUSION

Cancer due to high mortality and morbidity becomes a leading cause of death worldwide. World Health Organization (WHO) reported 7.6 million deaths in 2005 due to different types of cancer. In 2012, Cancer research in the UK estimated that approximately 14 million adult population were diagnosed with different types of cancer. During cancer progression epithelial cells lose their normal characteristics like cell-cell adhesion, controlled cell growth, etc. and behaves like mesenchymal cells. This transition state is defined as Epithelial to Mesenchymal transition (EMT), an important phenomenon takes place during embryonic development, organogenesis. This transition could also be studied at the molecular level. Expression of various transcriptional factors up-regulated while some get down-regulated. Expression of epithelial cell markers such as E-cadherin, plakoglobin and desmoplakin declined while expression of Vimentin, fibronectin, N-cadherin (mesenchymal cell markers) up-regulated. Metastasis is a multistep and complex biological process that may involve epithelial-mesenchymal transition (EMT), cell-cell contact and cytokines. Phenomenon of EMT plays a vibrant role in cancer metastasis. Various scientific studies confirmed the role of transcriptional factors in EMT induction. NF-κB stimulated transcription factors such as Snail, Twist, Zeb and many more which later act as an inducer of EMT. Additionally, Snail stabilization is supported by NF-κB and is also associated with invasive potential and metastasis of cancer cells. On the other hand, Smad pathways also facilitate activation of TGF-β which leads to phosphorylation of Smad3 and stimulation of the EMT process. When assessing the overall contributions of EMT to discrete steps of multi-stage cancer progression, the aggregate of EMT-associated changes, including stem cell properties, changed genomic stability, increased invasiveness and disseminating ability, avoidance of senescence and apoptosis, sensitivity to cytotoxic therapies and localized effects on the tumor-associated microenvironment, need to be taken into account. Regarding EMT, it is clear that different populations of tumor cells offering different degrees of EMT could be found in different types of cancers and these diverse populations exhibited different functional properties, the hybrid state of EMT is thought to associate with increased metastatic potential.

Recently, EMT has appeared to be the main driver of chemo-resistance in anticancer therapies. The biological reason behind this phenomenon needs to be elucidated most probably unusual EMT in carcinoma cells unlocks an innate dedifferentiation program integral to tissue repair, development and homeostasis. But these traditional therapies and medications have their own limitations which could not be neglected. Anticancer therapies could affect healthy cells and also exhibited cytotoxic effects and drug resistance. To overcome with these issues, there is an urgent need to develop an alternative and safe therapeutical approach which could prevent cancer progression. Medicinal plants or plant-derived drugs could be a better alternative as it possesses various secondary metabolites which exhibit potent bioactivities against various chronic diseases including cancer and EMT. Anticancer agents derived from the plant source have largely contributed to the development of new drugs. Discovery and development of phytochemicals/plant derived drugs shows a great promise for the future. Different plant extracts possess various bioactive compounds that exhibit broad spectrum against numerous diseases including cardiovascular disorders, cancer insurgence, immune dysfunction, diabetes and oxidative stress. Use of phyto-compounds against chronic disease drawn the attention of researchers towards it as it exhibits less cytotoxicity and could work as a synergistic drug with synthetic drugs. Finally, the basic understanding of mechanism which control EMT should be used to develop new therapeutic strategies to prevent tumor progression, metastasis and resistance in anticancer therapies.

REFERENCES

Aarthi, R. (2019). Brusatol-as potent chemotherapeutic regimen and its role on reversing EMT transition. *Journal of Pharmaceutical Sciences and Research*, *11*(5), 1753–1762.

Ackerknecht, E. H. (1973). *From the primitives to the twentieth century*. Academic Press.

Aiello, N. M., Brabletz, T., Kang, Y., Nieto, M. A., Weinberg, R. A., & Stanger, B. Z. (2017). Upholding a role for EMT in pancreatic cancer metastasis. *Nature*, *547*(7661), E7–E8. doi:10.1038/nature22963 PMID:28682339

Bierie, B., Pierce, S. E., Kroeger, C., Stover, D. G., Pattabiraman, D. R., Thiru, P., & Weinberg, R. A. (2017). Integrin-β4 identifies cancer stem cell-enriched populations of partially mesenchymal carcinoma cells. *Proceedings of the National Academy of Sciences of the United States of America*, *114*(12), E2337–E2346. doi:10.1073/pnas.1618298114 PMID:28270621

Brabletz, T. (2012). To differentiate or not—Routes towards metastasis. *Nature Reviews. Cancer*, *12*(6), 425–436. doi:10.1038/nrc3265 PMID:22576165

Buhrmann, C., Kunnumakkara, A. B., Popper, B., Majeed, M., Aggarwal, B. B., & Shakibaei, M. (2020). Calebin A Potentiates the Effect of 5-FU and TNF-β (Lymphotoxin α) against Human Colorectal Cancer Cells: Potential Role of NF-κB. *International Journal of Molecular Sciences*, *21*(7), 2393. doi:10.3390/ijms21072393 PMID:32244288

Cano, A., Pérez-Moreno, M. A., Rodrigo, I., Locascio, A., Blanco, M. J., del Barrio, M. G., & Nieto, M. A. (2000). The transcription factor snail controls epithelial–mesenchymal transitions by repressing E-cadherin expression. *Nature Cell Biology*, *2*(2), 76–83. doi:10.1038/35000025 PMID:10655586

Capasso, R., Izzo, A. A., Pinto, L., Bifulco, T., Vitobello, C., & Mascolo, N. (2000). Phytotherapy and quality of herbal medicines. *Fitoterapia*, *71*, S58–S65. doi:10.1016/S0367-326X(00)00173-8 PMID:10930714

Chou, L. F., Chen, C. Y., Yang, W. H., Chen, C. C., Chang, J. L., Leu, Y. L., & Wang, T. H. (2020). Suppression of Hepatocellular Carcinoma Progression through FOXM1 and EMT Inhibition via Hydroxygenkwanin-InducedmiR-320a Expression. *Biomolecules*, *10*(1), 20. doi:10.3390/biom10010020

Comijn, J., Berx, G., Vermassen, P., Verschueren, K., van Grunsven, L., Bruyneel, E., & Van Roy, F. (2001). The two-handed E box binding zinc finger protein SIP1 downregulates E-cadherin and induces invasion. *Molecular Cell*, *7*(6), 1267–1278. doi:10.1016/S1097-2765(01)00260-X PMID:11430829

Dai, G., Sun, B., Gong, T., Pan, Z., Meng, Q., & Ju, W. (2019). Ginsenoside Rb2 inhibits epithelial-mesenchymal transition of colorectal cancer cells by suppressing TGF-β/Smad signaling. *Phytomedicine*, *56*, 126–135. doi:10.1016/j.phymed.2018.10.025 PMID:30668333

Dattner, A. M. (2003). From medical herbalism to phytotherapy in dermatology: Back to the future. *Dermatologic Therapy*, *16*(2), 106–113. doi:10.1046/j.1529-8019.2003.01618.x PMID:12919112

De Craene, B., & Berx, G. (2013). Regulatory networks defining EMT during cancer initiation and progression. *Nature Reviews. Cancer*, *13*(2), 97–110. doi:10.1038/nrc3447 PMID:23344542

Deng, M., Liu, B., Song, H., Yu, R., Zou, D., Chen, Y., & Lv, Q. (2020). β-Elemene Inhibits the Metastasis of Multidrug-Resistant Gastric Cancer Cells Through miR-1323/Cbl-b/EGFR Pathway. *Phytomedicine*, *69*, 153184. doi:10.1016/j.phymed.2020.153184 PMID:32199253

Desai, A. G., Qazi, G. N., Ganju, R. K., El-Tamer, M., Singh, J., Saxena, A. K., & Bhat, H. K. (2008). Medicinal plants and cancer chemoprevention. *Current Drug Metabolism*, *9*(7), 581–591. doi:10.2174/138920008785821657 PMID:18781909

Falzon, C. C., & Balabanova, A. (2017). Phytotherapy: An introduction to herbal medicine. *Primary Care: Clinics in Office Practice*, *44*(2), 217–227. doi:10.1016/j.pop.2017.02.001 PMID:28501226

Farnsworth, N. R., Akerele, O., Bingel, A. S., Soejarto, D. D., & Guo, Z. (1985). Medicinal plants in therapy. *Bulletin of the World Health Organization*, *63*(6), 965. PMID:3879679

Feng, F., Cheng, P., Wang, C., Wang, Y., & Wang, W. (2019). Polyphyllin I and VII potentiate the chemosensitivity of A549/DDP cells to cisplatin by enhancing apoptosis, reversing EMT and suppressing the CIP2A/AKT/mTOR signaling axis. *Oncology Letters*, *18*(5), 5428–5436. doi:10.3892/ol.2019.10895 PMID:31612051

Firenzuoli, F., & Gori, L. (2007). Herbal medicine today: Clinical and research issues. *Evidence-Based Complementary and Alternative Medicine*, *4*(s1, S1), 37–40. doi:10.1093/ecam/nem096 PMID:18227931

Fischer, K. R., Durrans, A., Lee, S., Sheng, J., Li, F., Wong, S. T., & Schwabe, R. F. (2015). Epithelial-to-mesenchymal transition is not required for lung metastasis but contributes to chemoresistance. *Nature*, *527*(7579), 472–476. doi:10.1038/nature15748 PMID:26560033

Fridlender, M., Kapulnik, Y., & Koltai, H. (2015). Plant derived substances with anti-cancer activity: From folklore to practice. *Frontiers in Plant Science*, *6*, 799. doi:10.3389/fpls.2015.00799 PMID:26483815

Friedl, P., & Mayor, R. (2017). Tuning collective cell migration by cell–cell junction regulation. *Cold Spring Harbor Perspectives in Biology*, *9*(4), a029199. doi:10.1101/cshperspect.a029199 PMID:28096261

Ganesan, A. (2008). The impact of natural products upon modern drug discovery. *Current Opinion in Chemical Biology*, *12*(3), 306–317. doi:10.1016/j.cbpa.2008.03.016 PMID:18423384

Hajra, K. M., Chen, D. Y., & Fearon, E. R. (2002). The SLUG zinc-finger protein represses E-cadherin in breast cancer. *Cancer Research*, *62*(6), 1613–1618. PMID:11912130

Halberstein, R. A. (2005). Medicinal plants: Historical and cross-cultural usage patterns. *Annals of Epidemiology*, *15*(9), 686–699. doi:10.1016/j.annepidem.2005.02.004 PMID:15921929

Hamilton, A. C. (2004). Medicinal plants, conservation and livelihoods. *Biodiversity and Conservation*, *13*(8), 1477–1517. doi:10.1023/B:BIOC.0000021333.23413.42

Harvey, A. L. (2008). Natural products in drug discovery. *Drug Discovery Today*, *13*(19-20), 894–901. doi:10.1016/j.drudis.2008.07.004 PMID:18691670

Huang, R. Y., Wong, M. K., Tan, T. Z., Kuay, K. T., Ng, A. H. C., Chung, V. Y., & Sim, W. J. (2013). An EMT spectrum defines an anoikis-resistant and spheroidogenic intermediate mesenchymal state that is sensitive to E-cadherin restoration by a src-kinase inhibitor, saracatinib (AZD0530). *Cell Death & Disease*, *4*(11), e915–e915. doi:10.1038/cddis.2013.442 PMID:24201814

Javir, G., Joshi, K., Khedkar, V., & Rojatkar, S. (2020). 6 α-Hydroxy-4 [14], 10 [15]-guainadien-8β, 12-olide induced cell cycle arrest via modulation of EMT and Wnt/β-catenin pathway in HER-2 positive breast cancer cells. *The Journal of Steroid Biochemistry and Molecular Biology*, *197*, 105514. doi:10.1016/j.jsbmb.2019.105514 PMID:31678110

Jiang, Z., Cao, Q., Dai, G., Wang, J., Liu, C., Lv, L., & Pan, J. (2019). Celastrol inhibits colorectal cancer through TGF-β1/Smad signaling. *OncoTargets and Therapy*, *12*, 509–518. doi:10.2147/OTT.S187817 PMID:30666129

Jolly, M. K., Tripathi, S. C., Jia, D., Mooney, S. M., Celiktas, M., Hanash, S. M., & Levine, H. (2016). Stability of the hybrid epithelial/mesenchymal phenotype. *Oncotarget*, *7*(19), 27067–27084. doi:10.18632/oncotarget.8166 PMID:27008704

Jordan, N. V., Johnson, G. L., & Abell, A. N. (2011). Tracking the intermediate stages of epithelial-mesenchymal transition in epithelial stem cells and cancer. *Cell Cycle (Georgetown, Tex.)*, *10*(17), 2865–2873. doi:10.4161/cc.10.17.17188 PMID:21862874

Kim, S. R., Lee, E. Y., Kim, D. J., Kim, H. J., & Park, H. R. (2020). Quercetin Inhibits Cell Survival and Metastatic Ability via the EMT-Mediated Pathway in Oral Squamous Cell Carcinoma. *Molecules (Basel, Switzerland)*, *25*(3), 757. doi:10.3390/molecules25030757 PMID:32050534

Ko, Y. S., Lee, W. S., Panchanathan, R., Joo, Y. N., Choi, Y. H., Kim, G. S., & Kim, H. J. (2016). Polyphenols from artemisia annua L inhibit adhesion and EMT of highly metastatic breast cancer cells MDA-MB-231. *Phytotherapy Research*, *30*(7), 1180–1188. doi:10.1002/ptr.5626 PMID:27151203

Krebs, A. M., Mitschke, J., Losada, M. L., Schmalhofer, O., Boerries, M., Busch, H., & Brunton, V. G. (2017). The EMT-activator Zeb1 is a key factor for cell plasticity and promotes metastasis in pancreatic cancer. *Nature Cell Biology*, *19*(5), 518–529. doi:10.1038/ncb3513 PMID:28414315

Lamouille, S., Xu, J., & Derynck, R. (2014). Molecular mechanisms of epithelial–mesenchymal transition. *Nature Reviews. Molecular Cell Biology*, *15*(3), 178–196. doi:10.1038/nrm3758 PMID:24556840

Lee, C. H. (2019). Reversal of Epithelial–Mesenchymal Transition by Natural Anti-Inflammatory and Pro-Resolving Lipids. *Cancers (Basel)*, *11*(12), 1841. doi:10.3390/cancers11121841 PMID:31766574

Lin, X., Li, K., Yang, Z., Chen, B., & Zhang, T. (2020). Dulcitol suppresses proliferation and migration of hepatocellular carcinoma via regulating SIRT1/p53 pathway. *Phytomedicine*, *66*, 153112. doi:10.1016/j.phymed.2019.153112 PMID:31786318

Lin, H., Hao, Y., Wan, X., He, J., & Tong, Y. (2020). Baicalein inhibits cell development, metastasis and EMT and induces apoptosis by regulating ERK signaling pathway in osteosarcoma. *Journal of Receptors and Signal Transduction*, *40*(1), 49–57. doi:10.1080/10799893.2020.1713807 PMID:31948366

Liu, R., Wang, Q., Ding, Z., Zhang, X., Li, Y., Zang, Y., & Zhang, G. (2020). Silibinin Augments the Antifibrotic Effect of Valsartan Through Inactivation of TGF-β1 Signaling in Kidney. *Drug Design, Development and Therapy*, *14*, 603–611. doi:10.2147/DDDT.S224308 PMID:32103902

Liu, S. C., Huang, C. M., Bamodu, O. A., Lin, C. S., Liu, B. L., Tzeng, Y. M., & Chen, T. M. (2019). Ovatodiolide suppresses nasopharyngeal cancer by targeting stem cell-like population, inducing apoptosis, inhibiting EMT and dysregulating JAK/STAT signaling pathway. *Phytomedicine*, *56*, 269–278. doi:10.1016/j.phymed.2018.05.007 PMID:30668347

Liu, W. J. (Ed.). (2011). Traditional herbal medicine research methods: identification, analysis, bioassay, and pharmaceutical and clinical studies. John Wiley & Sons. doi:10.1002/9780470921340

Ma, Z., Yang, J., Yang, Y., Wang, X., Chen, G., Shi, A., Lu, L., Jia, S., Kang, X., & Lu, L. (2020). Rosmarinic acid exerts an anticancer effect on osteosarcoma cells by inhibiting DJ-1 via regulation of the PTEN-PI3K-Akt signaling pathway. *Phytomedicine*, *68*, 153186. doi:10.1016/j.phymed.2020.153186 PMID:32088353

Madsen, H. L., & Bertelsen, G. (1995). Spices as antioxidants. *Trends in Food Science & Technology*, *6*(8), 271–277. doi:10.1016/S0924-2244(00)89112-8

Marques da Fonseca, L., Jacques da Silva, L. R., Santos dos Reis, J., Rodrigues da Costa Santos, M. A., de Sousa Chaves, V., Monteiro da Costa, K., & de Alcântara-Pinto, D. C. (2020). Piperine Inhibits TGF-β Signaling Pathways and Disrupts EMT-Related Events in Human Lung Adenocarcinoma Cells. *Medicines (Basel, Switzerland)*, *7*(4), 19. doi:10.3390/medicines7040019 PMID:32276474

Nieto, M. A., Huang, R. Y. J., Jackson, R. A., & Thiery, J. P. (2016). EMT: 2016. *Cell*, *166*(1), 21–45. doi:10.1016/j.cell.2016.06.028 PMID:27368099

Ocaña, O. H., Córcoles, R., Fabra, Á., Moreno-Bueno, G., Acloque, H., Vega, S., & Nieto, M. A. (2012). Metastatic colonization requires the repression of the epithelial-mesenchymal transition inducer Prrx1. *Cancer Cell, 22*(6), 709–724. doi:10.1016/j.ccr.2012.10.012 PMID:23201163

Pastushenko, I., Brisebarre, A., Sifrim, A., Fioramonti, M., Revenco, T., Boumahdi, S., & De Clercq, S. (2018). Identification of the tumour transition states occurring during EMT. *Nature, 556*(7702), 463–468. doi:10.103841586-018-0040-3 PMID:29670281

Pérez-Moreno, M. A., Locascio, A., Rodrigo, I., Dhondt, G., Portillo, F., Nieto, M. A., & Cano, A. (2001). A new role for E12/E47 in the repression ofe-cadherin expression and epithelial-mesenchymal transitions. *The Journal of Biological Chemistry, 276*(29), 27424–27431. doi:10.1074/jbc.M100827200 PMID:11309385

Phillipson, J. D. (2001). Phytochemistry and medicinal plants. *Phytochemistry, 56*(3), 237–243. doi:10.1016/S0031-9422(00)00456-8 PMID:11243450

Puisieux, A., Brabletz, T., & Caramel, J. (2014). Oncogenic roles of EMT-inducing transcription factors. *Nature Cell Biology, 16*(6), 488–494. doi:10.1038/ncb2976 PMID:24875735

Qiu, J. (2007). Traditional medicine: A culture in the balance. *Nature, 448*(7150), 126–128. doi:10.1038/448126a PMID:17625539

Rasool Hassan, B. (2012). Medicinal plants (importance and uses). *Pharmaceutica Analytica Acta, 3*(10), e139. doi:10.4172/2153-2435.1000e139

Remacle, J. E., Kraft, H., Lerchner, W., Wuytens, G., Collart, C., Verschueren, K., & Huylebroeck, D. (1999). New mode of DNA binding of multi-zinc finger transcription factors: δEF1 family members bind with two hands to two target sites. *The EMBO Journal, 18*(18), 5073–5084. doi:10.1093/emboj/18.18.5073 PMID:10487759

Rios, J. L., & Recio, M. C. (2005). Medicinal plants and antimicrobial activity. *Journal of Ethnopharmacology, 100*(1-2), 80–84. doi:10.1016/j.jep.2005.04.025 PMID:15964727

Saini, R. K., Chouhan, R., Bagri, L. P., & Bajpai, A. K. (2012). Strategies of targeting tumors and cancers. *Journal of Cancer Research Updates, 1*(1), 129–152.

Salehi, B., Varoni, E. M., Sharifi-Rad, M., Rajabi, S., Zucca, P., Iriti, M., & Sharifi-Rad, J. (2019). Epithelial-mesenchymal transition as a target for botanicals in cancer metastasis. *Phytomedicine, 55*, 125–136. doi:10.1016/j.phymed.2018.07.001 PMID:30668422

Savagner, P. (2015). Epithelial–mesenchymal transitions: from cell plasticity to concept elasticity. Current Topics in Developmental Biology, (112), 273-300.

Schippmann, U. W. E., Leaman, D., & Cunningham, A. B. (2006). A comparison of cultivation and wild collection of medicinal and aromatic plants under sustainability aspects. *Frontis*, (17), 75-95.

Solecki, R. S. (1975). Shanidar IV, a Neanderthal flower burial in northern Iraq. *Sci, 190*(4217), 880–881. doi:10.1126cience.190.4217.880

Shakya, A. K. (2016). Medicinal plants: Future source of new drugs. *Int. J. Herb. Med., 4*(4), 59–64.

Sun, X., Chang, X., Wang, Y., Xu, B., & Cao, X. (2019). Oroxylin A Suppresses the Cell Proliferation, Migration, and EMT via NF-κB Signaling Pathway in Human Breast Cancer Cells. *BioMed Research International, 2019*, 2019. doi:10.1155/2019/9241769

Takano, S., Reichert, M., Bakir, B., Das, K. K., Nishida, T., Miyazaki, M., & Maitra, A. (2016). Prrx1 isoform switching regulates pancreatic cancer invasion and metastatic colonization. *Genes & Development, 30*(2), 233–247. doi:10.1101/gad.263327.115 PMID:26773005

Thiery, J. P., Acloque, H., Huang, R. Y., & Nieto, M. A. (2009). Epithelial-mesenchymal transitions in development and disease. *Cell, 139*(5), 871-890.

Thompson, E. W., & Newgreen, D. F. (2005). Carcinoma invasion and metastasis: A role for epithelial-mesenchymal transition? *Cancer Research, 65*(14), 5991–5995. doi:10.1158/0008-5472.CAN-05-0616 PMID:16024595

Tilburt, J. C., & Kaptchuk, T. J. (2008). Herbal medicine research and global health: An ethical analysis. *Bulletin of the World Health Organization, 86*(8), 594–599. doi:10.2471/BLT.07.042820 PMID:18797616

Tran, H. D., Luitel, K., Kim, M., Zhang, K., Longmore, G. D., & Tran, D. D. (2014). Transient SNAIL1 expression is necessary for metastatic competence in breast cancer. *Cancer Research, 74*(21), 6330–6340. doi:10.1158/0008-5472.CAN-14-0923 PMID:25164016

Tsai, J. H., Donaher, J. L., Murphy, D. A., Chau, S., & Yang, J. (2012). Spatiotemporal regulation of epithelial- mesenchymal transition is essential for squamous cell carcinoma metastasis. *Cancer Cell, 22*(6), 725–736. doi:10.1016/j.ccr.2012.09.022 PMID:23201165

Verma, S., & Singh, S. P. (2008). Current and future status of herbal medicines. *Veterinary World, 1*(11), 347–350. doi:10.5455/vetworld.2008.347-350

Wang, D. X., Zou, Y. J., Zhuang, X. B., Chen, S. X., Lin, Y., Li, W. L., Lin, Z. Q., & Lin, Z. (2017). Sulforaphane suppresses EMT and metastasis in human lung cancer through miR-616-5p-mediated GSK3β/β-catenin signaling pathways. *Acta Pharmacologica Sinica, 38*(2), 241–251. doi:10.1038/aps.2016.122 PMID:27890917

Wang, M., Chen, D. Q., Wang, M. C., Chen, H., Chen, L., Liu, D., Zhao, Y. Y., & Zhao, Y.-Y. (2017). Poricoic acid ZA, a novel RAS inhibitor, attenuates tubulo-interstitial fibrosis and podocyte injury by inhibiting TGF-β/Smad signaling pathway. *Phytomedicine, 36*, 243–253. doi:10.1016/j.phymed.2017.10.008 PMID:29157821

WHO. (2001). *Legal status of traditional medicine and complementary/alternative medicine: a worldwide review*. WHO.

Wichtl, M. (2004). Herbal drugs and phytopharmaceuticals: a handbook for practice on a scientific basis (No. Ed. 3). Medpharm GmbH Scientific Publishers.

Xu, Y., Lee, D. K., Feng, Z., Xu, Y., Bu, W., Li, Y., & Xu, J. (2017). Breast tumor cell-specific knockout of Twist1 inhibits cancer cell plasticity, dissemination, and lung metastasis in mice. *Proceedings of the National Academy of Sciences of the United States of America, 114*(43), 11494–11499. doi:10.1073/pnas.1618091114 PMID:29073077

Yang, J., & Weinberg, R. A. (2008). Epithelial-mesenchymal transition: At the crossroads of development and tumor metastasis. *Developmental Cell, 14*(6), 818–829. doi:10.1016/j.devcel.2008.05.009 PMID:18539112

Yang, J., Mani, S. A., Donaher, J. L., Ramaswamy, S., Itzykson, R. A., Come, C., & Weinberg, R. A. (2004). Twist, a master regulator of morphogenesis, plays an essential role in tumor metastasis. *Cell, 117*(7), 927–939. doi:10.1016/j.cell.2004.06.006 PMID:15210113

Yang, X., Zhang, Y., Huang, Y., Wang, Y., Qi, X., Su, T., & Lu, L. (2020). Evodiamine suppresses Notch3 signaling in lung tumorigenesis via direct binding to γ-secretases. *Phytomedicine, 68*, 153176. doi:10.1016/j.phymed.2020.153176 PMID:32045841

Yarnell, E., & Abascal, K. (2002). Dilemmas of traditional botanical research. *HerbalGram*, (55), 46-54.

Ye, X., Brabletz, T., Kang, Y., Longmore, G. D., Nieto, M. A., Stanger, B. Z., & Weinberg, R. A. (2017). Upholding a role for EMT in breast cancer metastasis. *Nature, 547*(7661), E1–E3. doi:10.1038/nature22816 PMID:28682326

Yu, M., Bardia, A., Wittner, B. S., Stott, S. L., Smas, M. E., Ting, D. T., Isakoff, S. J., Ciciliano, J. C., Wells, M. N., Shah, A. M., Concannon, K. F., Donaldson, M. C., Sequist, L. V., Brachtel, E., Sgroi, D., Baselga, J., Ramaswamy, S., Toner, M., Haber, D. A., & Maheswaran, S. (2013). Circulating breast tumor cells exhibit dynamic changes in epithelial and mesenchymal composition. *Science, 339*(6119), 580–584. doi:10.1126cience.1228522 PMID:23372014

Zhang, H., & Chen, J. (2018). Current status and future directions of cancer immunotherapy. *Journal of Cancer, 9*(10), 1773–1781. doi:10.7150/jca.24577 PMID:29805703

Zhang, J., Tian, X. J., Zhang, H., Teng, Y., Li, R., Bai, F., & Xing, J. (2014). TGF-β–induced epithelial-to-mesenchymal transition proceeds through stepwise activation of multiple feedback loops. *Science Signaling, 7*(345), ra91–ra91. doi:10.1126cisignal.2005304 PMID:25270257

Zhang, Z., Auyeung, K. K. W., Sze, S. C. W., Zhang, S., Yung, K. K. L., & Ko, J. K. S. (2020). The dual roles of calycosin in growth inhibition and metastatic progression during pancreatic cancer development: A "TGF-β paradox". *Phytomedicine, 68*, 153177. doi:10.1016/j.phymed.2020.153177 PMID:32106002

Zheng, X., Carstens, J. L., Kim, J., Scheible, M., Kaye, J., Sugimoto, H., & Kalluri, R. (2015). Epithelial-to-mesenchymal transition is dispensable for metastasis but induces chemoresistance in pancreatic cancer. *Nature, 527*(7579), 525–530. doi:10.1038/nature16064 PMID:26560028

Zhu, J., & Wen, K. (2018). Astragaloside IV inhibits TGF-β1-induced epithelial-mesenchymal transition through inhibition of the PI3K/Akt/NF-κB pathway in gastric cancer cells. *Phytotherapy Research, 32*(7), 1289–1296. doi:10.1002/ptr.6057 PMID:29480652

Liskova, A., Kubatka, P., Samec, M., Zubor, P., Mlyncek, M., Bielik, T., & Büsselberg, D. (2019). Dietary phytochemicals targeting cancer stem cells. *Molecules (Basel, Switzerland), 24*(5), 899. doi:10.3390/molecules24050899 PMID:30836718

Yen, C. H., Lai, C. C., Shia, T. H., Chen, M., Yu, H. C., Liu, Y. P., & Chang, F. R. (2018). Gynura divaricata attenuates tumor growth and tumor relapse after cisplatin therapy in HCC xenograft model through suppression of cancer stem cell growth and Wnt/β-catenin signalling. *Journal of Ethnopharmacology*, *213*, 366–375. doi:10.1016/j.jep.2017.07.019 PMID:28729225

Aravindan, S., Ramraj, S. K., Somasundaram, S. T., Herman, T. S., & Aravindan, N. (2015). Polyphenols from marine brown algae target radiotherapy-coordinated EMT and stemness-maintenance in residual pancreatic cancer. *Stem Cell Research & Therapy*, *6*(1), 182. doi:10.118613287-015-0173-3 PMID:26395574

Zubair, H., Azim, S., Ahmad, A., Khan, M. A., Patel, G. K., Singh, S., & Singh, A. P. (2017). Cancer chemoprevention by phytochemicals: Nature's healing touch. *Molecules (Basel, Switzerland)*, *22*(3), 395. doi:10.3390/molecules22030395 PMID:28273819

Kim, E. K., Choi, E. J., & Debnath, T. (2016). Role of phytochemicals in the inhibition of epithelial–mesenchymal transition in cancer metastasis. *Food & Function*, *7*(9), 3677–3685. doi:10.1039/C6FO00901H PMID:27507108

Pal, H. C., Sharma, S., Strickland, L. R., Katiyar, S. K., Ballestas, M. E., Athar, M., Elmets, C. A., & Afaq, F. (2014). Fisetin inhibits human melanoma cell invasion through promotion of mesenchymal to epithelial transition and by targeting MAPK and NFκB signaling pathways. *PLoS One*, *9*(1), e86338. doi:10.1371/journal.pone.0086338 PMID:24466036

Kin, R., Kato, S., Kaneto, N., Sakurai, H., Hayakawa, Y., Li, F., & Yokoyama, S. (2013). Procyanidin C1 from Cinnamomi Cortex inhibits TGF-β-induced epithelial-to-mesenchymal transition in the A549 lung cancer cell line. *International Journal of Oncology*, *43*(6), 1901–1906. doi:10.3892/ijo.2013.2139 PMID:24141365

Das, B., Sarkar, N., Bishayee, A., & Sinha, D. (2019, June). Dietary phytochemicals in the regulation of epithelial to mesenchymal transition and associated enzymes: A promising anticancer therapeutic approach. *Seminars in Cancer Biology*, *56*, 196–218. doi:10.1016/j.semcancer.2018.11.007 PMID:30472212

Lu, J. J., Bao, J. L., Chen, X. P., Huang, M., & Wang, Y. T. (2012). Alkaloids isolated from natural herbs as the anticancer agents. *Evidence-Based Complementary and Alternative Medicine*, *2012*, 2012. doi:10.1155/2012/485042 PMID:22988474

Lee, I. C., & Choi, B. Y. (2016). Withaferin-A—A natural anticancer agent with pleitropic mechanisms of action. *International Journal of Molecular Sciences*, *17*(3), 290. doi:10.3390/ijms17030290 PMID:26959007

Xu, J., Liu, D., Niu, H., Zhu, G., Xu, Y., Ye, D., & Zhang, Q. (2017). Resveratrol reverses Doxorubicin resistance by inhibiting epithelial-mesenchymal transition (EMT) through modulating PTEN/Akt signaling pathway in gastric cancer. *Journal of Experimental & Clinical Cancer Research*, *36*(1), 19. doi:10.118613046-016-0487-8 PMID:28126034

Wang, D. X., Zou, Y. J., Zhuang, X. B., Chen, S. X., Lin, Y., Li, W. L., Lin, Z. Q., & Lin, Z. (2017). Sulforaphane suppresses EMT and metastasis in human lung cancer through miR-616-5p-mediated GSK3β/β-catenin signaling pathways. *Acta Pharmacologica Sinica*, *38*(2), 241–251. doi:10.1038/aps.2016.122 PMID:27890917

Bhat, F. A., Sharmila, G., Balakrishnan, S., Arunkumar, R., Elumalai, P., Suganya, S., & Arunakaran, J. (2014). Quercetin reverses EGF-induced epithelial to mesenchymal transition and invasiveness in prostate cancer (PC-3) cell line via EGFR/PI3K/Akt pathway. *The Journal of Nutritional Biochemistry*, *25*(11), 1132–1139. doi:10.1016/j.jnutbio.2014.06.008 PMID:25150162

Zuo, J., Guo, Y., Peng, X., Tang, Y., Zhang, X., He, P., & Xu, D. (2015). Inhibitory action of pristimerin on hypoxia-mediated metastasis involves stem cell characteristics and EMT in PC-3 prostate cancer cells. *Oncology Reports*, *33*(3), 1388–1394. doi:10.3892/or.2015.3708 PMID:25571882

Chang, H. Y., Kao, M. C., Way, T. D., Ho, C. T., & Fu, E. (2011). Diosgenin suppresses hepatocyte growth factor (HGF)-induced epithelial–mesenchymal transition by down-regulation of Mdm2 and vimentin. *Journal of Agricultural and Food Chemistry*, *59*(10), 5357–5363. doi:10.1021/jf200598w PMID:21504235

Nambiar, D. K., Rajamani, P., & Singh, R. P. (2015). Silibinin attenuates ionizing radiation-induced pro-angiogenic response and EMT in prostate cancer cells. *Biochemical and Biophysical Research Communications*, *456*(1), 262–268. doi:10.1016/j.bbrc.2014.11.069 PMID:25446081

Schmid, P., Adams, S., Rugo, H. S., Schneeweiss, A., Barrios, C. H., Iwata, H., & Henschel, V. (2018). Atezolizumab and nab-paclitaxel in advanced triple-negative breast cancer. *The New England Journal of Medicine*, *379*(22), 2108–2121. doi:10.1056/NEJMoa1809615 PMID:30345906

Zhang, D., Liu, B., Cao, B., Wei, F., Yu, X., Li, G. F., & Wang, P. L. (2017). Synergistic protection of Schizandrin B and Glycyrrhizic acid against bleomycin-induced pulmonary fibrosis by inhibiting TGF-β1/Smad2 pathways and overexpression of NOX4. *International Immunopharmacology*, *48*, 67–75. doi:10.1016/j.intimp.2017.04.024 PMID:28476015

Section 4
Other Metabolic and Endocrine Disorders

Chapter 10
Efficacy of Herbal Medicine in Treating Metabolic and Endocrine Disorders

Chittipolu Ajaykumar
https://orcid.org/0000-0001-8243-3405
Vision College of Pharmaceutical Sciences and Research, Jawaharlal Nehru Technological University, Hyderabad, India

ABSTRACT

Metabolic syndrome is an interrelated cluster of pathogens such as obesity, impaired glucose tolerance, cancer, and insulin resistance leading to endocrinal disorders. In the 21st century, progression of the disease is rapid increases due to change in the lifestyle of humans having a chance to develop metabolic change, and in some cases, mutations occur, which drastically affects the endocrine functionality and subsequently causes syndrome X. In modern medicine, different medications are available but only to maintain the condition lifetime. For the complete cure, WHO focused on the traditional knowledge in 2004, using the herbal medicine to cure all metabolic aliments. According to ancient medical treatment, metabolic syndromes are completely curable. They divided the disease progression stages and formulated the different dosage forms. All the data obtained from the ancient herbal medicine treatment are not evidence-based. So, the researchers all around the world focused on the evidence-based proofs to confirm whether herbal medicine shows efficacy in curing the metabolic syndrome or not.

INTRODUCTION

Since ancient times, human and other animal societies have always depended on plants and their products as a portion of food for survival and curing ailments. Around 3300BC Indigenous groups of people developed knowledge about ethnomedicinal plant-based products through their skills to solve various problems and pandemic situations by practical experiences (Petrovska, 2012). At 3000BC Ayurveda showed up as a treatment for curing aliments and prevent diseases. Later Egyptian medicine, Chinese medicine, and Tibetian traditional treatments used plants as a source of medicines.

DOI: 10.4018/978-1-7998-4808-0.ch010

Experience-based practices typically are intended to prevent or cure specific diseases or symptoms in a comprehensive fashion, the ancient people have no scientific knowledge of diseases and treatments. The treatments were conducted based on the opportunities had around them. At some point increase the demand for scientific knowledge with the advancements of technology to believe that actually, the herbal medicine is beneficial (Schulz, et, al,2001).

In the 19th-century increase demand for allopathic medicine (modern medicine) because relying on the evidence of effectiveness when considering other medical treatments, with the advancement in industrial techniques both Europe and North America during the early 19th century the production of this medicines increased (Petrovska, 2012).

Allopathic medicinal system approach focuses on the specific region in the human body and exerts pharmacological properties to cure the particular aliments unlike, other techniques ancient technology failed to focus on the preventive measures of treatment. Even though the allopathic medicines are created based on the practical knowledge, almost 40% of the new drugs approved in North America from 1983 to 1994, were derived from herbal plants, and approximately 70% of the new chemical moieties reported between 1981 - 2006 (Newman and Cragg, 2007).

The increase in interest originated in the late quarter of the 20th century, researchers found out that synthetic agents come from technical advancements also have potential side effects alongside benefits. In the case of ayurvedic and other herbal medicine treatment, no side effects were reported, led the researchers towards herbal medicines in the treatment of many diseases (Sen, S., et.al, 2011) (Gurib-Fakim, A.2006). It is important to recognize the plant constituents which are still used today becoming the basis for many synthetic drugs. Due to these findings, researches focus has been shifted to herbal medicine in the treatment of many diseases.

The world health organization has attentive on the traditional knowledge associated with herbal medicine from the early 20th century about 80% of the world population had experience with plant-based medicine for curing primary health. Issues were raised at the same time on the effects of the allopathic medicine increase the possibilities for the developing new bioactive compounds to offer better safety and efficacy (Fokunang, C. N, 2011). The global market for herbal medicine and medicinal plants is estimated to be worth US$800 billion annually. Traditional medicines are continuously increasing due to features like safety and efficacy against diseases (Sheng-Ji, P.2001) (Odugbemi, T. (Ed.). (2008). In today's world, important to recognize a majority of clinical research on in 21st century is based on the herbal entities in addition to a tool of alternative medicine focusing on the efficacy and safety to standardize biomass and manufacturing processes. A recent survey shows the majority of clinical research on herbal medicines in the 21st century involves modernization and globalization, focusing on efficacy and safety (Jachak and Saklani, 2007).

Researchers concentrated on to create an evidence base for herbal medicine to know the exact statistics involved under curing the elements. Herbal drug development requires unique approaches like reverse pharmacology to create the new drug moieties. Reverse pharmacology selects the herbs already used in the traditional medicinal treatment and evaluated during exploratory clinical studies. Experimental studies can be carried to conclude analytical explanations for clinical activity (Vaidya, A. D., & Devasagayam, T. P. 2007). Now a day's Herbal medicine therapeutics follows the systematic approach, has more promising in the treatment of multi-target disease. For various chronic diseases including diabetes and cardiovascular conditions, endocrine disorders where long-term treatment is needed, the actual problems arise herbal medicine co-administration with modern medicines may pose a higher risk of adverse effects and hence sufficient evidence data of the safety is necessary, Such approaches as Safety

Pharmacology focused on the pharmacodynamics / pharmacokinetic relationship of a drug's adverse effects using continuously evolving methodology. Unlike toxicology, Safety on Pharmacology requires a regulatory to predict the risk of rare lethal events (Pugsley, et.al, 2008).

A survey report in the US 2004, states more than a third of American adults use alternative medicine (Voigt, 2006). The consumer has driven back to nature an impressive expansion of the market in the past decade. Worldwide sales of medicinal plants include crude extracts and products finished in 1999 was 15 billion US dollars, in 2002 23 billion US dollar market as per world bank the market shows a 5-15% growth rate. The current market holds 60 billion dollars in sales of crude and finished products expected to multiply this growth rate in the first half of the 21st century (Hussain, K., 2009).

In India, the practice of herbal medicine is continued from ancient periods, since it is the birthplace of the oldest herbal medicine technology, the availability of plant medicines is widespread in India still it holds good marketing over the modern medicine (Pandey, M. et.al,2013).

THE REGULATIONS AROUND THE WORLD ON HERBAL MEDICINE

In the USA, State and the federal levels are regulating herbal products, with distinct pathways establishment of a committed evaluation team in the FDA's Center for Drug Evaluation and Research (CDER, 2006) to facilitate the renovation from dietary supplements to the botanical drug. From the several years of debate, in 2004 the CDER published the "Guidance for Industry–Botanical Drug Products", opening a gateway to register herbal remedies like prescription drugs (U.S. Department of Health and human services, 2004) (RH, R. U. et.al, 2015). Unlike previous regulations, new guidelines provide a condensed registration passage the identification and purification of a single bioactive ingredient are not required for prescribing herbal medicine.

The guidelines allow well-validated herbal preparations were expedited to enter human studies. However, standards for manufacturing and clinical trials were remained unchanged (Zamiska, 2007). This policy shift led to the flow of the investigational new drug (IND) applications: In 2005 more than 250 natural product-related submissions were recorded. In 2006, a special extract from green tea approved as Veregen™(Polyphenon® E) ointment, for treating genital warts (Zamiska, 2007).

In Europe 2004 decided to place a directive on herbal medicines that came into force by 2005 called under The "European Directive on Traditional Herbal Medicinal Products" (Herb Society, 2004), this directive calls for the unified regulations across Europe on a collection of the traditional and over-the-counter herbal remedies with predetermined safety and quality standards. The UK Medicines and Healthcare Products Regulatory Agency has since issued detailed guidelines to permit registration under the directive of botanical products for treating some qualified indications. This was followed and approved the oA.Vogel® (Atrogel Arnica Gel) a traditional herb ointment for the symptomatic relief of muscular aches, bruises, stiffness, and swelling in 2006.

Germany and France In March 2004, they announced a registration procedure. According to the procedure, established medicines of all herbal products do not fulfil the requirements for classification. (i) Most of the Herbal plants contain one or more herbal ingredients, besides, contain vitamins or minerals is allowed only if their safety is well documented and their action is supplementary to that of the herb; (ii) In some specified cases applications are not harmful are supported adequately by the data on traditional use, and their pharmacological effects; and (iii) herbal medicines combination must have been used medicinally for at least 30 years and should be used at least for 15 years in the European Community (Ekor M. 2014).

The entire scientific enthusiastic are took a step forward a created the derived products from the herbal extracts. The products synthesized as derivatives from the medicinal plants follow regulations of the Therapeutic Goods Act 1989 in Australia. It states The Therapeutic Goods Administration is implementing the regulatory process into a two-sub system based on risks assessment: listed (low risk) and registered medicines (higher risk) (Bensoussan and Lewith, 2004) and production of the herbal medicines as other therapeutics must be manufactured under the same code of good manufacturing practice (Liu, Y., & Wang, M. W. 2008).

In India, the use of herbal medicine is continued from the ancient times in the names of Ayurveda, Naturopathy, Yoga, Unani, Siddha and Homoeopathy. Indians take herbals as daily as a food source to maintain a healthy life. Even placed a ministry on such technology came to existence from 2014 marketing the herbal medicine products under the name of ayuh working on the evidence-based herbal medicine technologies. Recently a group of PhD students take multiple plants and observe the effects on a particular disease. The observations remain unknown for their mechanisms of action. Without the proper proposed mechanism of action modern medicine not accept formulations in mainstream therapeutics. Even though the mechanism of action of these formulations were studied become easier to file a patent on such observations but such patents remain on-shelf forever only very few patents that succeeds in the market (Ekor M. 2014).

Modern medicine considers only an individual either in health or disease. Ayurveda elaborates progressive conversion from a healthy state to diseased state on a six-stage process of disease manifestation as Shatkriyakaal (Basisht G.2014) (Chauhan, A.et.al, 2017). These Shatkriyakaal or six stages permit the recognition and management of disease much before it progresses into evidently differentiated clinical symptoms understand the steps involved in the progression from health to Prameha using Shatkriyakaal (Patwardhan, B., 2005). Herbal drugs used to treat various long term diseases easily such as diabetes, cancer, thyroid and other diseases which are also termed as metabolic disorders because of the cause of such results from defects in the regular metabolic processes (Ghavi, F., et.al, 2019). Any system of medicine should prove its ability in all aspects to enter into the pharmaceutical market.

STANDARDIZATION OF HERBAL MEDICINE

The pharmaceuticals are prepared with a single chemical entity that deals with ailments and disorders in target cells, tissues, or organs, the herbal remedies lack scientific establishment fall into the realm of myth. To achieve sustained growth and acceptable by the pharmaceutical market, the need for solid scientific evidence is required to support the functionality of many botanical products. Due to the lack of scientific evidence, variable sources of biomass, unclear mechanism of action, unknown active ingredients, difficulties in quality and safety evaluation, etc., make difficult strategy to achieve scientific standardization (Mukherjee, P, 2010).

The steps involved in the standardization of biomass (Atanasov, A. G., 2015):

1. The authentification of raw materials (biomass): Identification of Plant species must be proper manner. The plant products such as place of the growth, harvesting period, storage period, climatic changes affect the pharmacological action even the genetic makeup of the herbal plant. Also, the

herbal extract should free from microbial and chemical contaminants, to overcome all the aspects herbal plants must grow in well-controlled systems.

2. A general claim of "safety" on herbal medicine based on a long history of use is considered spurious. The claims need to evaluate with appropriate methods such as extraction procedure which affect the herbal plant's activity, multiple chromatographic fingerprinting represent ideal characterization of plants.
3. Unlike modern medicine, there is no specific methodology for assuring the herbal content to confirm the difference between batch and manufacturing process (Wang and Ren, 2002).In modern medicine one single chemical entity characterized for evaluation in every step such as the safety and effectiveness of drugs in well-designed clinical studies. Herbal medicines also follow the protocols, as required by the FDA, will consider herbal medicine as the gold standard for all classes of medicine (Patwardhan and Gautam, 2005).
4. Problems faced by the herbal medicine in clinical trials: Drug formulations must remain the same for all patients in the same treatment group, uniform and consistent treatment. However, In herbal medicine is individual basis treatment each patient varies by herb selection, composition and dosage needed results to conduct the binding clinical trial between patients in the same group and between the different group making it impossible to work.

Making new way for the tremendous opportunity subsist both in developed and developing countries to include herbal medicine in the healthcare systems. Despite a long history of use with proven efficacy in a variety of pathological situations, herbal medicine required qualifying in comprehensive terms such as biomass authentification, process development, safety assessment chemical characterization, and efficacy evaluation to prescribe or OTC use. Solid scientific evidence needed for the functional claims essential to herbal medicine to be accepted by the mainstream pharmaceutical market.

METABOLIC DISORDERS

Metabolic syndrome is a multifactorial disease associated with a cluster of pathologies including impaired glucose tolerance, obesity, hypertriglyceridemia, and insulin resistance, collectively referred to as the metabolic syndrome (formerly known as syndrome X). In the United States and other developed countries 25–50% of the population facing metabolic syndrome complications. (Kaur, J. 2014) (Felizola, S. J. 2015). Due to the fact metabolic syndrome having a strong association with premature morbidity and mortality increase awareness directed towards prevention and subsequent in particular, the individual having greater risk for developing cardiovascular disease, cancer, and Type 2 diabetes (Ford, E. S., 2005)

Causes

The exact mechanisms of the complex pathways of metabolic syndrome are under investigation but linked to a condition called insulin resistance. Normally, your digestive system breaks the food into sugar. Insulin helps the sugar to enter into the cells to be used as fuel for an organism. In people with metabolic changes most likely insulin resistance, cells fail to respond normally to the insulin produced in pancreas and glucose can't enter the cells as easily. As a result, blood sugar levels rise will lead to serious issues like cardiac arrest and kidney damage. Causes of metabolic syndrome (Payab M., et.al,

Figure 1. Overview on Risk factors and associated diseases of metabolic disorders

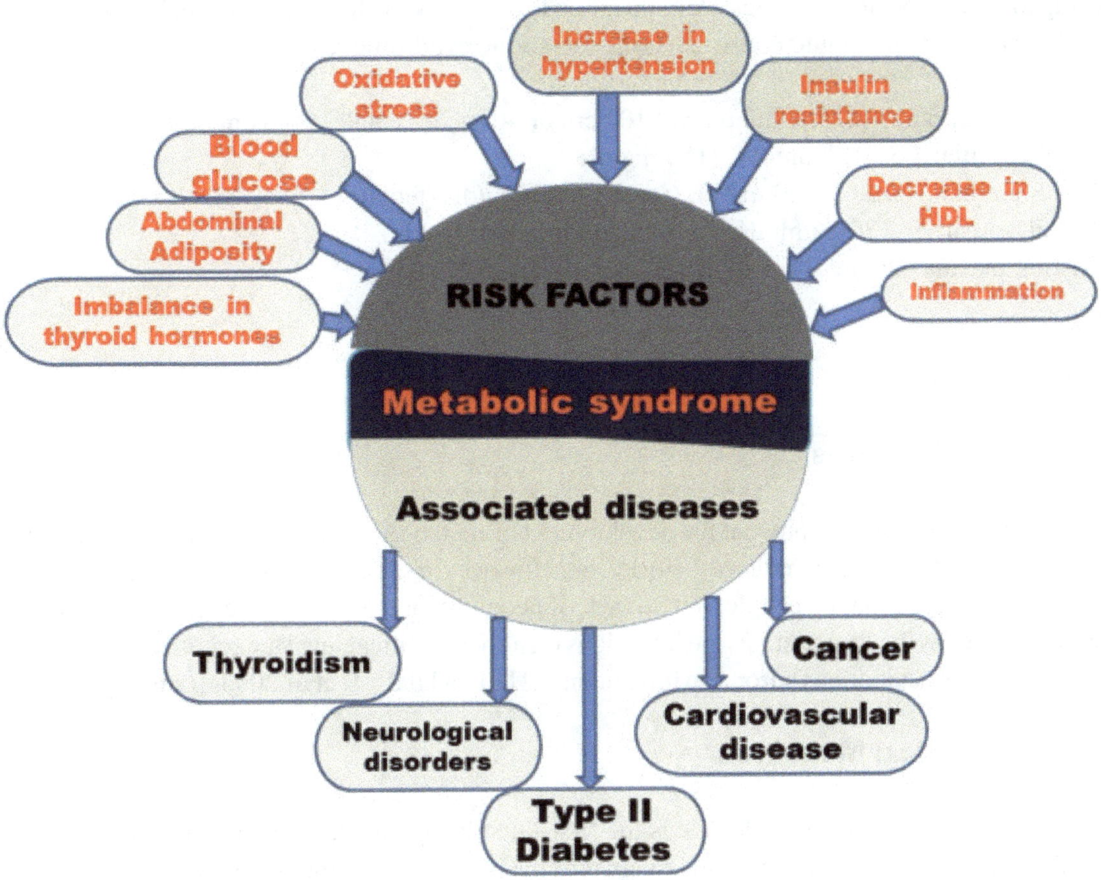

2020): Stress, Overweight, Sedentary lifestyle, Aging (Liu, y., et.al, 2019), Diabetes mellitus type 2, Alcohol intake, High calories food intake.

Sign and Symptoms

The main sign of the metabolic syndrome is central obesity (visceral, apple-shaped adiposity), overweight by the accumulation of adipose tissue particularly around the waist and trunk. Other signs include high blood pressure, impaired fasting glucose, elevated fasting serum triglyceride level, and decreased fasting serum HDL cholesterol, insulin resistance. Symptoms include if patient having a type -2 diabetes are increased blood sugar, excessive thirst, frequent urination especially in night fatigue and blurred vision. Patients with heart disease increase in high blood pressure early stages may have dull headaches, dizzy spells, or more nosebleeds.

Diagnostic Criteria

According to The US National Cholesterol Education Program, Adult Treatment Panel III (2001) requires at least three of the following to confirm having metabolic syndrome: [5]

- Central obesity: waist circumference ^{3} 102 cm or 40 inches (male), ^{3} 88 cm or 35 inches(female)
- Dyslipidemia: TG ^{3} 1.7 mmol/L (150 mg/dl)
- Dyslipidemia: HDL-C < 40 mg/dL (male), < 50 mg/dL (female)
- Blood pressure: ^{3} 130/85 mmHg (or treated for hypertension)
- Fasting plasma glucose: ^{3} 6.1 mmol/L (110 mg/dl)

TREATMENT FOR METABOLIC DISORDERS

1. Preventive Measures

Various strategies proposed to prevent the development of metabolic disorders, which include increased physical activity, a healthy and reduced-calorie diet. However, these potentially beneficial measures are effective in only a marginal of people, due to lack of acquiescence with lifestyle and diet changes. The International Obesity Taskforce states the intrusions on a sociopolitical level are required to moderate the development of the metabolic syndrome in inhabitants. (Hajian-Tilaki, K et.al,2013) (Gregory J. W. 2019).

2. Pharmacological Measures

In metabolic syndrome change of lifestyle is the first-line management, which includes Dietary intakes and physical activity. However, if in three to six months of efforts at remedying prove insufficient then drug treatment is required. The individual disorders that compose the metabolic syndrome are treated discretely because conditions are lined with other ailments in the body. ACE inhibitors and Diuretic agents may be used to treat hypertension.

Cholesterol maintenance drugs are used to raise the HDL levels if they are low and lower LDL cholesterol and triglyceride levels if they are elevated. Use of metformin and thiazolidinediones that decrease insulin resistance is becoming controversial; this treatment is not approved by the U.S. Food and Drug Administration. Weight-loss medications are used for obesity may result in weight loss. Restricting the overall dietary intake is more effective in reducing the most common symptoms of metabolic syndrome.

3. Treating Endocrine and Metabolic Disorders by Herbal Medicine

Different ancient herbal medicine systems were proposed treatment for the metabolic and endocrine disorders in which Ayurveda is oldest.

Ayurveda Concept of Metabolic Syndrome

According to Ayurveda Metabolic syndrome is a result of improper metabolism. Ayurveda treatment of metabolic syndrome divided into various stages based on ailment progression. The Initial stage of metabolic syndrome can be related with *medavaha srotodusti laxana* (obesity, Diabetes Mellitus), the middle stage or developed stage metabolic syndrome without complications can be compared with *Apathyanimittaja prameha* and the final stage or complicated stage of metabolic syndrome can be compared with *Updrava* of *Avaran*. In Ayurveda metabolism is considered the function of Agni. Various causes of metabolic syndromes like excessive calorie consumption, oily, heavy food, lack of exercise or physical exertion, sedentary lifestyle.

The main types of metabolic syndrome are obesity, diabetes and dyslipidemia. In Ayurveda, the initial stage or primary progression stage of metabolic syndrome can be compared with *medavaha Sroto dusti* above features have been mentioned as been the result of *Medavaha Sroto dusti*.

In the middle stage of metabolic syndrome turns in to type 2 diabetes mellitus and coronary artery diseases. So it can be said as the condition of *Sankara Vyadhi.*

In the later stage of the metabolic syndrome, the difficulty of specific diseases like acute pancreatitis, coronary artery disease due to hypertriglyceridemia, Diabetic retinopathy, nephropathy, neuropathy etc. due to diabetes mellitus and hypertensive cardiomyopathy, cerebral haemorrhage, hypertensive retinol and nephropathy caused due to hypertension, with the gradual evolution of the disease, it gets worsen conditions become difficult to treat. So, it is better to treat the disease before reaches to middle or later stage condition, *Acharya* Sushruta has mentioned *Shadvidha kriyakala* for early diagnosis of the disease so that treatment planned as early as possible and further progress of disease stopped.

Medavaha Sroto dusti is the initial stage of metabolic syndrome. So the nidan and *samprapti* of *medavaha srotasa dusti* can be helpful to understand Ayurveda Aspect of metabolic syndrome. For a complete understanding of metabolic syndrome as per Ayurveda perspective we can divide the condition of metabolic syndrome in three stages;

a. The Initial Stage of Metabolic Syndrome

Patients having a mild increase in waist circumferences, Prediabetes, Prehypertension and Mild dyslipidemia can be diagnosed as an initial stage of metabolic syndrome. Above condition of the initial stage of metabolic syndrome can be compared with *Medavaha sroto dusti laxana.*

i. *Hetu* (Causes): *Nidana* of *Medavaha Sroto Dusti:* Avyayama (Lack of exercise), Medyanam Ati Bhakshanat (Excessive eating of high calorie diet), Varuni Ati Sevana (Excessive drinking of alcohol), Divasvapna (Daytime sleep).
ii. *Linga* (Sign and Symptoms): Symptoms of medavaha sroto dusti include purvarupa of Prameha and Atishula Laxana.
    Atisthula Laxana: Loss of enthusiasm, excessive perspiration, weakness, excessive Appetite, loss of libido and difficulty in coitus, foul smell from the body, Excessive thirst, Reduced life span and quality of life.
    Purvarupa of Prameha: Numbness and burning insole and palm, throat and palate, Curling of the hairs, excessive thirst or increased desire for water, Dryness of mouth, Laziness, Attraction of ants toward urine and body, sweat tastes of mouth, burning and numbness in body parts, Accumulation of excretory products in the body, body smell, Turbid or vitiated urine, excessive sleep
iii. *Aushadha* (Treatment protocol): Treatment of *medavaha sroto dusti* shares similar principle of treatment for *Sthaulya*, like;

Chikitsa Sutra: *Kapha- medahara, Niruha basti and vatanulomaka Anna pana,* prepared with *Ruksh, Ushna* and *Tkshana Aushadha, Udvartana* (Dry massage by herbal medicines) by *Ruksha Aushadha*

iv. Herbal medicine used for treatment:

Guduchi: A valued herbal medicine acknowledged as *Tinospora cordifolia*. According to the myth, ancient gods created guduchi for immortality by churning Primordial Ocean; but modern science doesn't confirm any immortality properties but creating a potential medicine to cure stress and illness. Due to the presence of different classes of alkaloids, glycosides, steroids in Guduchi exert its activity.

Bhadramusta: Also known as *Cyperus scariosus*. It is a riverbed perennial herbaceous plant available majorly in Madhya Pradesh, India. Contain cineol copadiene, copaene, cyperol, cyperone, sugenol and beta-sitosterol which made herbal medicine to treat the muscle relaxant, fevers, digestive system disorders, and dysmenorrheal.

Triphala: It is the combination of Bibhitaki (*Terminalia bellirica*), Amalaki (*Emblica Officinalis*), and Haritaki (*Terminalia chebula*) which supports the bowel system; detoxify the body by removing the toxic materials.

Takrarista: It is one of the ayurvedic churna, consists thirteen different herbal medicine containing plant parts are ground separately on equal portions and mix with buttermilk or hot water while giving it to the patient about 3-6 grams two times a day reduce the bowel related problems and patients suffering from piles. Excess dose leads to gastritis so medical supervision is necessary.

Madhu: It is also called makshika. Madhu having different properties and also increase the medicinal qualities of herbal formulation. Honey consist of a wide range of vitamins, proteins, amino acids, enzymes, minerals and various other biological acids contribute properties such as used to treat hyperlipidemia, respiratory tract disorders, and good healing property. In Ayurveda, Madhu recognized as new and old new Madhu used as laxative purposes but old honey failed to show this property. The precautionary measures for taking honey compete the uses should not eat excess, avoid in summer, not to mix with hot foods and avoid during indigestion and don't mix with ghee in equal quantities.

Vidangadi Lauha: It is a mix of ten herbal medicines with metals such as mercury, sulphur and bhasma prepared from iron used in the formulation. Used in anorexia, helminthiasis, gastroenteritis, inflammatory disorders and abnormal colic pains. The self-medication was found to be dangerous, should continue for a limited period and accidental usage led to poisonous effects in case of children.

Vivaldi Panchamula kwath with honey: It is a mixture of six ingredients in all mixed in one portion saunf mixed in four portions along with honey. Shows astringent, antimicrobial, irritable bowel syndrome, anti-bacterial, antidiarrheals, digestive stimulant, anti-spasmodic, antihemorrhagic properties and also detoxifies Pitta Dosha, pacifies Vata Dosha and reduces Kapha Dosha. However also treat the colitis when it is given with the vanshlochan, praval pishti, mukka pishti.there were no side effects shown in any age patient, but in some cases cause constipation. Pregnant woman and lactating mother use kwath under supervision.

Agnimanth Svaras: It is an important herbal plant in Ayurveda belongs to the family ceodendrum phlomidis. It has cletodin, cerodendrin and clerosterol as constituents used to treat rheumatism, inflammation, reduce the severity of the haemorrhoids in gastrointestinal system and also having analgesic properties

Shilajit prayoga: Shilajit is a sticky like substance found under the rocks of the Himalayas mainly obtained from the slow decomposition of plants. It has a positive effect on healths such as it treats progressive memory loss disorder, Alzheimer, regulate the testosterone level, effective in the treatment of chronic fatigue syndrome (boost up the mitochondrial function), shilajit is rich in fulvic acid a good antioxidant and anti-inflammatory property which slow down the ageing process. Researchers found shilajit can overcome the high altitude sickness (condition include insomnia, pulmonary oedema, dementia and hypoxia), also cure iron deficiency anaemia, Improves the fertility and cardiac health. other effects like containing a high amount of minerals and meta constituents children should not prefer to use, contraindication in patients with sickle cell anaemia and hemochromatosis.

v. Pathyapathya:

Pathya (protocol): The protocol includes Daily exercise, Maximum use of Yava (Barely), Jirne Bhojana (restrict the food intake until complete digestion of previous food), and Purana Godhuma (Old Wheat) for food preparation which contain high fiber and less carbohydrates.

Aharam (diet): Avoid High-calorie diet, like fast foods; Fatty, heavy and oily food substances, Excessive and daily use of meat, Excessive use of milk/dairy products like curd, paneer, ghee, sweets and Avoiding excessive alcohol consumption also favours the decrease the metabolic syndromes severity.

b. The Middle Stage of Metabolic Syndrome

It can be compared with *Avaranajanya madhumeha* In *Ayurveda*. Sushruta has mentioned it as *Sthula pramehi.*

i. *Hetu*(Causes): Excessive indulgence of Snigdha, Guru, Amla and Lavana rasa as a dominant diet, Samashana, Nava Anna and pana, Excessive Seating on very comfortable seats, Lack of exercise, Excessive Sleep, Lack of Samshodhana of vitiated and accumulated dosha.

ii. *Linga*(Sign and Symptoms): The excessive escalation of Pitta and Shleshma leads to Avaran of Vata and obstructed Vata excrete Ojas with urine and the urine becomes like Madhu in taste and color and the condition is called *Madhumeha*. The patients feel symptoms of vatta, pitta and kapha frequently become shrunken due to excessive loss of Ojas in urine.

iii. Treatment:

Upakrma: In the condition of extreme *dosha Samshodhana* like *vamana* and *virechana* should be given. If Dosha is moderate Pachana and Vyayama drugs were used. Rukshana can be done with udavartana of powder of drugs having laghu, Ruksha and Kashaya, properties. After the completion of shodhana and Rukshana, Bruhana and Snehana should be performed.

iv. Herbal medicines:

Phalatrikadi Kwath: It is an eight different herbals combination (Amalaki, Haritaki .Vibhitaki, Guduchi, Katuki, Nimba, Bhunimba, Vasakataken from different portions like root, bark, leaves and fruit used in metabolic disorders. Mainly used in case sedentary lifestyle nonalcoholic fatty liver disease, Drug-induced hepatitis like paracetamol, viral hepatitis like B and C, anti-tubercular drugs. Some fevers like malaria and typhoid have a direct impact on liver tissues and also having antioxidant, immune-modulatory, choleretic, cholagogue activities.

Shows dose depended on precautions, Diabetic patients, pregnant women, lactating mothers and children should use under medical supervision.

Nisha Amalaki: It is the equal amount composition of amla (Emblica Officinalis), turmeric (Curcuma Longa L). Amla contains tannins, polyphenols, alkaloids, vitamins and minerals. Ellagic acid, emblicanin A & B, Gallic acid, quercetin, phyllembein, and turmeric contain curcuminoids, volatile oils and several proteins all these chemical constituents noticed biological activities. Nisha Amalaki used as ant hyperglycemic, insulin mimetic, Antidiabetic, and α-glucosidase inhibitory, α-Amylase inhibitory and antioxidant properties. It improves insulin sensitivity, increases the glucose uptake by skeletal muscles, according to herbal medicine technology in case of Diabetes as well as prevention of its complications microvascular- like diabetic nephropathy, retinopathy, neuropathy, gastropathy and macrovascular like atherosclerosis. There are no certain precautionary needed because used in daily bases food preparation, pregnant and lactating women and children below three years age should consult the doctor to use as a medication.

Ayaskruti: It is herbal medicine liquid preparation contains 50 different kind of ingredients formulated and form ayaskruti. Preparation involves a decoction of Asanadi Gana (23 herbs) is first prepared add to the decoction. Prepare Kalka of Vatsakadi Gana Drayas (22 herbs) is made independently and added to the decoction. The mixture poured into the honey and pepper and ghee smeared pot from inside and outside smeared with Laksha and cooked on the bundle of barley. Add the iron into decoction repeat heating and cooldown the iron sheets process repeated until the iron completely mixed with the decoction. close pot mouth with lid and ferment for one month then filter the contents. Ayaskruti used in various disease conditions includes metabolic syndrome problems urinary complications, insomnia, jaundice, insanity, epilepsy, oedema, anaemia, obesity, impaired digestive problems, phthisis, clean the body channels, control sugar levels and mobilization in type -2 diabetes. large doses cause stomach irritation and stomach upset, due to the involvement of many herbs should use under the medicinal supervision.

Khadir Rasayana: It is fermented decoction Rasayana it made by using Acacia Catechu (2kg), Cedrus Deodara(2kg), Psoralea Corylifolia(480gms), Berberis Aristata(800gm), Triphala (800gm), Water(81kg) and subject for heating up to 8th part then add 10 more ingredients and prepare it for fermentation up to 30-40 days filter it once the fermentation was completed. mainly used in case of leprosy, psoriasis, urticaria, dermatitis and lymph nodes, spleen enlargement, liver disorders, anaemia and tumours and cysts in the skin and also detoxify the blood and metabolic health improvement. There is only one common side effect noticed cause heartburn or burning sensation. Pregnant and lactating women should consult Ayurvedic specialist before taking medication.

Tuvaraka Rasayana: Tuvaraka herb has great importance in ancient herbal medicine source of the medicine is a seed. Tuvaraka Rasayana prepared by adding 768gm of tuvaraka added in the 2 litres of Acacia catechu and 128 gm of Hydnocarpus lauroifolia added heat in pot oil will be prepared. Oil should be kept in cow dung or hot ash store for 15 days before use. The prepared Rasayana used for the various skin disorders, urinary tract infections and wound healing, blood purifying properties. No serious side effects are reported but may cause vomiting and diarrhoea.

c. The Later Stage of Metabolic Syndrome

A complicated case of Avarana and Madhumeha. If Madhumeha not treated timely and properly, its complication likes developing carbuncles in vital parts and muscular area.

i. Upadrava of Avarana: Cardiac disease, Splenomegaly, Abscess, Tumour in Maha Srotasa and Diarrhea
ii. Treatment: If the patient facing difficulties due to avarana treated with Snigdha, Shroto shodhaka, Anabhishyandi, Vatanulomana and Kapha, pitta Aviruddha herbal medicine. It is long term treatment with a proper specialist in ayurvedic medicine.

4. Treatment for inulin resistant diabetes:

If a person with diabetes means decrease the capability in secretion of insulin in the body causes increased blood sugar levels. antihyperglycemic agent controls the blood sugar level but concerns all about the energy production which is caused by the insulin. So, the patients suffering from diabetes should take insulin as intravenous route only oral insulin tablets are failing to produce energy. To overcome this condition Maharshi Charaka wrote Charaka Samhita about diabetes

In detail include cause, signs and symptoms, treatment and maintenance.

According to Charaka Samhita, the cause of the disease is by the family background, laziness, lack of exercise are the primary reasons, excessive eating and over sleepy are the secondary reasons, and eating curd, milk products, fish, prawns, excessive eating of new rice, drinking rainwater, eating excessive jaggery sweets are other reasons to cause diabetes.

Treatment in Charaka Samhita

Aegle marmelos L., commonly known as bael, Bryophyllum pinnatum, also known as the air plant, Azadirachta indica, commonly known as neem, seeds of Gossypium herbaceum, commonly known as Levant cotton, Picrorhiza kurroa also known as kutki, seeds of Syzygium cumini, commonly known as Malabar plum most useful in treatment of diabetes.

a. Take 20gm of suvarna bhasma and rajitha bhasma added to a pot containing vanga bhasma, sisa bhasma, kantha bhasma 30gms each and rasa bhasma,abraka bhasma and pravala bhasma added 40 gms each then add cow milk, sugar cane and addasaramu (a liquid decoction) and levigate the mixture with elixirs of sandalwood, vetiver, kuruveru, turmeric. And juices of aratigadda and jasmine molle then Kasturi (musk deer) individually. It is best ayurvedic medicine written by Maharshi Charaka.
b. The bark of Erralodduga, thunga musthalu (cyperus rotundas), seeds of Chebulic myrobalan and *Gmelina Asiatica* L.(gummudu) are taken in equal quantity and made decoction with them and add Madhu(honey) before using the decoction.
c. Fruits of Malabar plum and Senna auriculata mixture are mixed well with the decoction made from the Ficus racemosa bark or root use twice in a day for diabetes and also control the excessive urination.

5. Treatment for Cancer

Cancer is an abnormal proliferation of cell growth; the metabolic outline observed in tumour cells often shows increased glucose and glutamine consumption, increased glycolysis rate, changes in the use of the metabolic enzymes, and secretion of lactate increased. Oncogenes and tumour suppressors are also discovered to have roles in cancer-associated changes in metabolism as well. The metabolic rate shifted to the equal to need of tumour cells reflect the rapid proliferative rate.

There are many treatments are available in modern medicine to fail to cure disease and scientists focused on the herbal medicine proved that plant-based medicines such as camptotheca, catharanthus, taxus species, nordihydroguaiaretic acid (Manda, G.et.al, 2020) and their derivatives exert therapeutic activity can control and cure the cancer ailment.

Herbal drugs used for cancer:

a. Take Vana Tulsi (Ocimum gratissimum) in 10 parts, Catharanthus roseus in 3parts are grounded well and add one ounce of Madhu two times in a day (early morning and before bed).
b. Gomutra (cow urine) 75ml two times a day, according to Charaka for collection of urine placed many conditions like should collect the urine between 10 pm to 4 am at first urination of cow, should collect at the middle of urination then subjected for the slight heating at low temperature along with the unboiled turmeric powder 5mg and filter for seven times under the cotton cloth store in a glass container can be used for 7 days when stored in a dark place at 25°C to prevent from the sunlight which causes increase the concentration of ammonia. The collected urine comes from a healthy cow and it should not be pregnant.
c. The bark of Tinospora cordifolia (neem tippa teeega) 5gms triturate along with the Azadirachta indica 100mg and soak the mixture in water for 12 hours then filter it. Take 5gm of aloe vera ground well and mixt with the filtered solution finally add one ounce of wheat gross elixir take one dose daily after three hours of Krishna Tulasi dose.
d. Take 2gm of Sheesham Leaves (Indian rosewood) (Dalbergia Sissoo), 200mg Ficus religiosa or sacred fig leaves, 200mg of garlic paste, 2 teaspoons of Cyperus Rotundus or Tunga Gaddalu leaves powder, 10mg of black pepper, 100mg of basil leaves powder to grind all of them until making into a paste and add drink along with juice or make a solid round pack then swallow. One dose daily subsequently after tippa teega dose mentioned earlier.
e. According to Charaka Samhita, continue this daily routine for 75days for curing any kind of cancer (metabolic disorder).
f. Food concern in the treatment is very high in the morning Sprawls and high fiber diet. In afternoon 250gms of cow curd along with 10mg of Krishna Tulasi along with vegetables and regular low quantity diet in the evening.

6. Treatment for Hypertension

Change in blood pressure is one of the cluster disorders from metabolic disorders.

a. Swarna suryavarthi rasa and Brihadhathre Chintamani rasa given along with yukthanupanam for one-day hypertension can be controlled.
b. Ginger, coriander and cumin as a cold decoction for 41 days.

c. Garlic with milk (10 drops of garlic with 1-ounce milk) use for 41 days along with blood pressure also cures paralysis.
d. Equal portions of levitated ginger and coriander one tablespoon dose three times a day control the blood pressure.

7. Treatment for Thyroid

The thyroid is an endocrine gland having butterfly shape located just above the caller's bone. Produces T_3, T_4 hormones regulate the body temperature, calorie consumption, heart rate, sweating and controls the digestive action according to herbal medicine technologies due to thyroid imbalance in body cause hyperthyroidism and hypothyroidism.

Hyperthyroidism is caused due to hyperactivity of thyroid gland results in excessive body heat, increased heart rate, accelerated pulse and hypermetabolic activity. signs and symptoms include Nervousness, irritability, sleeplessness, hyper excitement, difficulty in sitting quietly, rapid pulse, heart palpitations, low heat tolerance, flushed skin, increased appetite, weight loss, muscle fatigue and bulging eyes.

Treatment

Traditional herbal medicine used to treat hyperthyroidism by Lycopus spp-4parts, Leonurus cardiac – 2 parts, Scutellaria spp – 2 parts and crataegus spp – 1 part triturate make tp to 5ml dosage three times a day. If the patient also having insomnia Valeriana officinalis – 1part and passiflora incarnata – 1part made the 5-15ml tincture use it half an hour before sleep.

Hypothyroidism is caused due to the low activity of thyroid gland results slowdown in metabolism, fatigue, lack of energy, cold tolerance, severe constipation, heavy menstrual periods and weight gain. Slowed pulse, muscle aches, puffiness around the eyes, hair loss, sluggish reflexes and coarse skin.

Treatment

Hypothyroidism accelerates the development of atherosclerosis due to deposition of mucopolysaccharides in heart muscles further increase the coronary heart disease. A decoction of Ginkgo biloba, Allium sativum, crataegus spp in equal quantities used as cardiotonic for the hypothyroidism. Rumex Crispus, juglans cinerea herbs used to treat extreme constipation.

Humulus lupulus and Valeriana officinalis serve as neuro tonic mixture to treat the hypothyroidism. Artemisia vulgaris, Hypericum perforatum tinctures serve as antidepressant herbs Treatment for adrenal glands:

Adrenal glands are present on the top of each kidney deep in the back part of the abdomen. Each gland is organized to secrete different hormones place a crucial role in the homeostasis in the body regulate the alpha and beta receptors, peripheral resistance, facilitate the blood flow to brain, muscles and viscera, stimulate the transformation from glycogen to glucose, protein metabolism, maintain the mineral levels homeostasis. The disorder or improper function of adrenal glands accelerate the metabolic disorders

Treatment

Adrenal medulla: Siberian ginseng and other ginseng show a direct effect on the adrenal medulla and also serve as a nerve tonic. Other herbal medicines like ginseng, ashwagandha, skullcap, oats support and cure the disorder in the adrenal medulla.

Adrenal Cortex: Saponins containing species like Glycyrrhiza glabra (liquorice), wild yam (Dioscorea villosa) herbal medicine support and cure the adrenal cortex, regulate the rennin angiotensin system, electrolyte balance, regulate the urine volume.

DETECTION OF ADVERSE REACTIONS BY AYURVEDIC MEDICINES

A study was conducted on the 49-year-old man shows improved cognitive abilities after received therapy by Ginkgo biloba with a dose of 40 milligrams three times per day for 14 days but complained about the palpitations within the mouth and frequent ventricular premature sinus rhythm observed (Cianfrocca, C., et; al, 2002). The condition resolved after withdrawal of treatment. In 2011 allergic reactions in paediatric patients after inhaling the American ginseng reported (Erdle, S. C., et.al, 2018). Curcumin; an herbal medicine in turmeric was also reported to cause skin allergies (Chaudhari, S. P., et.al, 2015). Even though the severity of adverse effects was low when compared to the allopathic medicine the Detection of adverse reactions in herbal medicines is a major challenge. Accurate identification and monitoring of adverse reactions are not covered in herbal medicine technologies. So, the Methods related to study the herbal drugs safety problems not evolved adequately in any of the system (Ekor M., 2014). Even though the complete information related to herbal medicines exists in the stanzas of ancient treatises, which is not easily accessible to the modern world, confounding factors such as collecting reports in quality assurance and control in the manufacture of ayurvedic medicine for diagnosing the adverse reactions (Thatte, U., & Bhalerao, S., 2008). The informal manufacturing and selling herbal medicine on the local market in a small-scale is huge making it impossible to identify the adverse reactions of herbal medicine.

ASSESSMENT OF ADVERSE REACTIONS TO HERBAL MEDICINES

Causality assessment available for several scales, but when it comes to ayurvedic medicine is become a challenge for several reasons includes: The information of adverse effects is of herbal medicine is not in electronic form making difficult to access (Shetti, S., 2011). Most of the Ayurvedic formulations are multi-ingredient-fixed dose formulations rarely prescribed alone with multiple herbs and minerals not easy to predict and access the Pharmacokinetics and toxicokinetics (Thatte, U., & Bhalerao, S., 2008) (Shetti, S., 2011). There is no objective evidence reported on the adverse events of herbal medicine, dose-related responses are hardly measured and described. The causality analysis with ayurvedic medicines becomes most challenging aspects in performing. The person should be trained in both Ayurveda and pharmacovigilance to perform the casualty assessment (Thatte, U., & Bhalerao, S., 2008).

PREVENTION OF ADVERSE REACTIONS TO AYURVEDIC MEDICINES

The raised issue with veneration to herbal medicine is increasing reports on Adverse Drug Reagents this may be due to the increase in several people taking herbal products either as a medicine or as a nutritional supplemented. Such reports many times failed to identify the exact cause behind such events. Hence, the need for Pharmacovigilance implementation in herbal medicine technologies increased to make the system more scientific. The Pharmacovigilance is a ability to prevent the further adverse effects successfully by understanding the information collected, even though with collected data it is difficult to assess due to challenges faced at multiple levels (Suke, S. G., 2015). The difficulty in obtaining the herbal drug data of formulations, patients are aware of the adverse effects caused by herbal medicines and most importantly Communication between practitioners and policymakers of modern medicine and traditional medicine is not adequate (Ekor M. 2014) (Benzie, I. F. F.,2011).

As a matter of concern related to herbal medicine, the preventive measures would be the same when compared with the allopathic medicine because even though the treatment systems are different but treaties have remained the same include concern on administration, knowledge of the inappropriate drug, the examination of the patient, disease before prescription and prescription of expired medicines.

CONCLUSION

Undoubtedly, modern medicine assessed scientifically proved to provide overwhelming symptomatic relief. However, in long term treatment required disorders such as metabolic disorders like diabetes, thyroidal and obesity idiosyncrasy and dose-related toxicity are major obstacles Under these circumstances, WHO focused on the potential of herbal medicines converted into real-life treatment constituting an effective herbal-modern medicine interface. “Herbal medicine is natural and safe” and “modern medicine is harmful” according to embedded perceptions. Western medicine is tremendously strong in emergency clinical situations not in the long term run like endocrine and metabolic disorders. herbal medicine can’t use officially until 2004 new regulations are framed for herbal medicine treatment, to enter into the commercial market herbal drug should prove its efficacy and safety-related properties. Researchers focused on to create an evidence base for herbal medicine to know the exact statistics involved under curing the elements. Herbal drug development searches unique approaches like reverse pharmacology to create the new drug moieties. Reverse pharmacology selects the herbs already used in the traditional medicinal treatment and evaluated during exploratory clinical studies. Experimental studies can be carried to conclude analytical explanations for clinical activity. It would be difficult, but not impossible to provide incontestable confirmation to herbal medicine system. Due to its long term history reports on usage in several diseases, herbal medicines have the potential to use in long-term treatment. In a scientific context, however, critical questions raise about the standardization and clinical indications of herbals need to be answered through modern technical experiments and clinical trial studies. New standards need essential describing and testing methods, so both the systems used in parallel or tandem bypassing early stages of predictable western medicine models of drug discovery and development, the reverse pharmacology approach can straightforwardly test herbal medicines in controlled clinical trial situations, resulting in savings in time and money.

ACKNOWLEDGMENT

I would like to express my deep gratitude to Professor M. Sarangapani $_{\text{PhD, PGDBM,}}$ UCPSc, Kakatiya University and Professor G. Achaiah $_{\text{PhD,PDF,}}$ Principal, UCPSc, Kakatiya University for the patient guidance, enthusiastic encouragement and useful critiques of writing this chapter. I would also like to thank Dr Munija, vice-principal, Ms. ch. Manasa for their advice and assistance in keeping my progress on schedule.

I would also like to extend my thanks to the vision college of pharmaceutical sciences and research, pharmacy department for their help in offering me the resources in running the program.Finally, I wish to thank my parents for their support and encouragement throughout my study.

REFERENCES

Atanasov, A. G., Waltenberger, B., Pferschy-Wenzig, E. M., Linder, T., Wawrosch, C., Uhrin, P., Temml, V., Wang, L., Schwaiger, S., Heiss, E. H., Rollinger, J. M., Schuster, D., Breuss, J. M., Bochkov, V., Mihovilovic, M. D., Kopp, B., Bauer, R., Dirsch, V. M., & Stuppner, H. (2015). Discovery and resupply of pharmacologically active plant-derived natural products: A review. *Biotechnology Advances, 33*(8), 1582–1614. doi:10.1016/j.biotechadv.2015.08.001

Basisht, G. (2014). Exploring insights towards definition and laws of health in Ayurveda: Global health perspective. *Ayu, 35*(4), 351–355. doi:10.4103/0974-8520.158975

Bensoussan, A., & Lewith, G. T. (2004). Complementary medicine research in Australia: A strategy for the future. *The Medical Journal of Australia, 181*(6), 331–333. doi:10.5694/j.1326-5377.2004.tb06303.x

Benzie, I. F., & Wachtel-Galor, S. (Eds.). (2011). *Herbal medicine: biomolecular and clinical aspects.* CRC Press. doi:10.1201/b10787

Chaudhari, S. P., Tam, A. Y., & Barr, J. A. (2015). Curcumin: A contact allergen. *The Journal of Clinical and Aesthetic Dermatology, 8*(11), 43.

Chauhan, A., Semwal, D. K., Mishra, S. P., & Semwal, R. B. (2017). Ayurvedic concept of Shatkriyakala: Traditional knowledge of cancer pathogenesis and therapy. *Journal of Integrative Medicine, 15*(2), 88–94. doi:10.1016/S2095-4964(17)60311-X

Cianfrocca, C., Pelliccia, F., Auriti, A., & Santini, M. (2002). Ginkgo biloba-induced frequent ventricular arrhythmia. *Italian Heart Journal, 3*, 689–691.

Ekor, M. (2014). The growing use of herbal medicines: Issues relating to adverse reactions and challenges in monitoring safety. *Frontiers in Pharmacology, 4*, 177. doi:10.3389/fphar.2013.00177

Erdle, S. C., Chan, E. S., Yang, H., Vallance, B. A., Mill, C., & Wong, T. (2018). First-reported pediatric cases of American ginseng anaphylaxis and allergy. *Allergy, Asthma, and Clinical Immunology: Official Journal of the Canadian Society of Allergy and Clinical Immunology, 14*(1), 1–3.

Felizola, S. J. (2015). Ursolic acid in experimental models and human subjects: Potential as an anti-obesity/overweight treatment. *Cancer, 1*, 2.

Fokunang, C. N., Ndikum, V., Tabi, O. Y., Jiofack, R. B., Ngameni, B., Guedje, N. M., Tembe-Fokunang, E. A., Tomkins, P., Barkwan, S., Kechia, F., Asongalem, E., Ngoupayou, J., Torimiro, N. J., Gonsu, K. H., Sielinou, V., Ngadjui, B. T., Angwafor, F., 3rd, Nkongmeneck, A., Abena, O. M., Ngogang, J., … Kamsu-Kom. (2011). Traditional medicine: past, present and future research and development prospects and integration in the National Health System of Cameroon. *African Journal of Traditional, Complementary, and Alternative Medicines: AJTCAM, 8*(3), 284–295.

Ford, E. S., Ajani, U. A., & Mokdad, A. H. (2005). The metabolic syndrome and concentrations of C-reactive protein among US youth. *Diabetes Care, 28*(4), 878–881. doi:10.2337/diacare.28.4.878

Ghavi, F., Taghizadeh, M., Taebi, M., & Abdolahian, S. (2019). Effect of Foeniculum vulgare essence on symptoms of polycystic ovarian syndrome (PCOS): A randomized double-blind, Placebo-Controlled Trial. *Journal of Herbal Medicine, 17*, 100277. doi:10.1016/j.hermed.2019.100277

Gregory, J. W. (2019). Prevention of Obesity and Metabolic Syndrome in Children. *Frontiers in Endocrinology, 10*, 669. doi:10.3389/fendo.2019.00669

Gurib-Fakim, A. (2006). Medicinal plants: Traditions of yesterday and drugs of tomorrow. *Molecular Aspects of Medicine, 27*(1), 1–93. doi:10.1016/j.mam.2005.07.008

Hajian-Tilaki, K., & Heidari, B. (2013). A Comparison between International Obesity Task Force and Center for Disease Control References in Assessment of Overweight and Obesity Among Adolescents in Babol, Northern Iran. *International Journal of Preventive Medicine, 4*(2), 226–232.

Hussain, K., Majeed, M. T., Ismail, Z., Sadikun, A., & Ibrahim, P. (2009). Traditional and complementary medicines: Quality assessment strategies and safe usage. *Southern Med Review, 2*(1), 19–23.

Jachak, S. M., & Saklani, A. (2007). Challenges and opportunities in drug discovery from plants. *Current Science*, 1251–1257.

Kaur, J. (2014). A comprehensive review of metabolic syndrome. *Cardiology Research and Practice, 2014*, 943162. doi:10.1155/2014/943162

Liu, Y., & Wang, M. W. (2008). Botanical drugs: challenges and opportunities: contribution to Linnaeus Memorial Symposium 2007. *Life Sciences, 82*(9-10), 445–449. doi:10.1016/j.lfs.2007.11.007

Liu, Y., Weng, W., Gao, R., & Liu, Y. (2019). New Insights for Cellular and Molecular Mechanisms of Aging and Aging-Related Diseases: Herbal Medicine as Potential Therapeutic Approach. *Oxidative Medicine and Cellular Longevity, 2019*, 1–25. doi:10.1155/2019/4598167

Manda, G., Rojo, A. I., Martínez-Klimova, E., Pedraza-Chaverri, J., & Cuadrado, A. (2020). Nordihydroguaiaretic Acid: From Herbal Medicine to Clinical Development for Cancer and Chronic Diseases. *Frontiers in Pharmacology, 11*, 151. doi:10.3389/fphar.2020.00151

Mukherjee, P. K., Venkatesh, P., & Ponnusankar, S. (2010). Ethnopharmacology and integrative medicine - Let the history tell the future. *Journal of Ayurveda and Integrative Medicine, 1*(2), 100–109. doi:10.4103/0975-9476.65077

Newman, D. J., & Cragg, G. M. (2016). Natural products as sources of new drugs from 1981 to 2014. *Journal of Natural Products, 79*(3), 629–661. doi:10.1021/acs.jnatprod.5b01055

Pandey, M. M., Rastogi, S., & Rawat, A. K. S. (2013). Indian traditional ayurvedic system of medicine and nutritional supplementation. *Evidence-Based Complementary and Alternative Medicine, 2013*, 2013. doi:10.1155/2013/376327

Patwardhan, B., Warude, D., Pushpangadan, P., & Bhatt, N. (2005). Ayurveda and traditional Chinese medicine: A comparative overview. *Evidence-Based Complementary and Alternative Medicine*, *2*(4), 465–473. doi:10.1093/ecam/neh140

Payab, M., Hasani-Ranjbar, S., Shahbal, N., Qorbani, M., Aletaha, A., Haghi-Aminjan, H., & Abdollahi, M. (2020). Effect of the herbal medicines in obesity and metabolic syndrome: A systematic review and meta-analysis of clinical trials. *Phytotherapy Research*, *34*(3), 526–545. doi:10.1002/ptr.6547

Petrovska, B. B. (2012). Historical review of medicinal plants' usage. *Pharmacognosy Reviews*, *6*(11), 1. doi:10.4103/0973-7847.95849

Pugsley, M. K., Authier, S., & Curtis, M. J. (2008). Principles of safety pharmacology. *British Journal of Pharmacology*, *154*(7), 1382–1399. doi:10.1038/bjp.2008.280

RH, R. U. (2015). Traditional herbal medicine, pharmacognosy, and pharmacopoeial standards: a discussion at the crossroads. In Evidence-Based Validation of Herbal Medicine (pp. 45-85). Academic Press.

Schulz, V., Hänsel, R., & Tyler, V. E. (2001). *Rational phytotherapy: a physician's guide to herbal medicine*. Psychology Press. doi:10.1007/978-3-642-98093-0

Sen, S., Chakraborty, R., & De, B. (2011). Challenges and opportunities in the advancement of herbal medicine: India's position and role in a global context. *Journal of Herbal Medicine*, *1*(3-4), 67–75. doi:10.1016/j.hermed.2011.11.001

Sheng-Ji, P. (2001). Ethnobotanical approaches of traditional medicine studies: some experiences from Asia. *Pharmaceutical Biology, 39*(sup1), 74-79.

Shetti, S., Kumar, C. D., Sriwastava, N. K., & Sharma, I. P. (2011). Pharmacovigilance of herbal medicines: Current state and future directions. *Pharmacognosy Magazine*, *7*(25), 69. doi:10.4103/0973-1296.75905

Suke, S. G., Kosta, P., & Negi, H. (2015). Role of Pharmacovigilance in India: An overview. *Online Journal of Public Health Informatics*, *7*(2), e223. doi:10.5210/ojphi.v7i2.5595

Thatte, U., & Bhalerao, S. (2008). Pharmacovigilance of ayurvedic medicines in India. *Indian Journal of Pharmacology*, *40*(Suppl 1), S10–S12.

Vaidya, A. D., & Devasagayam, T. P. (2007). Current status of herbal drugs in India: An overview. *Journal of Clinical Biochemistry and Nutrition*, *41*(1), 1–11. doi:10.3164/jcbn.2007001

Voigt, K. (2006). Our look at global burgeoning Asian herbal industry. *The Wall Street Journal, 6*(11), 2006.

Zamiska, N. (2007). Dueling Therapies-Is a Shotgun Better Than a Silver Bullet? *Wall Street Journal,* p. B1.

ADDITIONAL READING

Bird, G., Press, C., Dc, R., & Autism, J. (2011). Ayurveda and Metabolic Diseases: The Whole is Greater than the Sum of the PartsAyurveda and Metabolic Diseases: The Whole is Greater than the Sum of the Parts. *Journal of Autism and Developmental Disorders*, 8–10.

Liu, Y., & Wang, M. W. (2008). Botanical drugs: Challenges and opportunities. Contribution to Linnaeus Memorial Symposium 2007. *Life Sciences*, *82*(9–10), 445–449. doi:10.1016/j.lfs.2007.11.007

KEY TERMS AND DEFINITIONS

Cancer: Growth of abnormal cells in the body from uncontrolled cell division.

Glucose Intolerance: Metabolic conditions result in higher blood glucose than normal blood glucose levels.

Herbal Medicine: Describes as an alternative and pseudoscientific medicine used for promoting health by using unpurified plant extracts.

Insulin Resistance: Inability caused in fat, muscles, and liver don't respond well to insulin thereby glucose in the blood failed to use for energy production.

Metabolic Syndrome: The disorders at metabolic state in the organism caused by genes and other lifestyle issues.

Obesity: Excess body fat has accumulated in the body to the extent that it may harm health. According to WHO, when body mass index (BMI) higher than 30% then considered as obesity.

Pharmacovigilance: A science relating to the collection, detection, assessment, monitoring, and prevention of adverse effects through pharmaceutical products.

Thyroidism: Imbalance in the production of thyroid hormone from the thyroid gland.

Chapter 11
Herbal Medicines for Thyroid Diseases

Bhawana Singh
Banaras Hindu University, India

Shyam Sundar
Institute of Medical Sciences, Banaras Hindu University, India

Ashish Shukla
Institute of Medical Sciences, Banaras Hindu University, India

ABSTRACT

Thyroid dysfunctions represent the most common endocrine disorders and a major healthcare issue throughout the globe. The drawbacks associated with the conventional treatment approaches calls upon for the need to explore alternative treatment strategies. Herbal medicinal approach has been used since ages; however, it is not acceptable by the clinicians. Currently, there is no scientific evidence for the efficacy of herbal medicines in patient management. The necessity to fight against adverse drug events, high treatment costs, and compliance issues is forcing the scientists to look upon for traditional herbal medicinal approaches. This chapter provides an overview of the efficacy of different herbal medicines and scientific evidence that necessitates their usage for improving thyroid functions. There remains a need for a careful and routine follow-up as a mandatory parameter before establishing herbal medicine as a global treatment approach.

BACKGROUND

The endocrine system is the network of glands that regulates several vital functions of the human body ranging from regulation of heart beat to reproduction. It consists of ten glands including the thyroid gland, adrenal gland, hypothalamus, islet cells of pancreas, pituitary gland, parathyroid gland, thymus, pineal gland, ovaries and testis. Even a slight hiccup can perturb the delicate balance of these glands leading to endocrine disorders that manifests in various forms. Usually these disorders have been characterized-

DOI: 10.4018/978-1-7998-4808-0.ch011

depending upon the amount of hormone (too much or too scanty) produced by these glands; secondly, depending upon the development of lesions/tumors in the endocrine system that may/may not affect hormone levels; thirdly, infection and fourthly, failure of gland to stimulate another. The imbalances in the hormone levels are kept in check by the feedback system, however, anomalous feedback system possess threat for managing the levels of hormones in the blood thus, leading to the development of disease that manifests depending upon the gland in question.

Thyroid gland constitutes an important component of endocrine system that regulates several physiological functions ranging from oxygen utilization, growth, development to cellular metabolism. The gland is located at the front of neck; secretes thyroxine (T4) and tri-iodothyronine (T3) that travels through the blood stream to orchestrate the basal metabolic rates, growth and development. Thyroid disorders symptoms ranges from tiredness, depression, constipation, abnormal weight gain/loss, sensitivity to cold temperature, brachycardia/tachycardia, tremors, diarrhea, irritability, anxiety, insomnia etc. Thyroid disorder is amongst the major and most common health disorders that affects the global community, with an estimate of 42 million cases in India (Unnikrishnan & Menon, 2011). According to projections of American Thyroid Association (ATA) more than 12 percent of Americans develop thyroid diseases during their life time. With an approximate number of 20 million thyroid cases; the female population possesses five to eight times higher risk of disease development than males(Sabra & Di Cristofano, 2019). There remains a growing concern for managing the thyroid diseases due to its increasing prevalence.

It has long been known that thyroid functions can be modulated by natural (present in water or foodstuffs) and/or synthetic (in medicines) compounds. Such compounds affecting the thyroid homeostasis are termed as the thyroid disruptors that exert their effect on either hormone synthesis, metabolism, signaling, transport and/or tumorigenesis that may trigger autoimmune process. Disease management involves the hormone replacement therapy, iodine therapy, surgery and/or anti-thyroid therapy depending upon the form of disorder. The available treatment approaches possess certain side effects including the muscular weakness, loss of appetite, hair fall etc.(Sabra & Di Cristofano, 2019). Furthermore, certain medications affect the thyroid functions while others may worsen the symptoms of hypo-/hyper-thyroidism; these issues call upon for organized patient care approach. These days research for alternative medicinal approach, with minimal side effects has gained momentum. This chapter gains an insight into the various thyroid dysfunctions, herbal medicinal approach and their mode of action for managing thyroid disorders.

VARIOUS THYROID DYSFUNCTIONS

Iodine deficiency has been considered as the most common cause of thyroid diseases throughout the world. Further there are significant evidences for the involvement of environmental factors that potentiates the risk for thyroid disorders. As discussed previously, there are several mechanisms in which thyroid functions are perturbed; pesticides, fungicides and insecticides have endocrine disruptors which directly hampers the thyroid functions by inhibiting the iodine uptake, interfering with receptor signaling, enzymes, gene expressions and transport proteins. Depending upon the different anomalies of thyroid functioning the thyroid dysfunctions can be broadly categorized into- goiter, hypothyroidism, hyperthyroidism (Grave's disease), thyroid cancer, thyroid nodules, thyroiditis (Hashimoto's thyroiditis) and thyroid hormone resistance. The disease management has been pretty straightforward however, inappropriate treatment, misdiagnosis, overdiagnosis sometimes possess the obstacle for disease management practices.

Goiter is an abnormal painless enlargement of thyroid gland which causes difficulty in breathing and swallowing. The disease manifests due to lack of iodine in diet, however, not all form of goiter manifests symptoms (tightness in throat, swelling in lower neck, coughing, hoarseness, difficulty in swallowing and breathing). It can be temporary problem which resolves without medical intervention or can be indication of chronic thyroid condition that needs medical attention. The enlargement of thyroid is generally associated with many thyroid diseases, increased signaling through TSH (thyroid stimulating hormone) receptors causes production of thyroid hormone which eventually increases the vascularity and thyroid hypertrophy (Stephen & Gary, 2014).Goiter does not represent a single medical condition instead it can be an indicator of autoimmune disorders.It also results from hypothyroidism, hyperthyroidism, Hashimoto's thyroiditis, cyanide poisoning, Grave's disease, goitrogen ingestion, thyroid hormone insensitivity, adverse drug reaction, thyroid neoplasm, acromegaly, thyroiditis etc.

Hypothyroidism, also termed as the underactive thyroid disease; thyroid gland does not produce enough thyroid hormones (T3 and T4). Since, thyroid hormone regulates the metabolism that exerts direct effect on heartbeat and body's temperature; in the absence of thyroid hormone metabolism slows down and reduces the ability of thyroid gland to produce the hormone. This leads to different manifestation of disease in the form of anxiety, depression, dry skin, brittle hair, fatigue, puffy face, edematous eyelids, greater sensitivity to cold temperature. Standard treatment option includes the daily medication of levothyroxine, that restores the hormone levels however, long term treatment is associated with decreased cholesterol levels and weight loss.

Hyperthyroidism is also termed as the overactive thyroid disease and often used synonymously to thyrotoxicosis, a medical condition with thyroid hormone excess.This form of disease is less common than the hypothyroidism. Usually the disease is the result of secondary manifestation to grave's disease, toxic multinodular goiter and toxic adenomas. Hyperthyroidism is characterized by exopthalmia, irritability, fatigue, increased basal metabolic rates (BMR), hyperactivity, dysphoria, tachycardia, weight loss, hyperactivity, increased appetite, diarrhea, polyuria and tremors (Association et al., 2011). Symptomatic treatment option for hyperthyroidism includes anti-thyroid drugs (methimazole, propylthiouracil), immediate relief with beta-blockers (propranolol, atenolol, metoprolol), radioactive iodine therapy and surgery. Anti-thyroid drugs suppress the WBCs production from the bone marrow (agranulocytosis), fever, sore throat and many infections, while, long term use of drug induces disease remission that calls for surgery. Although beta blockers nullify the effect of thyroid hormone and increases metabolism but do not alter the level of thyroid hormone and fails to treat patient depending on varying underlying causes of hyperthyroidism.

Thyroid nodules (benign) and cancer (malignant) are also termed as the colloid nodules, cysts, nodular thyroiditis; present in 5 percent of the population. These are solid or fluid filled lumps in the thyroid. Usually, it is not severe (only 1 percent of nodules are cancerous) and does not present symptoms but occasionally, they can be felt at the base of the neck and can cause shortness of breath and difficulty in swallowing. Upon confirmation of the benign nature of the nodule by thyroid nodule biopsy, observation is the most apt management practice. It includes routine thyroid blood tests, ultrasound and physical examination. Some nodules do not change over period of years thus, never require any treatment while, some nodules increase in size that needs other interventions as the surgery, ionizing radiation and sometimes thyroid hormone therapy (28191095).

According to National Cancer Institute (USA), each year there are 56,000 new thyroid cancer cases; with risk population of the females (risk ratio of 3:1 for Female: Male). The disease manifests aggressively in older population with approximately 1.2 percent of population that encounters thyroid cancer in their life time. The disease manifests without any obvious symptoms and present commonly with lump in the neck and voice hoarseness (less common). Although 75 percent of population has thyroid nodules, mostly it remains benign; however, the risk of the development of the thyroid cancer is higher in adolescents and children as compared to the adults. By the age of 80, approximately 90 percent population develops atleast one thyroid nodule(Haugen et al., 2016; Hegedus, Bonnema, & Bennedbaek, 2003).

Thyroid cancer can be categorized into four types: papillary and/or mixed papillary/follicular thyroid cancer (most common, incidence rate: 85 percent), follicular and/or hurthle cell thyroid cancer (incidence rate: approx. 10 percent), medullary thyroid cancer (incidence rate: approx. 3 percent), anaplastic thyroid cancer (incidence rate: approx.1percent). Upon thorough examination with high-resolution ultrasound for the benign/ malignant nature of the thyroid nodule/cancer, entire/partial surgical removal of thyroid gland is planned. In medullary cases, lymph nodes are removed while, in anaplastic thyroid cancer cases, tracheostomy is the treatment option. Upon surgical removal, patients are treated with personalized radioactive iodine and thyroid hormone pill (levothyroxine) for entire life (Hoang, 2010).

Hashimoto's thyroiditis is also termed as chronic lymphocytic thyroiditis, autoimmune thyroiditis, is the most common cause of hypothyroidism in USA. It is an autoimmune disease where body's immune system attacks its own cells and organs by producing anti-thyroid antibodies. Antibodies directly target the thyroid and damage the organ eventually causing inflammation and hypothyroidism. As the disease progresses thyroid gland enlarges and over the course of time the symptoms manifests as fatigue, weight gain, joint stiffness, constipation, sensitivity to cold temperature, puffy face/eyes, hair thinning, irregular menstrual cycle, brachycardia and difficulty in focusing. The disease is prevalent in females, commonly affects the age group of 30-50 years and in person with other auto immune diseases (B12 deficiency, gluten sensitivity, rheumatoid arthritis, diabetes, lupus and Addison's disease).

Not all hypothyroidism cases have Hashimoto's disease, if the disease manifests with hypothyroidism then levo-thyroxine therapy is known to restore normal thyroid functions(Pyzik, Grywalska, Matyjaszek-Matuszek, & Rolinski, 2015). Additionally, it is recommended for patient to undergo routine blood check-up for thyroid levels.

Reduced sensitivity to thyroid hormone is the impairment of the sensitivity to thyroid hormone due to decreased tissue sensitivity to thyroid hormone (or thyroid hormone resistance). This can be attributed to the germline mutation in the thyroid hormone receptor beta (THRB) gene, that eventually reduces the binding affinity for the thyroid hormone. Thus, serum TSH level are not altered despite the elevated levels of thyroid hormones (Dumitrescu & Refetoff, 2013; Sakurai et al., 1989; Weiss, Weinberg, & Refetoff, 1993). Common manifestation of the disorder includes goiter, hyperactive behavior, learning disability and sinus tachycardia however, the symptoms varies from patient to patient. The treatment involves the use of atenolol (β-adrenergic blocker) that relieves the sinus tachycardia and improves the symptoms related to hyperactivity. However, some frame shift mutation prevent the action of β-blockers(S. Y. Wu et al., 2006).Thyroid hormone cell membrane transporter defect is another major cause of thyroid hormone resistance. X-linked monocarboxylate transporter8 (MCT-8) has been the thyroid hormone (TH) transporter, mutation in the transporter leads to neurological complications. Further problems manifests in the form of truncal hypotonia, dystonia, flaccidity to limb rigidity that leads to spastic quadriplegia in later stages(Holden et al., 2005; Visser et al., 2009). Treatment option for MCT8 mutation have not been much explored, current strategy relies on the supportive measures by the use of braces to prevent the mal-position contractures. Dystonia can be improved with anticholinergics, L-DOPA, carbamazepine and lioresol, however, the treatment evidences have been established only with few cases. TH metabolism is also regulated by the selenoprotein iodothyronine deiodinases (Ds) thus any defect in the TH metabolism due to defective selenocysteine binding protein (SBP2) gene that affects the selenoprotein synthesis (including the Ds) led to poor growth, impaired mental and motor coordination, congenital myopathy (Azevedo et al., 2010).The growth abnormality due to reduced T3 generation can be managed by treating with L-T3(Di Cosmo et al., 2009). Selenomethionine administration has also been recommended for normalizing the level of selenium but unfortunately it has not shown efficacy in reverting the TH metabolic dysfunctions(Schomburg et al., 2009).

In summary, there are various thyroid dysfunctions which affect the mankind and the current treatment options have not been satisfactory since they suffer from one or the other limitations. These issues call upon for research for alternative treatment strategies, herbal approach (or phytomedicine) possesses minimal side effects and holds hopes for treatment of thyroid cases. Therefore, the bench side to bedside application of herbal formulations needs more attention.

HERBAL MEDICATION AND THYROID DISORDERS

Complementary and alternative medicine (CAM) has been defined as the branch of medicine that has not been certified as the standard care regimen for disease management. According to NIH, as the name implies, complementary medicine can be used along with standard medical treatment while, alternative medicine can be used to replace the standard treatment regimen. Phytomedicine (or herbal medicinal approach) is one of the different categories of CAM approaches which has recently gained scientific attention due to emerging scientific evidences for their biological potency against different diseases.

The need to use herbal medicinal approach for management of thyroid diseases emerged because this approach potentially helps in coping with the side effects of the existing chemotherapeutics and treatment options. It also helps in curing the disease alone and/or in combination with standard treatment regimen. This approach eases the stress and anxiety of medication and its related complications. Although diagnosis of thyroid disorders forces the individuals for standard treatment options initially however, they do not want to stick to it for life time thus, herbal approach provides economical, natural and minimal side effect-based treatment approach for disease management. Figure 1 provides a glimpse of different thyroid disorders and utility of herbal medication over conventional therapeutics.

In stark contrast to the synthetic drugs and/or thyroid hormone replacement therapy, herbal medicinal approach provides pharmacological option that helps to control the inflammation and autoimmune triggers. Herbal approach of thyroid dysfunction treatment involves the careful monitoring of the environmental and lifestyle factors contributing towards the disease and combating the disease using the herbal medication in combination with the diet, nutrient supplementation as well as conventional therapeutics. In this context we have tried to explore the different herbal treatment options and their benefits for thyroid disorders.

1. Herbal Medicines for Goiter

Iodine supplementation has been age-old prophylactic and therapeutic option for goiter however, the risks of development of cancer in long run, hypothyroidism, Grave's disease, limitations associated with iodine administration and restricted proximity made the herbal medicinal approach the choice for treatment. Traditional herbal medicinal approach has been extensively applied in management of thyroid disorder especially goiter due to their minimal side effects. Herbal medicines reinvigorate blood circula-

Figure 1. Representative illustration of different thyroid dysfunction, conventional disease management approaches and their side effects as compared to the herbal medicinal approach

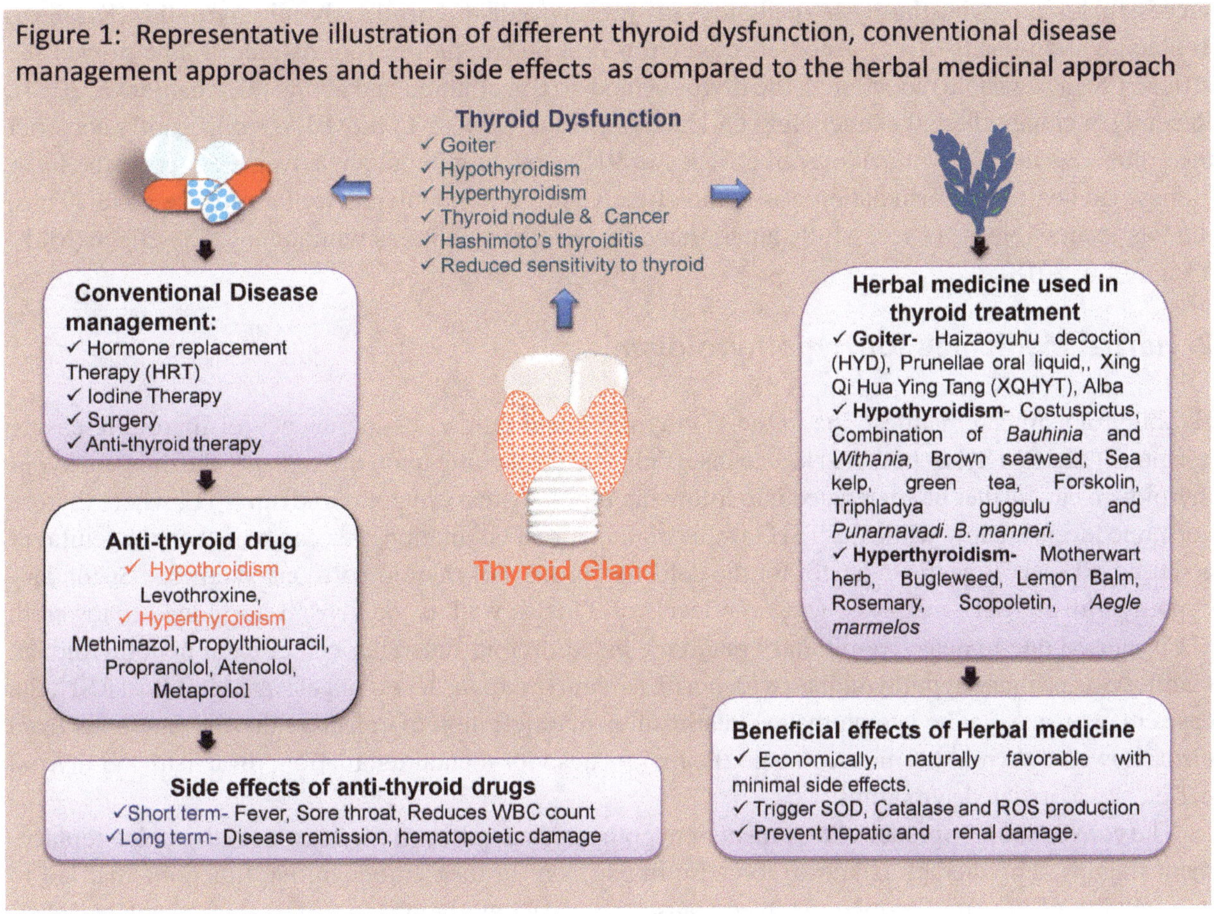

tion, eliminate the phelegm, soften and resolve the masses (Y. Zhang et al., 2016). Chinese traditional herbal medicine haizaoyuhu decoction (HYD) has been used for treating goiter since 500 years. The basic composition of the formulation was traced to be consisting of *Thallus Sargassi Pallidi, Thallus Laminariae Japonicae, RhizomaPinelliae Preparata, Bulbus Fritillariae Thunbergii, Pericarpium Citrus reticulata, RadixAngelicae Sinensis, Pericarpium Citri reticulata, Rhizoma Chan xiong, RadixAngelicae Pubescentis*, *Frutus Forsythiae Suspensae* and *Radix Glycyrrhiza* (Liu, Zhong, & Liu, 2015) . Iodine richness of the drug makes it top choice for treating 90 percent cases with iodine- deficiency without any side effects (Xiu et al., 2017). HYD has shown to trigger reactive oxygen species (ROS) production, decreases lipid peroxidation in thyroid therefore, it also protects against excess iodine induced organ damage (Poncin et al., 2008; Xiu et al., 2017).

The clinical effects of Prunellae oral liquid (POL) in combination with the conventional anti-thyroid medicine was superior in improving the thyroid functions and treating goiter as compared to the anti-thyroid medicine alone(K. Yang, Guo, & Wu, 2007).The high prevalence of thyroid disorders across the globe can be attributed to the iodine and selenium deficit. A herbal preparation of Alba was used in Ukrainian population where the treatment markedly reduced the thyroid volume and regained its normal function. The preparation significantly improved the TSH levels in short span of treatment and reduced the duration of treatment for thyrotoxicosis. In addition to its efficacy in goiter, this treatment was also successful for improving the thyroid pathology in hyperthyroidism as well as chronic thyroiditis (Kiseleva, Teplaia, & Kaminskii, 2012). Another research of oral preparation of root extract of alba proved the efficacy seen as visible reduction in the thyroid gland size in children and adults (Turchaninova, 2014). Recently, a chinese herbal extract Xing Qi Hua Ying Tang (XQHYT) proved to significantly constrict the goiter size in cases with an overall efficacy of 91.2 percent without any adverse effect on the liver, kidney and heart. The formulation was found effective for multinodular as well as diffuse goiter. Thus, the therapeutic regimen successfully ameliorated the disease symptoms without any side effects(M. L. Yang & Lu, 2018).

2. Herbal Medicines for Hypothyroidism

Hypothyroidism can manifest due to the (1) thyroid gland failure; (2) deficiency of thyroid releasing hormone (TRH), TSH or both; (3) iodine insufficiency. Depending upon the cause of the disease, hypothyroidism can further be segregated into following types: Primary hypothyroidism (PH), where thyroid hormone levels are low while the TSH level is high in blood circulation, this can be either congenital or acquired. PH serves as the indicator for the defective process of thyroid hormone synthesis. Secondary hypothyroidism (SH), manifests when the levels of TSH as well as the thyroid hormone are lowered. SH is caused due to defective pituitary gland mediated thyroid functions. Subclinical hypothyroidism manifests as primary hypothyroidism with normal serum thyroxine levels but elevated levels of TSH, the cases may or may not be symptomatic.Creatinism is manifestation of defective thyroid functions from birth. Lowered thyroid hormones remain the major cause for mental retardation, dwarfism and thyroid deficiency associated symptoms.

The conventional approach of treatment of hypothyroidism relies on the use of levothyroxine replacement therapy. The therapy is known to cause impairment in the neurocognitive functions that led to poor quality of life and life-long treatment causes poor patient compliance. Herbal approach and their bioactive constituents came up as suitable alternative for hypothyroidism. In this context, *Costuspictus* belonging to the family *Costaceae,* also termed as the insulin plant because of its utility for diabetes management has shown potential application for alleviating hypothyroidism. The concoction restores the normal thyroid levels and improved the thyroid profile. The formulation also known to abrogate inflammation, suppressed tissue oxidative stress, prevented hepatic and renal damage due to thyroid insufficiency (Ashwini, Bobby, Sridhar, & Cleetus, 2017).

Adaptogen based approach plays vital role in regulating various metabolic processes, counteract catabolic processes and increases oxygen consumption. Conversely, adaptogens have also shown potential effects in improving fatigue and debility. In subclinical hypothyroidism *Withania somnifera* (Ashwangandha), a conventional herbal medicine in Indian Ayurveda has shown potential in improving thyroid dysfunctions. The formulation efficiently elevated the serum TSH levels, T3 and T4 levels. Furthermore, the formulation proved to be safe enough for human consumption with fewer mild side effects (Sharma, Basu, & Singh, 2018). The combination of *Withania* (1.4g/kg body weight) along with *Bauhinia purpurea* (2.5mg/kg body weight) significantly improved the thyroid function and ameliorated diabetes induced hypothyroidism(Jatwa & Kar, 2009). Green tea has also been proven to improve the T3, T4 levels and results in marked reduction in pathological lesions that manifests as increased size and number of follicles (El Mgeed, Bstawi, Mohamed, & Gabbar, 2009). In addition to improving the thyroid function, the combination has also shown to improve hepatic glucose-6-phospahtase (G-6-Pase), exerted anti-peroxidative effects by dampening the hepatic lipid peroxidation and increased activity of antioxidant enzymes (Panda & Kar, 1999).

Seaweed have been amongst the top choices in the management of thyroid disorders due to their high iodine content. *Fucus vesiculosus* (or bladderwrack, brown seaweed) has shown thyroid stimulating property however, no safety, efficacy or clinical dosage evidences highlight its usage(Shilo & Hirsch, 1986). *Fucus versiculosus* and sea kelp (*Ascophyllum nodosum*) are known to be best sources of natural iodine however, excess intake is associated with thyroid overactivity.

Forskolin (derived from *Coleus forskohlli*) increased thyroid hormone production and its release. It activates the adenylate cyclase and induces cAMP mediated increase in the T3 and T4 levels(Laurberg, 1984). Another potential thyroid stimulator is the *Triphladya guggulu* that directly affects the thyroid gland without direct involvement of pituitary-TSH axis. Guggul (*Commiphora mukul*) possesses thyroid stimulating properties and helps in alleviating LDL levels in hypothyroidism cases. Guggulu (200mg/kg/day) treatment for thirty days stimulated the thyroid functions and exerted antiperoxidative and antioxidant effect by triggering the production of superoxide dismutase (SOD) and catalase (CAT) that helped to ameliorate hypothyroidism (Panda & Kar, 2005). The combination therapy of *Triphladya guggulu* with *Punarnavadi* showed improvement in hypothyroidism and circumvented the need of hormone replacement therapy in 80 percent of treated cases(Singh & Thakar, 2018). Interestingly, acupuncture based delivery of polyherbal medicine, MOK, has shown promising effects on improving the levels of T3 and T4 in hypothyroidism, increased the glucose levels while reducing the triglyceride, total cholesterol, alanine transaminase as well as low density lipoproteins in the hypothyroidism rats. Further, the treatment brought about histological improvement in the thyroid function in multiple ways including the normalization of hypothyroidism-induced thyroid hormone imbalance, stimulating the antioxidant pathway and fine-tuning the TH1/TH2 imbalance(Hwang et al., 2018).

Recent finding has highlighted for the role of Aloe in management of subclinical hypothyroidism by decreasing the autoimmune inflammation. The formulation effectively rescued the thyrocyte function and inhibited T4 deiodination thus, decreased the need for conversion of prohormone T4 into T3; markedly improving the thyroid functions(Metro, Cernaro, Papa, & Benvenga, 2018).

3. Herbal Medicines for Hyperthyroidism

Hyperthyroidism also termed as thyrotoxicosis that manifests due to excess circulating levels of thyroid hormones. It can manifest as a result several other thyroid anomalies including thyroditis, toxic adenoma and thyroid storm. Hyperthyroidism and subclinical hyperthyroidism follows a course of flaring-up and remission as seen with many other autoimmune disorders. It affects the quality of life and produces symptoms similar to adrenergic overactivity. Grave's disease is another common form of hyperthyroidism Conventional therapeutics for hyperthyroidism mediated by antibodies that stimulates TSH receptor, leading to excess secretion of thyroid hormone and thyroid hyperplasia that eventually results in diffuse goiter and hyperthyroidism. The disease is characterized by exopthalmos, ophthalmoplegia, conjunctival edema, thyroid dermopathy and moderate to severe ophthalmopathy. It manifests with many autoimmune disorders including type1 diabetes, rheumatoid arthritis and lupus.

Secondary hyperthyroidism is usually rare; caused due to pituitary pathology, where pituitary overrides the normal thyroid's instruction for hormone production. This leads to marked increase in the levels of the T3, T4 and TSH. Conversely, subclinical hyperthyroidism is condition where low levels of

TSH are accompanied with normal levels of T3 and T4. It is common in elderly population, caused by exogenous (grave's disease, thyroiditis, thyroid adenoma and toxic nodular goiter) and/or endogenous factors (excessive TSH suppressive therapy and TSH suppression during hormone therapy for hypothyroidism). It increases the risk of coronary heart diseases, bone fracture (due to decreased bone density) and dementia (Collet et al., 2014). The conventional treatment options rely on radioactive iodine therapy, anti-thyroid treatment (as methimazole), beta blockers and/or anti-inflammatory drugs (NSAIDs or corticosteroids) (Abraham, Avenell, McGeoch, Clark, & Bevan, 2010). Approximately 20-40 percent cases undergo remission after six months to fifteen years post-treatment with anti-thyroid therapy, furthermore, 50-60 percent cases relapses (Hoermann et al., 2002; Karmisholt et al., 2019; Struja et al., 2017). Anti-thyroid treatments are also associated with hematopoietic damage which is severe, seen in the form of agranulocytosis and pancytopenia, with life threatening consequences (Watanabe et al., 2012). Traditional herbal medicines have been found effective management of hyperthyroidism and its associated anomalies. Herbal formulation of *Leonurus cardia* (commonly known as motherwort herb), rich in flavonoid called quercetin, serves as an adjuvant for overactive thyroid especially against hyperthyroidism associated palpitation and anxiety (Wartofsky & Van Nostrand, 2016). Bugleweed (*Lycopus europaeus*) has been used as thyroid suppressor and widely accepted as the treatment option for mild hyperthyroidism. It has shown potential benefits by preventing thyroid stimulating antibodies in Grave's disease and abrogates the production of TSH, T4 deiodination and inhibits iodine metabolism. It has been recommended for symptomatic relief in hyperthyroidism associated palpitation, tachycardia and autonomic nervous system (Verma & Jameel, 2012).

Melissa officinalis (commonly called lemon balm or gladdening herb) has also been used for management of hyperthyroidism by blocking the TSH binding to the receptor. It also prevents production of cAMP and used for symptomatic relief from hyperthyroidism associated tachycardia, insomnia and hyperactivity. It is known to increase the production of T3,T4 and decreases the TSH levels by feedback inhibition. Another member of Laminaceae family, *Rosmarinus officinalis* (rosemary) is abundant in romarinic acid which has potential application for hyperthyroidism treatment. It affects TSH on receptor site, reduces the peripheral changes in T3 and abrogates antibodies effect on TSH receptor. Sage (*Salvia officinalis*), another member of this family exerts similar effects(Yarnell & Abascal, 2006).

Scopoletin, isolated from the *Aegle marmelos* (Bael/Shriphal) regulated hyperthyroidism by inhibiting the lipid peroxidation, increasing SOD as well as catalase activity. The formulation significantly inhibited the thyroid function and hyperglycemia without causing hepatic toxicity. It was suggested superior to the conventional anti-thyroid treatment (propylthiouracil) (Panda & Kar, 2006). Another study for the comparative evaluation of *Bacopa monnieri* (200mg/kg), *Aegle marmelos* (1g/kg) and *Aloe vera* (125mg/kg) established *A.marmelos* and *A.vera* decreased T3 concentration and effectively managed the symptoms of hyperthyroidism while, *B.monneri* was effective for hypothyroidism(Kar, Panda, & Bharti, 2002).

The active component of green tea *viz.* catechins, a class of flavonoids possesses beneficial health effects, also acts as anti-thyroid agent. Upon oral administration of pure catechin decreased thyroid peroxidase and 5'-deiodinase. The treatment also altered thyroid physiology marked by hypertrophy and/or hyperplasia of thyroid follicles, thus, exerted anti-thyroid effects by adversely affecting the thyroid function (Chandra & De, 2010). However, higher doses of dietary administration of catechins was found to be goiterogenic and induced thyroid lesions in rats which strengthened the anti-thyroid potential of the green tea (Sakamoto et al., 2001). Similarly, cutard apple (*Annona squamosa*) extract, with quercetin as the active ingredient, ameliorated hyperthyroidism by decreasing hepatic lipid peroxidation, SOD, catalase and reversing all effects associated with hyperthyroidism. The formulation proved to more potent in reinvigorating the thyroid function than the conventional anti-thyroid drug (propyl thiouracil) (Panda & Kar, 2007).

Conversely, *Aloe vera* gel (50 or 500mg/kg/day) potentially reduced the oxidative stress, lipid hydroperoxides, increased the levels of hepatic antioxidants and markedly improved the thyroid histology in hyperthyroidic mice. It appeared from the LC-MS/MS study that anti-thyroid potential was attributed majorly due to the phenolics in the formulation(Panda, Sharma, Khan, & Kar, 2020). Likewise, phenolic compound, chavibetol (20 mg/kg) from *Piper betel* leaf alleviated the thyrotoxicosis by normalizing the cellular antioxidants, thyroxine, T3, thyrotropin, thyroid peroxidase expression and preserved the integrity of thyroid tissue. The anti-thyroid potential of the drug was found to be comparable to the conventional anti-thyroid, propylthiouracil (Panda, Sharma, & Kar, 2019). Therefore, herbal approach for hyperthyroidism can be safe and efficacious measure for managing the thyroid dysfunctions.

4. Herbal Medicines for Thyroid Nodules (Benign) and Cancer (Malignant)

Thyroid nodules are discrete lesions which can be divided into cysts, inflammatory nodules, timorous nodules(benign or malignant) and manifests as proliferative nodular goiter(Surks et al., 2004). Mostly these nodules are asymptomatic, it becomes common problem with increasing age. Conversely, thyroid cancer is common endocrine neoplasm, with approximately 95 percent cancers emanating from thyroid follicular epithelial cells including the papillary thyroid carcinoma (PTC), follicular thyroid carcinoma (FTC), anaplastic thyroid cancer (ATC) and medullary thyroid cancer (MTC) from parafollicular cells in thyroid gland (Rusinek et al., 2017; Seib & Sosa, 2019). Current therapies (surgery, chemotherapy, radiofrequency ablation and physiotherapy) are effective but suffer from risk of recurrence, metastasis and other limitations. Herbal medicinal approach has been adopted in China to treat thyroid nodules; although the formulations are variable in composition but these are given depending upon the patient syndrome. Xanthohumol is a safe herbal option that promotes iodide uptake, inhibits proliferation and increases the sensitivity of radiotherapy for disease management (Cook, Luo, Ndiaye, Chen, & Kunnimalaiyaan, 2010; Vanhoecke et al., 2005). Chinese herbal medicines (CHM) are also amongst the top choices for managing thyroid nodules. CHM for thyroid nodules includes Milkvetch with no adverse events, however, firm evidences for effectiveness of formulation were not obtained. Similarly, *Codonopsis pilosula*, Pangolin scales, selfheal, Chinese Thorowax root, Nutgrass Galingale rhizome, seaweed, Laminaria tents, musk and figwort root also possess medicinal properties for managing thyroid nodules (Tan & Gharib, 1997; Wenxun Wu et al., 2014).

Epigallocatechin-3-gallate (EGCG) is polyphenolic from green tea, is an important phytoproduct that suppresses cancer growth by inhibiting proliferation, viability, angiogenesis and cell cycle progression. The formulation effectively reduced the phophorylated epidermal growth factor receptor (p-EGFR), RAS,p-RAF, p-MEK1/2, p-ERK1/2 signaling in PTC (30858760). Resverstol is another polyphenolic phytoalexin, known to inhibit multiple signaling pathways associated with carcinogenesis and invasiveness. It induced apoptosis, thyroid differentiation markers (TTF-1 and NIS) and reduces the markers associated with thyroid cancer stemness (aldehyde dehydrogenase, SOX2, OCT4 and NANOG). (Hardin et al., 2016; Kang, Youn, Hong, & Kim, 2011). Likewise, other polyphenolics as punicalagin and curcumin from *Curcuma longa* induces cell death and cell cycle arrest, holds potential for PTC (Cheng et al., 2018; L. Zhang et al., 2016). Curcumin also employs multiple routes as ROS activation, disruption of calcium homeostasis by activation of ER stress(L. Zhang, Cheng, Xu, Bao, & Yu, 2018) and inhibition of signaling pathways responsible for metastasis. When used in combination with extracts from *Spirulina* and *Boswellia* with curcumin effectively reduces the size of thyroid nodule and helps in regaining thyroid functions (Stancioiu et al., 2019).

Flavonoid administration has long been used in cancer treatment; the use of apigenin and flavokawain B inhibits proliferation, induces ROS-mediated apoptosis (DNA damage) and autophagy *via.* activation of AMPK/mTOR pathway (Hseu et al., 2019; L. Zhang et al., 2015). Similarly, icariin (from *Epimedium davidii*) has shown efficacy in treatment of thyroid cancer by inhibiting proliferation, cell migration and invasion (Fang, Xu, & Kong, 2019); myricetin also induces cell death by caspase-dependent mitochondrial dysfunctions (Ha, Jung, Kim, Bae, & Lee, 2017). Genistein from *Leguminosae* inhibits metastatic invasion PTC derived cell line (C. Zhang et al., 2019), while, silibinin arrests cell cycle, inhibits miRNA involved in PTC-tumorogenesis and cell migration in thyroid cancer(Jahanafrooz, Motamed, Rinner, Mokhtarzadeh, & Baradaran, 2018). Inactivation of Notch1 signaling pathway in ATC affects the thyrocyte proliferation and differentiation, Notch activator, hesperetin decreases ATC proliferation by inducing apoptosis and redifferentiation of ATC (Patel, Yu, Jaskula-Sztul, & Chen, 2014). Quercetin is also known inducer of apoptosis in PTC cells (Mutlu Altundag et al., 2014). Similarly, oral administration of chrysin (flavone) suppresses tumor growth in ATC by inducing apoptosis(X. M. Yu, Phan, Patel, Jaskula-Sztul, & Chen, 2013).Natural flavonoids are known inhibitors of thyroid peroxidase, myricetin, only known flavanoid that increased influx and decreased efflux of iodide. This effect of myricetin can be exploited for therapeutic benefit for treatment of thyroid carcinoma (Schroder-van der Elst, van der Heide, Romijn, & Smit, 2004).

Amongst terpenoids, paclitaxel (derived from *Taxus chinensis*) is preferred treatment for PTC cases with squamous cell carcinoma that serves as adjunctive therapy after surgery (Basnet, Pandita, Fullmer, & Sivapiragasam, 2017). Pseudolaric acid B (PAB) (derived from *Pseudolarix amabilis*) serves as anti-tubulin therapeutic option that inhibits proliferation, invasion and migration of cancer cells (J. Yu et al., 2015).

Ginsenosides are saponins with anti-tumor pharmacological effects; PPT-type ginsenosides that exerts cytotoxic effect on PTC. It is also known to suppress thyroid cancer proliferation, migration and invasion of PTC by upregulating connexin31 (Xu, Chen, Qi, Li, & Sun, 2018). Ginsenosides also inhibits Rho GTPase, Rac-1,VEGF and Cdc42 in metastatic thyroid cancers (W. Wu et al., 2018). Bioactive component from *Lithospermum erythrorhizon* termed as shikonin (2mg/kg) has been safe option that suppresses migration and invasion of PTC and induces apoptosis by targeting multiple signaling pathways (Q. Yang, Ji, Guan, Shi, & Hou, 2013; Y. Zhang, Sun, Huang, Zhao, & Zeng, 2018). Similarly, allicin inhibits proliferation of cancer and induces apoptosis and autophagy in cancer cells (Xiang, Zhao, Zhao, & Wang, 2018; Zou et al., 2016). Likewise, berberine induced apoptosis and inhibited PI3K/Akt as well as MAPK pathway for thyroid carcinoma intervention (Li, Wang, Sharvan, Gao, & Qu, 2017).

In summary, herbal formulation possess therapeutic effects for treating thyroid nodules and cancer however, further clinical researches are required for evaluating their safety and efficacies before adopting them as universal treatment option.

5. Herbal Medicines for Hashimoto's Thyroditis

Hashimoto's thyroiditis (HT) is an autoimmune thyroiditis where lymphocytes infiltrate the gland and produces auto-antibodies towards thyroglobulin and thyroid peroxidase. This leads to destruction of thyroid gland by blocking the enzyme required for hormone production, leading to development of goiter and eventually hypothyroidism. HT can manifest due to multiple factors-genetic, immunological and environmental(Pyzik et al., 2015). The conventional treatment strategy for HT due to thyroid hormone deficiency involves the hormone replacement therapy with synthetic thyroid hormone (levothyroxine).

Herbal medicinal approach for managing hypothyroidism can also be used in HT management. As mentioned above, herbal extracts from bladder wrack, guggul, *Curcuma longa*, *Vitex agnus-castus*, *Leonurus cardiac* and *Iris versicolor* can be beneficial for HT.

Withania somnifera is amongst the most preferred herbal medicine in HT; it inhibits NFκB thereby directly inhibiting the inflammation and autoimmune pathologies. *Aloe barbendensis* Miller juice is known to significantly improves the thyroid indices and thyroperoxidase autoantibodies. It is also known to rescue thyrocyte function, decreases the need for conversion of prohormone T4 into active T3 and inhibits T4 deiodination (Metro et al., 2018).

Additionally, in a trial, using *Nigella sativa* for HT treatment improved the thyroid status, reduced VEGF and ameliorated disease pathology (Farhangi, Dehghan, Tajmiri, & Abbasi, 2016). It is also known to improve the oxidative stress, endothelial dysfunction, serum lipid profiles and anthropometric features in HT cases and can be used in parallel with levothyroxine for managing HT related metabolic conditions (Farhangi, Dehghan, & Tajmiri, 2018; Farhangi & Tajmiri, 2020). Further, aconite-cake separated moxibustion in combination with oral administration of Euthyrox significantly improved thyroid functions, thyrotropin, T3 and T4 content as compared to Euthyrox alone (Xia et al., 2012).

Although hormone replacement therapy is the commonly used medication for HT and hypothyroidism but herbal drugs are known to boost immune system to tackle the thyroid disorders.

ISSUES, CONTROVERSIES, SOLUTION AND RECOMMENDATION

Instead of relying on western medical approaches recent years have experienced a swung towards the less intensive treatment options. The use of hormone replacement therapy, radioiodine, surgery, long-term disease management and sometimes more aggressive approaches than recommended by ATA guidelines increases the fear of patient's non-compliance and development of severe side effects. For example, the most potent risk associated with thyroid surgery includes the low calcium (secondary to hypoparathyroidism) and voice changes (due to vocal fold paralysis) while radioactive iodine therapy is associated with lacrimal and salivary gland damages, risk of cavities, primary malignancy (especially leukemia), bladder irritation, abdominal pain and early onset menopause. Similarly, hormone replacement therapy includes osteoporosis or fracture, arrhythemia and cognitive defects in elderly patients.

In context of anti-thyroid drugs as methimazole (MMI) or its precursor carbimazole (CMZ) and propylthiouracil, not much data is available about the remission rates. Both these thionamides inhibits the thyroid peroxidase mediated synthesis of thyroid hormone. During the time interval between the treatment and normalization of thyroid hormone levels, thyrotoxicosis is usually managed by beta-blockers. Unfortunately, beta blockers have threatening consequences on respiratory and/or circulatory system therefore, it is highly recommended to choose the patient for this therapy and it should be withdrawn when cases become euthyroid. Once thyroid functions are normalized it is logical to taper the dosage of these drugs depending upon the degree of thyroid dysfunction. This is important especially in context of MMI, where too low doses cannot retrieve an euthyroid state while, too high doses can result in iatrogenic hypothyroidism in cases with mild disease (Nakamura et al., 2007). It is noteworthy that adverse drug events are mainly associated with higher doses of MMI. Therefore, it becomes crucial to tailor the dose to achieve the clinical goal of normalizing the clinical parameters associated with thyroid. Since,

MMI and CMZ have long half life in circulation so, they are effective in single dose and might improve the compliance rates. In contrast to MMI and CMZ, PTU has shorter half life require two to three doses a day, depending upon the disease severity. The recent recommendation for the drug usage only in exceptional circumstances either for short duration for treating the cases experiencing severe side effects due to MMI/CMZ, owing to the suggested risk for development of hepatitis(Rivkees & Mattison, 2009).

Evidences from clinical follow-up have suggested for remission in 40-60% of cases after course of treatment; if the remission not appears after 12-18 months of treatment then it is safe for prolonged therapy with negligible chances of remission. However, there are other factors including age, thyroid volume, serum TSH receptor auto-antibodies, ethnicity and drug response that determine the disease remission(Kaguelidou et al., 2008; Leger & Carel, 2018). The issue of duration of treatment in children is a topic of controversy and needs further case studies.

Radioactive iodine therapy is usually the safe, efficacious and preferred treatment choice for Grave's disease associated hyperthyroidism however, approximately 90 percent cases complaint of permanent hypothyroidism that in turn require life-long hormone replacement therapy and routine monitoring of thyroid functions. Further, efficacy of the treatment is affected due to high TSH receptor auto-antibodies so in such cases surgery is preferred over iodine therapy. There are potential risks of deterioration of opthalmopathy in small percentage of subjects and usually anti-thyroid treatment has to be withdrawn before iodine therapy. Conversely, the therapy should be carefully administered to pregnant ladies.

Most of the clinicians do not recommend herbal medicines, essential oils or other alternative treatment strategies due to lack of scientific evidences. However, it has been used since thousands of years and recent decades have experiences a plethora of researches on the use of traditional herbal approaches for management of thyroid dysfunctions with negligible side effects. Traditional medicinal approach has been the cost effective and safe option that relives the symptoms, good compliance rates and provides the psychological satisfaction for using the safe and effective remedy for disease management. It can be used alone or in combination with the anti-thyroid drugs however, this issue needs further research to answer the controversies associated with the efficacy of traditional herbal medicinal approach.

FUTURE RESEARCH DIRECTION

The optimal disease management approach depends on number of criteria (age, clinical history, disease severity etc.) therefore, before starting the treatment there remains an urgent need of assessment of WBCs (to understand blood cells profile). The future relies on careful monitoring the drug dosage and tailoring it for development of individualized treatment approach. This will pave the way for better, safe and efficacious way to disease management with minimal adverse drug reaction. Additionally, varied immunological and genetic make-up of subjects highlights the need of tailoring the drug dosage to obtain better therapeutic efficacies. This will also be helpful in reducing the disease remission rates and inter-individual variability for drug tolerance. Additionally, the current advances in the genomics, proteomics as well as the metabolomics can further help the scientists to gain better insight into the disease intervention strategies.

CONCLUSION

Although the herbal approach of thyroid dysfunction management is not widely accepted however, it is the only measure to avoid the various side effects of conventional therapeutics. This calls upon for development of better research strategies for evaluating the beneficial effects of herbal medicines by using different *in vitro, in silico* as well as *in vivo* methodologies. The research output will pave a full-proved way for benchside to bedside application of the herbal medicines for thyroid dysfunctions. Thus, an integrated approach of combined efforts of the clinicians and scientists are required to make herbal medicine based treatment approach a trustworthy and certified treatment option for disease management.

REFERENCES

Abraham, P., Avenell, A., McGeoch, S. C., Clark, L. F., & Bevan, J. S. (2010). Antithyroid drug regimen for treating Graves' hyperthyroidism. *Cochrane Database of Systematic Reviews*, (1), CD003420. doi:10.1002/14651858.CD003420.pub4 PMID:20091544

Ashwini, S., Bobby, Z., Sridhar, M. G., & Cleetus, C. C. (2017). Insulin Plant (Costus pictus) Extract Restores Thyroid Hormone Levels in Experimental Hypothyroidism. *Pharmacognosy Research, 9*(1), 51–59. doi:10.4103/0974-8490.199766 PMID:28250654

Association, A. T., Hyperthyroidism, A. A. C. E. T., Thyrotoxicosis, O. C., Bahn, R. S., Burch, H. B., Cooper, D. S., ... Montori, V. M. (2011). Hyperthyroidism and other causes of thyrotoxicosis: Management guidelines of the American Thyroid Association and American Association of Clinical Endocrinologists. *Thyroid, 21*(6), 593–646. doi:10.1089/thy.2010.0417 PMID:21510801

Azevedo, M. F., Barra, G. B., Naves, L. A., Ribeiro Velasco, L. F., Godoy Garcia Castro, P., de Castro, L. C., Amato, A. A., Miniard, A., Driscoll, D., Schomburg, L., & de Assis Rocha Neves, F. (2010). Selenoprotein-related disease in a young girl caused by nonsense mutations in the SBP2 gene. *The Journal of Clinical Endocrinology and Metabolism, 95*(8), 4066–4071. doi:10.1210/jc.2009-2611 PMID:20501692

Basnet, A., Pandita, A., Fullmer, J., & Sivapiragasam, A. (2017). Squamous Cell Carcinoma of the Thyroid as a Result of Anaplastic Transformation from BRAF-Positive Papillary Thyroid Cancer. *Case Reports in Oncological Medicine, 4276435*, 1–4. Advance online publication. doi:10.1155/2017/4276435 PMID:29158933

Chandra, A. K., & De, N. (2010). Goitrogenic/antithyroidal potential of green tea extract in relation to catechin in rats. *Food and Chemical Toxicology, 48*(8-9), 2304–2311. doi:10.1016/j.fct.2010.05.064 PMID:20561943

Cheng, X., Yao, X., Xu, S., Pan, J., Yu, H., Bao, J., Guan, H., Lu, R., & Zhang, L. (2018). Punicalagin induces senescent growth arrest in human papillary thyroid carcinoma BCPAP cells via NF-kappaB signaling pathway. *Biomedicine and Pharmacotherapy, 103*, 490–498. doi:10.1016/j.biopha.2018.04.074 PMID:29677534

Collet, T. H., Bauer, D. C., Cappola, A. R., Asvold, B. O., Weiler, S., Vittinghoff, E., ... Thyroid Studies, C. (2014). Thyroid antibody status, subclinical hypothyroidism, and the risk of coronary heart disease: An individual participant data analysis. *The Journal of Clinical Endocrinology and Metabolism*, *99*(9), 3353–3362. doi:10.1210/jc.2014-1250 PMID:24915118

Cook, M. R., Luo, J., Ndiaye, M., Chen, H., & Kunnimalaiyaan, M. (2010). Xanthohumol inhibits the neuroendocrine transcription factor achaete-scute complex-like 1, suppresses proliferation, and induces phosphorylated ERK1/2 in medullary thyroid cancer. *American Journal of Surgery*, *199*(3), 315–318. doi:10.1016/j.amjsurg.2009.08.034 PMID:20226902

Di Cosmo, C., McLellan, N., Liao, X. H., Khanna, K. K., Weiss, R. E., Papp, L., & Refetoff, S. (2009). Clinical and molecular characterization of a novel selenocysteine insertion sequence-binding protein 2 (SBP2) gene mutation (R128X). *The Journal of Clinical Endocrinology and Metabolism*, *94*(10), 4003–4009. doi:10.1210/jc.2009-0686 PMID:19602558

Dumitrescu, A. M., & Refetoff, S. (2013). The syndromes of reduced sensitivity to thyroid hormone. *Biochimica et Biophysica Acta*, *1830*(7), 3987–4003. doi:10.1016/j.bbagen.2012.08.005 PMID:22986150

El Mgeed, A. A., Bstawi, M., Mohamed, U., & Gabbar, M. A. (2009). Histopathological and biochemical effects of green tea and/or licorice aqueous extracts on thyroid functions in male albino rats intoxicated with dimethylnitrosamine. *Nutrition & Metabolism*, *6*(1), 2. doi:10.1186/1743-7075-6-2 PMID:19138393

Fang, L., Xu, W., & Kong, D. (2019). Icariin inhibits cell proliferation, migration and invasion by down-regulation of microRNA-625-3p in thyroid cancer cells. *Biomedicine and Pharmacotherapy*, *109*, 2456–2463. doi:10.1016/j.biopha.2018.04.012 PMID:30551506

Farhangi, M. A., Dehghan, P., & Tajmiri, S. (2018). Powdered black cumin seeds strongly improves serum lipids, atherogenic index of plasma and modulates anthropometric features in patients with Hashimoto's thyroiditis. *Lipids in Health and Disease*, *17*(1), 59. doi:10.118612944-018-0704-x PMID:29587770

Farhangi, M. A., Dehghan, P., Tajmiri, S., & Abbasi, M. M. (2016). The effects of Nigella sativa on thyroid function, serum Vascular Endothelial Growth Factor (VEGF) - 1, Nesfatin-1 and anthropometric features in patients with Hashimoto's thyroiditis: A randomized controlled trial. *BMC Complementary and Alternative Medicine*, *16*(1), 471. doi:10.118612906-016-1432-2 PMID:27852303

Farhangi, M. A., & Tajmiri, S. (2020). The effects of powdered black cumin seeds on markers of oxidative stress, intracellular adhesion molecule (ICAM)-1 and vascular cell adhesion molecule (VCAM)-1 in patients with Hashimoto's thyroiditis. *Clinical Nutrition ESPEN*, *37*, 207–212. doi:10.1016/j.clnesp.2020.02.015 PMID:32359745

Ha, T. K., Jung, I., Kim, M. E., Bae, S. K., & Lee, J. S. (2017). Anti-cancer activity of myricetin against human papillary thyroid cancer cells involves mitochondrial dysfunction-mediated apoptosis. *Biomedicine and Pharmacotherapy*, *91*, 378–384. doi:10.1016/j.biopha.2017.04.100 PMID:28463801

Hardin, H., Yu, X. M., Harrison, A. D., Larrain, C., Zhang, R., Chen, J., Chen, H., & Lloyd, R. V. (2016). Generation of Novel Thyroid Cancer Stem-Like Cell Clones: Effects of Resveratrol and Valproic Acid. *American Journal of Pathology*, *186*(6), 1662–1673. doi:10.1016/j.ajpath.2016.02.003 PMID:27060227

Haugen, B. R., Alexander, E. K., Bible, K. C., Doherty, G. M., Mandel, S. J., Nikiforov, Y. E., ... Schlumberger, M. (2016). 2015 American Thyroid Association management guidelines for adult patients with thyroid nodules and differentiated thyroid cancer: The American Thyroid Association guidelines task force on thyroid nodules and differentiated thyroid cancer. *Thyroid*, *26*(1), 1–133. doi:10.1089/thy.2015.0020 PMID:26462967

Hegedus, L., Bonnema, S. J., & Bennedbaek, F. N. (2003). Management of simple nodular goiter: Current status and future perspectives. *Endocrine Reviews*, *24*(1), 102–132. doi:10.1210/er.2002-0016 PMID:12588812

Hoang, J. (2010). Thyroid nodules and evaluation of thyroid cancer risk. *Australasian Journal of Ultrasound in Medicine*, *13*(4), 33–36. doi:10.1002/j.2205-0140.2010.tb00177.x PMID:28191095

Hoermann, R., Quadbeck, B., Roggenbuck, U., Szabolcs, I., Pfeilschifter, J., Meng, W., Reschke, K., Hackenberg, K., Dettmann, J., Prehn, B., Hirche, H., & Mann, K. (2002). Relapse of Graves' disease after successful outcome of antithyroid drug therapy: Results of a prospective randomized study on the use of levothyroxine. *Thyroid*, *12*(12), 1119–1128. doi:10.1089/105072502321085225 PMID:12593726

Holden, K. R., Zuniga, O. F., May, M. M., Su, H., Molinero, M. R., Rogers, R. C., & Schwartz, C. E. (2005). X-linked MCT8 gene mutations: Characterization of the pediatric neurologic phenotype. *Journal of Child Neurology*, *20*(10), 852–857. doi:10.1177/08830738050200101601 PMID:16417886

Hseu, Y. C., Huang, Y. C., Thiyagarajan, V., Mathew, D. C., Lin, K. Y., Chen, S. C., Liu, J.-Y., Hsu, L.-S., Li, M.-L., & Yang, H. L. (2019). Anticancer activities of chalcone flavokawain B from Alpinia pricei Hayata in human lung adenocarcinoma (A549) cells via induction of reactive oxygen species-mediated apoptotic and autophagic cell death. *Journal of Cellular Physiology*, *234*(10), 17514–17526. doi:10.1002/jcp.28375 PMID:30847898

Hwang, J. H., Jung, H. W., Kang, S. Y., Kang, A. N., Ma, J. N., Meng, X. L., Hwang, M., & Park, Y. K. (2018). Therapeutic effects of acupuncture with MOK, a polyherbal medicine, on PTU-induced hypothyroidism in rats. *Experimental and Therapeutic Medicine*, *16*(1), 310–320. doi:10.3892/etm.2018.6190 PMID:29896255

Jahanafrooz, Z., Motamed, N., Rinner, B., Mokhtarzadeh, A., & Baradaran, B. (2018). Silibinin to improve cancer therapeutic, as an apoptotic inducer, autophagy modulator, cell cycle inhibitor, and microRNAs regulator. *Life Sciences*, *213*, 236–247. doi:10.1016/j.lfs.2018.10.009 PMID:30308184

Jatwa, R., & Kar, A. (2009). Amelioration of metformin-induced hypothyroidism by Withania somnifera and Bauhinia purpurea extracts in Type 2 diabetic mice. *Phytotherapy Research*, *23*(8), 1140–1145. doi:10.1002/ptr.2765 PMID:19170137

Kaguelidou, F., Alberti, C., Castanet, M., Guitteny, M. A., Czernichow, P., & Leger, J. (2008). Predictors of autoimmune hyperthyroidism relapse in children after discontinuation of antithyroid drug treatment. *The Journal of Clinical Endocrinology and Metabolism*, *93*(10), 3817–3826. doi:10.1210/jc.2008-0842 PMID:18628515

Kang, H. J., Youn, Y. K., Hong, M. K., & Kim, L. S. (2011). Antiproliferation and redifferentiation in thyroid cancer cell lines by polyphenol phytochemicals. *Journal of Korean Medical Science*, *26*(7), 893–899. doi:10.3346/jkms.2011.26.7.893 PMID:21738342

Kar, A., Panda, S., & Bharti, S. (2002). Relative efficacy of three medicinal plant extracts in the alteration of thyroid hormone concentrations in male mice. *Journal of Ethnopharmacology*, *81*(2), 281–285. doi:10.1016/S0378-8741(02)00048-X PMID:12065164

Karmisholt, J., Andersen, S. L., Bulow-Pedersen, I., Carle, A., Krejbjerg, A., & Nygaard, B. (2019). Predictors of Initial and Sustained Remission in Patients Treated with Antithyroid Drugs for Graves' Hyperthyroidism: The RISG Study. *Journal of Thyroid Research*, *5945178*, 1–9. Advance online publication. doi:10.1155/2019/5945178 PMID:30719273

Kiseleva, I. A., Teplaia, E. V., & Kaminskii, A. V. (2012). Application of herbal medicine alba in treatment of patients with the pathology of thyroid. *Likars'Ka Sprava*, (8), 116–119. PMID:23786024

Laurberg, P. (1984). Forskolin stimulation of thyroid secretion of T4 and T3. *FEBS Letters*, *170*(2), 273–276. doi:10.1016/0014-5793(84)81327-7 PMID:6327383

Leger, J., & Carel, J. C. (2018). Diagnosis and management of hyperthyroidism from prenatal life to adolescence. *Best Practice & Research. Clinical Endocrinology & Metabolism*, *32*(4), 373–386. doi:10.1016/j.beem.2018.03.014 PMID:30086864

Li, L., Wang, X., Sharvan, R., Gao, J., & Qu, S. (2017). Berberine could inhibit thyroid carcinoma cells by inducing mitochondrial apoptosis, G0/G1 cell cycle arrest and suppressing migration via PI3K-AKT and MAPK signaling pathways. *Biomedicine and Pharmacotherapy*, *95*, 1225–1231. doi:10.1016/j.biopha.2017.09.010 PMID:28931215

Liu, Y., Zhong, G., & Liu, H. (2015). Therapeutic effect of HaizaoYuhu decoction with/without seaweed and liquorice anti-drug combination on goiter rats in preferred dosage conditions. *Science and Technology Review*, *33*, 87-91.

Metro, D., Cernaro, V., Papa, M., & Benvenga, S. (2018). Marked improvement of thyroid function and autoimmunity by Aloe barbadensis miller juice in patients with subclinical hypothyroidism. *Journal of Clinical & Translational Endocrinology*, *11*, 18–25. doi:10.1016/j.jcte.2018.01.003 PMID:29527506

Mutlu Altundag, E., Mine Yilmaz, A., Kasaci, T., Corek, C., Taga, Y., & Suha Yalcin, A. (2014). The role of HSP90 in Quercetin-induced apoptosis in human papillary thyroid (B-CPAP) cancer cells. *Free Radical Biology & Medicine*, *75*(Suppl 1), S43. doi:10.1016/j.freeradbiomed.2014.10.797 PMID:26461378

Nakamura, H., Noh, J. Y., Itoh, K., Fukata, S., Miyauchi, A., & Hamada, N. (2007). Comparison of methimazole and propylthiouracil in patients with hyperthyroidism caused by Graves' disease. *The Journal of Clinical Endocrinology and Metabolism*, *92*(6), 2157–2162. doi:10.1210/jc.2006-2135 PMID:17389704

Panda, S., & Kar, A. (1999). Withania somnifera and Bauhinia purpurea in the regulation of circulating thyroid hormone concentrations in female mice. *Journal of Ethnopharmacology*, *67*(2), 233–239. doi:10.1016/S0378-8741(99)00018-5 PMID:10619390

Panda, S., & Kar, A. (2005). Guggulu (Commiphora mukul) potentially ameliorates hypothyroidism in female mice. *Phytotherapy Research, 19*(1), 78–80. doi:10.1002/ptr.1602 PMID:15798994

Panda, S., & Kar, A. (2006). Evaluation of the antithyroid, antioxidative and antihyperglycemic activity of scopoletin from Aegle marmelos leaves in hyperthyroid rats. *Phytotherapy Research, 20*(12), 1103–1105. doi:10.1002/ptr.2014 PMID:17078113

Panda, S., & Kar, A. (2007). Annona squamosa seed extract in the regulation of hyperthyroidism and lipid-peroxidation in mice: Possible involvement of quercetin. *Phytomedicine, 14*(12), 799–805. doi:10.1016/j.phymed.2006.12.001 PMID:17291737

Panda, S., Sharma, R., & Kar, A. (2019). Chavibetol corrects thyrotoxicosis through alterations in thyroid peroxidase. *Naunyn-Schmiedeberg's Archives of Pharmacology, 392*(5), 541–550. doi:10.100700210-018-01606-x PMID:30610248

Panda, S., Sharma, R., Khan, A., & Kar, A. (2020). Ameliorative effect of Aloe gel against L-T4-induced hyperthyroidism via suppression of thyrotropin receptors, inflammation and oxidative stress. *Molecular Biology Reports, 47*(4), 2801–2810. doi:10.100711033-020-05405-7 PMID:32242301

Patel, P. N., Yu, X. M., Jaskula-Sztul, R., & Chen, H. (2014). Hesperetin activates the Notch1 signaling cascade, causes apoptosis, and induces cellular differentiation in anaplastic thyroid cancer. *Annals of Surgical Oncology, 21*(S4, Suppl 4), S497–S504. doi:10.124510434-013-3459-7 PMID:24419754

Poncin, S., Gerard, A. C., Boucquey, M., Senou, M., Calderon, P. B., Knoops, B., Lengelé, B., Many, M.-C., & Colin, I. M. (2008). Oxidative stress in the thyroid gland: From harmlessness to hazard depending on the iodine content. *Endocrinology, 149*(1), 424–433. doi:10.1210/en.2007-0951 PMID:17884933

Pyzik, A., Grywalska, E., Matyjaszek-Matuszek, B., & Rolinski, J. (2015). Immune disorders in Hashimoto's thyroiditis: What do we know so far? *Journal of Immunology Research, 979167*, 1–8. Advance online publication. doi:10.1155/2015/979167 PMID:26000316

Rivkees, S. A., & Mattison, D. R. (2009). Ending propylthiouracil-induced liver failure in children. *The New England Journal of Medicine, 360*(15), 1574–1575. doi:10.1056/NEJMc0809750 PMID:19357418

Rusinek, D., Chmielik, E., Krajewska, J., Jarzab, M., Oczko-Wojciechowska, M., Czarniecka, A., & Jarzab, B. (2017). Current Advances in Thyroid Cancer Management. Are We Ready for the Epidemic Rise of Diagnoses? *International Journal of Molecular Sciences, 18*(8), 1817. Advance online publication. doi:10.3390/ijms18081817 PMID:28829399

Sabra, M. M., & Di Cristofano, A. (2019). *89th Annual Meeting of the American Thyroid Association*. Mary Ann Liebert, Inc.

Sakamoto, Y., Mikuriya, H., Tayama, K., Takahashi, H., Nagasawa, A., Yano, N., ... Aoki, N. (2001). Goitrogenic effects of green tea extract catechins by dietary administration in rats. *Archives of Toxicology, 75*(10), 591–596. doi:10.100700204-001-0286-6 PMID:11808919

Sakurai, A., Takeda, K., Ain, K., Ceccarelli, P., Nakai, A., Seino, S., Bell, G. I., Refetoff, S., & DeGroot, L. J. (1989). Generalized resistance to thyroid hormone associated with a mutation in the ligand-binding domain of the human thyroid hormone receptor beta. *Proceedings of the National Academy of Sciences of the United States of America*, *86*(22), 8977–8981. doi:10.1073/pnas.86.22.8977 PMID:2510172

Schomburg, L., Dumitrescu, A. M., Liao, X. H., Bin-Abbas, B., Hoeflich, J., Kohrle, J., & Refetoff, S. (2009). Selenium supplementation fails to correct the selenoprotein synthesis defect in subjects with SBP2 gene mutations. *Thyroid*, *19*(3), 277–281. doi:10.1089/thy.2008.0397 PMID:19265499

Schroder-van der Elst, J. P., van der Heide, D., Romijn, J. A., & Smit, J. W. (2004). Differential effects of natural flavonoids on growth and iodide content in a human Na*/I- symporter-transfected follicular thyroid carcinoma cell line. *European Journal of Endocrinology*, *150*(4), 557–564. doi:10.1530/eje.0.1500557 PMID:15080787

Seib, C. D., & Sosa, J. A. (2019). Evolving Understanding of the Epidemiology of Thyroid Cancer. *Endocrinology and Metabolism Clinics of North America*, *48*(1), 23–35. doi:10.1016/j.ecl.2018.10.002 PMID:30717905

Sharma, A. K., Basu, I., & Singh, S. (2018). Efficacy and Safety of Ashwagandha Root Extract in Subclinical Hypothyroid Patients: A Double-Blind, Randomized Placebo-Controlled Trial. *Journal of Alternative and Complementary Medicine (New York, N.Y.)*, *24*(3), 243–248. doi:10.1089/acm.2017.0183 PMID:28829155

Shilo, S., & Hirsch, H. J. (1986). Iodine-induced hyperthyroidism in a patient with a normal thyroid gland. *Postgraduate Medical Journal*, *62*(729), 661–662. doi:10.1136/pgmj.62.729.661 PMID:3748931

Singh, K., & Thakar, A. B. (2018). A clinical study to evaluate the role of Triphaladya Guggulu along with Punarnavadi Kashaya in the management of hypothyroidism. *Ayu*, *39*(1), 50–55. doi:10.4103/ayu.AYU_62_17 PMID:30595635

Stancioiu, F., Mihai, D., Papadakis, G. Z., Tsatsakis, A., Spandidos, D. A., & Badiu, C. (2019). Treatment for benign thyroid nodules with a combination of natural extracts. *Molecular Medicine Reports*, *20*(3), 2332–2338. doi:10.3892/mmr.2019.10453 PMID:31322200

Stephen, J. M., & Gary, D. H. (2014). *Pathophysiology of disease-an introduction to clinical medicine: Medical*. Academic Press.

Struja, T., Fehlberg, H., Kutz, A., Guebelin, L., Degen, C., Mueller, B., & Schuetz, P. (2017). Can we predict relapse in Graves' disease? Results from a systematic review and meta-analysis. *European Journal of Endocrinology*, *176*(1), 87–97. doi:10.1530/EJE-16-0725 PMID:27780830

Surks, M. I., Ortiz, E., Daniels, G. H., Sawin, C. T., Col, N. F., Cobin, R. H., ... Denke, M. A. (2004). Subclinical thyroid disease: Scientific review and guidelines for diagnosis and management. *Journal of the American Medical Association*, *291*(2), 228–238. doi:10.1001/jama.291.2.228 PMID:14722150

Tan, G. H., & Gharib, H. (1997). Thyroid incidentalomas: Management approaches to nonpalpable nodules discovered incidentally on thyroid imaging. *Annals of Internal Medicine*, *126*(3), 226–231. doi:10.7326/0003-4819-126-3-199702010-00009 PMID:9027275

Turchaninova, L. I. (2014). Experience of using phytopreparation Alba (root extract of the Potentilla alba) in complex treatment of thyroid pathology in children and adolescents. *Likars'Ka Sprava*, (3-4), 125–129. PMID:25286612

Unnikrishnan, A. G., & Menon, U. V. (2011). Thyroid disorders in India: An epidemiological perspective. *Indian Journal of Endocrinology and Metabolism, 15*(6, Suppl 2), S78–S81. doi:10.4103/2230-8210.83329 PMID:21966658

Vanhoecke, B. W., Delporte, F., Van Braeckel, E., Heyerick, A., Depypere, H. T., Nuytinck, M., ... Bracke, M. E. (2005). A safety study of oral tangeretin and xanthohumol administration to laboratory mice. *In Vivo (Athens, Greece), 19*(1), 103–107. PMID:15796161

Verma, K., & Jameel, K. (2012). Studies on traditional treatment of thyroid by the tribals of Chitrakoot district, Uttar Pradesh. *International Journal of Scientific Research (Ahmedabad, India), 3*, 2319–7064.

Visser, W. E., Jansen, J., Friesema, E. C., Kester, M. H., Mancilla, E., Lundgren, J., van der Knaap, M. S., Lunsing, R. J., Brouwer, O. F., & Visser, T. J. (2009). Novel pathogenic mechanism suggested by ex vivo analysis of MCT8 (SLC16A2) mutations. *Human Mutation, 30*(1), 29–38. doi:10.1002/humu.20808 PMID:18636565

Wartofsky, L., & Van Nostrand, D. (2016). *Thyroid cancer: a comprehensive guide to clinical management*. Springer. doi:10.1007/978-1-4939-3314-3

Watanabe, N., Narimatsu, H., Noh, J. Y., Yamaguchi, T., Kobayashi, K., Kami, M., Kunii, Y., Mukasa, K., Ito, K., & Ito, K. (2012). Antithyroid drug-induced hematopoietic damage: A retrospective cohort study of agranulocytosis and pancytopenia involving 50,385 patients with Graves' disease. *The Journal of Clinical Endocrinology and Metabolism, 97*(1), E49–E53. doi:10.1210/jc.2011-2221 PMID:22049174

Weiss, R. E., Weinberg, M., & Refetoff, S. (1993). Identical mutations in unrelated families with generalized resistance to thyroid hormone occur in cytosine-guanine-rich areas of the thyroid hormone receptor beta gene. Analysis of 15 families. *The Journal of Clinical Investigation, 91*(6), 2408–2415. doi:10.1172/JCI116474 PMID:8514853

Wu, S. Y., Cohen, R. N., Simsek, E., Senses, D. A., Yar, N. E., Grasberger, H., Noel, J., Refetoff, S., & Weiss, R. E. (2006). A novel thyroid hormone receptor-beta mutation that fails to bind nuclear receptor corepressor in a patient as an apparent cause of severe, predominantly pituitary resistance to thyroid hormone. *The Journal of Clinical Endocrinology and Metabolism, 91*(5), 1887–1895. doi:10.1210/jc.2005-2428 PMID:16464943

Wu, W., Yin, D., Yang, W., Kan, Q., Liu, Z., Ren, X., Zhai, C., & Zhang, S. (2014). Chinese herbal medicines for benign thyroid nodules in adults. *Cochrane Database of Systematic Reviews*, 3. doi:10.1002/14651858.CD010492.pub2 PMID:24596045

Wu, W., Zhou, Q., Zhao, W., Gong, Y., Su, A., Liu, F., Liu, Y., Li, Z., & Zhu, J. (2018). Ginsenoside Rg3 Inhibition of Thyroid Cancer Metastasis Is Associated with Alternation of Actin Skeleton. *Journal of Medicinal Food, 21*(9), 849–857. doi:10.1089/jmf.2017.4144 PMID:30136914

Xia, Y., Xia, M. Z., Li, Y., Liu, S. M., Ju, Z. Y., & He, J. S. (2012). Effect of aconite cake-separated moxibustion at Guanyuan (CV 4) and Mingmen (GV 4) on thyroid function in patients of Hashimoto's thyroiditis. *Zhongguo Zhenjiu, 32*(2), 123–126.

Xiang, Y., Zhao, J., Zhao, M., & Wang, K. (2018). Allicin activates autophagic cell death to alleviate the malignant development of thyroid cancer. *Experimental and Therapeutic Medicine, 15*(4), 3537–3543. doi:10.3892/etm.2018.5828 PMID:29545880

Xiu, L., Zhong, G., Liu, D., Chen, S., Liu, H., & Chen, F. (2017). Comparative efficacy and toxicity of different species of Sargassum in Haizao Yuhu Decoction in PTU-induced goiter rats. *Evidence-Based Complementary and Alternative Medicine, 2017*, 2017. doi:10.1155/2017/3526186 PMID:28713435

Xu, L., Chen, S. W., Qi, X. Y., Li, X. X., & Sun, Y. B. (2018). Ginsenoside improves papillary thyroid cancer cell malignancies partially through upregulating connexin 31. *The Kaohsiung Journal of Medical Sciences, 34*(6), 313–320. doi:10.1016/j.kjms.2017.12.006 PMID:29747774

Yang, K., Guo, K. Q., & Wu, H. Y. (2007). Clinical effect of Prunellae Oral Liquid on goiter with different thyroid function. *Zhongguo Zhong Xi Yi Jie He Za Zhi, 27*(1), 37–39. PMID:17302062

Yang, M. L., & Lu, B. (2018). Treatment of Goiter with Traditional Chinese Medicine Regimen Xing Qi Hua Ying Tang: A Clinical Study on 72 Patients with Multinodular and Diffuse Goiter. *Journal of Alternative and Complementary Medicine (New York, N.Y.), 24*(4), 374–377. doi:10.1089/acm.2017.0138 PMID:29215302

Yang, Q., Ji, M., Guan, H., Shi, B., & Hou, P. (2013). Shikonin inhibits thyroid cancer cell growth and invasiveness through targeting major signaling pathways. *The Journal of Clinical Endocrinology and Metabolism, 98*(12), E1909–E1917. doi:10.1210/jc.2013-2583 PMID:24106286

Yarnell, E., & Abascal, K. (2006). Botanical medicine for thyroid regulation. *Alternative and Complementary Therapies, 12*(3), 107–112. doi:10.1089/act.2006.12.107

Yu, J., Ren, P., Zhong, T., Wang, Y., Yan, M., Xue, B., Li, R., Dai, C., Liu, C., Chen, G., & Yu, X. F. (2015). Pseudolaric acid B inhibits proliferation in SW579 human thyroid squamous cell carcinoma. *Molecular Medicine Reports, 12*(5), 7195–7202. doi:10.3892/mmr.2015.4418 PMID:26460192

Yu, X. M., Phan, T., Patel, P. N., Jaskula-Sztul, R., & Chen, H. (2013). Chrysin activates Notch1 signaling and suppresses tumor growth of anaplastic thyroid carcinoma in vitro and in vivo. *Cancer, 119*(4), 774–781. doi:10.1002/cncr.27742 PMID:22991264

Zhang, C., Lv, B., Yi, C., Cui, X., Sui, S., Li, X., Qi, M., Hao, C., Han, B., & Liu, Z. (2019). Genistein inhibits human papillary thyroid cancer cell detachment, invasion and metastasis. *Journal of Cancer, 10*(3), 737–748. doi:10.7150/jca.28111 PMID:30719173

Zhang, L., Cheng, X., Gao, Y., Bao, J., Guan, H., Lu, R., Yu, H., Xu, Q., & Sun, Y. (2016). Induction of ROS-independent DNA damage by curcumin leads to G2/M cell cycle arrest and apoptosis in human papillary thyroid carcinoma BCPAP cells. *Food & Function, 7*(1), 315–325. doi:10.1039/C5FO00681C PMID:26442630

Zhang, L., Cheng, X., Gao, Y., Zheng, J., Xu, Q., Sun, Y., Guan, H., Yu, H., & Sun, Z. (2015). Apigenin induces autophagic cell death in human papillary thyroid carcinoma BCPAP cells. *Food & Function*, *6*(11), 3464–3472. doi:10.1039/C5FO00671F PMID:26292725

Zhang, L., Cheng, X., Xu, S., Bao, J., & Yu, H. (2018). Curcumin induces endoplasmic reticulum stress-associated apoptosis in human papillary thyroid carcinoma BCPAP cells via disruption of intracellular calcium homeostasis. *Medicine*, *97*(24), e11095. doi:10.1097/MD.0000000000011095 PMID:29901626

Zhang, Y., Li, Y., Mao, X., Yan, C., Guo, X., Guo, Q., Liu, Z., Song, Z., & Lin, N. (2016). Thyroid hormone synthesis: A potential target of a Chinese herbal formula Haizao Yuhu Decoction acting on iodine-deficient goiter. *Oncotarget*, *7*(32), 51699–51712. doi:10.18632/oncotarget.10329 PMID:27384475

Zhang, Y., Sun, B., Huang, Z., Zhao, D. W., & Zeng, Q. (2018). Shikonin Inhibites Migration and Invasion of Thyroid Cancer Cells by Downregulating DNMT1. *Medical Science Monitor*, *24*, 661–670. doi:10.12659/MSM.908381 PMID:29389913

Zou, X., Liang, J., Sun, J., Hu, X., Lei, L., Wu, D., & Liu, L. (2016). Allicin sensitizes hepatocellular cancer cells to anti-tumor activity of 5-fluorouracil through ROS-mediated mitochondrial pathway. *Journal of Pharmacological Sciences*, *131*(4), 233–240. doi:10.1016/j.jphs.2016.04.017 PMID:27177453

Chapter 12
Nutraceuticals:
An Approach Towards Safe and Effective Medications

Shalini Singh
University of Lucknow, India

Pushkar Singh Rawat
https://orcid.org/0000-0002-8679-5603
University of Lucknow, India

ABSTRACT

Nutraceutical is a unique grouping of two words, nutrition and pharmaceutical, which describes a food or food product that regularly provides health and medical benefits, including the prevention and cure of various diseases. Chemically, nutraceuticals contain a range of bioactive elements classified as polyphenolic compounds, isoprenoids, minerals, amino acid derivatives, carbohydrate derivatives, fatty acids and structural lipids, prebiotics, and probiotics. The majority of nutraceuticals have numerous beneficial and healing effects without any kind of side effects that keep their attention towards the consumer. The demand for nutraceuticals was increasing slowly due to a high risk of toxicity or adverse effect of drugs. Consequently, in such circumstances, nutraceuticals prove a safer approach for health management. Meanwhile, a few challenges were hindering the fame of nutraceuticals like lack of standardization and awareness, high pricing, marketing, and supply. This chapter mainly emphasizes the recent role of nutraceuticals in human health and its status in other nations.

1. INTRODUCTION

Scarcity of healthier foods was expanding gradually due to the population, pollution and adulteration in food items. All these factors create a great risk to human health and vegetation and raising a question in front of us how can we riddle out from this problem? The way of using grains has also changed with evolution in time. Natural foods have resulted in the deficiency of essential nutrients in human beings specifically due to modification in traditional methods used such as polishing of grains leads to loss of

DOI: 10.4018/978-1-7998-4808-0.ch012

essential nutrients and fibers that are very much required for the proper functioning of a healthy body. Along with this, the overall consumption of refined sugar and processed foods has also increased.

But somehow people have understood that along with taste, convenience, and value, health is an important subject of concern. Therefore the value of Nutritive food items has become a great concern. People in the developed world are aware of the fact that processed food is nutritionally deficient, so they would take vitamin supplements to compensate for the loss of nutrients. Now the trend has changed. Rather than going for pharmaceuticals, people prefer natural substitutes such as herbals. Ayurveda is the ancient Indian science of medicine, emphasis is given to the role of nutrition in health and disease. The term "nutraceutical," derived from the terms nutrition and pharmaceutical was coined in 1989 by Dr Stephen De Felice, (Chairman of the Foundation for Innovation in Medicine). It was the first time used in the United States to describe foods or food components that have the potential to cure specific disease conditions (Gupta et al., 2010). The term is intended for a nutritional supplement that is sold with the intent to treat or prevent disease and does not have any regulatory definition. Hence, a "nutraceutical" is any constituent that may be considered a food or part of food which provides medical or health benefits, encompassing, prevention and treatment of diseases. Isolated nutrients, dietary supplements, and diets to genetically engineered "designer" foods, herbal products, and processed foods such as cereals, soups, and beverages may be also included under the canopy of the term nutraceuticals (Nasri et al., 2014; Singh & Sinha, 2012).

Figure 1. The major properties of nutraceuticals

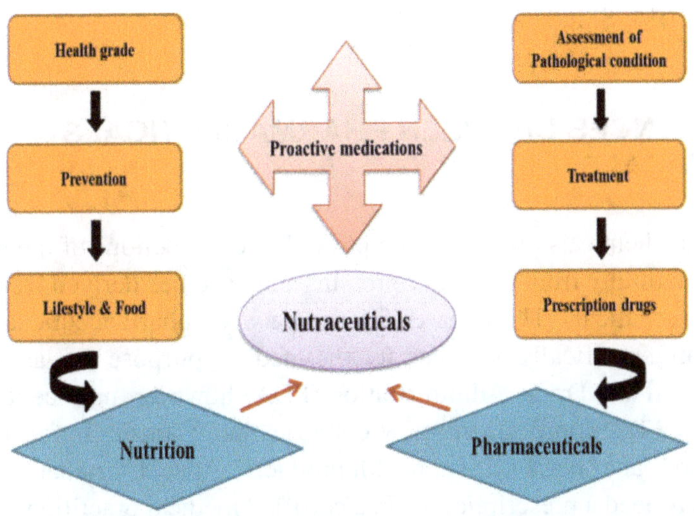

2. CONCEPT OF NUTRACEUTICALS

The nutrition required for health + Pharmaceuticals remedy for sickness/injury = Nutraceuticals preventative medical approach

The concept of a nutraceutical is confirmed to have a physiological benefit and provide protection against chronic disease (Zhao, 2008). A variety of products may be ranging in this thought is also included in the functional food category. However functional food is food where a new ingredient(s) (or more of an existing ingredient) has been added to food and the new product has an additional function (often one related to health promotion or disease prevention) (Gupta et al., 2010). With recent developments in cellular-level nutraceutical agents, researchers and medical practitioners are developing templates for integrating and assessing information from clinical studies on complementary and alternative therapies into responsible medical practices (Prietl et al., 2013). Peoples from all over the world participating in a debate on the regulation of traditional medicines from other systems of medicines like '*Ayurved, Unani, Siddha* and *Homeopathy, Chinese*', all of which have a herbal or natural source of origin. There are many civilizations like Indians, Egyptians, Chinese and Sumerians have provided evidence suggesting that foods can be effectively used as medicine to treat and prevent disease. Ayurveda, the 5000-year-old ancient Indian health science, mentioned the benefits of food for the therapeutic purpose (Wildman, 2016). The father of Western medicine, Hippocrates stated that 'Let food be your medicine and medicine be your food' to show the bonding between food and its impact over health. The popularity of Indian Ayurvedic therapies enhances the export opportunities for formulations based on ashwagandha, ginger, haldi, tulsi etc. Vitamin D will see the fastest growth in demand due to increasing clinical evidence of swine flu, cancer, and other preventive medicine benefits (Prietl et al., 2013). Global demand for herbal and non-herbal extracts is increasing continuously. Green tea for weight loss, acute kidney injury and cancer treatment, while *Ginkgo biloba* for improving cognitive function, has been widely used as nutraceuticals (Nasri et al., 2014; Shinde et al., 2014).

3. MAJOR DIFFERENCES BETWEEN PHARMACEUTICALS AND NUTRACEUTICALS

Pharmaceuticals are the chemicals that affect the physiological functions of the human body. Whereas the chemicals derived naturally from plants, or proteins and vaccines derived from animal sources may have referred to as nutraceuticals. The main difference between pharmaceuticals and nutraceuticals is that pharmaceuticals are specifically designed for the medical purpose and are subjected to the matter of approval from Food and Drugs Administration (FDA) however; nutraceuticals may do not need medical supervision, or FDA approval. In many countries like Canada nutraceuticals can be divided between 'functional food' and 'nutraceutical health products'. Apart from that as per the rules of FDA, pharmaceutical products need a prescription from a certified medical practitioner for purchase whereas selection of nutraceutical products is completely dependent on the individual.

4. NEED OF NUTRACEUTICALS

Peoples have started to take initiatives towards the use of nutraceuticals in their daily life due to a large number of health impacts. Likewise, one such problem is chronic diseases with reduced healing substitutes. Another fact stated that a greater number of the population are trying to plank out the effects of ageing and wish for improved medicine. However, the public belief in natural products is another reason for the increased demand for nutraceuticals.

5. CLASSIFICATION OF NUTRACEUTICALS

Nutraceuticals can be classified based on either their chemical nature, the type of food items or whether they are traditional or not (Patil, 2011).

1. *Based on the chemical constituents*: phenols, alkaloids, fibres, fatty acid, minerals, terpenes, etc.
2. *Traditional/nontraditional*: fruits, vegetables, fortified juices.
3. *Type of food items*: vitamins, minerals, dairy products.

Table 1. The constituents of nutraceuticals with examples

Compounds and its types	
Terpenoids	Carotenoids, saponins, tocotrienols, tocopherols, simple terpenes.
Phenolics	Coumarins, tannins, lignin, anthocyanins, isoflavones, flavones, flavonols
Protein and amino acid	Amino acids, allyl-S compound, capsaicinoids, isothiocyanates, indoles, folate, choline and yeast extract
Carbohydrate and its derivatives	Ascorbic acid, oligosaccharides, non-starch polysaccharides
Fatty acids and structural lipids	n-3 polyunsaturated fatty acid (n-3 PUFA), Conjugated linoleic acid (CLA), monounsaturated fatty acid (MUFA), sphingolipids, lecithin
Minerals	Ca, Se, K, Cu, Zn.
Microbials based products	Probiotics, yeast

6. FUNCTIONAL FOOD AS NUTRACEUTICAL COMPONENT

Functional food is the broad term which is especially used for such kind of food that has been associated with health benefits. The Institute of Medicine's Food and Nutrition Board (in the United States) has defined functional food as "any food and food ingredients that may provide a health benefit beyond the traditional nutrition that it contains". Whereas in the Japanese literature the term 'functional food' was introduced in 1984 to differentiate between a tertiary function of food from the primary and secondary function of nutrition. Functional food can be obtained from either plant or animal sources. It was thought that it is directly involved in modifying several physiological systems like digestive, immune, nervous, endocrine and circulatory systems (Aronson, 2017).

Table 2. Based on the literature survey and research findings, functional food component and its health benefits listed in Table 2 (Aronson, 2017; Li et al., 2003; Wildman, 2016)

Active Constituent	Source	Potential benefits
Dietary Fibers		
β-Glucan	Oats, barley	Reduce the risk of cardiovascular disease protect against heart disease and some cancers; lower LDL and total cholesterol fiber
Soluble fiber	Psyllium	Reduce the risk of cardiovascular disease; protect against heart disease and some cancers; lower LDL and total cholesterol
Insoluble fiber	Wheat bran	Reduce the risk of breast or colon cancer
Carotenoids		
α-Carotene/β-carotene	Carrots, fruits, vegetables	Neutralize free radicals, which may cause damage to cell
Lycopene	Tomato products (ketchup, sauces)	Reduce the risk of prostate cancer
Lutein	Green vegetables	Reduce the risk of muscular degeneration
Fatty Acids		
Conjugated linoleic acid	Salmon and other fish Oils, Cheese, meat products	Improve body composition; decrease the risk of certain cancers
Long-chain omega-3 fatty acids-DHA/EPA		Reduce the risk of cardiovascular disease Improve mental, visual functions
Phenolics		
Tannins (proanthocyanidins)	Cranberries and its products, cocoa, chocolate	Improve urinary tract health; reduce risk of cardiovascular disease, anticancer (Aronson, 2017)
Anthocyanidins	Fruits	Neutralize free radicals; reduce risk of cancer
Catechins	Tea	Neutralize free radicals; reduce risk of cancer
Flavones	Fruits/vegetables	Neutralize free radicals; reduce risk of cancer
Flavanones	Citrus fruit	Neutralize free radicals; reduce risk of cancer
Lignans	Flax, vegetables, rye,	Prevention of cancer, renal failure
Prebiotics/ Probiotics		
Lactobacillus Lactobacillus	Yogurt, other dairies	Improve the quality of intestinal microflora, gastrointestinal health
Fructo-oligosaccharides	Jerusalem artichokes, shallots, onion powder	Improve the quality of intestinal microflora, Gastrointestinal health
Stanly ester **Plant Sterols**		
tanol ester Corn, soy, wheat, wood oils Lower blood cholesterol levels by inhibiting cholesterol absorption Stanol ester Corn, soy, wheat, wood oils Lower blood cholesterol levels by inhibiting cholesterol absorption Stanol ester Corn, soy, wheat, wood oils Lower blood cholesterol levels by inhibiting cholesterol absorption Stanol ester Corn, soy, wheat, wood oils Lower blood cholesterol levels by inhibiting cholesterol absorption Stanol ester Corn, soy, wheat, wood oils Lower blood cholesterol levels by inhibiting cholesterol absorption Stanol ester Corn, soy, wheat, wood oils Lower blood cholesterol levels by inhibiting cholesterol absorption Stanol ester Corn, soy, wheat, wood oils Lower blood cholesterol levels by inhibiting cholesterol absorption Stanol ester Corn, soy, wheat, wood oils Lower blood cholesterol levels by inhibiting cholesterol absorption Stanol ester	Corn, soy, wheat, wood oil	Lower blood cholesterol levels by inhibiting cholesterol absorption lower blood cholesterol level by inhibiting cholesterol absorption
Soy phytoestrogens		
Soflavones: Daidzein, genistein	Soybeans and soy-based foods	Menopause symptoms, such as hot flashes; protect against heart disease and some cancers; lower LDL and total cholesterol

Functional foods are enriched during processing and then marketed as providing some benefit to consumers. Sometimes, additional complementary nutrients are added, such as vitamin D to milk or Iodine to table salt (Zhang et al., 2015). Health Canada defines functional foods as "ordinary food that has components or ingredients added to give it a specific medical or physiological benefit, other than a purely nutritional effect. In Japan entirely functional foods must meet three established requirements: foods should be (Hardy, 2000),

(1) Present in their naturally occurring form, instead of a capsule, tablet, or powder;
(2) Consumed in the diet as often as daily;
(3) Should regulate a biological process in hopes of preventing or controlling the disease.

PHYTOCHEMICALS

Phytochemicals also prove as one of the important components of nutraceuticals. These bioactive constituents sustain and promote health and occur at the intersection of food and pharmaceutical industries. Rather than, phytochemicals used as cofactors as well as inhibitors in a diverse group of enzymatic reactions. They play specific pharmacological effects in human healths as an anti-inflammatory, anti-allergic, antioxidants, antibacterial, antifungal, chemopreventive, hepatoprotective, neuroprotective, antiaging, anticancer and many other roles.

BACTERIAL AND ALGAL NUTRACEUTICAL PRODUCTS

Bacterial Nutraceuticals have been recognised for the physiological benefit of human health. Consumption of nutraceuticals shows a major claim in the reduction of certain chronic diseases e.g. diabetes, hypertension, immune-regulatory diseases etc. In general, antioxidants act as the major nutrient constituents in bacterial nutraceuticals which are known to be effective in the treatment and prevention of an extensive range of chronic illnesses. Some examples are phenolics or more accurately described as polyphenolics such as tocopherols and tocotrienols. Polyphenol antioxidants are generally believed to be contributory in combating oxidative stress in humans, a process associated with some cardiovascular and some neurodegenerative diseases. Lactic acid bacteria (LAB) are used all over the world in several industrial food fermentations (Siezen et al., 2002). LAB contributes to the fermentation processes primarily by the formation of lactic acid from the available carbon source that results in rapid acidification of the food raw-material. Although, Lactic acid bacteria can add some other characteristics in food like flavour, texture and nutrition.

Algae Nutraceuticals

1) Single Cell Protein: Spirullina, Chlorella.
2) Polyunsaturated fatty acids: Docosahexaenoic acid (DHA), Eicosapentaenoic Acid (EPA)
3) Carotenoids and Pigments: β-carotene, Lycopene, Lutein, Phycocyanin, Zeaxanthin, Fucoxanthin

Table 3. List of some important phytochemicals and their health benefits (Prakash & Gupta, 2009)

S.No	Phytochemical	Plant source	Benefit on Health
1	α linolenic acid	Flaxseed	Cancer prevention diminishes the risk of Coronary heart disease
2	Allicin	Onion, Garlic	Antifungal, antibacterial, hepatoprotective, antihypertensive, neuroprotective, hypolipidemic, anti-inflammatory, chemo-preventive, anticancer (Borghi & Cicero, 2017; Rafieian-kopaei, 2012)
3	Anthocyanins	Orange, purple corn, Cherry, Blackberry, raspberry, red grapes.	Anti-allergic, antioxidant, anti-inflammatory
4	Apigenin	Apple, artichoke, basil, celery, Cherry, grapes, nuts, parsley	Anti-inflammatory, antioxidant, chemo-preventive, induce apoptosis, inhibits ovarian and breast cancer, antispasmodic
5	Caffeic acid	Pear, basil oregano, artichoke	Anti-fatigue, anti-stress, anti-inflammatory
6	Carotene	Carrots, green leafy, pumpkin, red-orange, yellow vegetables	Anti-carcinogenic, enhances cytokines IL-1 secretion, TNF-α, cornea protection against UV light, stimulate DNA repair enzymes
7	Catechins	Tea	CNS stimulant, antioxidant, diuretic
8	Gallic acid	Strawberry, Mango, soy, tea	Anti-diabetic, antioxidant, anti-leukemia, anti-neoplastic, anti-inflammatory (Rafieian-kopaei, 2012)
9	Curcumin	Turmeric	Anti-inflammatory, chemo-preventive, antioxidant, antihypertensive (Rafieian-Kopaei et al., 2014)
10	Genistein	Alfa-alfa sprout, red clover	Phytoestrogen, antioxidant
11	Diosgenin	Fenugreek Seed	Hypo-lipidemic
12	Ferulic acid	Oats, rice, pineapple, peanut, orange	Protect against bone degeneration, menopausal symptoms, anticancer
13	Ellagic acid	cranberry, grapes, pecans, pomegranates, raspberry, strawberry, walnuts	Anticancer, antioxidant
14	Epigallocatechin gallate (EGCG)	Green tea	Antioxidant, anti-inflammatory (Forni et al., 2019; Niu et al., 2013)
15	Quercetin	Onion, grapes, berries, cherries, broccoli, citrus fruits	Antioxidant, antihypertensive, antiobesity, antihypercholesterolemic, antiatherosclerotic, anti-inflammatory (Anand David et al., 2016)

7. A VIEW TOWARDS CATEGORY OF FOOD PRODUCTS UNDER REGULATIONS

1) **Foods for Special Dietary Uses** (FSDU) (labelling regulated under NLEA, Nutrition Labelling & Education Act, of 1990). This component includes hypoallergenic foods, weight reduction foods, diabetics' foods, reduced-sodium foods and various infant formulas.
2) **Dietary Supplements** (Labelling Regulated Under DSHEA, Dietary Supplement Health and Education Act of 1994). Any product (other than tobacco) intended to supplement the diet that contains one or more of the following ingredients: a vitamin, mineral, herb or other botanical, an amino acid; a concentrate, metabolite, constituent, extract or combination of any of these ingredients. The classification of dietary supplements can be described under three major classes.
   a. Essential nutrients (includes vitamins, minerals, amino acids)

Table 4. Illustrates a major list of bacteria involved in the field of nutraceuticals. Apart from this algae have also played a potential role in the formation of nutraceutical products

Name of bacteria	Functional role	References
Streptococcus thermophilus	Provide folate in yoghurt.	(Kleerebezem et al., 2002)
Lactococcus lactis	Provide folate in cheese and butter (milk). Able to produce and excrete riboflavin.	(Siezen et al., 2002)
Lactobacillus reuteri	Involved in the production of a neutraceutical which is a cobalamin-like substance, especially in the presence of glycerol which is converted in this organisms to propanediol (and to hydroxypropionaldehyde, reuterin) through a cobalamin dependent enzymatic step.	(Taranto et al., 2003)
Leuconostoc mesenteroides	Ability to produce mannitol in the fermentation of fructose	(Soetaert et al., 1995)
Lactobacillus plantarum	Ability to produce sorbitol.	(Van Rooijen et al., 1991)
Lactobacillus casei and Bifidobacteria	Used as probiotics.	(Hickson et al., 2007)
Lactobacillus rhamnosus	Reduce the risk of antibiotic-associated diarrhoea; improve stool consistency during antibiotic therapy.	(Blaabjerg et al., 2017)
Lactobacillus delbrueckii	Provide the ability to tolerate more lactose.	(Silanikove et al., 2015)
Bifidobacterium infantis	Improved some symptoms of irritable bowel syndrome in women.	(Whorwell et al., 2006)
Lactobacillus	Play a role in immune function, cancer, antibiotic-associated diarrhoea, travellers' diarrhoea, pediatric diarrhoea, inflammatory bowel disease and irritable bowel syndrome.	(Siezen et al., 2002)

b. Herbal preparations
c. Glandular extracts

A supplement must be in "dosage forms such as capsules, tablets, liquids, powders, or soft gels and may not be represented as a conventional food or as a sole item of a meal or the diet" (Patil, 2011). Besides, dietary supplements must be labelled as supplements.

Dietary supplements and its functional role in the prevention of listed diseases are the following:

1. Folic acid with decreased risk of neural defects
2. Calcium with a lower risk of osteoporosis
3. Psyllium seed husk, soy protein, Omega-3 fatty acids, vitamin B (folic acid, B6, and B12) related to heart disease
4. The antioxidants, vitamin A, C, and E, are among the most commonly known nutrients which, in general, may be useful in the prevention of cancer and cerebrovascular disease.
5. The combination of vitamin E, C, and β-carotene has been useful in reducing LDL oxidation and subsequent atherosclerosis.
6. Combination of vitamin E, C, and β-carotene work synergistically to prevent oxidation of LDL in the following manner (Ng et al., 2008). Vitamin C scavenges aqueous radicals and regenerates α-tocopherol from the tocopheroxyl radical species;

a) Vitamin E, in the form of α-tocopherol, protects polyunsaturated fatty acids within the LDL particle, reduces platelet adhesion and inhibits smooth muscle cell proliferation and protein kinase C activity; and

b) β-carotene provides reserve antioxidant activity, especially in the arterial wall where low partial pressures of oxygen are found.

c) Supplementation with vitamin C may be beneficial in the management of asthma patients, and high dietary intake of vitamin E may prevent Parkinson's disease.

    3) **Medical Foods** (Exempt from most NLEA and DSHEA Labeling Requirements) fall under narrower scope than FSDU. Panaxytriol is a nutraceutical-based active constituent of Korean red ginseng and is reported to exhibit potent anti-tumour properties. Its activity may be in part due to its induction of phase II chemoprotective enzymes. Its unique properties may have important implications in cancer therapeutics (Ng et al., 2008).

8. NUTRACEUTICALS ROLE IN THE TREATMENT OF DISEASES

1) Role of Nutraceuticals in Neurological Diseases

Alzheimer's disease (AD) is the most common form of dementia that results in the degeneration of brain cells. There is no proper treatment for the disease and eventually leads to fatality. Most often, AD is diagnosed in people over 65 years of age, although the less-prevalent early-onset Alzheimer's can occur much earlier. There were 26.6 million patients worldwide in 2006 and is predicted to affect 1 in 85 people globally by 2050. Women are more affected in comparison to men, at a ratio of almost 2:1. Some evidence suggested that oxidative stress might be related to a number of neurodegenerative disorders including AD, Parkinson's disease (PD), and Huntington's disease (HD) (Klatte et al., 2003). Oxidative stress is enhanced through the ageing process along with the deficiency of dietary antioxidants. A vast number of studies have found a link between high dietary antioxidant intake and a reduced risk of AD which is actually vital because preventing disease is significantly easier than treating it. Antioxidants are found to be crucial in the treatment of almost all diseases because most chronic diseases carry an excessive promise of oxidative stress. Nutraceutical antioxidants such as curcumin, lutein, lycopene, turmerin and β-carotene may exert positive effects on specific diseases by combating oxidative stress (Glenville, 2006). Other research data showed that natural (herbal) therapeutics with anti-oxidative and anti-inflammatory plays an important role in neurons protection. Among these, the most promising are withanolides, caffeine, resveratrol, trigonelline, shogaol, curcumin, baicalein, wogonin, ginsenosides, tanshinones, picrosides, parthenolide, cannabinoids, Devil's claw and white willow bark, including Chinese formulations Renshen Shouwu and Shengmai San (Parvez, 2017). Several research papers presenting the encouraging effects of different nutraceutical plants such as *Zizyphus jujube*, *Lavandula officinalis* on AD, learning or memory (Nasri et al., 2014). An on-going study with vitamin E decelerates the progression of AD was reported. Another interesting neurological disease i.e. PD also related to the brain disorder that affects nerve damage in certain regions of the brain triggering muscle rigidity, shaking, and difficult walking (Losso, 2003). Research from Canada showed that vitamin E in food may be protective against Parkinson's disease (Anwar et al., 2007). Creatine appeared to modify Parkinson's disease features as measured by a decline in the clinical signs (Brower, 2005). Studies on glutathione are also focused out that help to determine its effect on nerve and its influence as an antioxidant. The appropriate long-term dosing, side-effects and the most effective method of administration are not yet clear. Nutritional supplements have shown some promising results in preliminary studies, it is important to remember that there is not sufficient scientific data to recommend them for Parkinson's disease at present. The patients should be cautioned that over-the-counter medications do have side effects and interactions with other drugs and are also expensive.

2) Role of Nutraceuticals in Cardiovascular Diseases

Over worldwide, the frequency of cardiovascular diseases CVD and the studies in this area is growing day by day. CVD is a term which is used for disorders of the heart and blood vessels and includes coronary heart disease (heart attack), peripheral vascular diseases, cerebrovascular disease (stroke), hypertension, heart failure, and so on. It is supposed that low consumption of vegetables and fruits are related to a high death rate in case of CVD whereas, the majority of the CVD is preventable also. Many studies have reported a protective role for a diet rich in vegetables and fruits against CVD (Bucher et al., 2002). Nutraceuticals in the form of vitamins, minerals, antioxidants, dietary fibres and omega-3 polyunsaturated fatty acids (n−3 PUFAs) together with physical exercise are recommended for prevention and treatment of CVD (Leray et al., 2001). Flavonoids are widely distributed in vegetables, onion, endives, cruciferous, grapefruits, apples, cherries, pomegranate, berries, black grapes, and red wine, and are available as flavones, flavanones and flavonols, playing a major role in prevention and curing the CVD (Sanders, 1994). Orange juice is one of the instances because the pulp of orange is a rich source of flavonoids (Iriti & Faoro, 2006). Hesperidin is a flavanone glycoside which is classified as a citrus bioflavonoid. *Citrus sinensis* and tangelos are the richest dietary sources of hesperidin. The peel and membranous parts of lemons and oranges have known for the highest hesperidin concentrations. Hesperidin is used for the treatment of venous insufficiency and haemorrhoids (Garg et al., 2001). However, herbal medications are generally employed for clinical purposes like in the treatment of cardiovascular conditions. As compared to conventional medications, herbal medications do not need clinical studies before their marketing or formal approval from regulatory agencies, and for this reason, their efficacy and safety are rarely proven. Herbal medications have become more prominent in cardiovascular medicine in contrast with the various medical specialities. The effects of the most promising compounds have undergone systematic evaluations as reported in the case of digoxin and digitoxin, derived from *Digitalis lanata* and *Digitalis purpurea*; reserpine, derived from *Rauwolfia serpentina* and originally used for the treatment of psychosis; and acetylsalicylic acid (aspirin), extracted from willow bark. Various studies reported some herbal medicines with a possible indication for the treatment of the following cardiovascular conditions: heart failure, thromboembolic disorders, coronary artery disease, hypertension, dyslipidemia and peripheral artery diseases. The majority of the herbal medications are including Asian ginseng (Panax ginseng), astragalus (Astragalus membranaceous), flaxseed oil (*Linum usitatissimum*), garlic (*Allium sativum*), ginkgo (*Ginkgo biloba*), grape (*Vitis vinifera*) seeds, green tea (*Camellia sinensis*), hawthorn (*Crataegus*), milk thistle (*Silybum marianum*), and soy (*Glycine max*). Flavonoid intake was significantly inversely associated with mortality from coronary heart disease and the incidence of myocardial infarction. Flavonoids in regularly consumed foods may reduce the risk of death from coronary heart disease, especially in elderly people. The rhizome of *Zingiber officinalis* is a common spice for various foods and beverages. It has a long history of medicinal use and has a positive effect on CVD. Ginger has potent antioxidant and anti-inflammatory activities and recently it has been recommended for various diseases including hypertension and palpitation. This plant has a good protective effect on the toxicity of synthetic drugs, too. Phytosterols compete with dietary cholesterol by blocking the uptake as well as facilitating its excretion from the body. Hence, they have the potential to reduce the morbidity and mortality of CVD (Bucher et al., 2002). Phytosterols occur in most plant species and although green and yellow vegetables contain significant amounts of sterols, their seeds concentrate them. Buckwheat seeds possess phytosterols, flavonoids, flavones, proteins and thiamine-binding proteins, etc., Buckwheat proteins lower blood cholesterol and hypertension.

Dietary fibres have also cholesterol-lowering property with beneficial effects in the prevention and alleviation of CVD and diabetes (Anderson et al., 2009; Glore et al., 1994). Fatty acids of the omega-3 series (n−3 fatty acids) present in fish are dietary components affecting plasma lipids and the CVD, like arrhythmias (Leray et al., 2001; Stoll et al., 1999). Octacosanol, present in whole grains, fruits and leaves of many plants, has lipid-lowering property, with no side-effects.

3) Role of Nutraceuticals in Cancer

Cancer has appeared as a main public health problem in developing as well as developed countries. As per the World Cancer Report, the cancer rates are increasing and it would be 15 million new cases in the year 2020 i.e., a rise in 50%. A healthy lifestyle and diet can help in the prevention of cancer. Plants rich in daidzein, biochanin, isoflavones and genistein, also prevent prostate cancer cell growth. Natural and dietary nutraceuticals may have anticancer activities, like carotenoids that have the ability to stimulate gap-junctional communication, in vitro, through amplification of "connexin 43", or flavonoids, which modulate phase I and II xenobiotic detoxification, or vitamin E that inhibits protein kinase C, a critical enzyme in tumour progression of some types of cancer (Aggarwal et al., 2010). Due to the unsaturated nature of lycopene, it is reflected as a potent antioxidant and a singlet oxygen quencher. Lycopene concentrates in the prostate, testes, skin and adrenal where it protects against cancer. The association between carotenoids and cancer prevention heightened the importance of vegetable and fruits in the human diet. Lycopene contained vegetables and fruits exert cancer-protective effect via a decrease in oxidative stress and damage to DNA. Lycopene is one of the main carotenoids and is found exclusively in tomatoes, guava, pink grapefruit, watermelon and papaya. Antioxidant activity of Beta-carotene (β-carotene) has strong potential to inhibit cancer and other diseases. Alpha-carotene has also 50–54% of the antioxidant activity of β-carotene, while epsilon carotene has 42–50% of the antioxidant activity. β-carotene found in yellow, orange, and green leafy vegetables and fruits such as tomatoes, lettuce, oranges, sweet potatoes, broccoli, cantaloupe, carrots, spinach, and winter squash have anticancer activity (Sreejayan & Rao, 1994). Chronic inflammation is associated with high cancer risk. Chronic inflammation is also associated with immune-suppression, which is a risk factor for cancer. Ginseng is an example of an anti-inflammatory molecule that targets many of the key players in the inflammation-to-cancer sequence. Nowadays, phytochemicals with cancer-preventive properties have been on high attention. Chemopreventive components in fruits and vegetables, among other beneficial health effects, have potential anticarcinogenic and antimutagenic activities (Bucher et al., 2002). A broad range of phytopharmaceuticals with a claimed hormonal activity, called "phytoestrogens," is recommended for the prevention of prostate and breast cancers (Limer & Speirs, 2004). Citrus fruit flavonoids are able to protect against cancer by acting as antioxidants. Soy foods are a unique dietary source of isoflavones, the polyphenolic phytochemicals exemplified by epigallocatechin gallate from tea, curcumin from curry and soya isoflavones possess cancer chemopreventive properties. Soybean seems to offer protection against breast, uterine, lung, colorectal, and prostate cancers. Saponins are reported to possess antimutagenic and antitumor activities and might lower the risk of human cancers, by preventing cancer cells from growing. Saponins are phytochemicals which can be found in peas, soybeans, and some herbs with names indicating foaming properties such as soapberry, soapwort and soapbark. They are also present in tomatoes, potatoes, alfalfa, spinach, and clover. Commercial saponins are extracted mainly from *Yucca schidigera* and *Quillaja saponaria* (Li et al., 2003). Tannins also scavenge harmful free radicals and detoxify carcinogens. Tannins present in grapes, lentils, tea, blackberries, blueberries and cranberries are a proven anticarcinogen is used in alternative medicine and to prevent cancer. Ellagic acid, present in walnuts, pecans, strawberries, cranberries, pomegranates and red raspberry seeds, is an anticancer agent (Sahu, 2002). Pectin is a soluble fibre found in apples has been shown to prevent prostate cancer metastasis by inhibiting the cancer cells from adhering to other cells in the body. Several studies have shown that pectin decreases serum cholesterol levels. Naturally occurring phenolic acid derivatives are reported to possess potential anticancer properties. Phenolic compounds such as curcumin, gallic acids, ferulic and caffeic acid are reported to possess anticancer activity (Nasri et al., 2014). Glucosinolates and their hydrolysis products, including indoles and isothiocyanates, and high intake of cruciferous vegetables have been associated with a lower risk of colorectal and lung cancer. Bio-transformation products of glucosinolates include dithiol thiones, isothiocyanates, and sulforaphane. They block the enzymes that promote tumour growth, particularly in liver, colon, lung, breast, stomach and oesophagus. The sulphur compounds, in garlic, have been found to boost the immune system and reduce atherogenesis and platelet stickiness and cancer. The use of garlic as an anticancer agent has long been established. The allyl sulfur compounds derived from garlic have also important anti-proliferate activity against human cancers. Diallyl sulfide and diallyl disulfide induce apoptosis in non-small cell lung cancer cells and in prostate cancer and breast cancer cells. With our increased understanding of the chemistry and biology of nutraceuticals, the nutraceutical research will shift more into the area of chemoprevention. Sulforaphane, rich in broccoli is a potent phase 2 enzyme inducer. It produces D-glucarolactone, a significant inhibitor of breast cancer. Sulforaphane is an antioxidant and stimulator of natural detoxifying enzymes. Sulforaphane has been reported to reduce the risk of breast cancer and prostate cancer (Asadi-Samani et al., 2014; Tamadon et al., 2013). Curcumin is a polyphenol derived from the plant *Curcuma longa*, commonly called turmeric. Curcumin has been reported to possess antioxidative, anticarcinogenic, and anti-inflammatory properties (Sreejayan & Rao, 1994). Consumption of fruits and vegetables having cysteine, glutathione, selenium, Vitamin E, Vitamin C, lycopene, and various phytochemicals elevates the levels of antioxidative capacity. However, more investigations are needed to determine their beneficial effects in cancer prevention or treatment. Large scale clinical trials suggest that some agents such as green tea, Vitamins D and E, selenium, lycopene, soy, anti-inflammatory and inhibitors of 5 α -reductase are effective in preventing prostate cancer. Cancer was not prevented by β-carotene, N-acetylcysteine, α-tocopherol, retinol, retinyl palmitate, or isotretinoin in smokers. On-going trials may help define new avenues for chemoprevention. Several studies have shown the values of alternative and complementary medicine as an adjuvant to chemotherapy or radiotherapy. In the case of prostate cancer patients, complementary therapy is one of the reliable and useful supportive measures. Majority of the studies have shown a preventive role for nutraceuticals in cancer, however, more elaborate studies are needed.

9. REVERSE PHARMACOLOGY

In recent times, some of the important visionaries and scientists have stimulated the concept of 'Reverse Pharmacology' in India by using research strategies linked with *Ayurvedic* drugs (Patwardhan et al., 2008). In other way the nutraceutical products i.e. several phytoconstituents lead to the drug discovery by using reverse pharmacology. Here the traditional knowledge inspired reverse pharmacology and reversing the routine "laboratory to clinic" progress of discovery into "clinics to laboratories". Consequently 'Reverse Pharmacology' proved successful in the development of formulations many natural drugs like 1) *Saraca indica* for dysfunctional uterine bleeding 2) *Panchvalkal (5 plants combination)* for burns and infected wounds 3) *Commiphora mukul* in Phase I trial in volunteers 4) Volatile essential oils of spices for antimicrobial activity 5) *Mucuna pruriens* for Parkinson's disease 6) *Curcuma longa* for cancer prevention and urticaria 7) *Commiphora mukul* for rheumatoid arthritis 8) *Arogyawardhani,* the *Picrorrhiza kurroa* for hepatitis and 9) *Rubia cordifolia* for eczema and many more. The approach towards "Reverse Pharmacology" seems to have been established all over the world. Willcox et al. have reviewed the development of anti-malarial drugs by using Reverse Pharmacology approach from herbal sources (Willcox et al., 2011). Nutraceutical antioxidants and other compounds like Aged garlic extract, Angelica gigas, curcumin, Cinnamon, lutein, Piperine, lutein, lycopene, Ursolic acid, turmerin, ginger and β-carotene have a positive effect on specific diseases by combating oxidative stress (Wildman, 2016; Borghi & Cicero, 2017). These growing trends in nutraceutical practices are because of the ability of these compounds to postpone the development of dementias such as Alzheimer's disease (Glenville, 2006).

10. STATUS OF NUTRACEUTICALS IN INDIA AS COMPARED TO OTHER COUNTRIES

India is a developing country therefore we do not get so much success in the awareness program of nutraceutical products concerning other countries. But the food habits of Indian people include many compounds of nutraceuticals like ginger, turmeric, aloe vera, tulsi etc. With such approaches in 2005, several committees like Standing Committee of Parliament on Agriculture have highlighted the requirement for a single regulatory body and integrated law. This result to signed and include the Indian Food Safety Standard Bill 2005 into the law that emerges as a major impact on the Indian food processing industry. The two main objectives of the Indian Food Safety and Standard Act which came into enforcement in 2006: to introduce a single act relating to food and to provide for the scientific development of the food processing industry. The Food Safety and Standard Act 2006 comprise 12 chapters in which chapter IV, Article 22 of the act addresses nutraceutical, functional food, and dietary supplements. With that it regulates these products such that anyone can manufacture, sell, or distribute or import these products. The products include novel foods, genetically modified articles of food, irradiated food, organic food and food for special dietary uses, functional food, nutraceuticals and health supplements, whereas Articles 23 and 24 address the packaging and labelling of food and restriction of advertisement regarding foods (Prakash & Gupta, 2009). The Food Safety and Standard Act still need to be considerably more functional with an organization and appropriate leadership is required to match the international standards of the United States and Europe. A significant augmentation is necessary for the act to have a large impact on the Indian functional food and nutraceutical industry like the Dietary Supplements Health Education Act (DSHEA) 1994 has had on the dietary supplement industry in the United States.

The passing of this act in India is a significant first step, but much more has to happen to eliminate the confusing overlap with old laws and regulations. Yet, in India, functional foods/nutraceutical are not categorized separately as in the United States, Europe and Japan. And also, the concept of functional food has somewhat different connotations in different countries (Patil, 2011). In Japan, for example, functional foods are defined based on their use of natural ingredients (Chaturvedi et al., 2011). In India, these functional foods can include herbal extracts, spices, fruits and nutritionally improved foods or food products with added functional ingredients.

Table 5. Some popular commercialized nutraceutical products in the worldwide market.

Products	Category	Manufacturer
Glucose-D	Energy drink	Dabur
GRD®	Nutritional supplement	Zydus Cadila Ltd., Ahmedabad, India
Omega woman	Immune supplement	Wassen, Surrey, U.K.
Proteinex®	Protein Supplement	Pfizer Ltd., Mumbai, India
Maltova, Boost, Horlicks,	Health food drink	GSK
Yakult	Health food drink	Yakult Danone India (P) Ltd. and Yakult Honsha, Japan
Calcirol D-3®	Calcium supplement	Cadila Healthcare Ltd., Ahmedabad, India
Bournvita	Chocolate beverage	Cadbury
Coral calcium	Calcium supplement	Nature's answer, Hauppauge, NY, USA
PNer plusTM	Neuropathic pain supplement	NeuroHelp, San Antonia, Texas, USA

List of Food Regulations Act in India

- Export (Quality Control and Inspection) Act 1963
- Solvent Extracted Oil Control Order 1967
- The Insecticide Act 1968
- Meat Food Products Order 1973
- Prevention of Food Adulteration Act (PFA) 1954 rules (Ministry of Health and Family Welfare) with last amendments in 1986
- Bureau of Indian Standards Act 1986
- Environmental Protection Act 1986
- Nutrition Labeling & Education Act 1990
- Milk and Milk Products Order 1992
- The Infant Milk Substitutes Feeding Bottles and Infant Food (Regulation of
- Production, Supply) Act 1992 and Rules 1993
- Food Product Order 1995
- Agriculture Produce Act
- Essential Commodities Act 1995 (Ministry of Food and Consumers Affairs)
- Industrial license
- Vegetable Oil Product Control order 1998

- The Food Safety and Standards Act 2006

11. CONCLUSION

Nutraceuticals have the potential to play a key role in healthy and safe ingestion by giving a positive impact on the prevention and treatment of many diseases. Therefore, we can imagine that the upcoming era will be devoted to nutraceuticals. The herbal medication i.e. also a part of nutraceuticals create an important role in various deadly diseases related to cancer, neurological and cardiovascular. New molecules (Drugs) used for the curing of various diseases are very difficult to discover and more expensive, hence many pharmaceutical companies are now trying to prepare nutraceutical products. Moreover, side-effect by many drugs is also one of the serious problems. Increasing changes towards preventive therapies and positive pricing situation in pharma retail chain are some other factors which are responsible for rapid growth in the marketing of nutraceutical products. Apart from this the belief of consumers about the harmless and least toxic effects of "food-like substances" compared to conventional pharmaceuticals also enhances the uses of nutraceuticals. So all these concern grow a very huge market of nutraceutical products. With this subject, the review also focuses on the food regulation laws in India and its impact on other nations. In comparison to previous years, the rules and laws related to food products are improved but the awareness about the nutraceutical products are not more satisfactory. On the other side, regulations are also one of the factors that needed to ensure quality, efficacy and safety of herbal medicines. So, there is a need to explore the health benefits of nutraceuticals and make the world healthier.

ABBREVIATIONS

FDA, Food and Drugs Administration; n-3 PUFA, n-3 polyunsaturated fatty acid; CLA, Conjugated linoleic acid; MUFA, monounsaturated fatty acid; LDL, Low-density lipoprotein; FSDU, Foods for Special Dietary Uses; NLEA, Nutrition Labeling & Education Act; DSHEA, Dietary Supplement Health and Education Act; DHA, Docosahexaenoic acid; EPA, Eicosapentaenoic Acid

ACKNOWLEDGEMENT

The central library and internet facilities provided by the University of Lucknow, Lucknow, are gratefully acknowledged.

REFERENCES

Aggarwal, B. B., Sundaram, C., Prasad, S., & Kannappan, R. (2010). Tocotrienols, the vitamin E of the 21st century: Its potential against cancer and other chronic diseases. Biochemical Pharmacology. https://doi.org/ doi:10.1016/j.bcp.2010.07.043

Anand David, A. V., Arulmoli, R., & Parasuraman, S. (2016). Overviews of biological importance of quercetin: A bioactive flavonoid. Pharmacognosy Reviews, 10(20). https://doi.org/ doi:10.4103/0973-7847.194044

Anderson, J. W., Baird, P., Davis, R. H., Ferreri, S., Knudtson, M., Koraym, A., Waters, V., & Williams, C. L. (2009). Health benefits of dietary fiber. Nutrition Reviews. https://doi.org/ doi:10.1111/j.1753-4887.2009.00189.x

Anwar, F., Latif, S., Ashraf, M., & Gilani, A. H. (2007). Moringa oleifera: A food plant with multiple medicinal uses. Phytotherapy Research. https://doi.org/ doi:10.1002/ptr.2023

Aronson, J. K. (2017). Defining 'nutraceuticals': neither nutritious nor pharmaceutical. British Journal of Clinical Pharmacology. https://doi.org/ doi:10.1111/bcp.12935

Asadi-Samani, M., Bahmani, M., & Rafieian-Kopaei, M. (2014). The chemical composition, botanical characteristic and biological activities of Borago officinalis: A review. *Asian Pacific Journal of Tropical Medicine*. Advance online publication. doi:10.1016/S1995-7645(14)60199-1 PMID:25312125

Blaabjerg, S., Artzi, D. M., & Aabenhus, R. (2017). Probiotics for the prevention of antibiotic-associated diarrhea in outpatients—A systematic review and meta-analysis. Antibiotics. https://doi.org/ doi:10.3390/antibiotics6040021

Borghi, C., & Cicero, A. F. G. (2017). Nutraceuticals with a clinically detectable blood pressure-lowering effect: a review of available randomized clinical trials and their meta-analyses. British Journal of Clinical Pharmacology. https://doi.org/ doi:10.1111/bcp.12902

Brower, V. (2005). A nutraceutical a day may keep the doctor away. *EMBO Reports*. Advance online publication. doi:10.1038j.embor.7400498 PMID:16065061

Bucher, H. C., Hengstler, P., Schindler, C., & Meier, G. (2002). N-3 polyunsaturated fatty acids in coronary heart disease: A meta-analysis of randomized controlled trials. American Journal of Medicine. https://doi.org/ doi:10.1016/S0002-9343(01)01114-7

Chaturvedi, S., Sharma, P. K., Garg, V. K., & Bansal, M. (2011). Role of nutraceuticals in health promotion. *International Journal of Pharm Tech Research.*

Forni, C., Facchiano, F., Bartoli, M., Pieretti, S., Facchiano, A., D'Arcangelo, D., Norelli, S., Valle, G., Nisini, R., Beninati, S., Tabolacci, C., & Jadeja, R. N. (2019). Beneficial role of phytochemicals on oxidative stress and age-related diseases. BioMed Research International (Vol. 2019). https://doi.org/ doi:10.1155/2019/8748253

Garg, A., Garg, S., Zaneveld, L. J. D., & Singla, A. K. (2001). Chemistry and pharmacology of the Citrus bioflavonoid hesperidin. Phytotherapy Research. https://doi.org/ doi:10.1002/ptr.1074

Glenville, M. (2006). Nutritional supplements in pregnancy: Commercial push or evidence based? Current Opinion in Obstetrics and Gynecology. https://doi.org/ doi:10.1097/GCO.0b013e328010214e

Glore, S. R., Van Treeck, D., Knehans, A. W., & Guild, M. (1994). Soluble fiber and serum lipids: A literature review. Journal of the American Dietetic Association. https://doi.org/ doi:10.1016/0002-8223(94)90099-X

Gupta, S., Chauhan, D., Mehla, K., Sood, P., & Nair, A. (2010). An overview of nutraceuticals: Current scenario. *Journal of Basic and Clinical Pharmacy*. PMID:24825966

Hardy, G. (2000). Nutraceuticals and functional foods: Introduction and meaning. *Nutrition (Burbank, Los Angeles County, Calif.)*. Advance online publication. doi:10.1016/S0899-9007(00)00332-4 PMID:10906598

Hickson, M., D'Souza, A. L., Muthu, N., Rogers, T. R., Want, S., Rajkumar, C., & Bulpitt, C. J. (2007). Use of probiotic Lactobacillus preparation to prevent diarrhoea associated with antibiotics: Randomised double blind placebo controlled trial. *British Medical Journal*. Advance online publication. doi:10.1136/bmj.39231.599815.55 PMID:17604300

Iriti, M., & Faoro, F. (2006). Grape phytochemicals: A bouquet of old and new nutraceuticals for human health. *Medical Hypotheses*. Advance online publication. doi:10.1016/j.mehy.2006.03.049 PMID:16759816

Klatte, E. T., Scharre, D. W., Nagaraja, H. N., Davis, R. A., & Beversdorf, D. Q. (2003). Combination therapy of donepezil and vitamin E in Alzheimer disease. *Alzheimer Disease and Associated Disorders*. Advance online publication. doi:10.1097/00002093-200304000-00010 PMID:12794389

Kleerebezem, M., Boels, I. C., Groot, M. N., Mierau, I., Sybesma, W., & Hugenholtz, J. (2002). Metabolic engineering of Lactococcus lactis: The impact of genomics and metabolic modelling. *Journal of Biotechnology*. Advance online publication. doi:10.1016/S0168-1656(02)00132-3 PMID:12141987

Leray, C., Wiesel, M. L., Freund, M., Cazenave, J. P., & Gachet, C. (2001). Long-chain n-3 fatty acids specifically affect rat coagulation factors dependent on vitamin K relation to peroxidative stress. *Arteriosclerosis, Thrombosis, and Vascular Biology*. Advance online publication. doi:10.1161/01.ATV.21.3.459 PMID:11231929

Li, H., Wang, Z., & Liu, Y. (2003). Review in the studies on tannins activity of cancer prevention and anticancer. Zhong yao cai = Zhongyaocai = Journal of Chinese Medicinal Materials.

Limer, J. L., & Speirs, V. (2004). Phyto-oestrogens and breast cancer chemoprevention. Breast Cancer Research. https://doi.org/ doi:10.1186/bcr781

Losso, J. N. (2003). Targeting excessive angiogenesis with functional foods and nutraceuticals. *Trends in Food Science & Technology*. Advance online publication. doi:10.1016/S0924-2244(03)00156-0

Nasri, H., Baradaran, A., Shirzad, H., & Kopaei, M. R. (2014). New concepts in nutraceuticals as alternative for pharmaceuticals. *International Journal of Preventive Medicine*. PMID:25709784

Ng, F., Yun, H., Lei, X., Danishefsky, S. J., Fahey, J., Stephenson, K., Flexner, C., & Lee, L. (2008). (3R,9R,10R)-Panaxytriol: A molecular-based nutraceutical with possible application to cancer prevention and treatment. *Tetrahedron Letters*. Advance online publication. doi:10.1016/j.tetlet.2008.09.169 PMID:20011028

Niu, Y., Na, L., Feng, R., Gong, L., Zhao, Y., Li, Q., Li, Y., & Sun, C. (2013). The phytochemical, EGCG, extends lifespan by reducing liver and kidney function damage and improving age-associated inflammation and oxidative stress in healthy rats. *Aging Cell, 12*(6). Advance online publication. doi:10.1111/acel.12133 PMID:23834676

Parvez, M. K. (2017). Natural or Plant Products for the Treatment of Neurological Disorders: Current Knowledge. *Current Drug Metabolism*. Advance online publication. doi:10.2174/1389200218666170710190249 PMID:28699506

Patil, C. S. (2011). Current Trends and Future Prospective of Nutraceuticals in Health Promotion. *BIOINFO Pharmaceutical Biotechnology, 1*(1), 1–7. https://bioinfopublication.org/viewhtml.php?artid=BIA0000894

Patwardhan, B., Vaidya, A., Chorghade, M., & Joshi, S. (2008). Reverse Pharmacology and Systems Approaches for Drug Discovery and Development. *Current Bioactive Compounds*. Advance online publication. doi:10.2174/157340708786847870

Prakash, D., & Gupta, K. R. (2009). The Antioxidant Phytochemicals of Nutraceutical Importance. *The Open Nutraceuticals Journal*. Advance online publication. doi:10.2174/1876396000902010020

Prietl, B., Treiber, G., Pieber, T. R., & Amrein, K. (2013). Vitamin D and immune function. Nutrients. https://doi.org/ doi:10.3390/nu5072502

Rafieian-kopaei, M. (2012). Medicinal plants and the human needs. Journal of HerbMed Pharmacology. https://doi.org/ doi:10.1016/S2222-1808(14)60708-8

Rafieian-Kopaei, M., Nasri, H., Sahinfard, N., Rafieian, M., Rafieian, S., & Shirzad, M. (2014). Turmeric: A spice with multifunctional medicinal properties. *Journal of HerbMed Pharmacology*.

Sahu, S. C. (2002). Dual role of organosulfur compounds in foods: A review. *Journal of Environmental Science and Health. Part C, Environmental Carcinogenesis & Ecotoxicology Reviews*. Advance online publication. doi:10.1081/GNC-120005388 PMID:12734054

Sanders, M. E. (1994). Lactic Acid Bacteria as Promoters of Human Health. Functional Foods. https://doi.org/ doi:10.1007/978-1-4615-2073-3_14

Shinde, N., Bangar, B., Deshmukh, S., & Kumbhar, P. (2014). Nutraceuticals: A review on current status. Research Journal of Pharmacy and Technology.

Siezen, R. J., Kok, J., Abee, T., & Schaafsma, G. (2002). Lactic acid bacteria: Genetics, metabolism and applications. *International Journal of General and Molecular Microbiology*. doi:10.1023/A:1020685028897

Silanikove, N., Leitner, G., & Merin, U. (2015). The interrelationships between lactose intolerance and the modern dairy industry: Global perspectives in evolutional and historical backgrounds. Nutrients. https://doi.org/ doi:10.3390/nu7095340

Singh, J., & Sinha, S. (2012). Classification, Regulatory Acts and Applications of Nutraceuticals for Health. *International Journal of Pharma and Bio Sciences, 2*(1), 177–187.

Soetaert, W., Schwengers, D., Buchholz, K., & Vandamme, E. J. (1995). A wide range of carbohydrate modifications by a single micro-organism: Leuconostoc mesenteroides. Progress in Biotechnology. https://doi.org/ doi:10.1016/S0921-0423(06)80116-4

Sreejayan, & Rao, M. N. A. (1994). Curcuminoids as Potent Inhibitors of Lipid Peroxidation. *The Journal of Pharmacy and Pharmacology*, *46*(12), 1013–1016. doi:10.1111/j.2042-7158.1994.tb03258.x PMID:7714712

Stoll, A. L., Severus, W. E., Freeman, M. P., Rueter, S., Zboyan, H. A., Diamond, E., Cress, K. K., & Marangell, L. B. (1999). Omega 3 fatty acids in bipolar disorder: A preliminary double-blind, placebo-controlled trial. *Archives of General Psychiatry*. Advance online publication. doi:10.1001/archpsyc.56.5.407 PMID:10232294

Tamadon, M. R., Baradaran, A., & Rafieian-Kopaei, M. (2013). Antioxidant and kidney protection; differential impacts of single and whole natural antioxidants. *Journal of Renal Injury Prevention*. Advance online publication. doi:10.12861/jrip.2014.14 PMID:25340165

Taranto, M. P., Vera, J. L., Hugenholtz, J., De Valdez, G. F., & Sesma, F. (2003). Lactobacillus reuteri CRL1098 produces cobalamin. *Journal of Bacteriology*. Advance online publication. doi:10.1128/JB.185.18.5643-5647.2003 PMID:12949118

Van Rooijen, R. J., Van Schalkwijk, S., & De Vos, W. M. (1991). Molecular cloning, characterization, and nucleotide sequence of the tagatose 6-phosphate pathway gene cluster of the lactose operon of Lactococcus lactis. *Journal of Biological Chemistry*.

Whorwell, P. J., Altringer, L., Morel, J., Bond, Y., Charbonneau, D., O'Mahony, L., Kiely, B., Shanahan, F., & Quigley, E. M. M. (2006). Efficacy of an encapsulated probiotic Bifidobacterium infantis 35624 in women with irritable bowel syndrome. *The American Journal of Gastroenterology*. Advance online publication. doi:10.1111/j.1572-0241.2006.00734.x PMID:16863564

Wildman, R. E. C. (2016). Handbook of Nutraceuticals and Functional Foods. Handbook of Nutraceuticals and Functional Foods, Second Edition. https://doi.org/ doi:10.1201/9781420006186

Willcox, M. L., Graz, B., Falquet, J., Diakite, C., Giani, S., & Diallo, D. (2011). A reverse pharmacology approach for developing an anti-malarial phytomedicine. Malaria Journal. https://doi.org/ doi:10.1186/1475-2875-10-S1-S8

Zhang, Y. J., Gan, R. Y., Li, S., Zhou, Y., Li, A. N., Xu, D. P., Li, H. B., & Kitts, D. D. (2015). Antioxidant phytochemicals for the prevention and treatment of chronic diseases. Molecules. https://doi.org/ doi:10.3390/molecules201219753

Zhao, J. (2008). Nutraceuticals, Nutritional Therapy, Phytonutrients, and Phytotherapy for Improvement of Human Health: A Perspective on Plant Biotechnology Application. *Recent Patents on Biotechnology*. Advance online publication. doi:10.2174/187220807779813893 PMID:19075834

KEY TERMS AND DEFINITIONS

Bioactive Compound: It is a compound that affects a living organism, tissue/cell.

Cancer: Cancer is a group of diseases involving abnormal cell growth with the potential to invade or spread to other parts of the body.

Dementia: Dementia is a collective term used to describe various symptoms of cognitive declines, such as forgetfulness. It is a symptom of several underlying diseases and brain disorders.

Functional Food: A functional food is a food claimed to have an additional function (often one related to health-promotion or disease prevention) by adding new ingredients or more of existing ingredients.

Glandular Therapy: Glandular therapy (GT) refers to the practice of using whole animal tissues to support or promote the healthy functioning of a body's internal organs. Glandular tissues contain vitamins, minerals, enzymes, peptides, nucleotides, and other nutrients, specific to each organ.

Pharmacology: It is a branch of pharmaceutical sciences which is concerned with the study of a drug or medication action, where a drug can be broadly or narrowly defined as any man-made, natural, or endogenous (from within the body) molecule which exerts a biochemical or physiological effect on the cell, tissue, organ, or organism.

Chapter 13
Nutraceuticals for Management of Metabolic Disorders

Monica Premi
Manipal Academy of Higher Education, UAE

Vikas Bansal
Jaipur National University, India

ABSTRACT

Human wellness and health are predominately governed by the consumption of nutritive foods. Modern approaches such as healthy diet, modified lifestyle, and switching to natural products (nutraceuticals) instead of pharmaceuticals are recommended to counteract the metabolic abnormalities. Globally, usage of nutraceuticals has increased in recent years. Nutraceuticals provide better therapeutic opportunity with lesser-known side effects. Nutraceuticals are the products obtained from foods (dietary supplements, isolated nutrients, and herbal products) that aid physiological effect in the body by promoting health benefits beyond basic nutrition. Many researchers claimed nutraceuticals are effective in improving health and wellness by curing metabolic disorder and thus increasing life expectancy. Clinically, nutraceuticals target the pathogenesis of metabolic disorders and their complications and positively harmonize different clinical and biochemical outcomes. This review highlights the beneficial effects of the popular nutraceuticals in managing metabolic disorders.

1. INTRODUCTION

1.1 Nutraceuticals

Dr. Stephen Defelice introduced the term "Nutraceutical" in 1989, which was derived from words "Nutrition" (food) and "Pharmaceutical" (drug) (Brower, 1998). According to Defelice, nautraceuticals are the foods or part of it that have health-promoting benefits or medicinal properties in preventing or treatment of metabolic disorders (Trottier et al., 2010). Father of medicine "Hippocrates" said, "let food be your medicine" the ideology behind this was to mainly focus on prevention rather than treatment of

DOI: 10.4018/978-1-7998-4808-0.ch013

diseases. Usually, nutraceuticals are also referred to as multifunctional foods, functional food and dietary supplements, etc. Functional foods are the food that claim to have health-giving additives either by incorporating new ingredients or from existing ingredients. It can be defined as foods that usually have a positive impact on an individual's health besides providing basic necessary nutritional requirements. These foods are also known as FOSHU (Foods for specific health uses) (Kalra, 2003).

Figure 1. Basic theory of nutraceuticals

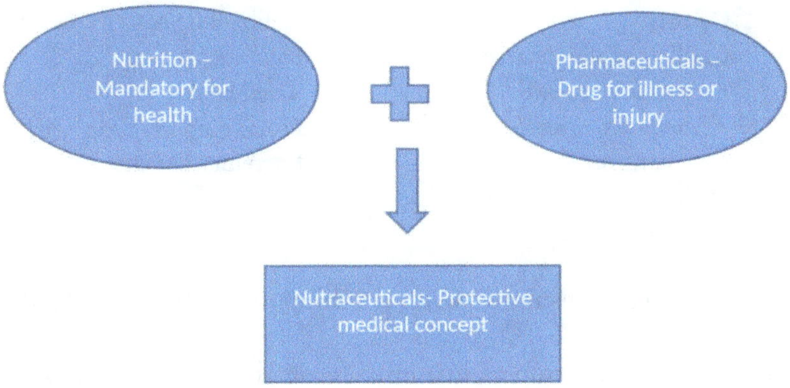

1.2 Nutraceutical Principle

Dietary supplement, health and education act (DSHEA, 1994) defined dietary supplements are the dietary products which are specifically designed to supplement the diet. It usually contains one of the following dietary ingredients such as herb, mineral, vitamin, amino acid or botanical either in extracted or concentrated form, which is consumed in liquid, tablet or pill form (Zeisel, 1999). It is generally labelled as "dietary supplements" (FDA/CFSAN, 1994), it cannot be consumed as a sole meal or conventional food. As per DSHEA Act 1994, the firms are whole sole liable for ensuring the legal safety requirements of their dietary supplements before marketing to safeguard that they meet up all specifications of DSHEA (Unites state Pharmacopeia USP, 2006).

In simple words, Nutraceuticals can be defined as a "food substance that has both nutritive as well pharmaceutical properties that help to promote health benefits by preventing metabolic disorders" whereas, functional foods are described as "food products that are consumed as a part of a routine diet to attain health benefits in addition to basic nutritional properties".

1.3 Nutraceuticals Benefits

- No side effect
- Increase healthful effects
- Usually have natural dietary supplements
- Amend medical condition by improving health values
- Readily available at nominal price

Figure 2. Benefits of Nutraceuticals

Nutraceuticals

Disease prevention
- -Stress management
- -Cancer
- -Obesity
- -Cardiovascular disease
- -Parkinson's disease
- -Alzheimer's disease
- -Osteoarthritis
- -Diabetes

Health Promotion
- -Reproductive health
- -Gastrointestinal health
- -Antioxidant activity
- -Stem cell growth
- -Renal health
- -Prolonging life span
- -Excretory health

Many researchers linked the relationship between consumption of healthful food and prevention of multiple degenerative diseases.

Nutritional therapy is a remedial process that utilizes nutraceutical or dietary products to improve human health. This concept is based on facts that foods not only just provide energy and nutrients but it could also promote health benefits.

As per nutritional therapy and nutraceutical theory, the target goal of preventing degenerative diseases is achieved by using the efficacy of nutraceuticals and dietary products in building up healthy digestion, detoxify the body, preventing deficiencies of vitamins and minerals. Phytonutrients are essential plant chemicals or nutrients that have selective biological properties in promoting health benefits (Zhao, 2007).

1.4 Biological Role of Phytochemicals

1. Act as a substrate for biochemical reactions.
2. Act as cofactors and inhibitors in enzymatic reactions.
3. Act as absorbents that can eliminate and bind to an undesirable constituent in the intestine.
4. It increases the stability or absorption of essential nutrients required by the body.
5. Act as selective growth factor and fermentation substrate for retaining beneficial (good) bacteria.
6. Act as selective inhibitors for destructive bacteria (Intestinal).
7. Act as scavengers of toxic chemicals from the body.
8. Act as ligands that antagonize or agonize intracellular receptors (Dillard & German, 2000).

1.5 Classification of Nutraceuticals

Nutraceuticals are classified based on its mechanism of action, natural food source and chemical nature of the products (Table 1).

The natural food substances used as nutraceuticals are (Kalia 2005; Kokate et al., 2002): Dietary fibre, prebiotics, probiotics, polyunsaturated fatty acids, antioxidant vitamins, polyphenols and spices.

Broadly, nutraceuticals are classified into two major groups (Pandey et al. 2010): Potential nutraceutical and established nutraceutical.

Most of the nutraceuticals are kept in the category of "potential nutraceutical". But a potential nutraceutical could be turned to establish nutraceutical once its scientific clinical database related to its health benefits are obtained.

Table 1. Classification of nutraceuticals (Hueda, 2020)

	Classification	
Nutraceuticals	Chemical nature	Fatty acids, carotenoids, flavonoids, phenols, plant sterols, pre/probiotics, glucosinolates, dietary fibres, phytoestrogens
	Food availability	-Traditional: Chemical constituents (Herbal, phytochemicals and nutrient), probiotics microorganism, nutraceuticals enzymes -Non-traditional: Fortified nutraceuticals, recombinant nutraceuticals
	Mechanism of action	Antioxidant activity, anti-cancer, anti-inflammatory, positive impact on lipid profile, osteogenetic

1.5.1 Dietary fibres (DFs)

Technically, dietary fibres (roughage) are the edible portion of plant material that cannot be hydrolyzed by human digestive enzymes, but partial or completed fermentation by gut microflora. Chemically, dietary fibres are plant-based carbohydrate polymers having a degree of polymerization not lower than 3 that are resistant to digestion and absorption by the microflora of the small intestine. Dietary fibre includes polysaccharides (Non-starch) and other associated plant components such as oligosaccharides, cellulose, lignin, beta-glucans, resistance starch and dextrin. It is commonly found in whole grains, beans, legumes, nuts, oats, fruits and vegetables etc.

Based on water solubility, dietary fibres are classified into two components:

a. Insoluble dietary fibres (IDFs) – are not soluble in water. IDFs remain inert to the fermentation process in the colon (upper GI tract), but some type of IDFs such as resistant starch is fermented by digestive enzymes in the colon. It includes cellulose, hemicellulose and lignins. These fibres are known as bulking fibres as it provide bulk to the stool.

b. Soluble dietary fibres (SDFs) – are soluble in water. These fibres are also known as prebiotic fibres, as readily fermented by the gut microflora in the colon into gases and by-products such as short-chain fatty acids. It includes gums, mucilages, pectin and some hemicellulose. It increases the viscosity and delays emptying of the stomach, which further extends the feeling of stomach fullness.

Collectively, both IDFs and SDFs are known as non-starch polysaccharides.

Many researchers found that SDFs has a positive impact on human immunity (Watzl et al. 2005). Recommended dietary intake (RDI) for adults ranges from 20-35 g/day (Pilch 1987) and for children is 14 g/1,000 Kcal (Anderson et al. 2009). Many studies reveals that excessive consumption of dietary fibres leads to diarrhoea, decreased absorption of vitamins, minerals and proteins (Das et al., 2012; Saibil, 1989).

1.5.2 Polyunsaturated fatty acids (PUFAs)

PUFAs are also known as "essential fatty acids (EFAs)" or "beneficial fats" as they play a significant role in various biological functions. As human cannot metabolize EFAs therefore, it is crucial to obtain it from dietary substances (Escott-Stump & Mahan, 2000).

PUFAs are of two types:

a. Omega-3 PUFAs (n-3) - It mainly consists of alpha-linolenic acid (ALA), docosahexaenoic acid (DHA) and eicosapentaenoic acid (EPA). ALA is a precursor for DHA and EPA. Main source of DHA and EPA are fatty fishes like salmon, tuna, mackerel and fish oil. As per the Institute of Medicine, the richest source of ALA are flaxseed, canola, nuts (walnuts), soybean and seeds (black currant) (IOM, 2002).
b. Omega-6 PUFAs (n-6) – It mainly consist of linoleic acid (LA), arachidonic acid (ARA) and gamma-linolenic acid (GLA). Vegetables such as safflower, soybean, sunflower and corn contains a significant amount of LA whereas, animals products such as eggs, poultry and meat are a good sources of ALA.

The prevalence of clinical studies indicates that increased intake of omega-3 fatty acids is directly associated with a lesser risk of premature birth (PMB) (Ciesielski, 2019; Bernardi, 2012) and diabetes (Connor, 2000). Because of these studies, nowadays all infant formula is fortified with DHA and ARA, which closely imitate the mother's milk. FDA recommends a daily intake of DHA and EPA maximum of 3 g/day and not more than 2 g/day for dietary supplements (US FDA, 2014).

1.5.3 Probiotics

Probiotics are defined as live microbes which when administered/consumed in appropriate amounts it confers the beneficial health effects on the host by repairing intestinal microflora (FAO/WHO, 2001). The concept of transforming large intestine harmful microorganism with beneficial microorganism [Bacillus bulgaricus (Hord, 2008)] was laid by Russian scientist Metchinkoff (1907).

Generally, probiotics contain the following good microorganism:

a. Lactobacilli (L. casei, L. acidophilus, L. bulgaricus, L. delbruecki).
b. Gram positive cocci (S. thermophiles, L. lactis).
c. Bifidobacteria (B. adolescentis, B. bifidun, B. thermophilum).

Currently, probiotics are readily available in different forms like liquid, granule, gel, powder and capsules (Govender, 2014; Suvarna & Boby, 2005). Particular probiotics are used to cure the problems associated with the gastrointestinal tract such as acute diarrhoea, lactose intolerance (LI) and side effects related to antibiotics (Antibiotic-associated diabetes, AAD) (Markowiak & Slizewska, 2017). An effectual probiotic owns characteristics like non-toxic, non-pathogenic, maintain good viability, adherence to intestinal epithelial cell producing anti-bacterial compounds (Suvarna & Boby, 2005). Many researchers validate that usage of probiotics reduces the risk associated with peptic ulcers, allergy, cancer, asthma, urinary tract infections (UTIs) and ear infections (Lenoir-Wijnkoop et al., 2007, Geier et al., 2006; Lesbros-Pantoflickov et al., 2007).

1.5.4 Prebiotics

Prebiotics are specialized dietary fibres from plants that effectively facilitate the host by selectively modifying the metabolism or composition of gut microflora (Macfarlane et al., 2006). Oligosaccharides are the major source of prebiotics that are not digested by humans specifically, galactans and fructans because of its specific structure. Oligosaccharides behave as prebiotics by stimulating the activity and growth of beneficial gut microflora (Lactobacillus and Bifidobacterium Sp.), thus aid in the metabolism (Pandey et al., 2015; Hord, 2008). An effectual prebiotic should own characteristics like resistance to stomach acid, easily fermentable by beneficial gut microflora and does not get absorbed in the upper GI tract (Kuo, 2013).

Raw oats, unrefined barley and wheat, vegetables like artichoke, banana, chicory roots, tomato, yacon root and jerusalem, soybean and breast milk are good source of non- digestible oligosaccharides (Pandey et al., 2015). An RDI of 5-20 g of oligosaccharide and insulin stimulate the proliferation of bifidobacteria microflora (Das et al., 2012). But, excessive consumption of non-digestible oligosaccharides leads to abdominal distension, diarrhoea and bloating (Guarner, 2005).

1.5.5 Selenium

Selenium is a vital trace mineral that plays a very important role in many body functions such as reproduction, protection against reactive oxygen species (ROS) toxicity (cancer protection), thyroid hormone regulation, prevention in cognitive decline, and regulation of cells redox state. The richest source of selenium is Brazil nut, it contains 68-81 mcg that meets the RDA for adults that is 55mg as per FDA (NIH, 2020).

Deficiency of selenium generates sever biochemical changes which lead to serious disease of the heart muscle (Keshan disease) that mainly affects the child and young women (Sunde, 2006). It also plays a significant role in male fertility, kashin-beck (osteoarthritis) disease, aggravate iodine deficiency and deepen cretinism risk in infants (Sunde, 2006; Sunde, 2010).

Selenium is a basic element of selenoprotein/ selenoenzyme that plays an essential role as antioxidants in the form of glutathione peroxidase and thioredoxin reductase. Glutathione peroxidase plays a very important role in cell defence mechanism against oxidative stress from reactive nitrogen species (RNS) and reactive oxygen species (ROS). Pentose phosphate pathway (PPP) reinforce glutathione peroxidase (selenium-containing enzymes) aids in erythrocytes defence against haemolysis.

As per Food and Nutrition Board of U.S Institute of Medicine (IOM, 2000), recommended dietary allowance (RDA) for adults is 55 µg Se per day and for children is 20 µg Se per day. Excessive intake of selenium (>100 µg per day) leads to a disease known as "Selenosis", that may cause hair loss, fatigue, irritability, garlic breath odour, GI upset, mild nerve damage and white blotchy nails (Goldhaber, 2003).

1.5.6 Antioxidants

Antioxidants such as vitamin C, vitamin E and carotenoids are also called as "antioxidant vitamins". Antioxidant vitamins work either independently or synergistically in the prevention of several degenerative diseases that leads to cardiovascular disease, cancer and cataracts (Zhang, 2015).

A rich resource of these antioxidant vitamins are fruits and vegetables like guava, grape, pomegranate and berries that act as free radical scavengers and defend cells against damage (Mangnaris et al., 2014). Moreover, by-product waste like peel and seeds obtained from fruits and vegetables processing units are a

Figure 3. Effect of reactive oxygen species on health and various disease

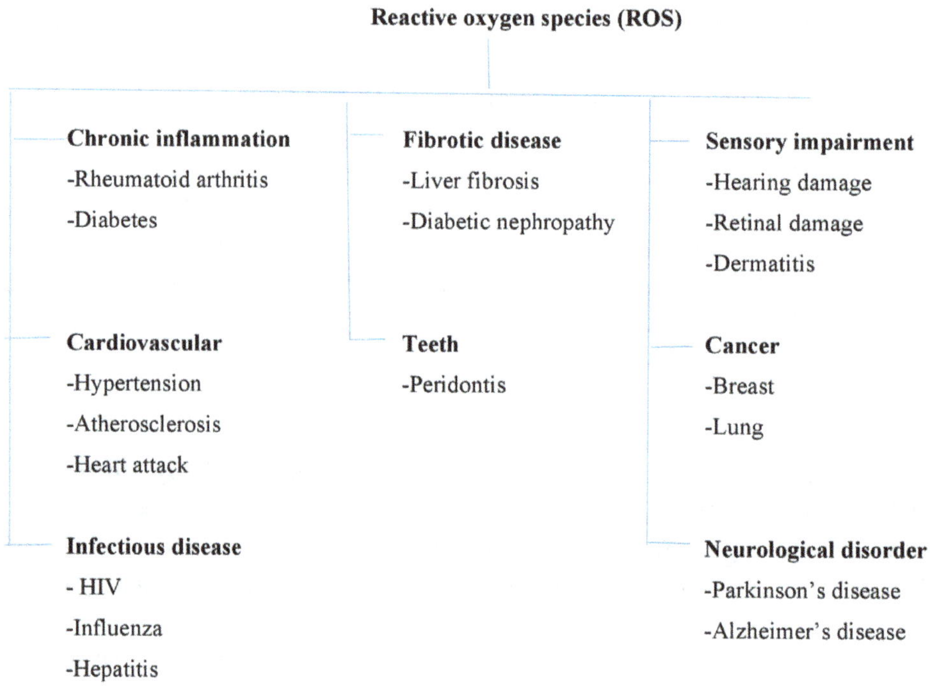

rich source of bioactive compounds such as kaempferol, chlorogenic, gallic acid, catechin and epicatechin (Deng et al., 2012). Bioactive compounds that are specifically responsible for antioxidant properties in plant-based food substances are polyphenols and carotenoids. For instance, myricetin, β-carotene, kaempferol and quercetin are the principal bioactive compounds found in gooseberry (Zhang et al., 2013).

Vitamin E is a fat-soluble chain splitting antioxidant compound found in the human body which consists of tocopherols and tocotrienols. It mainly acts as an "antioxidant" that scavenge free radicals that may damage cells and thus protecting the lipid oxidation of biological membrane (Meydani, 2000). It strengthens the body's immune system by fighting against infections, maintain the health of eyes, brain and skin. Besides, having anti-oxidative properties it also has anti-inflammatory and anti-atherogenic properties (Hadi et al., 2018). Many clinical studies have shown the significant inhibitory effect of vitamin E on liver disease like nonalcoholic steatohepatitis (NASH) (El Hadi et al., 2018; Larion and Khurana, 2018; Pacana and Sanyal, 2012).

Vitamin E and selenium has a symbiotic role in preventing the lipid peroxidation. Similar to vitamin E, vitamin C also donates hydrogen atom to lipid radicals and scavenge singlet oxygen and protect reactive species. Carotenoids such as β-carotene, zeaxanthin, lutein and lycopene are termed as chain splitting antioxidant as they are very effective in quenching singlet oxygen without formation of oxidizing compounds in biological membranes. At low oxygen concentration, β-carotene entraps free radicals present in membranes. Hence, β-carotene also has synergistic antioxidant activity with vitamin E (Das et al., 2012).

1.5.7 Polyphenols

Polyphenols are naturally occurring plant secondary metabolites, which are associated in defence mechanism against ultraviolet radiation (UV), stress, pathogens or reactive oxygen species.

Figure 4. Classification of polyphenols

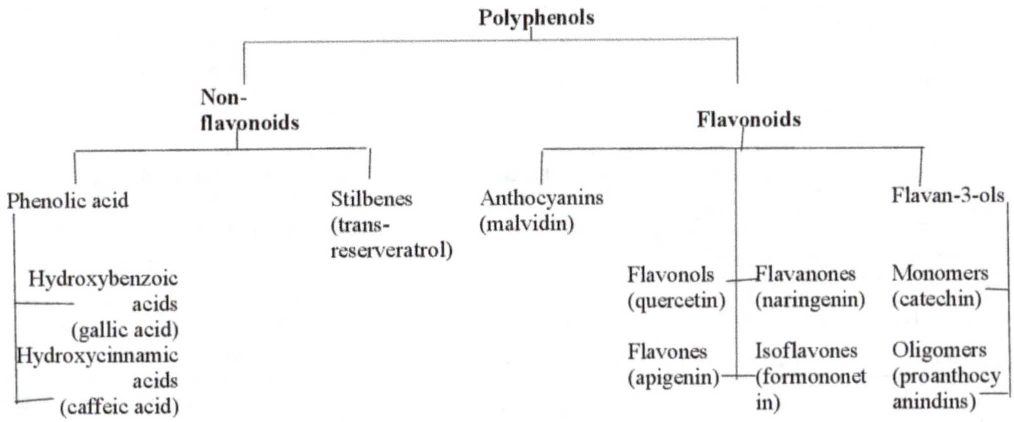

Figure 5. Possible mechanism for anti-cancer effect by dietary polyphenols

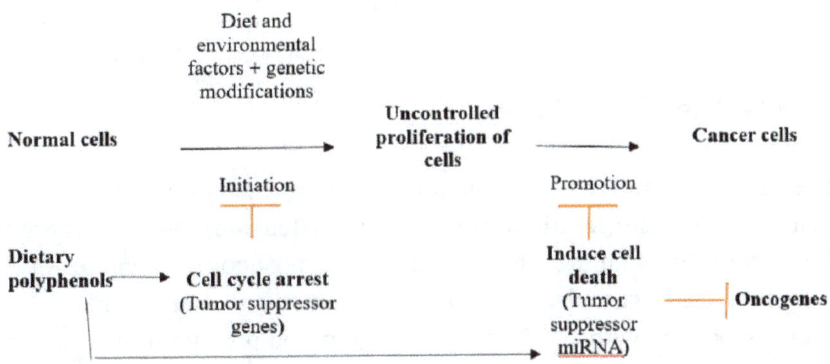

Polyphenols are the largest group of phytochemicals that performs different protective action against metabolic disease (Alissa and fern, 2012). Nearly 8,000 distinct types of polyphenols are identified, among those flavonols, flavanones, flavan-3-ols, flavones and anthocyanins are most important. Phenolic compounds and flavonoids are two most commonly appearing polyphenols found in foods. According to in-vitro studies, polyphenols also affect different cellular process such as apoptosis, gene expression, intercellular signalling, platelet aggregation (Duthie et al., 2003; Das et al., 2012). Other than these, many epidemiologic studies reveal that polyphenols have a positive impact on many disorders such as cancer, neurodegenerative disease, obesity, diabetes and cardiovascular disease (Singh et al., 2011; Corny et al., 2018).

1.6 Nutraceuticals in the Prevention and Treatment of Disease

Nutraceuticals play a significant role in inhibiting the number of disease outbreak and reduce disease aggravation. These bioceutical also defend against different non-communicable disease, arrest the ageing process, expand life expectancy and maintains usual physiological body functions.

Table 2. Potential role of nutraceuticals in the prevention of metabolic disorders (Dutta et al. 2018)

Nutraceuticals	Metabolic disorder	Reference
Flavonoids, quercetin, allicin	Cardiovascular disease	Cicero & Colletti (2016); Wildman (2007); Ramaa et al. (2006);
Ginseng, β-carotene, sulfur compounds	Cancer	Sabita & Trygve (2012); Wargovich et al. (2010)
ω-3 fatty acids, catechins, soy isoflavones	Type 2 diabetes	Nasri et al. (2014); Stephen (2012)
Capsaicin, conjugated linolenic acid, vitamin C, caffeine	Obesity	Kaur et al. (2015)
Glucosamine, collagen hydrolysate, curcumin	Osteoarthristis	Agarwal (2017); Bohlooli et al. (2012)
Pro-anthocyanidins, flavonoids, polyphenols,	Oral disease	Varani & Iriti (2016); Janczarek et al. (2016)
Polyphenols, Vitamin D & E, inosine, phytoestrogens	Parkinson's disease	Lama et al. (2020)
Curcumin, folic acid, β-carotene, lycopene	Alzheimer's disease	Kennedy (2016); Ji & Zhang (2008); Klatte et al. (2003)
Flavanoids, curcumin, lutein, ascorbic acid, carotenoids	Eye disorder	Varani & Iritis (2016)
Adaptogens	Stress management	Kalra (2003)

1.6.1 Cardiovascular Diseases (CVDs)

Cardiovascular disease is a class of disease generally affecting the blood vessels and heart. It includes heart attack (coronary heart disease), high blood pressure (hypertension), stroke (cerebrovascular disease), peripheral vascular disease, heart failure, etc. It is one of the most common causes of death for humans (CDC, 2019). Most of the cardiovascular diseases are prevented and manageable.

Major risk factors associated with CVDs are diet, high blood pressure (BP), smoking, lack of exercise, high low-density lipoproteins (LDL), age, and genetic conditions. Many studies show the direct correlation of lower intake of fruits and vegetables with high mortality rates due to CVD (Wang et al., 2014; Rissanen et al., 2003). It was reported by several researchers that fruits and vegetables rich diet has a protective role against many diseases (Salvin & Lloyd, 2012; Hu & Willett, 2002). Nutraceuticals such as quercetin, flavonoids, flavones, flavones, antioxidants, vitamins and minerals present in apples, cruciferous vegetables, cherries, onion, blackberries prevent the risk associated with CVDs. These compounds inhibit the angiotensin converting enzyme (ACE) activity and cyclooxygenase pathway

Figure 6. Health benefits of gingerol

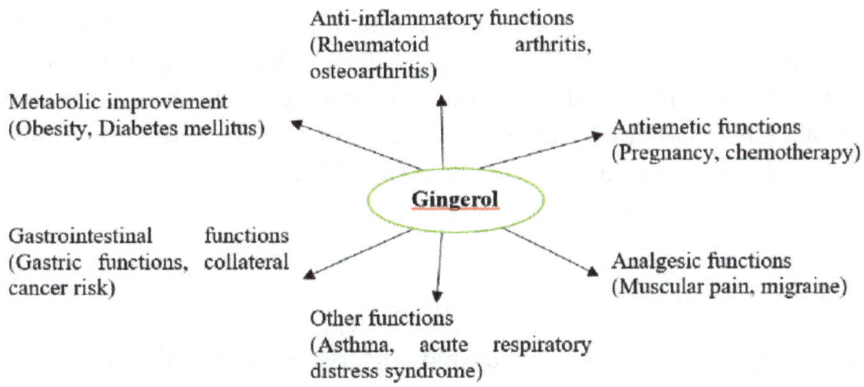

Figure 7. Role of garlic as an anti-cardiovascular agent (Alves et al., 2019)

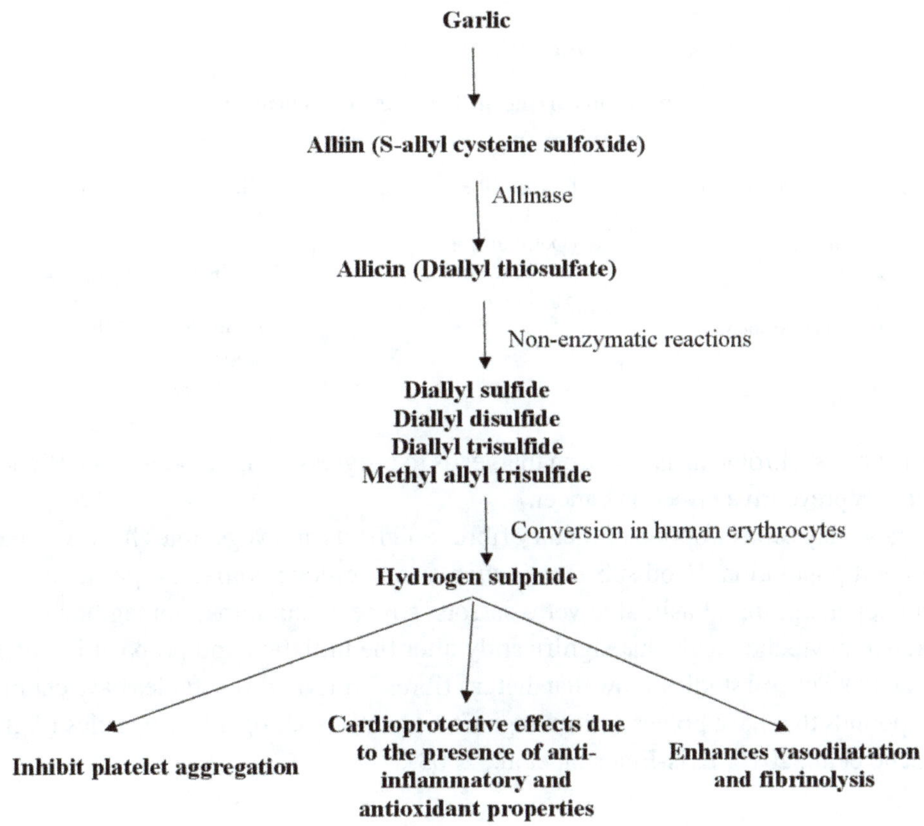

which is responsible for high BP. Apart, form nutraceuticals also prevents aggregation of platelets and stickiness (Dutta et al., 2018).

Polyphenols particularly flavonoids insulate vascular system and rejuvenate tiny capillaries that transfer oxygen and essential nutrients to all cells. Gingerol, a major bioactive compound of ginger which is responsible for providing health benefits. This compound has strong antioxidant and anti-inflammatory properties that help to prevent palpitation and hypertension.

Polyphenols such as anthocyanins, flavans, resveratrol and flavonols are present in grapes modulate oxidative stress, inflammation and LDL cholesterol. It also modifies cellular signalling and metabolism that significantly diminish arterial diseases (Wildmen, 2007). Allicin, dominate bioactive compound present in garlic. It primarily contains sulphur as the main component that reduces cholesterol and blood pressure (Shang et al., 2019). Omega-3 fatty acids are recommended for arrhythmias treatment as it has lipid-lowering effects (Ramaa et al., 2006). Development of CVDs could be prevented by lipid-lowering bioceuticals together with proper lifestyle.

1.6.2 Cancer

Cancer is the second largest cause of death in developing countries (Zainni et al., 2015). Herbal nutraceuticals retains anti-carcinogenic and anti-mutagenic functions. Lycopene and carotenoids are powerful antioxidants against cancer. These phytochemicals scavenge singlet oxygen and reduces cellular oxidative stress. Nutraceuticals prevents the factors responsible for damaging cellular DNA and impeding DNA transcription in tumour cells. Ginseng, an herbal supplement contains anti-inflammatory and antioxidant

Figure 8. Anti-cancer phytochemicals (Wong, 2012)

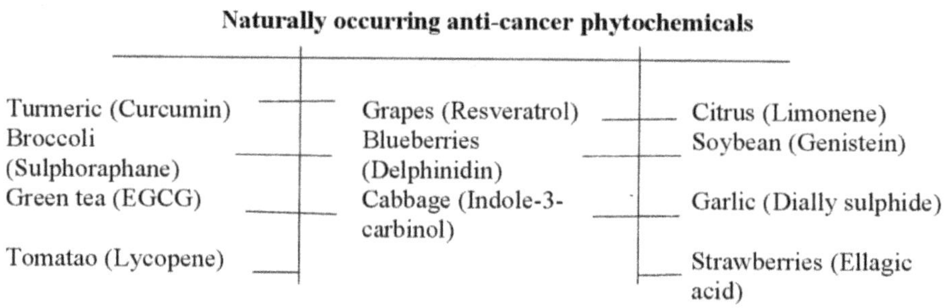

molecules which arrest chronic inflammation that leads to progression in tumour cells. Bioactive dietary compounds have a preventive effect on cancer.

Therefore, nowadays consumption of dietary fibres and fruits and vegetables have attracted attention among the general population. Food substances such as tea, onions, tomatoes, garlic, olive oil, honey, berries, chilli peppers, grapes, basil, aloe vera, carrots, soybean, curcuma, pomegranate and rosemary contains bioactive phytochemicals that significantly alter the initiation and propagation of carcinogens (Zainni et al., 2015). Several studies show that dietary fibres, fruits and vegetables have chemopreventive bioactive compounds that have potent anti-mutagenic and anti-carcinogenic properties (Aghajanpour et al., 2017; Panche et al., 2016; Kris-Etherton et al., 2003).

β-carotene and lycopene are type of carotenoids widely dispersed among fruits and vegetables. These pigmented bioactive compounds plays a significant role in human health as they possess numerous biological properties like antioxidant, anti-inflammatory and anticancer. Cruciferous vegetables such as cabbage, cauliflower, kale, broccoli, brussel sprouts etc. also contains nutraceuticals with anti-cancer properties that prevent abnormal cell growth. It specifically block the enzymes responsible for tumour growth and suppresses cancer progression. Foods rich in sulfur compounds such as onion, garlic etc. helps to build up the immune system, it lowers platelet aggregation and thus reduces atherosclerosis (Shang et al., 2019). Recently, researchers noted that herbal nutraceuticals have potential to prevent metastatic proliferation of cancer cells as they contain anti-tumor agents (Nasri et al., 2014; Wargovich et al., 2010).

Table 3. Nutraceuticals and its mechanism of action for the prevention and treatment of cancer (Arora and Jaglan, 2016)

	Nutraceuticals	**Sources**	**Mechanism of action**
Nutraceuticals for prevention and treatment of cancer	Carotenoids	-β-carotene -Lycopene -Lutein -Zeaxanthin	- Inhibits cell proliferation and differentiation -DNA methylation for gene expression - Inhibits efflux transporters - Protect DNA from damage - Reduces toxicity of chemotherapeutic drugs - Reduces metastases
	Dietary fibres	-Soluble and insoluble fibres	
	Prebiotics/ Probiotics	-Yogurt -Fermented milk -Pickles -Garlic -Tubers -Banana	
	Vitamins and minerals	-Vitamin A, D & E -Vitamin C - Carotenoids -Folic acid	
	Fatty acids	-ω-3fatty acids -Lecithin -Conjugated linoleic acid	
	Phenolic compounds	-Catechins -Quercetin -Gallic acid -Resveratrol -Curcumin	

1.6.3 Diabetes

Diabetes mellitus is a metabolic syndrome growing epidemic due to exceptionally high blood glucose levels due to defects in either insufficient insulin production or insulin action or both (American diabetes association, 2009). Many abnormalities are associated with diabetes such as alter carbohydrate and lipid metabolism and also it significantly influence individual physically as well as mentally (Sharma et al., 2016).

Nutraceuticals such as herbal dietary supplements contains essential bioactive compounds and exhibits therapeutic properties against diabetes. So, nowadays nutraceuticals are used as an effective alternative against pharmaceutical drugs for type 2 diabetes treatment (Nasri et al., 2014; Raut et al., 2013). Common antioxidants such as catechins and lipoic acid and few spices such as cinnamon and fenugreek are very effective against diabetic retinopathy, nephropathy and neuropathy. Bioactive molecules like omega-3 fatty acids, soy isoflavones and nutrients such as Vitamin D, calcium, chromium and magnesium reduces diabetes prevalence as these molecules favors insulin sensitivity, bring blood sugar normal and decrease glucose tolerance. Moreover, in patients with insulin resistance caffeic acid helps to decrease high plasma glucose levels. Epigallocatechin-3-gallate (EGCG), a potent anti-diabetic catechin derived from green tea has beneficial effects in lowering the fasting and postprandial glucose level and rectify insulin resistance (Fu et al., 2017). Also, fruits like pomegranate and watermelon manage metabolism and carry glucose from the blood to the cells (Stephen, 2012).

Figure 9. Role of EGCG against obesity and Type 2 diabetes (Casanova et al., 2019)

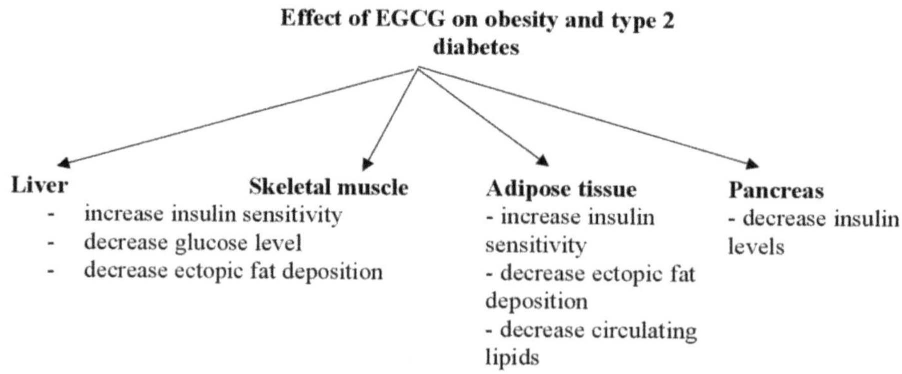

1.6.4 Obesity

Obesity is a complex chronic metabolic disease described as abnormal or excessive body fat accumulation. Nutraceuticals such as psyllium, capsaicin and conjugated linoleic acid effective against obesity (Nasri et al., 2014). Herbal products and dietary supplements such as vitamin C, caffeine, chitosan, green tea, fenugreek, bottle guard, fenugreek emits leptin and cytokines (IL-1,6) and helps to decreases body weight and manage food intake. These products significantly lower LDL and total cholesterol (Kaur et al., 2015).

1.6.5 Osteoarthritis

Osteoarthritis is the largest chronic joint disorder affecting millions of people globally. It's a multifactorial disorder where protective cartilage degrades (Mora et al., 2018). Joint pain decreases an individual's physical activity that further leads to weight gain problem and energy imbalance (Kumar et al., 2013).

Nutraceuticals such as curcumin, diacerein, chondroitin sulfate, collagen hydrolysate, glucosamine are used to mitigate osteoarthritis symptoms (Sacco et al., 2013). Fish oil is effective against joint disorder, as it contains anti-inflammatory agents such as omega-3 fatty acids, docosahexaenoic acid (DHA) and eicosapentaenoic acid (EPA) that reduces gene expression and inflammation signals and suppress proliferation of lymphocyte (Castrogiovanni et al., 2016). Olive oil appliance recovers patients from stiffness, swelling and pain and helps in cartilage recovery (Bohlooli et al., 2012). Nutritional supplementation of chondroitin sulfate and glucosamine sulfate protects joints from stiffness and pain (Castrogiovanni et al., 2016).

1.6.6 Dental Disorder

Odonto nutraceutical is a new terminology, which shows pleiotropic phytotherapeutic agents for dental care as it organizes at different biochemical and molecular targets (Gonzalez-Vallinas et al., 2013). These substances are bioactive compounds which prevent dental disorder. Odonto nutraceuticals such as grapes, cocoa seed extracts and green tea are excellent source flavonoids, proanthocyanidins and polyphenols. It performs a definite function against multifactorial and complex oral disease. Probiotics perform preventive action against dental caries, halitosis, gingivitis, malodour and periodontitis (Janczarek et al., 2016). Aloe vera gel is particularly used for the treatment of dental lichen planus disorder and also alleviate individual pain and mucosal wound (Nair et al., 2016).

1.6.7 Alzheimer's Disorder

Alzheimer's disorder is an inevitable, progressive brain disease that moderately damaged memory and thinking skill and ultimately, the capacity to accomplish simple tasks. This disorder is also recognized as senile dementia. Utilization of nutraceuticals slacken the progression of the disorder. Nutraceuticals such as curcumin, beta-carotene, lavandula extract, lutein and lycopene exhibits antioxidant properties that prevent oxidative stress and combat neuronal damage. These bioactive compounds setback the dementia development (Klatte et al., 2003). Many studies show that augmentation of B-complexes such as B12 and folic acid prevent the progression of this brain disorder by decreasing levels of homocysteine (Kennedy, 2016; Ji & Zhang, 2008).

1.6.8 Parkinson's Disorder

Parkinson's disorder is a progressive nervous system that affects movement. Worldwide, it's the second most reappearing ageing-related neurodegenerative disorder. This disease is related to the loss of dopamine-producing brain cells due to neurodegeneration. Many herbals and phytochemicals such as vitamin A, C and D, co-enzyme Q10, crocin, epigallocatechin-3-gallate (EGCG), gallic acid, unsaturated fatty acid, resveratrol and quercetin exerts antioxidants properties and shows improvement in neurobehavioral defects by preventing apoptosis of dopamine neuron (Lama et al., 2020). The Mucuna pruriens seed extract exhibits anti-parkinsonian activity by limiting neuroinflammatory activities (Ghaffari et al., 2018). Traditional herbal nutraceutical Bacopa monniera (Brahmi), is used as a brain tonic to treat a person suffering from Parkinson's disorder. Besides, promoting neurological and cognitive functions, brahmi also helps to boost circulation to the brain, improves mood, rejuvenate brain cells and mental peace (Agarwal, 2017).

1.6.9 Eyes Disorder

Diet rich in nutraceuticals seems to be advantageous for age-related macular degeneration. Bioactive compounds such as vitamin E, DHA, carotenoids, lutein, coenzyme Q10, and flavonoids are very effective against cataracts and presbyopia as it possess antioxidant properties. Spirulina, soy isoflavones and melatonin are very beneficial in controlling macular degeneration. Fruits and vegetables and rice bran contain zeaxanthin and lutein that helps it improve eyesight and also decreases the chances of cataract occurring. Essential fatty acids such as omega 3,6,9 helps in the management of eye health (Varani & Iritis, 2016).

1.6.10 Stress Management

Stress is a physical and emotional strain that is a risk to our health. Stress is associated with many health issues such as anxiety, depression, high blood pressure, diabetes, asthma, heart problems etc. The herbal bioactive compound known as adaptogens are used as a protective measure against chronic stress. These compounds keep balancing reaction between stress and mental illness. Also, it buildup resistance of an organism to harmful effects and it leads to a hike in an emotional act that further rescue from stressful conditions (Kalra, 2003). Ashwagandha, ginseng, rhodiola, centella asiatica and bacopa are commonly used as adaptogens as they stimulate the formation of stress suppressing heat shock protein 70 (HSP-70). It also balances the physical process, increases resistance to environmental stress, promotes homeostasis, improve sleep, decrease depress and anxiety and recovers secondary memory (Dutta et al., 2018; Kalra, 2003).

2. NEW CHALLENGES IN NUTRACEUTICAL MARKET

Although the nutraceutical market survived for several years, yet it is tough to predict the future of the nutraceutical market because of the different challenges such as less innovation, country regulation and difficult in health claim validation. However, many countries have legal health claim regulation but still, the process has not emerged in acceptance for the use of these health claims (El Sohaimy, 2012). Also, the approval of health claims is difficult in some countries like the USA and Japan. Several parameters such as validation of biomarker, the dose-response curve for setting definite dosage and adverse effects that would augment a health claim are not robust in these regions. Moreover, the nutraceutical market still remains more as a theoretical idea rather than a reality because it regroup food supplements (Daliri and Lee, 2015). It's a very challenging task to prove scientific evidence of nutraceutical for its health benefits. For health improvement biomarkers are not easily recognized and also clinical trials are too length process that rarely give strong affirmation of definite dosage. Therefore, nutraceutical production companies have to consider these physiological factors as developing a food product with legal health claims is not at all cinch. For nutraceuticals, another challenging area is the lack of quality control that may lead to serious consequences as it increases the risk to the consumer. As there is no specific quality control process for nutraceuticals, adulteration and other impurities simply remain undetected in the formulations (Patil, 2011).

3. FUTURE PERSPECTIVES

As per the discussion in previous sections, it's very much clear that the few of the aforementioned compounds have promising results to clinical conditions. Nowadays, even healthcare companies also understand the fact how importantly nutrients affects consumer's health. Therefore, they are in search of adopting the combination of nutrition and medical care to ensure a holistic approach towards consumers. Currently, medical care is only concern towards the province of drugs, whereas nutrition deals as a product for health life being. In future, it is apprehended work will be executed on how medicine and nutrition will interact and complement each other. Scientific researchers are in the process of validating the safety and effectiveness of new nutraceutical products that may further promote the technology and nutraceuticals market. There is vast potential to develop specific food by utilizing various promising techniques such as imaging technology, nutrigenomics and converging techniques for targeted population groups with specific metabolic disorders (Da Costa, 2017). New tailoring approach of food and nutrition researchers may further lead to the development of functional foods required for optimal health benefits. Due to increased consumer awareness related to nutraceuticals, its growth is expected globally. However, the concern over the term "naturalness" may boost the global regulations but the concern about safety aspects mainly due to overseas production could suppress its growth (Daliri and Lee, 2015).

4. CONCLUSION

Unhealthy eating habits are often associated with anxiety and stress which leads to various degenerative disease with age. Many researchers have linked consumption of nutraceuticals with prevention of multiple degenerative diseases. Nutraceutical is a nutritional therapy that is used to improve overall human health. Nutraceuticals such as β-carotene, conjugated linolenic acid, vitamin C, polyphenols, flavanoids, curcumin plays a potential role in the prevention of metabolic disorders. Health-conscious consumers are adopting nutraceuticals over pharmaceuticals to prevent oxidative stress with no side effects. Nutraceuticals contains bioactive compounds that prevent metabolic disorders and enhance physical and mental health. Nutraceuticals is the latest trend in the market that connects a new generation of medicine with health.

Many epidemiologic studies reveal the positive impact of nutraceuticals on many degenerative disorders such as cancer, neurodegenerative disease, obesity, diabetes and cardiovascular disease. Food substances such as tea, onions, tomatoes, garlic, olive oil, honey, berries, chilli peppers, grapes, basil, aloe vera, carrots, soybean, curcuma, pomegranate and rosemary contains bioactive compounds helps to strengthen immune system.

REFERENCES

Agarwal, S. (2017). *Nutraceuticals and osteoarthritis. Leading pharmaceutical consultant.* http://www.drsanjayagrawal.com

Aghajanpour, M., Nazer, M. R., Obeidavi, Z., Akbari, M., Ezati, P., & Kor, N. M. (2017). Functional foods and their role in cancer prevention and health promotion: A comprehensive review. *American Journal of Cancer Research, 7*(4), 740–769. PMID:28469951

Alissa, E. M., & Ferns, G. A. (2012). Functional foods and nutraceuticals in the primary prevention of cardiovascular diseases. *Journal of Nutrition and Metabolism, 2012*, 1–16. doi:10.1155/2012/569486 PMID:22570771

Alves, Q.L., Camardo, S.B., & Silva, D.F. (2019). Role of nutraceuticals in the prevention and treatment of hypertension and cardiovascular diseases. *Journal of Hypertension and Management, 5*, 37.

American Diabetes Association. (2009). Diagnosis and classification of diabetes mellitus. *Diabetes Care, 32*(supplement 1), S62–S67. doi:10.2337/dc09-S062 PMID:19118289

Anderson, J. W., Baird, P., Davis, R. H. Jr, Ferreri, S., Knudtson, M., Koraym, A., ... Williams, C. L. (2009). Health benefits of dietary fiber. *Nutrition Reviews, 67*(4), 188–205. doi:10.1111/j.1753-4887.2009.00189.x PMID:19335713

Arora, D., & Jaglan, S. (2016). Nanocarriers based delivery of nutraceuticals for cancer prevention and treatment: A review of recent research developments. *Trends in Food Science & Technology, 54*, 114–126. doi:10.1016/j.tifs.2016.06.003

Bernardi, J. R., & Escobar, R. S. (2012). Fetal and neonatal levels of omega-3: Effect on neurodevelopment, nutrition and growth. *The Scientific World Journal.*

Bohlooli, S., Jastan, M., Nakhostin-Roohi, B., Mohammadi, S., & Baghari, Z. (2012). A pilot double-blinded, randomized, clinical trial of topical virgin olive oil versus piroxicam gel in osteoarthritis of the knee. *Journal of Clinical Rheumatology; Practical Reports on Rheumatic & Musculoskeletal Diseases, 18*(2), 99–101. doi:10.1097/RHU.0b013e31824a47b5 PMID:22334264

Brower, V. (1998). Nutraceuticals: Poised for a healthy slice of the healthcare market? *Nature Biotechnology, 16*(8), 728–731. doi:10.1038/nbt0898-728 PMID:9702769

Casanova, E., Salvado, J., Crescenti, A., & Gibert-Ramos, A. (2019). Epigallocatechin gallate modulates muscle homeostasis in type 2 diabetes and obesity by targeting energetic and redox pathways: A narrative review. *International Journal of Molecular Sciences, 20*(3), 532. doi:10.3390/ijms20030532 PMID:30691224

Castrogiovanni, P., Trovato, F. M., Loreto, C., Nsir, H., Szychlinska, M. A., & Musumeci, G. (2016). Nutraceutical supplements in the management and prevention of osteoarthritis. *International Journal of Molecular Sciences, 17*(12), 2042. doi:10.3390/ijms17122042 PMID:27929434

CDC. (2019). *Heart disease facts. Division for heart disease and stroke prevention*. National Center for Chronic Disease prevention and Health Promotion.

Cicero, A. F., & Colletti, A. (2016). Combination of phytomedicines with different lipid lowering activity for dyslipidemia management: The available clinical data. *Phytomedicine, 23*(11), 1113–1118. doi:10.1016/j.phymed.2015.10.011 PMID:26621556

Ciesielski, T. H., Bartlett, J., & Williams, S. M. (2019). Omega-3 polyunsaturated fatty acid intake norms and preterm birth rate: A cross-sectional analysis of 184 countries. *BMJ Open, 9*(4), e027249. doi:10.1136/bmjopen-2018-027249 PMID:31005937

Connor, W. E. (2000). Importance of n-3 fatty acids in health and disease. *The American Journal of Clinical Nutrition, 71*(1Supplement), 171S–175S. doi:10.1093/ajcn/71.1.171S PMID:10617967

Cory, H., Passarelli, S., Szeto, J., Tamez, M., & Mattei, J. (2018). The role of polyphenols in human health and food systems: A mini-review. *Frontiers in Nutrition, 5*, 87. doi:10.3389/fnut.2018.00087 PMID:30298133

Da Costa, J. P. (2017). A current look at nutraceuticals- Key concepts and future prospects. *Trends in Food Science & Technology, 62*, 68–78. doi:10.1016/j.tifs.2017.02.010

Daliri, E.B.-M., & Lee, B.H. (2015). Current trends and future perspectives on functional foods and nutraceuticals. *Microbiology Monographs*, 221-244.

Das, L., Bhaumik, E., Raychaudhuri, U., & Chakraborty, R. (2012). Role of nutraceuticals in human health. *Journal of Food Science and Technology, 49*(2), 173–183. doi:10.100713197-011-0269-4 PMID:23572839

Deng, G. F., Shen, C., Xu, X. R., Kuang, R. D., Guo, Y. J., Zeng, L. S., ... Li, H. B. (2012). Potential of fruit wastes as natural resources of bioactive compounds. *International Journal of Molecular Sciences, 13*(7), 8308–8323. doi:10.3390/ijms13078308 PMID:22942704

Dillard, C. J., & German, J. B. (2000). Phytochemicals: Nutraceuticals and human health. *Journal of the Science of Food and Agriculture, 80*(12), 1744–1756. doi:10.1002/1097-0010(20000915)80:12<1744::AID-JSFA725>3.0.CO;2-W

Duthie, G. G., Gardner, P. T., & Kyle, J. A. M. (2003). Plant polyphenols: Are they the new magic bullet? *The Proceedings of the Nutrition Society, 62*(3), 599–603. doi:10.1079/PNS2003275 PMID:14692595

Dutta, S., Ali, K. M., Dash, S. K., & Giri, B. (2018). Role of nutraceuticals on health promotion and disease prevention: A review. *Journal of Drug Delivery and Therapeutics, 8*(4), 42–47. doi:10.22270/jddt.v8i4.1759

El Hadi, H., Vettor, R., & Rossato, M. (2018). Congenital vitamin E deficiency. In V. R. Preedy & V. B. Patel (Eds.), *Handbook of famine, starvation, and nutrient deprivation* (pp. 1–18). Basel, Switzerland: Springer International Publishing AG. doi:10.1007/978-3-319-40007-5_86-1

El Sohaimy, S. A. (2012). Functional foods and nutraceuticals-modern approach to food science. *World Applied Sciences Journal, 20*, 691–708.

Escott-Stump, E., & Mahan, L. L. (2000). *Krause's food, nutrition and diet therapy*. Philadelphia: WB Saunders Company.

FAO/WHO. (2001). *Report on joint FAO/WHO expert consultation on evaluation of health and nutritional properties of probiotics in food including powder milk with live lactic acid bacteria*. Author.

FDA/CFSAN. (1994). *Food and Drug Administration website*. Dietary Supplement Health and Education Act. http://vm.cfsan.fda.gov/~dms/dietsupp.html

Fu, Q., Li, Q., Lin, X., Qiao, R., Yang, R., Li, X., ... Liang, Y. (2017). Antidiabetic effects of tea. *Molecules (Basel, Switzerland), 22*(5), 849. doi:10.3390/molecules22050849 PMID:28531120

Geier, M. S., Butler, R. N., & Howarth, G. S. (2006). Probiotics, prebiotics and synbiotics: A role in chemoprevention for colorectal cancer. *Cancer Biology & Therapy*, *5*(10), 1265–1269. doi:10.4161/cbt.5.10.3296 PMID:16969130

Ghaffari, F., Moghadd, M. A. H., & Zare, M. (2018). Neuroprotective effect of quercetin nanocrystal in a 6-hydroxydopamine model of Parkinson disease: Biochemical and behavioral evidence. *Basic and Clinical Neuroscience*, *9*(5), 317–324. doi:10.32598/bcn.9.5.317 PMID:30719246

Gonzalez-Vallinas, M., Gonzalez-Castejon, M., Rodriguez Casado, A., & Ramírez de Molina, A. (2013). Dietary phytochemicals in cancer prevention and therapy: A complementary approach with promising perspectives. *Nutrition Reviews*, *71*(9), 585–599. doi:10.1111/nure.12051 PMID:24032363

Govender, M., Choonara, Y. E., Kumar, P., Toit, L. C., Vuuren, S. V., & Pillay, V. (2014). A review of the advancements in probiotic delivery: Conventional vs. non-conventional formulations for intestinal flora supplementation. *Journal of the American Association of Pharmaceutical Scientists*, *15*(1), 29–43. PMID:24222267

Guarner, F. (2005). Inulin and oligofructose: Impact on intestinal disease and disorders. *British Journal of Nutrition*, *93*(S1Supplement), S61–S65. doi:10.1079/BJN20041345 PMID:15877897

Hord, N. G. (2008). Eukaryotic microbiotic crosstalk: Potential mechanism for health benefits of prebiotics and probiotics. *Annual Review of Nutrition*, *28*(1), 215–231. doi:10.1146/annurev.nutr.28.061807.155402 PMID:18489258

Hu, F. B., & Willett, W. C. (2002). Optimal diets for prevention of coronary heart disease. *Journal of the American Medical Association*, *288*(20), 25692578. doi:10.1001/jama.288.20.2569 PMID:12444864

Hueda, M. C. (2020). *Introductory chapter: Nutraceuticals as an alternative to maintain a healthy life-style, nutraceuticals- past, present and future*. IntechOpen. doi:10.5772/intechopen.89875

IOM. (2000). Selenium. In Dietary reference intakes for vitamin C, vitamin E, selenium and carotenoids. Food and Nutrition Board, Institute of Medicine. National Academy Press.

IOM. (2002). *Dietary reference intakes for energy, carbohydrate, fiber, fat, fatty acids, cholesterol, protein and amino acids*. Institute of Medicine.

Janczarek, M., Bachanek, T., Mazur, E., & Chalas, R. (2016). The role of probiotics in prevention of oral diseases. Postepy Higiency I. *Medycyna Doswiadczalna*, *70*(0), 850–885. PMID:27594560

Ji, H., & Zhang, H. (2008). Multipotent natural agents to combat Alzheimer's disease. Functional spectrum and structural features. *Acta Pharmacologica Sinica*, *29*(2), 143–151. doi:10.1111/j.1745-7254.2008.00752.x PMID:18215342

Kalia, A. N. (2005). *Textbook of industrial pharmacognocy*. New Delhi: CBS Publisher and Distributor.

Kalra, E. K. (2003). Nutraceuticals-Definition and introduction. *American Association of Pharmaceutical Scientists*, *5*(3), 27–28.

Kaur, G., Mukundan, S., Wani, V., & Kumar, M. S. (2015). Nutraceuticals in the management and prevention of metabolic syndrome. *Austin Journal of Pharmacology and Therapeutics*, *3*, 1–6.

Kennedy, D. O. (2016). B vitamins and the brain: Mechanism, dose and efficacy- A review. *Nutrients*, *8*(2), 68. doi:10.3390/nu8020068 PMID:26828517

Klatte, E. T., Scharre, D. W., Nagaraja, H. N., Davis, R. A., & Beversdorf, D. Q. (2003). Combination therapy of donepezil and vitamin E in Alzheimer disease. *Alzheimer Disease and Associated Disorders*, *17*(2), 113–116. doi:10.1097/00002093-200304000-00010 PMID:12794389

Kokate, C. K., Purohit, A. P., & Gokhale, S. B. (2002). *Nutraceutical and cosmaceutical* (21st ed.). Pune, India: Pharmacognosy, Nirali Prakashan.

Kris-Etherton, P. M., Hecker, K. D., Bonanome, A., Coval, S. M., Binkoski, A. E., Hilpert, K. F., ... Etherton, T. D. (2003). Bioactive compounds in foods: Their role in the prevention of cardiovascular disease and cancer. *The American Journal of Medicine*, *113*(Supplement 9B), 71S–88S. doi:10.1016/S0002-9343(01)00995-0 PMID:12566142

Kumar, R., Singh, G., Krishan, P., Kumari, P., Rizwi, S. I., & Gautam, S. P. (2013). Nutraceuticals: A boom to medical industry. *Pharmaceutical Sciences*, *2*, 1–8.

Kuo, S. M. (2013). The interplay between fiber and the intestinal microbiome in the inflammatory response. *Advances in Nutrition*, *4*(1), 16–28. doi:10.3945/an.112.003046 PMID:23319119

Lama, A., Pirozzi, C., Avagliano, C., Annunziata, C., Mollica, M.P., Calignano, A., Meli, R., & Raso, G.M. (2020). Nutraceuticals: An integrative approach to starve Parkinson's disease. *Brain, Behavior and Immunity- Health, 2*, 100037.

Larion, S., & Khurana, S. (2018). Clinical studies investigating the effect of vitamin E therapy in patients with NASH. *Clinics in Liver Disease*, *11*(1), 16–21. doi:10.1002/cld.687 PMID:30992781

Lenoir-Wijnkoop, I., Sanders, M. E., Cabana, M. D., Caglar, E., Corthier, G., Rayes, N., ... Timmerman, H. M. (2007). Probiotic and prebiotic influence beyond the intestinal tract. *Nutrition Reviews*, *65*(11), 469–489. doi:10.1111/j.1753-4887.2007.tb00272.x PMID:18038940

Lesbros-Pantoflickova, D., Corthesy-Theulaz, I., & Blum, A. L. (2007). Helicobacter pylori and probiotics. *The Journal of Nutrition*, *137*(3), 812S–818S. doi:10.1093/jn/137.3.812S PMID:17311980

Macfarlane, S., Macfarlane, G. T., & Cummings, J. H. (2006). Review article: Prebiotics in the gastrointestinal tract. *Alimentary Pharmacology & Therapeutics*, *24*(5), 701–714. doi:10.1111/j.1365-2036.2006.03042.x PMID:16918875

Manganaris, G. A., Goulas, V., Vicente, A. R., & Terry, L. A. (2014). Berry antioxidants: Small fruits providing large benfits. *Journal of the Science of Food and Agriculture*, *94*(5), 825–833. doi:10.1002/jsfa.6432 PMID:24122646

Markowiak, P., & Slizewska, K. (2017). Effects of probiotics, prebiotics and synbiotics on human health. *Nutrients*, *9*(9), 1021. doi:10.3390/nu9091021 PMID:28914794

Metchinkoff, E. (1907). *The prolongation of life*. New York: Putmans Sons.

Meydani, M. (2000). Effect of functional food ingredients: Vitamin E modulation of cardiovascular diseases and immune status in the elderly. *The American Journal of Clinical Nutrition*, *71*(6), 1665S–1668S. doi:10.1093/ajcn/71.6.1665S PMID:10837312

Mora, J. C., Przkora, R., & Cruz-Almeida, Y. (2018). Knee osteoarthritis: Pathophysiology and current treatment modalities. *Journal of Pain Research*, *11*, 2189–2196. doi:10.2147/JPR.S154002 PMID:30323653

Nair, G. R., Naidu, G. S., Jain, S., Nagi, R., Makkad, R. S., & Jha, A. (2016). Clinical effectiveness of aloe vera in the management of oral mucosal diseases- A systematic review. *Journal of Clinical and Diagnostic Research: JCDR*, *10*(8), ZE01–ZE07. PMID:27656587

Nasri, H., Baradaran, A., Shirzad, H., & Rafieian-Kopaei, M. (2014). New concepts in nutraceuticals as alternative for pharmaceuticals. *International Journal of Preventive Medicine*, *5*(12), 1487–1499. PMID:25709784

NIH. (2020). *Selenium, Health professional fact sheet*. National Institute of Healths, Office of Dietary Supplements.

Pacana, T., & Sanyal, A. J. (2012). Vitamin E and non-alcoholic fatty liver disease. *Current Opinion in Clinical Nutrition and Metabolic Care*, *15*(6), 641–648. doi:10.1097/MCO.0b013e328357f747 PMID:23075940

Panche, A. N., Diwan, A. D., & Chandra, S. R. (2016). Flavonoids: An overview. *Journal of Nutritional Science*, *5*, e47. doi:10.1017/jns.2016.41 PMID:28620474

Pandey, K. R., Naik, S. R., & Vaki, B. V. (2015). Probiotics, prebiotics and synbiotics- A review. *Journal of Food Science and Technology*, *52*(12), 7577–7587. doi:10.100713197-015-1921-1 PMID:26604335

Pandey, M., Verma, R. K., & Saraf, S. A. (2010). Nutraceuticals: New era of medicine and health. *Asian Journal of Pharmaceutical and Clinical Research*, *3*, 11–15.

Patil, C. S. (2011). Current trends and future prospective of nutraceuticals in health promotion. *BIOINFO Pharmaceutical Biotechnology*, *1*(1), 1–7.

Pilch, S. M. (1987). Physiologic effects and health consequences of dietary fiber. Life Science Research Office, Federation of American Societies for Experimental Biology.

Ramaa, C. S., Shirode, A. R., Mundada, A. S., & Kadam, V. J. (2006). Nutraceuticals- An emerging era in the treatment and prevention of cardiovascular diseases. *Current Pharmaceutical Biotechnology*, *7*(1), 15–23. doi:10.2174/138920106775789647 PMID:16472130

Raut, A., Bichile, L., Chopra, A., Patwardhan, B., & Vaidya, A. (2013). Comparative study of amrutbhallataka and glucosamine sulphate in osteoarthritis: Six months open label randomized controlled clinical trial. *Journal of Ayurveda and Integrative Medicine*, *4*(4), 229–236. doi:10.4103/0975-9476.123708 PMID:24459390

Rissanen, T. H., Voutilainen, S., Virtanen, J. K., Venho, B., Vanharanta, M., Mursu, J., & Salonen, J. T. (2003). Low intake of fruits, berries and vegetables in associated with excess mortality in men: The Kuopio ischaemic heart disease risk factor (KIHD) study. *The Journal of Nutrition*, *133*(1), 199–204. doi:10.1093/jn/133.1.199 PMID:12514290

Sabita, N. S., & Trygve, O. T. (2012). The role of nutraceuticals in chemoprevention and chemotheraphy and their clinical outcomes. *Journal of Oncology*, *64*, 1–23.

Sacco, S. M., Horcajada, M. N., & Offord, E. (2013). Pytonutrients for bone health during ageing. *British Journal of Clinical Pharmacology*, *75*(3), 697–707. doi:10.1111/bcp.12033 PMID:23384080

Saibil, F. (1989). Diarrhea due to fiber overload. *The New England Journal of Medicine*, *320*(9), 599. doi:10.1056/NEJM198903023200920 PMID:2536897

Shang, A., Cao, S., Xu, X., Gan, R., Tang, G., Corke, H., ... Li, H. (2019). Bioactive compounds and biological functions of garlic (*Allium sativum* L.). *Foods*, *8*(7), 246. doi:10.3390/foods8070246 PMID:31284512

Sharma, R., Amin, H., & Prajapati, P. K. (2016). Comparative lipid profile of type 2 obese diabetics and obese non-diabetics: A hospital based study from hilly terrains of Mandi, Himachal Pradesh. *International Journal of Health & Allied Sciences*, *5*(1), 63–64. doi:10.4103/2278-344X.173876

Singh, A., Holvoet, S., & Mercenier, A. (2011). Dietary polyphenols in the prevention and treatment of allergic diseases. *Clinical and Experimental Allergy*, *41*(10), 1346–1359. doi:10.1111/j.1365-2222.2011.03773.x PMID:21623967

Slavin, J. L., & Lloyd, B. (2012). Health benefits of fruits and vegetables. *Advances in Nutrition*, *3*(4), 506–516. doi:10.3945/an.112.002154 PMID:22797986

Stephen, D. (2012). A report of national nutraceutical center. Nutaceuticals India. *Webinar*, *2012*, 1–22.

Sunde, R. A. (2006). Selenium. In B. Bowman & R. Russell (Eds.), *Present knowledge in nutrition* (9th ed., pp. 480–497). Washington, DC: International Life Science Institute.

Sunde, R. A. (2010). Selenium. In *Encyclopedia of Dietary Supplements* (2nd ed., pp. 711–718). London: Informa Healthcare. doi:10.1201/b14669-82

Suvarna, V. C., & Boby, V. U. (2005). Probiotics in human health: A current assessment. *Current Science*, *88*, 1744–1748.

Trottier, G., Bostrom, P. J., Lawrentschul, N., & Fleshner, N. E. (2010). Nutraceuticals and prostate cancer prevention: A current review. *Nature Reviews. Urology*, *7*(1), 21–30. doi:10.1038/nrurol.2009.234 PMID:19997071

Unites State Pharmacopeia (USP). (2006). *The regulation of dietary supplements*. http://www.usp.org/pdf/EN/USPVerified/dietarySupplementRegulation.pdf

US FDA. (2014). *Summary of qualified health claims subject to enforcement discretion*. Author.

Varani, E. M., & Iriti, M. (2016). Odonto nutraceuticals: Pleioyropic photo therapeutic agents for oral health. *Pharmaceuticals*, *9*(1), 10–13. doi:10.3390/ph9010010

Wang, X., Ouyang, Y., Liu, J., Zhu, M., Zhao, G., Bao, W., & Hu, F. B. (2014). Fruit and vegetable consumption and mortality from all causes, cardiovascular disease, and cancer: Systematic review and dose-response meta-analysis of prospective cohort studies. *British Medical Journal*, *349*(jul29 3), g4490. doi:10.1136/bmj.g4490 PMID:25073782

Wargovich, M. J., Morris, J., Brown, V., Ellis, J., Logothetis, B., & Weber, R. (2010). Nutraceutical use in late-stage cancer. *Cancer and Metastasis Reviews*, *29*(3), 503–510. doi:10.100710555-010-9240-5 PMID:20714787

Watzl, B., Girrbach, S., & Roller, M. (2005). Inulin, oligofructose and immunomodulation. *British Journal of Nutrition*, *93*(S1), 49–55. doi:10.1079/BJN20041357 PMID:15877895

Wildman, R. E. C. (2007). *Nutraceuticals and functional foods*. New York: CRC Press.

Wong, K. V. (2012). Nutritional perspective about prostate cancer disparity between the west and the rest of the world. *Food Science and Technology Letters*, *3*(1), 14–19.

Zanini, S., Marzotto, M., Giovinazzo, F., Bassi, C., & Bellavite, P. (2015). Effects of dietary components on cancer of the digestive system. *Critical Reviews in Food Science and Nutrition*, *55*(13), 1870–1885. doi:10.1080/10408398.2012.732126 PMID:24841279

Zeisel, S. H. (1999). Rehulations of "Nutraceuticals". *Science*, *285*(5435), 1853–1855. doi:10.1126cience.285.5435.1853 PMID:10515789

Zhang, Y. J., Deng, G. F., Xu, X. R., Wu, S., Li, S., & Li, H. B. (2013). Chemical components and bioactivities of cape gooseberry (*Physalis peruviana*). *International Journal of Food Nutrition and Safety*, *3*, 15–24.

Zhang, Y. J., Gan, R., Li, S., Zhou, Y., Li, A., Xu, D., & Li, H. (2015). Antioxidants phytochemicals for the prevention and treatment of chronic diseases. *Molecules (Basel, Switzerland)*, *20*(12), 21138–21156. doi:10.3390/molecules201219753 PMID:26633317

Zhao, J. (2007). *Nutraceuticals, nutritional therapy, phytonutrients and phototherapy for improvement of human health: A perspective on Plant Biotechnology Application*. Bentham Science Publishers. http://www.benthamscience.com/biot/samples/biot1-1/Zhao.pdf

Chapter 14
Pharmacology and Therapeutic Applications of Resveratrol

Bui Thanh Tung
VNU University of Medicine and Pharmacy, Vietnam National University, Hanoi, Vietnam

ABSTRACT

Resveratrol (3,5,4'-trihydroxy-trans-stilbene) is a non-flavonoid polyphenolic compound belonging to the stilbene group which is the main compound found in grapes. Resveratrol has shown a wide range of preventive and therapeutic alternatives against several diseases including distinct types of cancer, heart disease, stroke, diabetes, obesity, inflammation, antioxidant. It is a highly efficient treatment, which might be due to the three hydroxyl groups in its structure. Consumption of resveratrol has been shown to improve health status and has the positive effect of treatment of many diseases. Moreover, it has been demonstrated that resveratrol possesses the potential of lifespan extension in various organism and animal models. However, the long-term use of resveratrol may have some adverse effects and should be studied deeper. This chapter will outline some pharmacological effects of resveratrol.

BACKGROUND

Name: Resveratrol
Different name: 3,4',5-stilbenetriol; 3,5,4'-trihydroxystilbene; trans-resveratrol-3-O-sulfate; trans-resveratrol; cis-resveratrol; resveratrol-3-sulfate.

Resveratrol has been known since 1939, when the Japanese by chance extracted the rhizomes of the "Veratrum" (Arichi et al., 1982). Its chemical texture was published in the "Journal of Japanese Chemistry Association" and was named Resveratrol, meaning "resorcinol from Veratrum". Resveratrol is a white powder, a molecular weight of 228.35, which is one of the simplest phenolic compounds from plants. Resveratrol is a substance found in at least 70 types of plants, most commonly found in foods, including grapes, peanuts, pineapple, strawberry, etc. (Figure 1). Resveratrol has a ring structure composed of many hydroxy acids (Figure 2). Hydroxy groups can be oxidized to promote antioxidant activity, provide for resveratrol stronger antioxidant activity than vitamin C, E, and glutathione (Sobolev & Cole, 1999).

DOI: 10.4018/978-1-7998-4808-0.ch014

THE POTENTIAL OF RESVERATROL IN CARDIOVASCULAR DISEASE TREATMENT

Cardiovascular diseases (CVDs) are considered to be the most common cause of the death in the global

Figure 1. Examples of fruits and food rich in resveratrol

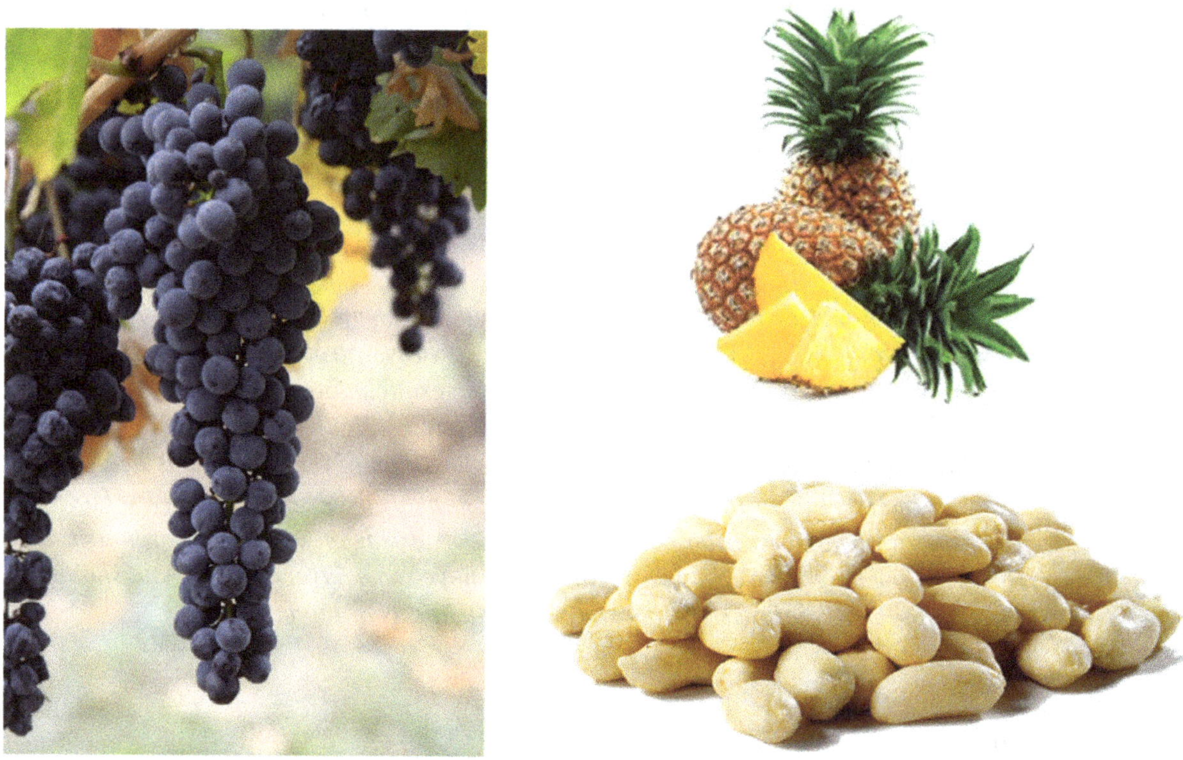

Figure 2. The structure of the trans-cis of resveratrol

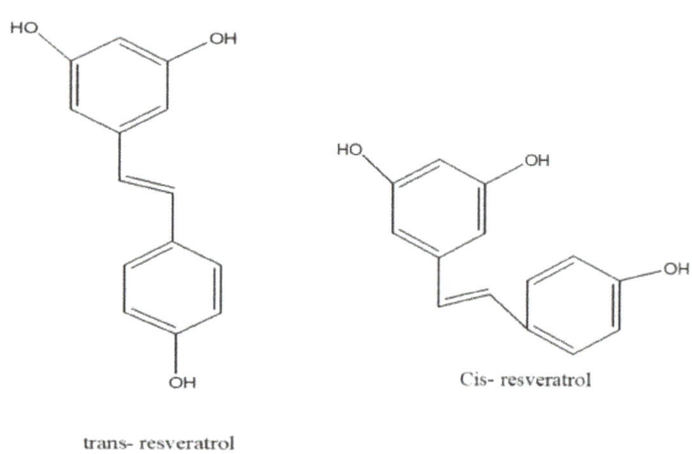

population and account for much treatment expenditures. The cardiovascular protection of resveratrol are associated with multiple molecular targets and which can lead to the development of novel therapeutic strategies for atherosclerosis, ischemia/reperfusion, metabolic syndrome, and heart failure, so on…

Hypertension

Hypertension is a chronic medical condition that is showed by sustained arterial blood pressure elevation. Several investigators have demonstrated that resveratrol can lower BP in experimental animal models of hypertension with the molecular target of sirtuins and SIRT1 (Figure 3). With regard to its endothelium-dependent effects, resveratrol supplementation has been shown to improve flow-mediated vasodilation, a surrogate for endothelial function, in several animal models (Pearson et al., 2008; Rush, Quadrilatero, Levy, & Ford, 2007; Soylemez, Sepici, & Akar, 2009; Toklu et al., 2010). Resveratrol increases the bioavailability of nitric oxide (NO) by increasing endothelial nitric oxide synthase (eNOS) expression to show the vasodilatory effects (Leikert et al., 2002; Wallerath et al., 2002). Three isoforms of NO synthase (NOS), eNOS, neuronal NOS (nNOS), and inducible NOS (iNOS) could mediated level of NO (Calvert & Lefer, 2009). eNOS plays important role in cardiovascular physiology because it regulates vascular tone via the release of NO in the vascular endothelium (Calvert & Lefer, 2009). It has been showed that resveratrol involves the effects of resveratrol on silent information regulator 1 (SIRT1), AMP-activated protein kinase (AMPK), and reactive oxygen species (ROS) to increasing the NO bioavailability. SIRT1 is a class III histone deacetylase which stimulates the NO production by deacetylating eNOS at lysine residues(Arunachalam, Yao, Sundar, Caito, & Rahman, 2010). Resveratrol activates SIRT1 then mediates both activity and expression of eNOS (Csiszar et al., 2009). It has been shown that resveratrol activates AMPK to stimulate NO production (Dolinsky et al., 2013).AMPK, a major regulator of energy metabolism (Nagendran, Waller, & Dyck, 2013), also regulates NO bioavailability via eNOS. AMPK phosphorylatea and activatea eNOS on serine 1177, resulting in a subsequent increase in NO production (Z.-P. Chen et al., 1999). In addition to the involvement of SIRT1 and AMPK in mediating the endothelium-dependent vasodilatory effects, resveratrol has been shown to enhance NOS activity by increasing tetrahydrobiopterin (BH4) levels, a cofactor necessary for proper function of NOS (Carrizzo et al., 2013).

Atherosclerosis

Atherosclerosis refers to the thickening of the artery due to the build up of plaque in the form of low density lipoprotein (LDL) in the arterial wall. The substance is changed by oxidation, inflammation, invasion of macrophages and then formed lots of foam cells, they intruded into the smooth muscle cells, and production of fibrin and extracellular matrix. All of this is the cause of the formed atherosclerosis plaques (Berliner et al., 1995). Several animal studies have shown that resveratrol can lower plasma levels of total and LDL cholesterol, as well as triglycerides, and increase the level of HDL cholesterol. The major mechanism is via increased the cholesterol 7α-hydroxylase (CYP7A1) expression (an enzyme is encoded by the CYP7A1 gene), which leads to be increasingly bile acid synthesis and secretion, thus lowering the plasma level of total and LDL cholesterol (Q. Chen, Wang, Ma, & Zhai, 2012). In addition, resveratrol has also been evidenced by many studies that it increases the LDL receptors expression in hepatocytes in vitro, thereby increasing the uptake of LDL by hepatic cells which id independent of AMPK pathway (Yashiro, Nanmoku, Shimizu, Inoue, & Sato, 2012). The quest for resveratrol effects

Figure 3. Proposed anti-hypertensive effect of resveratrol. Resveratrol showed its anti-ischemic effects through activation of AMP-activated protein kinase (AMPK), endothelial nitric oxide synthase (eNOS), and vascular endothelial growth factor (VEGF), and inhibition of reactive oxygen species (ROS) and atherosclerosis

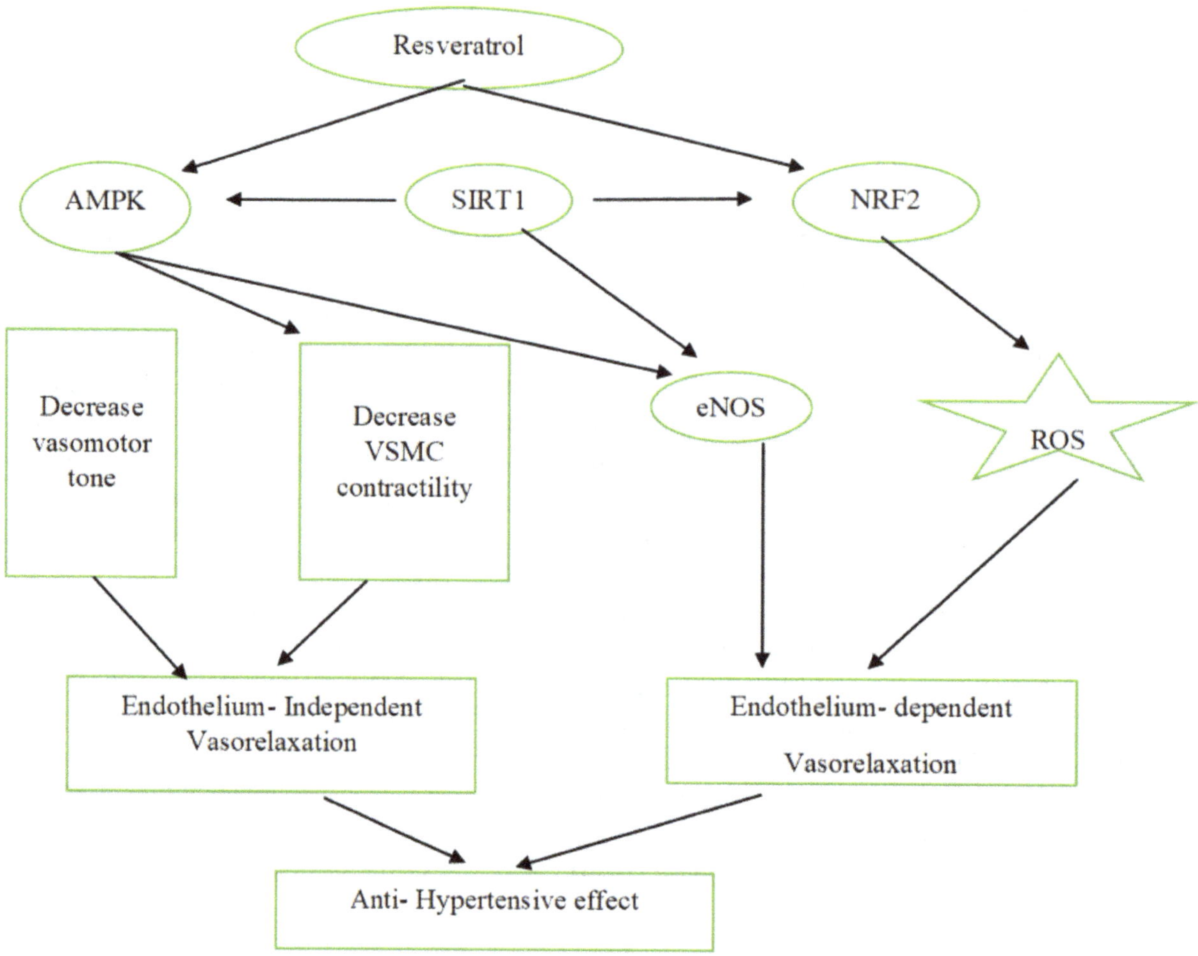

involved with atherosclerosis and jumped to conclusions that resveratrol will be capable of interfering with steps in the pathogenesis of atherosclerosis (Matos et al., 2012; Rocha et al., 2009; Z. Wang et al., 2005).

Arrhythmia

Arrhythmia refers to irregular heartbeat which may be either fast or slow. The mechanism anti-arrhythmic of resveratrol has been attributed to Ca^{2+}channel antagonism and KATP channel opening. It is also significantly shorten the action potential duration and the peak L-type Ca^{2+}current in guinea-pig ventricular myocytes (Y.-R. Chen et al., 2008; Liew, Stagg, MacLeod, & Collins, 2005; Zhang et al., 2006). The potential coronary syndrome treatment of resveratrol is studied by Tomes et al., in 2013 (Tomé-Carneiro et al., 2013). The resveratrol treatment is used with doses: 8mg/ 6 months and 16mg/ next 6 months, which increased the adiponectin and reduced the plasminogen activator inhibitor-1 (Tomé-Carneiro et al.,

2013). Another clinical study regarding atherosclerosis, which may contribute to make people the risk of CVDs, is gotten treatment by resveratrol (Bentzon, Otsuka, Virmani, & Falk, 2014). With being 8mg/day resveratrol in grape extract lead to decrease about 20% LDL and reduce for 4.5% LDL-cholesterol.

CANCER

Cancer is a group of diseases involving abnormal cell growth with the potential to invade to other parts of the body. More and more tumors become resistant to chemotherapy (chemoresistance) and radiotherapy (radioresistance) and this methods cause the side effects, which has become a major hurdle in cancer therapy. Several studies have showed that resveratrol can directly inhibit the proliferation and viability of cancer cell in a dose and time dependent manner in vitro. It is shown to be involved in growth inhibition, cell cycle arrest, and apoptosis in several human cancer cell lines.

Breast Cancer

A number of researchers have considered the anticarcinogenic effects of resveratrol in breast cancer (He, Wang, Zhu, Orloff, & Eng, 2011; Miksits et al., 2009; Scarlatti, Maffei, Beau, Codogno, & Ghidoni, 2008). Resveratrol could inhibit human breast cancer cell proliferation and promote cell death through multiple pathways including apoptosis, cell cycle arrest in the S phase. Resveratrol was demonstrated to induce cell death in both caspase-3 sensitive (MCF-7^{casp-3}) and caspase-3 insensitive (MCF-7^{vc}) human breast cancer cells. In addition, resveratrol stimulated autophagy by activating noncanonical (Beclin-1 independent) routes in both cell lines. The major molecular mechanism involved resveratrol-induced autophagy was associated with the suppression of Akt/protein kinase B (PKB) phosphorylation and mammalian target of rapamycin (mTOR)/S6K signaling pathway. A study had shown (He et al., 2011) that resveratrol and rapamycin combination could be a novel combinatorial strategy for breast cancer therapy. The result of this research was resveratrol significantly potentiate the anticancer activity of mTOR inhibitor rapamycin by suppressing rapamycin-induced AKt signaling pathway in MDA-MB-231, MCF-7, and BT-549 human breast cancer cells (He et al., 2011; Scarlatti et al., 2008).

Prostate Cancer

Prostate cancer is the most common cancer in men. It affects the prostate gland, the gland that produces some of the fluid in semen and plays a role in urine control in men. Prostate cancer cells possess large amounts of calcium channels that mediate multiple cellular processes such as cell proliferation, tumorigenesis, and migration (Monteith, Davis, & Roberts-Thomson, 2012; Prevarskaya, Skryma, & Shuba, 2011). Based on the modulation of calcium homeostasis, researchers tend to find effective treatment for this disease. Many studies have shown that resveratrol could inhibit cell proliferation, survival of prostate cancer PC-3 and DU145 cells via downregulation of stromal interaction molecular 1 (STIM1) which acts as calcium sensor in endoplasmic reticulum (ER). Resveratrol treatment reduced the STIM1 expression, thereby, inhibiting the interaction of STIM1 and transient receptor potential channel 1 (TRPC1), which could attenuate Ca^{2+} entry and induce prostate cancer cell death (Selvaraj, Sun, Sukumaran, & Singh, 2016). A mechanism against prostate cancer of resveratrol was to induce autophagic cell death through activation of AMP-activated protein kinase (AMPK) and inhibition of Akt/mTOR pathway (Selvaraj et al., 2016).

Liver Cancer

Liver cancer, or hepatocellular carcinoma (HCC), is one of the most deadly forms of cancer, and its incidence has been increasing worldwide. Multiple studies in rats have used diethylnitrosamine (DENA) injection followed by tumor promotion with phenobarbital to induce HCC in the animals. Resveratrol supplementation also caused an increase in hepatic expression of NFE2-related factor 2 (*Nrf2* (*Nfe212*) (Bishayee, Barnes, Bhatia, Darvesh, & Carroll, 2010). Increased expression of *Nfr2*, a transcription factor involved in the expression of antioxidant genes, suggests that resveratrol may exert an antioxidant effect in the liver of DENA-injected animals.

INFLAMMATION DISEASE

In biology, Inflammation is defined that a part of the complex biological response of body tissues to harmful stimuli, such as pathogens, damaged cells, or irritants,and is a protective response involving immune cells, blood vessels, and molecular mediators (Ferrero-Miliani, Nielsen, Andersen, & Girardin, 2007). Chronic inflammatory disease has been considered as the cause of many human diseases. The inflammatory processes might induce DNA mutations in cells via oxidative or nitrosative stress, which can influence normal cell functions and consequently lead to cancer (Chang, Lin, Peng, Day, & Hung, 2015). The NO have known to play an important role in aging oxidative stress in the form of high super oxide concentration leads to the impairment of mitochondrial NO synthesis and its inactivation. Resveratrol can enhance eNOS and NO bioavailability. In experiments, resveratrol prevents the production of free radicals, increase hemoxygenase-1 and glutamate cysteine ligase mRNA expression and Nrf2 activation, enhances reduced to oxidized ratio of glutathione. A other study, it was demonstrated that resveratrol significantly suppressed inflammation markers such as inducible nitric oxide synthase (iNOS), cyclooxygenase-2 (COX-2), and tumor necrosis factor-α (TNF-α) in dextran sulfate sodium (DSS) mouse model of colitis (Chang et al., 2015).

OBESITY

Obesity is a medical condition in which excess body fat has accumulated to the extent that it may have a negative effect on health based on their body mass index (BMI). Resveratrol has potential as an anti-obesity agent via downregulation of adipogenic processes (Chang et al., 2015; Kim, Jin, Choi, & Park, 2011). The obesity treatment was the dose-dependent of resveratrol. In an experiment: inducing obese mice model via a high- fat diet (HFD) and the supplement of resveratrol (1-30mg/kg/BW) for 10 weeks lead to reduce body weight significantly and prevented lipid deposition in adipose tissues, liver (Chang et al., 2015). When resveratrol was used with 30mg/kg/day dose, it made the expressions of genes increase significantly such as: miR-129, miR-328-5p, miR-539-5p (The miR-539-5p expression was enhanced lead to reduce in SP1 protein).Another study conducted showed that resveratrol suppressed adipogenic differentiation in 3T3-L1 adipose tissue cells via downregulating both peroxisome proliferator-activated receptor gamma (PPARγ) and perilipin proteins expression, which are two key regulators of adipogenesis and lipogenesis (Chang et al., 2015). Resveratrol effectively reduced the body weight gain, the weight of visceral adipose tissues, plasma triacylglycerol, free fatty acid, glucose, TNF-α, and monocyte chemoattractant protein-1 (MCP-1) through mechanism downregulation of galanin-mediated signaling modulators (GalR1, GalR2, PKCδ, Cyc-D, E2F1, and p-ERK) and the expression of adipogenic genes (PPARγ, C/EBPα, SREBP1c, LXR, FAS, LPL, aP2, and Leptin) (Kim et al., 2011).

AGING

Aging is a multifactorial process lead to limit and go down functional cells, tissues and organisms. The usage of resveratrol on lifespan extension has been shown in various organism and animal models (Kasiotis, Pratsinis, Kletsas, & Haroutounian, 2013; Pan, Lai, Tsai, Wu, & Ho, 2012). Majority reports suggested that the mechanism in regard to longevity promotion by resveratrol is involved to calorie restriction. Resveratrol helped increase DNA stability and prolonged 70% lifespan of budding yeast *Saccharomyces cerevisiae* via activating Sir2 (Pan et al., 2012), in which Sir2 is one of member of the sirtuin family induced by energy restriction, mimicking the effects of calorie restriction. A study was designed with "two groups of rats in late middle age (21 months age) chosen for study" (Kodali et al., 2015) within four weeks treated with resveratrol. Research was analyzed based on the level neurogenesis quantification, astrocyte hypertrophy and activation of microglia in the hippocampus. Resveratrol has ability to easy cross the blood-brain. It helps promote angiogenesis, oxidative stress inhibition, decrease mitochondrial dysfunction and extend longevity without adverse side effects.

NEURODEGENERATIVE DISEASES

In *in vitro* models, resveratrol has been demonstrated a protecting role against aging and play a therapeutic role within neurodegenerative disorder disease such as: epilepsy, Alzheimer's disease (AD), Parkinson's disease (PD), Huntington's disease (HD), amyotrophic lateral sclerosis (ALS), and nerve injury(Rocha-González, Ambriz-Tututi, & Granados-Soto, 2008). The effect of resveratrol on aging and neurodegenerative diseases might involve with AMPK, SIRT1, and PGC-1α pathway. The therapeutic potential of resveratrol in neurodegenerative disorders is supported by multiple studies demonstrating neuroprotective effects of resveratrol in different cell culture and *in vitro* systems (Vingtdeux, Dreses-Werringloer, Zhao, Davies, & Marambaud, 2008) such as: reducing oxidative damage, improving vascular function, promoting the activity of neurotrophic factors.

Alzheimer's disease (AD) is a neurodegenerative disorder characterized by the accumulation of β-amyloid peptides (Aβ) and neurofibrillary tangles (NFTs) in the brain, widespread cortical neuronal loss, and progressive memory impairment. However, the exact pathophysiological mechanism have still needed to elucidate lead to get lots of failures treatment. There are two types of medications for this disease treatment: cholinesterase inhibitors and N-methyl-D-aspartate receptor antagonists-which can decrease symptom. Targeting molecular mechanisms of resveratrol for Alzheimer's disease may be a viable treatment approach. It can help attenuate AD dementia by modulating β-amyloid (Aβ) neuropathology via the inhibition of both Aβ generation and abnormal Aβ oligomerization and based on the promotion of Aβ clearance and by modulating tau neuropathology through the inhibition of abnormal tau phosphorylation and tau aggregation (Ho et al., 2009; Ho et al., 2013; Howells et al., 2011; J. Wang et al., 2010; J. Wang et al., 2008). A study had been reported that the resveratrol dose of 50mg/kg/day/24 months will reduce the protein levels of TNFα, IL1β in AD of male mice (Gocmez et al., 2016).

However, resveratrol is extremely low bioavailability and metabolized rapidly, it has been suggested that some of its metabolites may be responsible for its biological activity in vivo (Wenzel, Soldo, Erbersdobler, & Somoza, 2005). The major metabolites of resveratrol are resveratrol-3-sulfate and resveratrol-3-O-glucuronide (Howells et al., 2011; Karuppagounder et al., 2009; Vingtdeux et al., 2010).. A study showed (Karthick, Periyasamy, Jayachandran, & Anusuyadevi, 2016) that the dose of 20mg/kg body weight for resveratrol will improve spatial learning performance, decrease significantly stress markers as nitrite, MDA levels through increasing antioxidant status.

CONCLUSION

In general, resveratrol can treatment of chronic disorders such as heart disease, stroke, cancer, diabetes, obesity, etc. and give us lots of beneficial effects on improving health status with their lesser side effects, cost. It acts as a chemopreventive agent due to its pharmacological potential to cure multiple human diseases such as cancer, diabetes, obesity; Hungtington's, Parkinson's and Alzheimer's disease. Resveratrol also works as an antioxidant by promoting nitric oxide production, suppressing platelet aggregation and enhancing high- density lipoprotein cholesterol. In conclusion, this chapter has shown that resveratrol can be a helpful supplementary medicine for the prevention and treatment of different diseases, especially it has been originally nature, safe and lower cost compared to cancer drugs.

REFERENCES

Arichi, H., Kimura, Y., Okuda, H., Baba, K., Kozawa, M., & Arichi, S. (1982). Effects of stilbene components of the roots of Polygonum cuspidatum Sieb. et Zucc. on lipid metabolism. *Chemical & Pharmaceutical Bulletin, 30*(5), 1766–1770. doi:10.1248/cpb.30.1766 PMID:7116511

Arunachalam, G., Yao, H., Sundar, I. K., Caito, S., & Rahman, I. (2010). SIRT1 regulates oxidant-and cigarette smoke-induced eNOS acetylation in endothelial cells: Role of resveratrol. *Biochemical and Biophysical Research Communications, 393*(1), 66–72. doi:10.1016/j.bbrc.2010.01.080 PMID:20102704

Bentzon, J. F., Otsuka, F., Virmani, R., & Falk, E. (2014). Mechanisms of plaque formation and rupture. *Circulation Research, 114*(12), 1852–1866. doi:10.1161/CIRCRESAHA.114.302721 PMID:24902970

Berliner, J. A., Navab, M., Fogelman, A. M., Frank, J. S., Demer, L. L., Edwards, P. A., ... Lusis, A. J. (1995). Atherosclerosis: basic mechanisms: oxidation, inflammation, and genetics. *Circulation, 91*(9), 2488–2496. doi:10.1161/01.CIR.91.9.2488 PMID:7729036

Bishayee, A., Barnes, K. F., Bhatia, D., Darvesh, A. S., & Carroll, R. T. (2010). Resveratrol suppresses oxidative stress and inflammatory response in diethylnitrosamine-initiated rat hepatocarcinogenesis. *Cancer Prevention Research (Philadelphia, Pa.), 3*(6), 753–763. doi:10.1158/1940-6207.CAPR-09-0171 PMID:20501860

Calvert, J. W., & Lefer, D. J. (2009). Myocardial protection by nitrite. *Cardiovascular Research*, *83*(2), 195–203. doi:10.1093/cvr/cvp079 PMID:19251721

Carrizzo, A., Puca, A., Damato, A., Marino, M., Franco, E., Pompeo, F., ... Trimarco, V. (2013). Resveratrol improves vascular function in patients with hypertension and dyslipidemia by modulating NO metabolism. *Hypertension*, *62*(2), 359–366. doi:10.1161/HYPERTENSIONAHA.111.01009 PMID:23753407

Csiszar, A., Labinskyy, N., Pinto, J. T., Ballabh, P., Zhang, H., Losonczy, G., ... Zhang, C. (2009). Resveratrol induces mitochondrial biogenesis in endothelial cells. *American Journal of Physiology. Heart and Circulatory Physiology*, *297*(1), H13–H20. doi:10.1152/ajpheart.00368.2009 PMID:19429820

Chang, C.-C., Lin, K.-Y., Peng, K.-Y., Day, Y.-J., & Hung, L.-M. (2015). Resveratrol exerts anti-obesity effects in high-fat diet obese mice and displays differential dosage effects on cytotoxicity, differentiation, and lipolysis in 3T3-L1 cells. *Endocrine Journal*, EJ15–EJ0545. PMID:26698690

Chen, Q., Wang, E., Ma, L., & Zhai, P. (2012). Dietary resveratrol increases the expression of hepatic 7α-hydroxylase and ameliorates hypercholesterolemia in high-fat fed C57BL/6J mice. *Lipids in Health and Disease*, *11*(1), 56. doi:10.1186/1476-511X-11-56 PMID:22607622

Chen, Y.-R., Yi, F.-F., Li, X.-Y., Wang, C.-Y., Chen, L., Yang, X.-C., ... Cai, J. (2008). Resveratrol attenuates ventricular arrhythmias and improves the long-term survival in rats with myocardial infarction. *Cardiovascular Drugs and Therapy*, *22*(6), 479–485. doi:10.100710557-008-6141-8 PMID:18853243

Chen, Z.-P., Mitchelhill, K. I., Michell, B. J., Stapleton, D., Rodriguez-Crespo, I., Witters, L. A., ... Kemp, B. E. (1999). AMP-activated protein kinase phosphorylation of endothelial NO synthase. *FEBS Letters*, *443*(3), 285–289. doi:10.1016/S0014-5793(98)01705-0 PMID:10025949

Dolinsky, V. W., Chakrabarti, S., Pereira, T. J., Oka, T., Levasseur, J., Beker, D., ... Lopaschuk, G. D. (2013). Resveratrol prevents hypertension and cardiac hypertrophy in hypertensive rats and mice. *Biochimica et Biophysica Acta (BBA)-. Molecular Basis of Disease*, *1832*(10), 1723–1733. doi:10.1016/j.bbadis.2013.05.018 PMID:23707558

Ferrero-Miliani, L., Nielsen, O.H., Andersen, P.S., & Girardin, S.E. (2007). Chronic inflammation: Importance of NOD2 and NALP3 in interleukin-1β generation. *Clinical and Experimental Immunology*, *147*(2), 227–235. PMID:17223962

Gocmez, S. S., Gacar, N., Utkan, T., Gacar, G., Scarpace, P. J., & Tumer, N. (2016). Protective effects of resveratrol on aging-induced cognitive impairment in rats. *Neurobiology of Learning and Memory*, *131*, 131–136. doi:10.1016/j.nlm.2016.03.022 PMID:27040098

He, X., Wang, Y., Zhu, J., Orloff, M., & Eng, C. (2011). Resveratrol enhances the anti-tumor activity of the mTOR inhibitor rapamycin in multiple breast cancer cell lines mainly by suppressing rapamycin-induced AKT signaling. *Cancer Letters*, *301*(2), 168–176. doi:10.1016/j.canlet.2010.11.012 PMID:21168265

Ho, L., Chen, L. H., Wang, J., Zhao, W., Talcott, S. T., Ono, K., ... Percival, S. S. (2009). Heterogeneity in red wine polyphenolic contents differentially influences Alzheimer's disease-type neuropathology and cognitive deterioration. *Journal of Alzheimer's Disease*, *16*(1), 59–72. doi:10.3233/JAD-2009-0916 PMID:19158422

Ho, L., Ferruzzi, M. G., Janle, E. M., Wang, J., Gong, B., Chen, T.-Y., ... Talcott, S. T. (2013). Identification of brain-targeted bioactive dietary quercetin-3-O-glucuronide as a novel intervention for Alzheimer's disease. *The FASEB Journal, 27*(2), 769–781. doi:10.1096/fj.12-212118 PMID:23097297

Howells, L. M., Berry, D. P., Elliott, P. J., Jacobson, E. W., Hoffmann, E., Hegarty, B., ... Gescher, A. J. (2011). Phase I randomized, double-blind pilot study of micronized resveratrol (SRT501) in patients with hepatic metastases—Safety, pharmacokinetics, and pharmacodynamics. *Cancer Prevention Research (Philadelphia, Pa.), 4*(9), 1419–1425. doi:10.1158/1940-6207.CAPR-11-0148 PMID:21680702

Karthick, C., Periyasamy, S., Jayachandran, K. S., & Anusuyadevi, M. (2016). Intrahippocampal administration of ibotenic acid induced cholinergic dysfunction via NR2A/NR2B expression: Implications of resveratrol against Alzheimer disease pathophysiology. *Frontiers in Molecular Neuroscience, 9*, 28. doi:10.3389/fnmol.2016.00028 PMID:27199654

Karuppagounder, S. S., Pinto, J. T., Xu, H., Chen, H.-L., Beal, M. F., & Gibson, G. E. (2009). Dietary supplementation with resveratrol reduces plaque pathology in a transgenic model of Alzheimer's disease. *Neurochemistry International, 54*(2), 111–118. doi:10.1016/j.neuint.2008.10.008 PMID:19041676

Kasiotis, K. M., Pratsinis, H., Kletsas, D., & Haroutounian, S. A. (2013). Resveratrol and related stilbenes: Their anti-aging and anti-angiogenic properties. *Food and Chemical Toxicology, 61*, 112–120. doi:10.1016/j.fct.2013.03.038 PMID:23567244

Kim, S., Jin, Y., Choi, Y., & Park, T. (2011). Resveratrol exerts anti-obesity effects via mechanisms involving down-regulation of adipogenic and inflammatory processes in mice. *Biochemical Pharmacology, 81*(11), 1343–1351. doi:10.1016/j.bcp.2011.03.012 PMID:21439945

Kodali, M., Parihar, V. K., Hattiangady, B., Mishra, V., Shuai, B., & Shetty, A. K. (2015). Resveratrol prevents age-related memory and mood dysfunction with increased hippocampal neurogenesis and microvasculature, and reduced glial activation. *Scientific Reports, 5*(1), 8075. doi:10.1038rep08075 PMID:25627672

Leikert, J. F., Räthel, T. R., Wohlfart, P., Cheynier, V., Vollmar, A. M., & Dirsch, V. M. (2002). Red wine polyphenols enhance endothelial nitric oxide synthase expression and subsequent nitric oxide release from endothelial cells. *Circulation, 106*(13), 1614–1617. doi:10.1161/01.CIR.0000034445.31543.43 PMID:12270851

Liew, R., Stagg, M. A., MacLeod, K. T., & Collins, P. (2005). The red wine polyphenol, resveratrol, exerts acute direct actions on guinea-pig ventricular myocytes. *European Journal of Pharmacology, 519*(1-2), 1–8. doi:10.1016/j.ejphar.2005.06.017 PMID:16102748

Matos, R. S., Baroncini, L.A., Précoma, L. B., Winter, G., Lambach, P.H., Caron, E.Y., . . . Précoma, D.B. (2012). Resveratrol causes antiatherogenic effects in an animal model of atherosclerosis. *Arquivos Brasileiros de Cardiologia, 98*(2), 136–142. doi:10.1590/S0066-782X2012005000006 PMID:22231915

Miksits, M., Wlcek, K., Svoboda, M., Kunert, O., Haslinger, E., Thalhammer, T., ... Jäger, W. (2009). Antitumor activity of resveratrol and its sulfated metabolites against human breast cancer cells. *Planta Medica, 75*(11), 1227–1230. doi:10.1055-0029-1185533 PMID:19350482

Monteith, G. R., Davis, F. M., & Roberts-Thomson, S. J. (2012). Calcium channels and pumps in cancer: Changes and consequences. *The Journal of Biological Chemistry*, *287*(38), 31666–31673. doi:10.1074/jbc.R112.343061 PMID:22822055

Nagendran, J., Waller, T. J., & Dyck, J. R. B. (2013). AMPK signalling and the control of substrate use in the heart. *Molecular and Cellular Endocrinology*, *366*(2), 180–193. doi:10.1016/j.mce.2012.06.015 PMID:22750050

Pan, M.-H., Lai, C.-S., Tsai, M.-L., Wu, J.-C., & Ho, C.-T. (2012). Molecular mechanisms for anti-aging by natural dietary compounds. *Molecular Nutrition & Food Research*, *56*(1), 88–115. doi:10.1002/mnfr.201100509 PMID:22083941

Pearson, K. J., Baur, J. A., Lewis, K. N., Peshkin, L., Price, N. L., Labinskyy, N., ... Perez, E. (2008). Resveratrol delays age-related deterioration and mimics transcriptional aspects of dietary restriction without extending life span. *Cell Metabolism*, *8*(2), 157–168. doi:10.1016/j.cmet.2008.06.011 PMID:18599363

Prevarskaya, N., Skryma, R., & Shuba, Y. (2011). Calcium in tumour metastasis: New roles for known actors. *Nature Reviews. Cancer*, *11*(8), 609–618. doi:10.1038/nrc3105 PMID:21779011

Rocha-González, H. I., Ambriz-Tututi, M., & Granados-Soto, V. (2008). Resveratrol: A natural compound with pharmacological potential in neurodegenerative diseases. *CNS Neuroscience & Therapeutics*, *14*(3), 234–247. doi:10.1111/j.1755-5949.2008.00045.x PMID:18684235

Rocha, K. K. R., Souza, G. A., Ebaid, G. X., Seiva, F. R. F., Cataneo, A. C., & Novelli, E. L. B. (2009). Resveratrol toxicity: Effects on risk factors for atherosclerosis and hepatic oxidative stress in standard and high-fat diets. *Food and Chemical Toxicology*, *47*(6), 1362–1367. doi:10.1016/j.fct.2009.03.010 PMID:19298841

Rush, J. W. E., Quadrilatero, J., Levy, A. S., & Ford, R. J. (2007). Chronic resveratrol enhances endothelium-dependent relaxation but does not alter eNOS levels in aorta of spontaneously hypertensive rats. *Experimental Biology and Medicine, 232*(6), 814-822.

Scarlatti, F., Maffei, R., Beau, I., Codogno, P., & Ghidoni, R. (2008). Role of non-canonical Beclin 1-independent autophagy in cell death induced by resveratrol in human breast cancer cells. *Cell Death and Differentiation*, *15*(8), 1318–1329. doi:10.1038/cdd.2008.51 PMID:18421301

Selvaraj, S., Sun, Y., Sukumaran, P., & Singh, B. B. (2016). Resveratrol activates autophagic cell death in prostate cancer cells via downregulation of STIM1 and the mTOR pathway. *Molecular Carcinogenesis*, *55*(5), 818–831. doi:10.1002/mc.22324 PMID:25917875

Sobolev, V. S., & Cole, R. J. (1999). trans-Resveratrol content in commercial peanuts and peanut products. *Journal of Agricultural and Food Chemistry*, *47*(4), 1435–1439. doi:10.1021/jf9809885 PMID:10563995

Soylemez, S., Sepici, A., & Akar, F. (2009). Resveratrol supplementation gender independently improves endothelial reactivity and suppresses superoxide production in healthy rats. *Cardiovascular Drugs and Therapy*, *23*(6), 449–458. doi:10.100710557-009-6198-z PMID:19809869

Toklu, H. Z., Şehirli, Ö., Erşahin, M., Süleymanoğlu, S., Yiğiner, Ö., Emekli-Alturfan, E., ... Şener, G. (2010). Resveratrol improves cardiovascular function and reduces oxidative organ damage in the renal, cardiovascular and cerebral tissues of two-kidney, one-clip hypertensive rats. *The Journal of Pharmacy and Pharmacology*, *62*(12), 1784–1793. doi:10.1111/j.2042-7158.2010.01197.x PMID:21054406

Tomé-Carneiro, J., Gonzálvez, M., Larrosa, M., Yáñez-Gascón, M. J., García-Almagro, F. J., Ruiz-Ros, J. A., ... Espín, J. C. (2013). Grape resveratrol increases serum adiponectin and downregulates inflammatory genes in peripheral blood mononuclear cells: A triple-blind, placebo-controlled, one-year clinical trial in patients with stable coronary artery disease. *Cardiovascular Drugs and Therapy*, *27*(1), 37–48. doi:10.100710557-012-6427-8 PMID:23224687

Vingtdeux, V., Dreses-Werringloer, U., Zhao, H., Davies, P., & Marambaud, P. (2008). Therapeutic potential of resveratrol in Alzheimer's disease. *BMC Neuroscience*, *9*(S2), S6. doi:10.1186/1471-2202-9-S2-S6 PMID:19090994

Vingtdeux, V., Giliberto, L., Zhao, H., Chandakkar, P., Wu, Q., Simon, J. E., ... Davies, P. (2010). AMP-activated protein kinase signaling activation by resveratrol modulates amyloid-β peptide metabolism. *The Journal of Biological Chemistry*, *285*(12), 9100–9113. doi:10.1074/jbc.M109.060061 PMID:20080969

Wallerath, T., Deckert, G., Ternes, T., Anderson, H., Li, H., Witte, K., & Förstermann, U. (2002). Resveratrol, a polyphenolic phytoalexin present in red wine, enhances expression and activity of endothelial nitric oxide synthase. *Circulation*, *106*(13), 1652–1658. doi:10.1161/01.CIR.0000029925.18593.5C PMID:12270858

Wang, J., Fivecoat, H., Ho, L., Pan, Y., Ling, E., & Pasinetti, G. M. (2010). The role of Sirt1: At the crossroad between promotion of longevity and protection against Alzheimer's disease neuropathology. *Biochimica et Biophysica Acta (BBA)-. Proteins and Proteomics*, *1804*(8), 1690–1694. doi:10.1016/j.bbapap.2009.11.015 PMID:19945548

Wang, J., Ho, L., Zhao, W., Ono, K., Rosensweig, C., Chen, L., ... Pasinetti, G. M. (2008). Grape-derived polyphenolics prevent Aβ oligomerization and attenuate cognitive deterioration in a mouse model of Alzheimer's disease. *The Journal of Neuroscience*, *28*(25), 6388–6392. doi:10.1523/JNEUROSCI.0364-08.2008 PMID:18562609

Wang, Z., Zou, J., Cao, K., Hsieh, T.-C., Huang, Y., & Wu, J. M. (2005). Dealcoholized red wine containing known amounts of resveratrol suppresses atherosclerosis in hypercholesterolemic rabbits without affecting plasma lipid levels. *International Journal of Molecular Medicine*, *16*(4), 533–540. PMID:16142383

Wenzel, E., Soldo, T., Erbersdobler, H., & Somoza, V. (2005). Bioactivity and metabolism of trans-resveratrol orally administered to Wistar rats. *Molecular Nutrition & Food Research*, *49*(5), 482–494. doi:10.1002/mnfr.200500003 PMID:15779067

Yashiro, T., Nanmoku, M., Shimizu, M., Inoue, J., & Sato, R. (2012). Resveratrol increases the expression and activity of the low density lipoprotein receptor in hepatocytes by the proteolytic activation of the sterol regulatory element-binding proteins. *Atherosclerosis*, *220*(2), 369–374. doi:10.1016/j.atherosclerosis.2011.11.006 PMID:22153697

Zhang, Y., Liu, Y., Wang, T., Li, B., Li, H., Wang, Z., & Yang, B. (2006). Resveratrol, a natural ingredient of grape skin: Antiarrhythmic efficacy and ionic mechanisms. *Biochemical and Biophysical Research Communications*, *340*(4), 1192–1199. doi:10.1016/j.bbrc.2005.12.124 PMID:16406237

Chapter 15
Dysbiosis, Small Intestinal Bacterial Overgrowth, and Chronic Diseases:
A Translational Approach

Ana Rita Silva
Centro de Investigação Interdisciplinar Egas Moniz, Portugal

Maria Alexandra Bernardo
Centro de Investigação Interdisciplinar Egas Moniz, Portugal

Maria Fernanda Mesquita
Centro de Investigação Interdisciplinar Egas Moniz, Portugal

José Vaz Patto
Instituto Português de Reumatologia, Portugal

Pedro Moreira
Faculdade de Ciências da Nutrição e Alimentação, Universidade do Porto, Portugal

Patrícia Padrão
Faculdade de Ciências da Nutrição e Alimentação, Universidade do Porto, Portugal

Maria Leonor Silva
Centro de Investigação Interdisciplinar Egas Moniz, Portugal

ABSTRACT

Dysbiosis is characterized by an alteration in quantity and quality of intestinal microbiota composition. In the presence of dysbiosis, enterocytes will have difficulty in maintaining the integrity of the mucosal barrier, leading to increased intestinal permeability. These events are recognised to be linked to several chronic diseases. One of the consequences of dysbiosis is the manifestation of small intestinal bacte-

DOI: 10.4018/978-1-7998-4808-0.ch015

rial overgrowth (SIBO), which is associated to a variety of chronic diseases. Single food nutrients and bioactive molecules, food additives, pre- and probiotics, and different dietary patterns may change the composition of the intestinal microbiota. Low FODMAPs diet has been a reference in SIBO treatment. This chapter intends to describe how the intestinal microbiota, dysbiosis, and SIBO can be related; to define dysbiosis food and nutrients influence; and to offer some nutritional therapy strategies for applying the low FODMAPs protocol, enabling better adherence by patients in order to increase their wellbeing.

1. INTRODUCTION

Microbiota corresponds to the community of microorganisms that inhabit a specific environment of the human body. It can be found in skin, genito-urinay tract, mouth and intestine. Each microbiota is composed of bacteria that varies not only according to its environment, but also throughout individual's life. Regarding to human gastrointestinal tract, there are approximately 100 trillions of bacteria, classified according to phyla, classes, orders, families, genus and species. There are more than 1000 different species identified [1]. They are clustered in six phyla, namely *Firmicutes, Bacteroidetes, Actinobacteria, Verrucomicrobia, Proteobacteria* and *Fusobacteria.* Approximately 60% of the bacteria belong to the *Bacteroidetes* and *Firmicutes* phyla [2, 3]. For each of these phyla, there are several classes of bacteria.

Gut mucosa consists of an external intestinal barrier and an inner immunological barrier. Intestinal barrier is composed by commensal gut microbiota, mucous layer and intestinal monolayer. It is responsible for two fundamental functions for the individual's survivance: allowing nutrients absorption and defending the entry of foreign molecules to the organism. The inner layer barrier consists in immune cells organized in Gut-associated lymphoid tissue (GALT). GALT depends on the dendritic cells and the M-cells present in the Payer's patches to interact with luminal antigens [4]. The interaction between commensal bacteria and mucosal immune system is essential for immune function.

Integrity of these structures is necessary for maintenance of normal intestinal barrier function. The microbiota produces bacteriocins and short-chain fatty acids (SCFA), including butyrate, acetate and propionate, which inhibit the pathogenic growth of microorganisms; and defensins, which control bacteriocins and SCFA. On the other hand, the mucosal immune system produces immunoglobulin A (IgA), preventing pathogenic bacteria from entering in the epithelium [5].

There is a mutual benefit between the microbiota and host organism during homeostasis. While prebiotics ingested by the individual are the necessary substrate for its growth, bacteria provide maintenance of mucosal barrier integrity; synthesis of vitamins B (B1, B2, PP, biotin, pantothenic acid, folate, and B12) and K, amino acids, neurotransmitters (e.g. serotonin) and SCFA; promote a better absorption of other vitamins and minerals; promote lymphocyte maturation; and prevent entry of pathogens [5, 6].

After being produced by bacteria, SCFA are released in the intestinal lumen, quickly absorbed and used as energy mainly by colonocytes, specially butyrate. In its turn, acetate and propionate may be carried into the bloodstream and become available to a variety of different organs [7]. SCFA regulate countless processes, regarding to appetite and weight management; inflammatory responses from immune system; lipid oxidation; and thermogenesis in brown adipose tissue. In fact, butyrate is crucial to tissue barrier function, epigenetic regulation, immune-regulation, colonic integrity and homeostasis, intestinal transit and satiety [8]. During homeostasis, SCFA produce lactic acid and gases, namely carbon dioxide (CO_2), hydrogen (H^+) and methane (NH_4), which will lower the intestine pH and allowing the production of energy.

On the other hand, the deregulation of intestinal microbiota and SCFA production may be changed, and therefore the products of their metabolism will consequently be compromised. Inversely, the SCFA overproduction will promote an increase in concentration of lactic acid and gases causing flatulence and bloating [9]. Types and amounts of SCFA depend on the composition of microbiota.

2. DYSBIOSIS AND INTESTINAL PERMEABILITY

Microbial programming begins in utero, and the composition of the microbiota is modulated by multiple factors including mode of delivery, gestational age, perinatal antibiotic exposure, feeding practices, environment, genetics, age, stress, diseases, and lifestyle, namely physical activity and diet quality and quantity (Rautava et al., 2012). Eating habits influence the gut bacterial structure and function during different time frames, including daily circadian rhythms of sleep-wakefulness and feeding-fasting cycle, and throughout the human lifespan (Zmora et al., 2019).

A westernized dietary pattern rich in ultra-processed products, trans-fatty acids, sugars and refined flour, along with stress and physical inactivity, is known to be associated with changes in the intestinal microbiota (Brown et al., 2012; Hawrelak & Myers, 2004). This promote alterations in the metabolism of bacteria and their overgrowth, with release of potentially toxic metabolites, such as endotoxins, hydrogen sulfide, phenols, ammonia and indoles. The intestinal mucosa is exposed to these metabolites, with harmful effects on the mucosa itself and host health (Hawrelak & Myers, 2004).

Considering that changes in the microbiota composition are common, and its flexibility is considered normal, how can dysbiosis be defined? The critical differential factor is the host's response to changes in the microbiota composition. Dysbiosis is then a qualitative and quantitative change in the intestinal microbiota composition (Lin & Zhang, 2017), in such a way that it induces an inflammatory response on the part of the host to the change in the microbiota composition compromising microbiota function. Dysbiosis lead to an increase of intestinal permeability, in which the intestine becomes more permeable to foreign and pathological agents (Cerf-Bensussan & Gaboriau-Routhiau, 2010; Frazier et al., 2011).

There is currently no specific biomarker to determine dysbiosis. However, in the last decades some alterations considered standard have been identified, in particular:

1- Reduction in overall microbial diversity of corresponding symbiotic community. Specifically, a depletion of obligate anaerobic bacteria such as *Bacteroides* and *Ruminococcus* spp., and conversely an increase in facultative anaerobes including *Enterobacteriaceae* (i.e. *E. Coli, Klebsiella* and *Proteus*) (Pham & Lawley, 2014);
2- Preferential loss of organisms considered beneficial to human health and increase in *pathobionts*, i.e. members of the normal commensal microbiota, with the potential to cause pathology. This may translate in a reduction of *Firmicutes* and increase of *Proteobacteria* (Chang et al., 2008; Lepage et al., 2011; Manichanh, 2006).

As a functional consequence of the loss of microbiota diversity, there appears to be a reduction in SCFA production, which compromises the metabolism stability.

2.1. Description and Triggering Factors

Increased intestinal permeability, defined by the destruction of tight-junctions and adherent-junctions, proteins that enable the enterocytes junction allowing the integrity of the intestinal mucosa, may arise as a result of dysbiosis. Its destruction increases the possibility of unwanted molecules entering the systemic circulation, including larger peptides, bacteria and lipopolysaccharides (LPS), triggering a pathological inflammation that harms the immune system. If prolonged over time, it can lead to the development of autoimmune diseases and immunodeficiency (Cerf-Bensussan & Gaboriau-Routhiau, 2010; Fasano, 2012a; Glaros, 2013). Intestinal hyperpermeability may be triggered by ingestion of gliadin (Hollon et al., 2015), alcohol (Draper et al., 1983; Leclercq et al., 2014), increased bile acids concentration (Pendyala et al., 2012), zinc deficit (Finamore et al., 2008), vitamin D deficit (Cantorna et al., 2004) and non-steroid antiinflammatoy drugs (NSAIDs) (Sigthorsson et al., 1998).

Regarding gliadin, a gluten constituent protein present in wheat, rye and barley, it is particularly related to the recognition of LPS by the TLR4, which causes consequent activation of the Nuclear Factor kappa B (NFkB) signalling pathway, promoter of inflammatory cytokine expression (Hollon et al., 2015), namely Tumor Necrosis Factor Alpha (TNF-α) and Interleukine-1 (IL-1) (Bosshart & Heinzelmann, 2007; Nahid et al., 2015). Increased intestinal permeability caused by gliadin can be identified by increased serum zonulin, a protein whose expression appears to be activated by gliadin, which binds to Protease Activated Receptor 2 (PAR2) and Epithelial Growth Factor Membrane Receptors (EGFR), inducing the destruction of tight-junctions (Fasano, 2012b).

Changes in barrier function are also related to an increase in TNF-α, IL-1β and IL-13, expressed in chronic low-grade intestinal inflammation (Clauw, 2009). Measurements over 0.3 mg/dL of serum ultra-sensitive Reactive C Protein (usCRP) reveals low-grade inflammation (Pearson et al., 2003; Ridker, 2016).

Chronic inflammation appears to result from an inadequate immune response as a result of genetic predisposition, as well as changes in the intestinal microbiota. On the other hand, an insufficient response to a stimulus of a bacterium results in an insufficient immune response to pathogens (Bischoff et al., 2014).

2.2. Influence of Food and Nutrients on Dysbiosis

Single food components, salt, food additives, pre- and probiotics, and different dietary patterns may change the composition of the intestinal microbiota [4]. Human intestine microbiota plasticity can respond efficiently and rapidly to external variable, as confirmed by changes in the microbiota composition detected within 24 hours, in a clinical trial that compared high-fat low-fiber and low-fat high-fiber controlled diets (Walker et al., 2011). However, short- and long-term dietary interventions differently impact the intestinal microbiota composition (Quercia et al., 2014; Wu et al., 2011).

Combining information from two reviews [4, 36], although further double-blind human intervention studies are still needed, there is already enough information to indicate that there are some modulating dietary factors in the composition of the intestinal microbiota.

2.2.1. Carbohydrates and Gut Microbiota

Carbohydrates can be categorized as digestible and non-digestible molecules. Digestible carbohydrates are enzymatically degraded and released as glucose in bloodstream. Indigestible carbohydrates are resistant starch and dietary fibers, which could be fermentable in colon and soluble in water, or insoluble and non-fermentable. Prebiotics are fermentable dietary fibers, that allow better development and activity of bacteria in the intestinal microbiota, especially in the colon (de Vrese & Schrezenmeir, 2008).

Beneficial effect of prebiotics on health has been widely recognized (Anderson et al., 2009; Kaczmarczyk et al., 2012; Veronese et al., 2018), particularly oligosaccharides, such as fructooligosaccharides (FOS) and inulin, present in bananas, onions, garlic, leeks, asparagus, chicory, yacon potatoes; gel-forming fibers, such as guar gum and psyllium husk; beta-glucan present in oat; and the resistant starch present in the green banana (Stipanuk, 2013). Several studies have pointed out the effectiveness of increased prebiotics intake in changes in intestinal microbiota composition. Several animal models and humans trials with inflammatory bowel disease (IBD) have reported that supplementation of some types of dietary fibre can prolong remission and reduce lesions of the intestinal mucosa during the progression of the disease (Pituch-Zdanowska et al., 2015). Additionally, a study points to a reduction in *Firmicutes* and an increase in *Bacteroides* with a diet rich in prebiotics, which in turn improve glucose sensitivity, inflammation and oxidative stress (Pimentel et al., 2012).

2.2.2. Proteins in Gut Microbiota

Fermentation of amino acids occurs in distal colon mainly by *Firmicutes, Bacteroides* and *Proteobacteria*.

Animal-based protein, particularly from red meat and dairy products, may lead to an increase of bile tolerant anaerobic bacteria, such as *Bacteroides, Alistipes* and *Bilophila*, which promotes an increase in Trimethylamine N-oxyde (TMAO) (David et al., 2014), associated with increased risk for cardiovascular disease (Kanitsoraphan et al., 2018; Roncal et al., 2019). In fact, proteolitic excessive fermentation produces a decrease in SCFA, and an increase in potentially toxic substrates, such as ammonia, nitrosamines and TMAO. Additionally, the intake of animal protein is also associated with an increase in hydrogen-sulfide by sulfate-reducing bacteria, and a decrease in *Bifidobacterium* (Singh et al., 2017), which increases the risk of IBD.

On the other hand, the intake of plant-based protein seems to have a beneficial impact on the intestinal microbiota. Humans clinical trials where pea protein has been used have promoted an increase in commensal *Bifidobacterium* and *Lactobacillus*, and a decrease in pathogenic *Bacteroides fragilis* and *Clorstridium perfringens* (Swiatecka, 2011). In fact, vegetarians and vegan microbiota composition differs from omnivores. Some studies showed higher ratio of *Bacteroides/Prevotella, along with higher occurrence of Bacteroides thetaiotaomicron, Clostridium clostridioforme, Klebsiella pneumoniae, and Faecalibacterium prausnitzii* and low occurrence of *Clostridium cluster* and *Bilophila wadsworthia* in vegetarians and vegans [4, 52, 53]. However, the effects of phenolic compounds should be taken into account, as these components increase the abundance of beneficial bacteria such as *Bifidobacterium and Lactobacillus*.

2.2.3. Lipids in Gut Microbiota

Lipids can be characterized in three classes: saturated, monounsaturated and polyunsaturated fatty acids. Saturated fatty acids are found mainly in animal fats, such as meat and dairy products. High fat diet, specially saturated fat, is associated to dysbiosis. In western diets, the intake of saturated fat is particularly high, and associated with a reduced intake of fiber. Diets high in saturated fat and in low fiber contribute to metabolic endotoxemia (Fuke et al., 2019). High saturated fat diet stimulates production of sulphate-reducing bacteria, such as *Bilophila wadsworthia*. These bacteria may reduce dissulfide bonds in mucus, causing alteration in mucus layer stability and consequent inflammation (Devkota & Chang, 2015; Gruber et al., 2013).

Monounsaturated fatty acids (MUFA) are found in olive oil, olives and avocado. A systematic review showed that high MUFA diet has no effect on microbiota composition, distribution or *Bacteroides-Firmicutes* ratio. However, MUFA were positively correlated with *Parabacteroides*, *Provetella*, and *Enterobacteriaceae* family, and low *Bifidobacterium genus* (Wolters et al., 2019).

Polyunsaturated fatty acids (PUFA) include n-3 and n-6 families. The n-3 PUFA are found in some fish, such as sardines, mackerel and salmon, in nuts, flaxseeds and sea algae, such as kelp. The n-6 PUFA are found in sunflower, corn and soybean oil.

The n-3 PUFA exert a beneficial effect in intestine, by restoring *Firmicutes-Bacteroides* ratio and increasing *Lachnospiraceae* family, both associated to increase of butyrate SCFA (Noriega et al., 2016). In the past, the n-6:n-3 ratio has enjoyed widespread use and was set at and ideal value of 1:1; however, this metric has both theoretical and practical difficulties, and is now outmoded (Harris, 2018). Nevertheless, in most industrialized countries with a westernized diet, this ratio is sometimes used to describe values between 10:1 and 50:1, which correlate to increased risk to cardiovascular and chronic disease (Simopoulos, 2008), increased intestinal permeability and metabolic endotoxemia (Kaliannan et al., 2015). In this sense, it is essential to promote a greater intake of n-3 PUFA, considering simultaneously a delicate balance with n-6 PUFA.

2.2.4. Vitamins and Minerals in Gut Microbiota

Some vitamins can be synthesized by the intestinal microbiota, namely thiamine, riboflavin, niacin, biotin, pantothenic acid, folate, cobalamin and vitamin K. *Bacteroidetes, Fusobacteria and Proteobacteria* are primarily responsible for the synthesis of these vitamins [4].

Additionally, some micronutrients are essential for intestinal health. Zinc may contribute to the host defence by maintaining the membrane barrier. An *in vitro* study where zinc deprivation was induced, revealed a disruption of membrane barrier integrity that led to an upregulation of chemokines, which plays a role in neutrophil migration and inflammatory development. It was seen an increase in the migration of neutrophils and secretion of IL-8, epithelial neutrophil activating peptide-78, and growth-regulated oncogene-a, alterations that were not found when culture medium was replete with zinc (Finamore et al., 2008). Several researchers point to zinc therapeutic effect, through the maintenance of the enterocytic barrier (Skrovanek, 2014). Therefore, its adequate nutritional supply must be taken into account.

Iron is another mineral with an important impact on the intestine, whose availability influences microbiota composition. Constante *et al.* demonstrated in mice that a heme-rich diet decreased microbiota diversity, having promoted an increase in the concentration of *Proteobacteria* and decreased *Firmicutes* [4].

Regarding vitamin D, there has been increase evidence of its antibacterial effect. Vitamin D induces the expression of cathelicidin antimicrobial peptide (CAMP) gene, which plays a critical role in innate immune defence and enhances barrier function (Reitsma et al., 2014). In experimental studies, Kong *et al.* demonstrated that activated vitamin D, 1,25-dihydroxy vitamin D (1,25(OH)2D3) increase tight junction (TJ) proteins, zonula occludens and E-cadherin (Kong et al., 2008), which suggest its importance in maintenance of the mucosal barrier. Jin *et al.* suggested that vitamin D receptors (VDR) status could influence the mice intestinal microbiota both taxonomic and functional levels. The authors advocated that VDR is crucial for the maintenance of microbial homeostasis. In humans, a reduction in the production of 1,25(OH)2D3 or in the expression of VDR may lead to gut inflammation and an increase in *Proteobacteria* colonization. This leads to an alteration in the balance of the microbiota composition, inducing dysbiosis (Tabatabaeizadeh, 2018). Additionally, in IBD patients, vitamin D has a recognized positive effect, by modulating the gut microbiome and increasing the abundance of potentially beneficial bacterial strains (Sun, 2018).

2.2.5. Redox Activity in Gut Microbiota

Several studies demonstrate the antioxidants effects in gut microbiota composition. In the carotenoid family, lutein significantly promotes the growth of *Bifidobacteria* and *Lactobacillus*, and a decrease in *Bacteroides* and *Clostridium*, in humans (Molan et al., 2014). On the other hand, quercetin supplementation significantly improved the *Firmicutes-Bacteroides* ratio, and inhibited the growth of bacteria associated with obesity, such as *Erysipelotrichaceae, Bacillus* spp. and *Eubacterium cylindroides*, in mice fed with high-sugar high-fat diet (Etxeberria et al., 2015). Also anthocyanines, which have a known anti-inflammatory effect against colorectal cancer significantly stimulates growth of *Bifidubacterium* spp., *Lactobacillus* and *Enterococcus* spp. (Hidalgo et al., 2012).

However, a study suggested that the anti-inflammatory effects of beta-carotene were mediated by the gut microbiota (Karlsson et al., 2012). Also with regard to phenolic compounds, a similar effect occurs, as the intestinal microbiota is able to modulate probiotic activity and influence its bioavailability (Ozdal et al., 2016). These facts suggest that an intestinal dysbiosis environment may remove less nutrient absorption and interfere with its antioxidant and anti-inflammatory activity.

2.2.6. Food Additives in Gut Microbiota

Ultra-processed foods frequently have emulsifiers in its composition, such as lecithins and mono- and diglycerides of fatty acids. These molecules may increase bacterial translocation across epithelial, promoting systemic inflammation and altering microbiota composition (Chassaing et al., 2015). Emulsifiers intake is associated to a decrease in diversity of microbiota composition, a decrease in *Bacteroides* and an increase in *Verrumicrobia*, specifically *Akkermansia muciniphila* and *Proteobacteria*, leading to dysbiosis and chronic gut inflammation (Chassaing et al., 2015; Chassaing et al., 2017).

Regarding to non-caloric artificial sweeteners, a systematic review showed an alteration in gut microbiota composition after ingestion of these molecules, particularly in respect to saccharin and aspartame (Spencer et al., 2016). Although data is scarce, studies have found similar results, both in animal (mice) and human models. After ingesting 50-100mg of sodium saccharin (NaS), there was an increase in the number of anaerobic bacteria, namely *Bacteroides and Clostridiales*, and a decrease in *Lactobacilus* (Spencer et al., 2016). A cohort study conducted by Suez and colleagues found a positive correlation between NaS and central obesity, Hemoglobin A1C and impaired glucose tolerance in 381 non-obese individuals who reported regular consumption of artificial sweeteners. One hundred and seventy-one randomly selected individuals showed intestinal microbiota changes, particularly an increase in *Enterobacteriaceae, Deltaproteobacteria and Actinobacteria phylum (Suez et al., 2014).* Regarding to steviol glycosides, there are no reported consistent microbial changes (Spencer et al., 2016).

Another molecule present in westernized countries diet, are designated advanced glycation end-products (AGEs). AGEs form during heating and processing of food products. It is vastly known its impact on increasing risk for chronic diseases (Clarke et al., 2016), inflammation (Van Puyvelde et al., 2014), oxidative stress and insulin resistance (Kellow & Savige, 2013). Additionally, limiting AGE intake may lead to a decrease in inflammation and chronic diseases related to inflammatory status (Van Puyvelde et al., 2014). In peritoneal dialysis patients, dietary AGE restriction altered the bacterial gut microbiota with a significant reduction in *Prevotella copri* and *Bifidobacterium animalis* and increased *Alistipes indistinctus*, *Clostridium citroniae*, *Clostridium hathewayi*, and *Ruminococcus gauvreauii* relative abundance (Yacoub et al., 2017). However, there is conflicting evidence regarding the impact of dietary AGEs on gut microbiota reshaping (Snelson & Coughlan, 2019).

2.2.7. Dietary Patterns in Gut Microbiota

If nutrients and bioactive food molecules influences the composition of the intestinal microbiota, then the differences in dietary patterns will have to manifest themselves significantly in the intestine. Table 1 illustrates the effect of different dietary patterns on microbiota and health.

The composition of the microbiome of modern civilizations with different lifestyles mimics the evolution between bacteria and the human host (Quercia et al., 2014). In a study carried out by Quercia and colleagues, six population groups, namely from Hazda, Malawi, Burkina Faso, Italy (adults and children) and the USA, were investigated with regard to their lifestyle and eating habits and composition of the intestinal microbiota. USA and Italy follow a western diet, based on farinaceous, refined sugar, saturated and trans fat, and high meat consumption, and have a sedentary and stressful lifestyle. Burkina Faso and Malawi inhabitants have a traditional rural African diet that is rich in starch, fibers, and plant foods. Hadza is a tribe from Tanzania, whose lifestyle remains the same as that of their ancestors, eating game meat, tubers, fruits and berries. Investigators identified a great variety in the composition of the microbiota between the various communities. Specifically, there was a higher abundance of *Ruminococcaceae* distinguishing for the Hadza hunter-gatherers, the emergence of *Clostridiales* and *Prevotella* in rural Malawi and Burkina Faso populations, and the dominance of the *Faecalibacterium* in Western populations (Quercia et al., 2014; Schnorr et al., 2014).

Other study compared the intestinal microbiota composition of European individuals with the one from Burkina Faso individuals, where the diet is based on millet, local vegetables and a low intake of animal fat and protein. It was found that individuals from Burkina Faso had a higher concentration of *Provetella* and *Xilanibacter*, and a decrease in *Proteobacteria,* compared to European individuals (De Filippo et al., 2010).

Intestinal microbiota composition of individuals from Venezuela, Malawi and United States was compared. It was found that, regardless of age, the composition of the microbiota of individuals from Venezuela and Malawi was similar. Individuals from United States showed less diversity of intestinal microbiota, with a reduction in *Provetella* and an increase in bile tolerant bacteria such as *Alistipes, Bilophila* and *Bacteroides*, and a decrease in *Firmicutes* (Yatsunenko et al., 2012).

Table 1. Dietary pattern, microbiota composition and health consequences.

Diet	Microbiota composition	Molecular and metabolic modifications	Health consequences
Vegan / Vegetarian diet	↓ Bifidobacteria ↑ Clostridium clostridioforme ↓ Clostridium cluster XIV ↑ Klebsiella pneumoniae ↓ Bilophila ↑ Bacteroides/Prevotella ↑ Bacteroidetes	Unkown	Unkown
Mediterranean diet	↑ Bifidobacteria ↑ Lactobacillus ↓ Clostridium ↑ Lachnospiraceae ↓ Enterobacteria ↑ Bacteroidetes	↑ SCFA production ↑ Microbiota diversity and stability ↑ Antiinflammatory citokine expression (IL10, IL22)	Prevention of metabolic diseases (Schwingshackl & Hoffmann, 2014)
Western diet	↓ Bifidobacteria ↑ Ruminococcus torques ↓ Roseburia ↓ Eubacterium rectale ↓ Ruminococcus bromii ↓ Lactobacillus ↑ Enterobacteria ↑ Bilophila ↑ Alistipes ↓ Prevotella ↑ Bacteroides ↑ Akkermansia	↓ SCFA production ↓ Microbiota diversity ↑ Profinflammatory citokine expression (IL17, TNFα, IFNγ) ↑ Endotoxins, hidrogen sulfide, phenols, ammonia, índoles	Increased risk of metabolic diseases (obesity; cardiovascular disease; diabetes mellitus type II) (Statovci et al., 2017)
Low FODMAPs diet	↓ Bifidobacteria ↓ Ruminococcus gravus ↓ Clostridium ↓ F. prausnitzii ↓ Akkermansia	↓ Microbiota diversity and abundance	If applied for over 6 weeks period: Possible weight loss (O'Keeffe et al., 2018); Deficit of antioxidants (flavonoids, carotenoids, vitamin C, phenolic acid and anthocyanins) (Bellini et al., 2020)

Legend: SCFA – Short Chain Fatty Acids; FODMAPs – Fermentable oligo-, di- and monosaccharides and polyols; IL - Interleukine

These differences come from diets composition of these populations. Westernized diet is rich in saturated fat, sugar, refined flours, food additives and AGEs, and low in antioxidant compounds, fibers and n-3 PUFA. This diet lead to an increase in bacteria of *Clostridium innocuum, Catenibacterium mitsuokai* and *Enterococcus*, and a decrease in *Bifidobacteria* spp. The increase in the ingestion of n-6 PUFA from sunflower oil, also common in westernized diet, promotes the reduction of *Firmicutes*, and the increase of *Actinobacteria* and *Proteobacteria*. On the other hand, the consumption of whole grains and fibers is associated with an increase in *Bifidobacteria longum, Bifidobacteria breve* and *Bifidobacteria theyaiotaomicron*, and a decrease in *Mycobacterium* and *Enterobacteriaceae* (Brown et al., 2012).

In the Mediterranean diet, whose concept was created to mimic the food of the inhabitants of Greece, Crete and southern Italy in the 1960s, the consumption of fruit, vegetables, olive oil, nuts, whole grains and fish is promoted. Thus, this diet translates into a high intake of fiber, antioxidants, PUFA and MUFA, being low in saturated fat, sugar and food additives. These characteristics improved *Firmicutes-Bacteroides* ratio and increased *Bifidobacterium* and SCFA production (De Filippis et al., 2016; Garcia-Mantrana et al., 2018; Mitsou et al., 2017).

In addition to the dietary aspects, it is important to remember that there are other factors that negatively influence the intestinal microbiota composition, such as physical inactivity, chronic stress, abuse of antibiotics and exposure to xenobiotics, such as tobacco and pollution.

2.2.8. Probiotics in Gut Microbiota

According to Food and Agriculture Organization (FAO), probiotics are defined as live microorganisms that, when administered in the adequate amounts, exert health benefits on the host (WHO, 2006). Probiotics act to restore microbial balance, optimizing its metabolic, protective and structural functions (Fedorak & Madsen, 2004). Some examples are yogurt, kefir and kombucha. Additionally, it can be taken as a supplement, in which case they must present a significant phyla diversity, especially *Firmicutes* and *Bacteroides* (Ashraf & Shah, 2014; Gill & Prasad, 2008; Lomax & Calder, 2009; Perdigon et al., 1995; Purchiaroni, 2013; Yan & Polk, 2011).

The effectiveness of probiotics is proven for a wide variety of pathologies. In IBD, the use of probiotics has been extensively studied, with several meta-analyses that affirm its effectiveness, especially in ulcerative colitis (UC) (Ganji-Arjenaki & Rafieian-Kopaei, 2018; Jia et al., 2018; Shen et al., 2014).

The effect of probiotic supplementation alone on Helicobacter Pylori (H. Pylori) eradication are minimal, although they suggest a direct and positive role (Losurdo et al., 2018). Nevertheless, the use of probiotics has been suggested as an adjunct to the usual medical therapy for the treatment of H. Pylori, with very interesting results not only with regard to the effectiveness of the antibiotic in the complete eradication of the bacteria, but also in the replacement of the intestinal microbiota (Losurdo et al., 2018).

In respect to oral health, literature suggests that probiotics usage could be beneficial due to its ability to decrease the colony forming units counts of the oral pathogens. However, randomized clinical trials with long-term follow-up periods are needed to confirm their efficacy in reducing the prevalence/incidence of oral infectious diseases (Seminario-Amez, 2017). Additionally, other systematic reviews demonstrate the beneficial effects of probiotics in Non-Alcoholic Fat Liver Disease (NAFLD) (Loman et al., 2018) and neurological diseases like Depression (Huang et al., 2016).

Regarding safety of probiotic usage, some studies indicate that some adverse effects may arise, particularly sepsis, fungemia and gastrointestinal ischemia. These effects are usually one-off and mostly in critically ill patients in intensive care units, critically sick infants, post-operative and hospitalized patients and patients with immune-compromised complexity (Didari et al., 2014). Some authors advocate taking prebiotics and probiotics in a combined way, thus taking advantage of the synergy between them created (de Vrese & Schrezenmeir, 2008).

2.3. Dysbiosis in Chronic Diseases

Dysbiosis seems to be associated to systemic and chronic metabolic diseases. However, the mechanism by which dysbiosis and the progression of chronic diseases are related remains unclear. There are two probable situations that occur in a very common way, and that, individually or in combination, can explain this connection: low-grade inflammation and bacterial translocation.

Many authors describe the presence of low-grade inflammation in many different chronic diseases, like rheumatoid arthritis, cystic fibrosis, psoriasis, periodontitis, diabetes mellitus type 2 and obesity.

The inflammatory process develops in the presence of an inflammatory stimulus, such as trauma or infection. Local macrophages are activated, which produce IL-1β and TNF-α. These two cytokines bind to endothelial cell receptors, inducing the inflammatory response. At the molecular level, within the macrophage, transcription factors bind to DNA promoting the expression of pro-inflammatory molecules. In case of NFkB signalling pathway, this protein is found outside the nucleus inhibited by IkBα. The inflammatory stimulus leads to an increase in kinases that destroy IkBα, releasing NFkB, which binds to DNA and increases the inflammatory cytokine outflow. These cytokines, namely IL-1β, IL-6 and TNF-α, are released into endothelial cells, where in addition to promoting local inflammation, they will destroy endothelial IkBα, releasing NFkB to express more proteins, such as Thelper (Th) 1, Th2 and Th17, and Tregulators (Treg) lymphocytes, selectins, Vascular cell adhesion protein 1 (VCAM-1) and Ciclo-oxigenase-2 (COX-2), amplifying the inflammatory response (Groschwitz & Hogan, 2009; Round & Mazmanian, 2009). The more extensive or systemic the inflammatory stimulus, the greater the production of pro-inflammatory molecules (Groschwitz & Hogan, 2009).

COX-2, being responsible for the metabolism of arachidonic acid, promotes an increase in Prostaglandines E_2 (PGE_2), which in turn increases intestinal permeability (Jang et al., 2020). Enterocytes themselves increase the production of PGE_2, so that intestinal hyperpermeability allows macrophages to enter and carry out its process. However, this same increase in permeability allows the occurrence of bacterial translocation and/or bacterial products, such as LPS, peptidoglycans, muramyl-dipeptides and bacterial DNA. This mechanism occurs across gut mucosal barrier to mesenteric lymph nodes, liver, spleen, kidney and bloodstream (Deitch, 1990), which justifies the manifestation of dysbiosis in numerous chronic diseases.

The association of dysbiosis with IBD including UC and chron's disease (CD), has been demonstrated (Carding et al., 2015; Ferreira et al., 2014). Several authors describe that bacterial alterations in the composition of intestinal microbiota strongly correlate with disease status (Gevers et al., 2014; Hold, 2014; Orel & Kamhi Trop, 2014; Sturm & Duffy, 2012).

However, there are other chronic conditions whose patients have changes in the intestinal microbiota composition such as, metabolic syndrome (Brown et al., 2012; Ferreira et al., 2014), diabetes mellitus type 2(Khan et al., 2016), atherosclerosis (Jonsson & Backhed, 2017) and obesity (Khan et al., 2016). The difference in gut microbiota of obese and non-obese individuals have been vastly reported (Andoh et al., 2016). In fact, a western diet has been shown to decrease beneficial bacteria (Singh et al., 2017). From a sociological and behavioural perspective, some authors suggest that SCFA would have a protective role against obesity, since they regulate hormones related to appetite control as previously mentioned, such as peptide YY (PYY), glucagon-Like peptide-1 (GLP-1) and leptin. In the presence of dysbiosis, the production of SCFA may be reduced, and as a consequence there may be a disturbance in the regulation of these hormones, further aggravating the individual's behaviour in an attempt to control his disease (Kumari & Kozyrskyj, 2017).

Several rheumatological diseases, namely ankilosing spondylitis (Costello et al., 2015), systemic sclerosis, rheumatoid arthritis (Scher & Abramson, 2011), psoriasis and fibromyalgia (FM), present alterations in the composition of the intestinal microbiota. In a study by Malatji and colleagues, several metabolites were identified in the urine of FM patients, by Hydrogen nuclear magnetic resonance spectroscopy (^{1}H NMR), suggesting changes in the intestinal microbiota, namely: 1) hyperuric acid, increased in the presence of reflux or hepatic detoxification; 2) 2-hydroxyisobutyrate acid, associated with the presence of *Faecalibacterium Prausnitzii*, a commensal bacteria; 3) lactic acid. On the other hand, they also identified taurine, succinate acid and TMAO as being the responsible metabolites for differentiation between patients of this pathology and the control group, also indicators of intestinal microbiome alteration (Malatji et al., 2017). Additionally, some therapeutic strategies developed with the aim of normalizing the microbiota have shown positive results (Zhong et al., 2018). In patients with Cystic Fibrosis, taking probiotics showed an improvement in respiratory function (Li & Somerset, 2014). However, effectiveness is still too limited to realize their application in the clinic.

Finally, the relationship between the brain and the intestine is already well documented. Many hormones and peptides produced in the intestine, such as PYY, and others such as leptin, ghrelin and insulin, can influence neurological function. The Brain Derived Neurotrophic Factor (BDNF) produced in the brain, modulates metabolic functions such as appetite suppression and insulin sensitivity. (Gomez-Pinilla, 2008). Several authors report an alteration of the intestinal microbiota and the presence of dysbiosis in patients with neuropsychiatric diseases and central nervous system (CNS) disruption (Kelly et al., 2015; Petra et al., 2015), such as depression (Clapp et al., 2017), schizophrenia (Szeligowski et al., 2020), attention-deficit hypersensitivity disorder (Richarte et al., 2018) and autism spectrum disorders (Li et al., 2017).

3. SMALL INTESTINAL BACTERIAL OVERGROWTH

During homeostasis, microorganisms are distributed throughout the entire gastrointestinal tract, from the mouth to the anus. This distribution varies qualitatively and quantitatively in each environment. In the stomach, duodenum and proximal jejunum are found between 10^1 and 10^3 colonyforming units (CFU) of bacteria per mL; in distal jejunum and ileum between 10^4 and 10^7 CFU/mL; and in the colon between 10^{11} and 10^{12} CFU/mL (O'Hara & Shanahan, 2006). In the presence of dysbiosis, one of three situations may occur: a migration of bacteria from the colon to the duodenum and proximal jejunum; an excessive proliferation of bacteria already present in the duodenum; or the appearance and subsequent proliferation of a nefarious bacteria in this region of the intestine (Bures, 2010). If we find ourselves in this scenario, we will probably be at the Small Intestine Bacterial Overgrowth (SIBO) demonstration.

3.1. Description and Triggering Factors

SIBO is defined as an increase in the number and/or alteration in the type of bacteria in the upper gastrointestinal tract (Bures, 2010). This situation leads to an alteration in intestinal track motility, often reflected in diarrhoea, constipation or to an alternation between the two. In addition to these symptoms, a variety of clinical complaints such as abdominal pain, bloating, flatulence, lack of energy and weight loss, are also common (Grace et al., 2013). As a result, the nutrients absorption can be compromised. The activity of brush border enzymes disaccharidase and hydrolase will be inhibited, which leads to a decrease in digestion and absorption of carbohydrates. In addition, the deconjugation of bile acids by bacteria may results in malabsorption of fat and liposoluble vitamins, such as vitamin A, D and E (Adike & DiBaise, 2018; Bures, 2010). In contrast, levels of vitamin K, a fat-soluble vitamin, are usually normal (Adike & DiBaise, 2018). Vitamin B12 deficiency may result from inhibition of normal B12 absorption by anaerobic organisms, and by the consumption of this vitamin within the intestinal lumen by enteric facultative microbes before it could be absorbed. Iron and vitamin B1 and B3 deficiencies have also been described in the setting of SIBO, although the mechanisms are not known (Adike & DiBaise, 2018; Bures, 2010).

Prevention of bacterial overgrowth is possible through several endogenous defence mechanisms of our organism, namely gastric acid secretion, intestinal motility, intact ileocecal valve, immunoglobulins within intestinal secretion and bacteriostatic properties of pancreatic and biliary secretion. Besides dysbiosis caused by an inadequate life style, aetiology of SIBO is associated with disorders of protective antibacterial mechanisms (e.g. immunodeficiency syndromes), imbalances in gastrointestinal enzyme production (e.g. achlorhydria, pancreatic exocrine insufficiency), anatomical abnormalities (e.g. small intestinal obstruction, diverticulosis, development of fistulae, surgical blind loop, loss of competence of the ileocecal valve) and/or motility disorders (e.g. scleroderma, autonomic neuropathy in diabetes mellitus, post-radiation enteropathy, small intestinal pseudo-obstruction). In some patients more than one factor may be involved (Bures, 2010).

3.2. SIBO in Chronic Diseases

The assessment of prevalence of SIBO in chronic diseases is difficult to do, mainly because tests used for the diagnosis of SIBO vary considerably in the still few studies carried out. However, the studies and systematic reviews that exist, despite their limitations, reveal significant results for the prevalence of SIBO in several chronic diseases.

Obesity could be a predisposing factor for SIBO, and several studies suggest an increased risk of developing SIBO in obese individuals compared to non-obese individuals. A meta-analysis found that the risk of SIBO was almost two times higher among individuals with obesity compared to individuals without obesity, however there was no statistical significance. Nevertheless, the risk increased to threefold and reached statistical significance when only studies from Western countries were included (Wijarnpreecha, 2019). Authors suggest two possible mechanisms to explain this observation. Firstly, the increased risk of gut dysmotility seen in individuals with obesity. Obesity negatively affects bowel motility by markedly increasing the occurrence of clustered contractions in the small intestine, which consequently could affect propulsive motility and therefore affect the bacteria natural life cycle, resulting in accumulation of bacteria (Madrid et al., 2011). This phenomenon, also seen in other pathologies, such as cirrhosis, portal hypertension, pancreatitis and IBD, have shown similar disruptions in the Migrating Motor Complex (MMC), resulting in the ineffective sweeping of bacteria from the proximal bowel into the colon (Pimentel et al., 2002). The second explanation is related to alteration of gut microbiota and consequent dysbiosis, which has been seen in obese patients (Sun et al., 2018; Wijarnpreecha, 2019).

IBD is associated with physiological phenomena of alteration of enzyme activity, loss of intestinal mucosa integrity and the presence of dysbiosis, which makes patients with this pathology more predisposed to the development of SIBO. A systematic review with meta-analysis identified a statistically significant prevalence of SIBO of 22.3% ($p<0.05$) in patients with IBD, 14.3% ($p<0.05$) in patients with UC and 25.4% ($p<0.05$) in patients with CD (Shah et al., 2019), which is corroborates within another systematic review (Ganji-Arjenaki & Rafieian-Kopaei, 2018). It was also found that loss of ileocecal valve (due to previous ileocecal resection) and/or large entero-enteric and enterocolic fistulae are important predisposing factors in IBD (Bures, 2010; Ganji-Arjenaki & Rafieian-Kopaei, 2018; Shah et al., 2019).

The prevalence of SIBO in patients with Irritable Bowel Syndrome (IBS) is 38% ($p<0.05$) (Chen et al., 2018), which is specially significant in this population.

With regard to Celiac Disease, although some authors point to the presence of SIBO in some patients (Bures, 2010), a meta-analysis that there is no significant relationship (Diwakarla et al., 2017).

Regarding Chronic Liver Disease (CLD), there is a consistent and statistically significant increase of SIBO in patients with the disease, with an Odds Ratio (OR) for SIBO in CLD of 7.15% ($p<0.05$). Particularly, in Non-Alcoholic Fat Liver Disease (NAFLD), the prevalence of SIBO is 33.5% ($p<0.05$), comparing to healthy control (7.3%, $p<0.05$). Studies have shown that patients with NAFLD and SIBO had significant higher blood endotoxin concentration compared with control. Additionally, TLR expression and serum TNFα and IL-8, which correlate with TRL-4 expression, were significantly higher in these patients. SIBO-associated increased intestinal permeability and endotoxemia results in activation of TLR signalling, that plays an important role in NAFLD and progression to Non-Alcoholic Steatohepatitis (NASH). On its turn, in Cirrhosis, the prevalence of SIBO is 40.1% ($p<0.05$), comparing to healthy control (7.3%, $p<0.05$) (Shah et al., 2017).

Chronic Pancreatitis (CP) is characterized by inflammatory and destructive functional changes in pancreas. There are some predictor factors to SIBO development, such as fat malabsorption, diabetic neuropathy, proton pump inhibitor (PPI) drugs use, alcohol intake and surgical procedures. A meta-analysis reveals an OR for SIBO in CP of 4.1 ($p<0.05$) (Capurso et al., 2016), which suggest a significant prevalence of SIBO in these patients. In respect to Systemic Sclerosis (SSc), the prevalence of SIBO range 30 to 62% (Pittman et al., 2018). Other studies associate the persistence of the FM symptoms with the presence of SIBO (Marsh et al., 2016; Othman et al., 2008; Pimentel, 2004), in particular the intensity of pain, as SIBO appears to increase the exposure of immune system cells to antigens in the intestinal lumen, thereby causing immune modulation (Malatji et al., 2017).

Additionally, SIBO seems to be present in others manifestations, such as dyspepsia, rosacea, restless legs syndrome, hypothyroidism, Parkinson's disease, diabetes, coronary artery disease, and abdominal surgery (e.g., hysterectomy, gastrectomy, cholecystectomy, and colectomy). However, the prevalence of SIBO in patients with these associated conditions is highly variable, with a range between 4% and 79% (Rao & Bhagatwala, 2019).

3.3. Influence of Food and Nutrients on SIBO

Conventional therapy involves the prescription of antibiotics, usually broad-spectrum Rifaximin, often applied 8-8h for 7 days. However, antibiotic therapy is not associated with a complete improvement in clinical symptoms, which leads to the very common need to repeat the prescription after 1 month (Ganji-Arjenaki & Rafieian-Kopaei, 2018). Additionally, the association of the antibiotic use and abuse with development of dysbiosis is well known (Jernberg et al., 2007; Jernberg et al., 2010). This often result in intolerance to treatment, *Clostridium dificile* infection and increase in antibiotic resistance (Adike & DiBaise, 2018; Ganji-Arjenaki & Rafieian-Kopaei, 2018; Sheehan et al., 2015; Ungaro et al., 2014).

Other strategy for SIBO treatment includes the introduction of probiotics. A meta-analysis verified that probiotics supplementation could effectively decontaminate SIBO, decrease H_2 concentration, and relieve abdominal pain, but were ineffective in preventing SIBO (Zhong et al., 2017). However, it has been verified that the intervention of probiotics can lead to the opposite result of the expected, with the exacerbation of the symptoms. It is possible that the effectiveness of using probiotics depends on the type of bacteria present in the product, and whether or not they are combined with prebiotics. Many probiotics on the market contain FOS, which are saccharides more fermentable by bacteria and that could therefore cause a worsening of symptoms. However the composition of the supplements used is not specified.

The intervention must always be individualized. Nutritional support is essential, mainly due to the possibility of nutritional deficits that SIBO entails (Bures, 2010). One of the most used nutritional approaches is the application of a diet low in fermentable oligo-, di- and monosaccharides and polyols (FODMAPs) foods.

Low FODMAPs Diet is a two-phase diet, characterized by avoidance of slowly absorbed or nondigestible short-chain carbohydrates (i.e. FODMAPs) for a period of between 4 and 6 weeks, followed by a slow reintroduction of well tolerated food. FODMAPs are a large class saccharides mainly absorbed in the colon, forming H_2 and CH_4 as a consequence of its metabolism by bacteria. The total daily intake of FODMAPs in a habitual diet ranges from 15 grams to 30 grams per day (Bellini et al., 2020). However, in the presence of an overgrowth of bacteria in the duodenum and proximal jejunum, this metabolism will generate flatulence, bloating and abdominal pain, classic SIBO symptoms (Marsh et al., 2016). Table 2 show the food alterative for Low FODMAPs diet.

Table 2. Food alternatives poor in FODMAPs - adapted from Hill et. al., 2017 (Hill et al., 2017)

FODMAPs	Foods high in FODMAPs	Suitable alternatives low in FODMAPs
Excess of Fructose	Fruits: apple, peach, mango, pear, pea, watermelon, preserves Honey sweeteners: fructose, corn syrup Large total dose of fructose: concentrated sources of fruit, large portions of fruit, dried fruit, fruit juice	Fruits: banana, melon, grape, grapefruit, melon, kiwi, lemon, lime, orange, passion fruit, papaya, raspberry, blueberry, strawberry, pineapple Honey substitutes: maple syrup Sweeteners: any sweeteners, except polyols
Lactose	Milk: regular and low-fat cow, goat, and sheep milk; ice cream Yogurts: regular and low-fat yogurts Cheeses: soft and fresh cheeses	Milk: lactose-free milk, rice milk Ice cream substitutes: gelato, sorbet Yogurts: lactose-free yogurts Cheeses: hard cheeses
Oligosaccharides (fructans and/or galactans)	Vegetables: artichoke, asparagus, beet, broccoli, Brussels sprouts, cabbage, fennel, garlic, leeks, okra, onion, pea, shallot Cereals: rye and wheat cereals (for example, biscuit, bread, couscous, biscuit, pasta) Legumes: baked beans, chickpeas, lentils, red beans Fruit: watermelon	Vegetables: bamboo root, spinach, carrot, celery, pak choy cabbage, cucumber, chives, corn, eggplant, green beans, lettuce, pumpkin, chard Cereals: bread / cereals gluten-free and spelled products Fruit: tomato
Polyols	Fruits: apple, apricot, avocado, cherry, lychee, nectarine, peach, pear, plum, watermelon Vegetables: cauliflower, mushroom, pea Sweeteners: isomalt, maltitol, mannitol, sorbitol, xylitol, and other sweeteners ending in "-ol"	Fruits: banana, blueberry, melon, grape, grapefruit, melon, kiwi, lemon, lime, orange, passion fruit, papaya, raspberry Sweeteners: glucose, sugar (sucrose), other artificial sweeteners that do not end in "-ol"

The FODMAPs mechanism of action is linked to the stimulation of mechanoreceptors as a response to luminal distension from a combination of increased luminal water content from the osmotic effect, especially in the small intestine, and from the release of H_2 and NH_4 from the bacterial fermentation of saccharides (Hill et al., 2017). Such stimulation can lead to ascending messages that might be interpreted as abdominal pain or bloating; reflex responses to the diaphragm and anterior abdominal wall, leading to increased abdominal distension; and effects on motility with potential change in bowel habits (Bellini et al., 2020; Hill et al., 2017). Additionally, there could occur an excessive production of SCFA, which could lead to visceral sensitivity and high-amplitude propagated colonic contractions, thus accelerating intestinal transit (Bellini et al., 2020).

In this context, limiting the intake of the most fermentable carbohydrates will potentially alleviate the symptoms, by reducing the formation of gases. There is still insufficient evidence to consider Low FODMAPs Diet a legitimate first-line therapy, mainly because most of the studies carried out are of low quality, with short durations, small number of patients and inappropriate comparator placebo groups (Hill et al., 2017).

A positive effect of Low FODMAPs Diet in gastrointestinal manifestations, specially in IBS has been suggested. IBS patients are probably the population where more clinical trials have been performed on a diet low in FODMAPs. In a randomized placebo-controlled trial, 104 IBS patients carried out a Low FODMAPs Diet or a placebo diet for four weeks, similar in amount of food restriction and in difficulty of implementation. Patients on the Low FODMAPs Diet had a significantly symptom relief (61%, $p < 0.05$) and a significant improvement in the results of the disease assessment questionnaire Irritable Bowel Syndrome Severity Scoring System (IBS-SSS) compared to placebo ($p < 0.001$) (Staudacher et al., 2017). Additionally, a meta-analysis showed a significant improvement in the quality of life questionnaires (IBS-QOL) and in IBS-SSS, as well as in symptoms such as bloating and abdominal pain, supports the efficacy of a low FODMAP diet in the treatment of functional gastrointestinal symptoms (Marsh et al., 2016).

Although there are no studies carried out with the application of Low FODMAPs Diet in other pathologies, the presence of SIBO in diseases such as NAFLD, CP and SSc, among others, suggests that this intervention could be beneficial in these patients. In fact, a four week Low FODMAPs Diet clinical trial implemented in 38 FM patients showed a significant improvement in pain, fatigue, gastric pain, mobility and gastrointestinal symptoms (Marum et al., 2016).

The composition of the intestinal microbiota is sensitive to several aspects, not only with regard to dietary habits but also general lifestyle components. The association of dysbiosis is the promotion of low-grade inflammation and the development of chronic diseases is, as we have seen, a reality.

REFERENCES

Adike, A., & DiBaise, J. K. (2018). Small Intestinal Bacterial Overgrowth: Nutritional Implications, Diagnosis, and Management. *Gastroenterology Clinics of North America, 47*(1), 193–208. doi:10.1016/j.gtc.2017.09.008 PMID:29413012

Anderson, J. W., Baird, P., Davis, R. H. Jr, Ferreri, S., Knudtson, M., Koraym, A., ... Williams, C. L. (2009). Health benefits of dietary fiber. *Nutrition Reviews, 67*(4), 188–205. doi:10.1111/j.1753-4887.2009.00189.x PMID:19335713

Andoh, A., Nishida, A., Takahashi, K., Inatomi, O., Imaeda, H., Bamba, S., ... Kobayashi, T. (2016). Comparison of the gut microbial community between obese and lean peoples using 16S gene sequencing in a Japanese population. *Journal of Clinical Biochemistry and Nutrition, 59*(1), 65–70. doi:10.3164/jcbn.15-152 PMID:27499582

Ashraf, R., & Shah, N. P. (2014). Immune system stimulation by probiotic microorganisms. *Critical Reviews in Food Science and Nutrition, 54*(7), 938–956. doi:10.1080/10408398.2011.619671 PMID:24499072

Bellini, M., Tonarelli, S., Nagy, A. G., Pancetti, A., Costa, F., Ricchiuti, A., ... Rossi, A. (2020). Low FODMAP Diet: Evidence, Doubts, and Hopes. *Nutrients*, *12*(1), 148. doi:10.3390/nu12010148 PMID:31947991

Biesalski, H. K. (2016). Nutrition meets the microbiome: Micronutrients and the microbiota. *Annals of the New York Academy of Sciences*, *1372*(1), 53–64. doi:10.1111/nyas.13145 PMID:27362360

Bischoff, S. C., Barbara, G., Buurman, W., Ockhuizen, T., Schulzke, J.-D., Serino, M., ... Wells, J. M. (2014). Intestinal permeability--a new target for disease prevention and therapy. *BMC Gastroenterology*, *14*(1), 189. doi:10.118612876-014-0189-7 PMID:25407511

Bosshart, H., & Heinzelmann, M. (2007). Targeting bacterial endotoxin: Two sides of a coin. *Annals of the New York Academy of Sciences*, *1096*(1), 1–17. doi:10.1196/annals.1397.064 PMID:17405910

Brown, K., DeCoffe, D., Molcan, E., & Gibson, D. L. (2012). Diet-induced dysbiosis of the intestinal microbiota and the effects on immunity and disease. *Nutrients*, *4*(8), 1095–1119. doi:10.3390/nu4081095 PMID:23016134

Bures, J. (2010). Small intestinal bacterial overgrowth syndrome. *World Journal of Gastroenterology*, *16*(24), 2978–2990. doi:10.3748/wjg.v16.i24.2978 PMID:20572300

Cantorna, M. T., Zhu, Y., Froicu, M., & Wittke, A. (2004). Vitamin D status, 1,25-dihydroxyvitamin D3, and the immune system. *The American Journal of Clinical Nutrition*, *80*(6Suppl), 1717S–1720S. doi:10.1093/ajcn/80.6.1717S PMID:15585793

Capurso, G., Signoretti, M., Archibugi, L., Stigliano, S., & Delle Fave, G. (2016). Systematic review and meta-analysis: Small intestinal bacterial overgrowth in chronic pancreatitis. *United European Gastroenterology Journal*, *4*(5), 697–705. doi:10.1177/2050640616630117 PMID:27733912

Carding, S., Verbeke, K., Vipond, D. T., Corfe, B. M., & Owen, L. J. (2015). Dysbiosis of the gut microbiota in disease. *Microbial Ecology in Health and Disease*, *26*(0), 26191. doi:10.3402/mehd.v26.26191 PMID:25651997

Cerf-Bensussan, N., & Gaboriau-Routhiau, V. (2010). The immune system and the gut microbiota: Friends or foes? *Nature Reviews. Immunology*, *10*(10), 735–744. doi:10.1038/nri2850 PMID:20865020

Chang, J. Y., Antonopoulos, D. A., Kalra, A., Tonelli, A., Khalife, W. T., Schmidt, T. M., & Young, V. B. (2008). Decreased diversity of the fecal Microbiome in recurrent Clostridium difficile-associated diarrhea. *The Journal of Infectious Diseases*, *197*(3), 435–438. doi:10.1086/525047 PMID:18199029

Chassaing, B., Koren, O., Goodrich, J. K., Poole, A. C., Srinivasan, S., Ley, R. E., & Gewirtz, A. T. (2015). Dietary emulsifiers impact the mouse gut microbiota promoting colitis and metabolic syndrome. *Nature*, *519*(7541), 92–96. doi:10.1038/nature14232 PMID:25731162

Chassaing, B., Van de Wiele, T., De Bodt, J., Marzorati, M., & Gewirtz, A. T. (2017). Dietary emulsifiers directly alter human microbiota composition and gene expression ex vivo potentiating intestinal inflammation. *Gut*, *66*(8), 1414–1427. doi:10.1136/gutjnl-2016-313099 PMID:28325746

Chen, B., Kim, J. J.-W., Zhang, Y., Du, L., & Dai, N. (2018). Prevalence and predictors of small intestinal bacterial overgrowth in irritable bowel syndrome: A systematic review and meta-analysis. *Journal of Gastroenterology*, *53*(7), 807–818. doi:10.100700535-018-1476-9 PMID:29761234

Clapp, M., Aurora, N., Herrera, L., Bhatia, M., Wilen, E., & Wakefield, S. (2017). Gut microbiota's effect on mental health: The gut-brain axis. *Clinics and Practice*, *7*(4), 987. doi:10.4081/cp.2017.987 PMID:29071061

Clarke, R. E., Dordevic, A., Tan, S., Ryan, L., & Coughlan, M. (2016). Dietary Advanced Glycation End Products and Risk Factors for Chronic Disease: A Systematic Review of Randomised Controlled Trials. *Nutrients*, *8*(3), 125. doi:10.3390/nu8030125 PMID:26938557

Clauw, D. J. (2009). Fibromyalgia: An overview. *The American Journal of Medicine*, *122*(12Suppl), S3–S13. doi:10.1016/j.amjmed.2009.09.006 PMID:19962494

Conlon, M. A., & Bird, A. R. (2014). The impact of diet and lifestyle on gut microbiota and human health. *Nutrients*, *7*(1), 17–44. doi:10.3390/nu7010017 PMID:25545101

Costello, M. E., Ciccia, F., Willner, D., Warrington, N., Robinson, P. C., Gardiner, B., ... Brown, M. A. (2015). Brief Report: Intestinal Dysbiosis in Ankylosing Spondylitis. *Arthritis & Rheumatology (Hoboken, N.J.)*, *67*(3), 686–691. doi:10.1002/art.38967 PMID:25417597

David, L. A., Maurice, C. F., Carmody, R. N., Gootenberg, D. B., Button, J. E., Wolfe, B. E., ... Turnbaugh, P. J. (2014). Diet rapidly and reproducibly alters the human gut microbiome. *Nature*, *505*(7484), 559–563. doi:10.1038/nature12820 PMID:24336217

De Filippis, F., Pellegrini, N., Vannini, L., Jeffery, I. B., La Storia, A., Laghi, L., ... Ercolini, D. (2016). High-level adherence to a Mediterranean diet beneficially impacts the gut microbiota and associated metabolome. *Gut*, *65*(11), 1812–1821. doi:10.1136/gutjnl-2015-309957 PMID:26416813

De Filippo, C., Cavalieri, D., Di Paola, M., Ramazzotti, M., Poullet, J. B., Massart, S., ... Lionetti, P. (2010). Impact of diet in shaping gut microbiota revealed by a comparative study in children from Europe and rural Africa. *Proceedings of the National Academy of Sciences of the United States of America*, *107*(33), 14691–14696. doi:10.1073/pnas.1005963107 PMID:20679230

de Vrese, M., & Schrezenmeir, J. (2008). Probiotics, prebiotics, and synbiotics. *Advances in Biochemical Engineering/Biotechnology*, *111*, 1–66. doi:10.1007/10_2008_097 PMID:18461293

Deitch, E. A. (1990). Bacterial translocation of the gut flora. *The Journal of Trauma*, *30*(12Suppl), S184–S189. doi:10.1097/00005373-199012001-00037 PMID:2254980

Devkota, S., & Chang, E. B. (2015). Interactions between Diet, Bile Acid Metabolism, Gut Microbiota, and Inflammatory Bowel Diseases. *Digestive Diseases (Basel, Switzerland)*, *33*(3), 351–356. doi:10.1159/000371687 PMID:26045269

Didari, T., Solki, S., Mozaffari, S., Nikfar, S., & Abdollahi, M. (2014). A systematic review of the safety of probiotics. *Expert Opinion on Drug Safety*, *13*(2), 227–239. doi:10.1517/14740338.2014.872627 PMID:24405164

Diwakarla, S., Fothergill, L. J., Fakhry, J., Callaghan, B., & Furness, J. B. (2017). Heterogeneity of enterochromaffin cells within the gastrointestinal tract. *Neurogastroenterology and Motility*, *29*(6), e13101. doi:10.1111/nmo.13101 PMID:28485065

Draper, L. R., Gyure, L. A., Hall, J. G., & Robertson, D. (1983). Effect of alcohol on the integrity of the intestinal epithelium. *Gut*, *24*(5), 399–404. doi:10.1136/gut.24.5.399 PMID:6840613

Etxeberria, U., Arias, N., Boqué, N., Macarulla, M. T., Portillo, M. P., Martínez, J. A., & Milagro, F. I. (2015). Reshaping faecal gut microbiota composition by the intake of trans-resveratrol and quercetin in high-fat sucrose diet-fed rats. *The Journal of Nutritional Biochemistry*, *26*(6), 651–660. doi:10.1016/j.jnutbio.2015.01.002 PMID:25762527

Fasano, A. (2012a). Zonulin, regulation of tight junctions, and autoimmune diseases. *Annals of the New York Academy of Sciences*, *1258*(1), 25–33. doi:10.1111/j.1749-6632.2012.06538.x PMID:22731712

Fasano, A. (2012b). Intestinal permeability and its regulation by zonulin: Diagnostic and therapeutic implications. *Clinical Gastroenterology and Hepatology*, *10*(10), 1096–1100. doi:10.1016/j.cgh.2012.08.012 PMID:22902773

Fedorak, R. N., & Madsen, K. L. (2004). Probiotics and the management of inflammatory bowel disease. *Inflammatory Bowel Diseases*, *10*(3), 286–299. doi:10.1097/00054725-200405000-00018 PMID:15290926

Ferreira, C. M., Vieira, A. T., Vinolo, M. A. R., Oliveira, F. A., Curi, R., & Martins, F. S. (2014). The central role of the gut microbiota in chronic inflammatory diseases. *Journal of Immunology Research*, *2014*, 689492. doi:10.1155/2014/689492 PMID:25309932

Finamore, A., Massimi, M., Conti Devirgiliis, L., & Mengheri, E. (2008). Zinc deficiency induces membrane barrier damage and increases neutrophil transmigration in Caco-2 cells. *The Journal of Nutrition*, *138*(9), 1664–1670. doi:10.1093/jn/138.9.1664 PMID:18716167

Frazier, T. H., DiBaise, J. K., & McClain, C. J. (2011). Gut microbiota, intestinal permeability, obesity-induced inflammation, and liver injury. *JPEN. Journal of Parenteral and Enteral Nutrition*, *35*(5Suppl), 14S–20S. doi:10.1177/0148607111413772 PMID:21807932

Fuke, N., Nagata, N., Suganuma, H., & Ota, T. (2019). Regulation of Gut Microbiota and Metabolic Endotoxemia with Dietary Factors. *Nutrients*, *11*(10), 2277. doi:10.3390/nu11102277 PMID:31547555

Ganji-Arjenaki, M., & Rafieian-Kopaei, M. (2018). Probiotics are a good choice in remission of inflammatory bowel diseases: A meta analysis and systematic review. *Journal of Cellular Physiology*, *233*(3), 2091–2103. doi:10.1002/jcp.25911 PMID:28294322

Garcia-Mantrana, I., Selma-Royo, M., Alcantara, C., & Collado, M. C. (2018). Shifts on Gut Microbiota Associated to Mediterranean Diet Adherence and Specific Dietary Intakes on General Adult Population. *Frontiers in Microbiology*, *9*, 890. doi:10.3389/fmicb.2018.00890 PMID:29867803

Gevers, D., Kugathasan, S., Denson, L. A., Vázquez-Baeza, Y., Van Treuren, W., Ren, B., ... Xavier, R. J. (2014). The treatment-naive microbiome in new-onset Crohn's disease. *Cell Host & Microbe*, *15*(3), 382–392. doi:10.1016/j.chom.2014.02.005 PMID:24629344

Gill, H., & Prasad, J. (2008). Probiotics, immunomodulation, and health benefits. *Advances in Experimental Medicine and Biology*, *606*, 423–454. doi:10.1007/978-0-387-74087-4_17 PMID:18183940

Glaros, T. G. (2013). Causes and consequences of low grade endotoxemia and inflammatory diseases. *Frontiers in Bioscience (Scholar Edition)*, *5*(2), 754–765. doi:10.2741/S405 PMID:23277084

Gomez-Pinilla, F. (2008). Brain foods: The effects of nutrients on brain function. *Nature Reviews. Neuroscience*, *9*(7), 568–578. doi:10.1038/nrn2421 PMID:18568016

Grace, E., Shaw, C., Whelan, K., & Andreyev, H. J. N. (2013). Review article: Small intestinal bacterial overgrowth--prevalence, clinical features, current and developing diagnostic tests, and treatment. *Alimentary Pharmacology & Therapeutics*, *38*(7), 674–688. doi:10.1111/apt.12456 PMID:23957651

Groschwitz, K. R., & Hogan, S. P. (2009). Intestinal barrier function: Molecular regulation and disease pathogenesis. *The Journal of Allergy and Clinical Immunology*, *124*(1), 3–20, quiz 21–22. doi:10.1016/j.jaci.2009.05.038 PMID:19560575

Gruber, L., Kisling, S., Lichti, P., Martin, F.-P., May, S., Klingenspor, M., ... Haller, D. (2013). High fat diet accelerates pathogenesis of murine Crohn's disease-like ileitis independently of obesity. *PLoS One*, *8*(8), e71661. doi:10.1371/journal.pone.0071661 PMID:23977107

Harris, W. S. (2018). The Omega-6:Omega-3 ratio: A critical appraisal and possible successor. *Prostaglandins, Leukotrienes, and Essential Fatty Acids*, *132*, 34–40. doi:10.1016/j.plefa.2018.03.003 PMID:29599053

Hawrelak, J. A., & Myers, S. P. (2004). The causes of intestinal dysbiosis: A review. *Alternative Medicine Review*, *9*(2), 180–197. PMID:15253677

Hevia, A., Delgado, S., Sánchez, B., & Margolles, A. (2015). Molecular Players Involved in the Interaction Between Beneficial Bacteria and the Immune System. *Frontiers in Microbiology*, *6*, 1285. doi:10.3389/fmicb.2015.01285 PMID:26635753

Hidalgo, M., Oruna-Concha, M. J., Kolida, S., Walton, G. E., Kallithraka, S., Spencer, J. P. E., ... de Pascual-Teresa, S. (2012). Metabolism of anthocyanins by human gut microflora and their influence on gut bacterial growth. *Journal of Agricultural and Food Chemistry*, *60*(15), 3882–3890. doi:10.1021/jf3002153 PMID:22439618

Hill, P., Muir, J. G., & Gibson, P. R. (2017). Controversies and Recent Developments of the Low-FODMAP Diet. *Gastroenterology & Hepatology*, *13*(1), 36–45. PMID:28420945

Hold, G. L. (2014). Role of the gut microbiota in inflammatory bowel disease pathogenesis: What have we learnt in the past 10 years? *World Journal of Gastroenterology*, *20*(5), 1192–1210. doi:10.3748/wjg.v20.i5.1192 PMID:24574795

Hollon, J., Puppa, E., Greenwald, B., Goldberg, E., Guerrerio, A., & Fasano, A. (2015). Effect of gliadin on permeability of intestinal biopsy explants from celiac disease patients and patients with non-celiac gluten sensitivity. *Nutrients*, *7*(3), 1565–1576. doi:10.3390/nu7031565 PMID:25734566

Huang, R., Wang, K., & Hu, J. (2016). Effect of Probiotics on Depression: A Systematic Review and Meta-Analysis of Randomized Controlled Trials. *Nutrients*, *8*(8), 483. doi:10.3390/nu8080483 PMID:27509521

Jang, Y., Kim, M., & Hwang, S. W. (2020). Molecular mechanisms underlying the actions of arachidonic acid-derived prostaglandins on peripheral nociception. *Journal of Neuroinflammation*, *17*(1), 30. doi:10.118612974-020-1703-1 PMID:31969159

Jernberg, C., Löfmark, S., Edlund, C., & Jansson, J. K. (2007). Long-term ecological impacts of antibiotic administration on the human intestinal microbiota. *The ISME Journal*, *1*(1), 56–66. doi:10.1038/ismej.2007.3 PMID:18043614

Jernberg, C., Löfmark, S., Edlund, C., & Jansson, J. K. (2010). Long-term impacts of antibiotic exposure on the human intestinal microbiota. *Microbiology*, *156*(Pt 11), 3216–3223. doi:10.1099/mic.0.040618-0 PMID:20705661

Jia, K., Tong, X., Wang, R., & Song, X. (2018). The clinical effects of probiotics for inflammatory bowel disease: A meta-analysis. *Medicine; Analytical Reviews of General Medicine, Neurology, Psychiatry, Dermatology, and Pediatries*, *97*(51), e13792. doi:10.1097/MD.0000000000013792 PMID:30572537

Jonsson, A. L., & Backhed, F. (2017). Role of gut microbiota in atherosclerosis. *Nature Reviews. Cardiology*, *14*(2), 79–87. doi:10.1038/nrcardio.2016.183 PMID:27905479

Kaczmarczyk, M. M., Miller, M. J., & Freund, G. G. (2012). The health benefits of dietary fiber: Beyond the usual suspects of type 2 diabetes mellitus, cardiovascular disease and colon cancer. *Metabolism: Clinical and Experimental*, *61*(8), 1058–1066. doi:10.1016/j.metabol.2012.01.017 PMID:22401879

Kaliannan, K., Wang, B., Li, X.-Y., Kim, K.-J., & Kang, J. X. (2015). A host-microbiome interaction mediates the opposing effects of omega-6 and omega-3 fatty acids on metabolic endotoxemia. *Scientific Reports*, *5*(1), 11276. doi:10.1038rep11276 PMID:26062993

Kanitsoraphan, C., Rattanawong, P., Charoensri, S., & Senthong, V. (2018). Trimethylamine N-Oxide and Risk of Cardiovascular Disease and Mortality. *Current Nutrition Reports*, *7*(4), 207–213. doi:10.100713668-018-0252-z PMID:30362023

Karlsson, F. H., Fåk, F., Nookaew, I., Tremaroli, V., Fagerberg, B., Petranovic, D., ... Nielsen, J. (2012). Symptomatic atherosclerosis is associated with an altered gut metagenome. *Nature Communications*, *3*(1), 1245. doi:10.1038/ncomms2266 PMID:23212374

Kasubuchi, M., Hasegawa, S., Hiramatsu, T., Ichimura, A., & Kimura, I. (2015). Dietary gut microbial metabolites, short-chain fatty acids, and host metabolic regulation. *Nutrients*, *7*(4), 2839–2849. doi:10.3390/nu7042839 PMID:25875123

Kellow, N. J., & Savige, G. S. (2013). Dietary advanced glycation end-product restriction for the attenuation of insulin resistance, oxidative stress and endothelial dysfunction: A systematic review. *European Journal of Clinical Nutrition*, *67*(3), 239–248. doi:10.1038/ejcn.2012.220 PMID:23361161

Kelly, J. R., Kennedy, P. J., Cryan, J. F., Dinan, T. G., Clarke, G., & Hyland, N. P. (2015). Breaking down the barriers: The gut microbiome, intestinal permeability and stress-related psychiatric disorders. *Frontiers in Cellular Neuroscience*, *9*, 392. doi:10.3389/fncel.2015.00392 PMID:26528128

Khan, M. J., Gerasimidis, K., Edwards, C. A., & Shaikh, M. G. (2016). Role of Gut Microbiota in the Aetiology of Obesity: Proposed Mechanisms and Review of the Literature. *Journal of Obesity, 2016*, 7353642. doi:10.1155/2016/7353642 PMID:27703805

Kong, J., Zhang, Z., Musch, M. W., Ning, G., Sun, J., Hart, J., ... Li, Y. C. (2008). Novel role of the vitamin D receptor in maintaining the integrity of the intestinal mucosal barrier. *American Journal of Physiology. Gastrointestinal and Liver Physiology*, *294*(1), G208–G216. doi:10.1152/ajpgi.00398.2007 PMID:17962355

Kumari, M., & Kozyrskyj, A. L. (2017). Gut microbial metabolism defines host metabolism: An emerging perspective in obesity and allergic inflammation. *Obesity Reviews*, *18*(1), 18–31. doi:10.1111/obr.12484 PMID:27862824

Leclercq, S., Matamoros, S., Cani, P. D., Neyrinck, A. M., Jamar, F., Stärkel, P., ... Delzenne, N. M. (2014). Intestinal permeability, gut-bacterial dysbiosis, and behavioral markers of alcohol-dependence severity. *Proceedings of the National Academy of Sciences of the United States of America*, *111*(42), E4485–E4493. doi:10.1073/pnas.1415174111 PMID:25288760

Lepage, P., Häsler, R., Spehlmann, M. E., Rehman, A., Zvirbliene, A., Begun, A., ... Schreiber, S. (2011). Twin study indicates loss of interaction between microbiota and mucosa of patients with ulcerative colitis. *Gastroenterology*, *141*(1), 227–236. doi:10.1053/j.gastro.2011.04.011 PMID:21621540

Li, L., & Somerset, S. (2014). The clinical significance of the gut microbiota in cystic fibrosis and the potential for dietary therapies. *Clinical Nutrition (Edinburgh, Lothian)*, *33*(4), 571–580. doi:10.1016/j.clnu.2014.04.004 PMID:24767984

Li, Q., Han, Y., Dy, A. B. C., & Hagerman, R. J. (2017). The Gut Microbiota and Autism Spectrum Disorders. *Frontiers in Cellular Neuroscience*, *11*, 120. doi:10.3389/fncel.2017.00120 PMID:28503135

Lin, L., & Zhang, J. (2017). Role of intestinal microbiota and metabolites on gut homeostasis and human diseases. *BMC Immunology*, *18*(1), 2. doi:10.118612865-016-0187-3 PMID:28061847

Loman, B. R., Hernández-Saavedra, D., An, R., & Rector, R. S. (2018). Prebiotic and probiotic treatment of nonalcoholic fatty liver disease: A systematic review and meta-analysis. *Nutrition Reviews*, *76*(11), 822–839. doi:10.1093/nutrit/nuy031 PMID:30113661

Lomax, A. R., & Calder, P. C. (2009). Probiotics, immune function, infection and inflammation: A review of the evidence from studies conducted in humans. *Current Pharmaceutical Design*, *15*(13), 1428–1518. doi:10.2174/138161209788168155 PMID:19442167

Losurdo, G., Cubisino, R., Barone, M., Principi, M., Leandro, G., Ierardi, E., & Leo, A. D. (2018). Probiotic monotherapy and Helicobacter pylori eradication: A systematic review with pooled-data analysis. *World Journal of Gastroenterology*, *24*(1), 139–149. doi:10.3748/wjg.v24.i1.139 PMID:29358890

Madrid, A. M., Poniachik, J., Quera, R., & Defilippi, C. (2011). Small intestinal clustered contractions and bacterial overgrowth: A frequent finding in obese patients. *Digestive Diseases and Sciences*, *56*(1), 155–160. doi:10.100710620-010-1239-9 PMID:20431947

Malatji, B. G., Meyer, H., Mason, S., Engelke, U. F. H., Wevers, R. A., van Reenen, M., & Reinecke, C. J. (2017). A diagnostic biomarker profile for fibromyalgia syndrome based on an NMR metabolomics study of selected patients and controls. *BMC Neurology, 17*(1), 88. doi:10.118612883-017-0863-9 PMID:28490352

Manichanh, C. (2006). Reduced diversity of faecal microbiota in Crohn's disease revealed by a metagenomic approach. *Gut, 55*(2), 205–211. doi:10.1136/gut.2005.073817 PMID:16188921

Marsh, A., Eslick, E. M., & Eslick, G. D. (2016). Does a diet low in FODMAPs reduce symptoms associated with functional gastrointestinal disorders? A comprehensive systematic review and meta-analysis. *European Journal of Nutrition, 55*(3), 897–906. doi:10.100700394-015-0922-1 PMID:25982757

Marum, A. P., Moreira, C., Saraiva, F., Tomas-Carus, P., & Sousa-Guerreiro, C. (2016). A low fermentable oligo-di-mono saccharides and polyols (FODMAP) diet reduced pain and improved daily life in fibromyalgia patients. *Scandinavian Journal of Pain, 13*(1), 166–172. doi:10.1016/j.sjpain.2016.07.004 PMID:28850525

Matijasic, B. B., Obermajer, T., Lipoglavšek, L., Grabnar, I., Avguštin, G., & Rogelj, I. (2014). Association of dietary type with fecal microbiota in vegetarians and omnivores in Slovenia. *European Journal of Nutrition, 53*(4), 1051–1064. doi:10.100700394-013-0607-6 PMID:24173964

Mitsou, E. K., Kakali, A., Antonopoulou, S., Mountzouris, K. C., Yannakoulia, M., Panagiotakos, D. B., & Kyriacou, A. (2017). Adherence to the Mediterranean diet is associated with the gut microbiota pattern and gastrointestinal characteristics in an adult population. *British Journal of Nutrition, 117*(12), 1645–1655. doi:10.1017/S0007114517001593 PMID:28789729

Molan, A. L., Liu, Z., & Plimmer, G. (2014). Evaluation of the effect of blackcurrant products on gut microbiota and on markers of risk for colon cancer in humans. *Phytotherapy Research, 28*(3), 416–422. doi:10.1002/ptr.5009 PMID:23674271

Nahid, M. A., Satoh, M., & Chan, E. K. (2015). Interleukin 1beta-Responsive MicroRNA-146a Is Critical for the Cytokine-Induced Tolerance and Cross-Tolerance to Toll-Like Receptor Ligands. *Journal of Innate Immunity, 7*(4), 428–440. doi:10.1159/000371517 PMID:25896300

Noriega, B. S., Sanchez-Gonzalez, M. A., Salyakina, D., & Coffman, J. (2016). Understanding the Impact of Omega-3 Rich Diet on the Gut Microbiota. *Case Reports in Medicine, 2016*, 3089303. doi:10.1155/2016/3089303 PMID:27065349

O'Hara, A. M., & Shanahan, F. (2006). The gut flora as a forgotten organ. *EMBO Reports, 7*(7), 688–693. doi:10.1038j.embor.7400731 PMID:16819463

O'Keeffe, M., Jansen, C., Martin, L., Williams, M., Seamark, L., Staudacher, H. M., ... Lomer, M. C. (2018). Long-term impact of the low-FODMAP diet on gastrointestinal symptoms, dietary intake, patient acceptability, and healthcare utilization in irritable bowel syndrome. *Neurogastroenterology and Motility, 30*(1), e13154. doi:10.1111/nmo.13154 PMID:28707437

Orel, R., & Kamhi Trop, T. (2014). Intestinal microbiota, probiotics and prebiotics in inflammatory bowel disease. *World Journal of Gastroenterology, 20*(33), 11505–11524. doi:10.3748/wjg.v20.i33.11505 PMID:25206258

Othman, M., Aguero, R., & Lin, H. C. (2008). Alterations in intestinal microbial flora and human disease. *Current Opinion in Gastroenterology*, *24*(1), 11–16. doi:10.1097/MOG.0b013e3282f2b0d7 PMID:18043226

Ozdal, T., Sela, D. A., Xiao, J., Boyacioglu, D., Chen, F., & Capanoglu, E. (2016). The Reciprocal Interactions between Polyphenols and Gut Microbiota and Effects on Bioaccessibility. *Nutrients*, *8*(2), 78. doi:10.3390/nu8020078 PMID:26861391

Pearson, T. A., Mensah, G. A., Alexander, R. W., Anderson, J. L., Cannon, R. O. III, Criqui, M., ... Vinicor, F. (2003). Markers of inflammation and cardiovascular disease: application to clinical and public health practice: A statement for healthcare professionals from the Centers for Disease Control and Prevention and the American Heart Association. *Circulation*, *107*(3), 499–511. doi:10.1161/01.CIR.0000052939.59093.45 PMID:12551878

Pendyala, Walker, & Holt. (2012). A high-fat diet is associated with endotoxemia that originates from the gut. *Gastroenterology, 142*(5), 1100-1101.

Perdigon, G., Alvarez, S., Rachid, M., Agüero, G., & Gobbato, N. (1995). Immune system stimulation by probiotics. *Journal of Dairy Science*, *78*(7), 1597–1606. doi:10.3168/jds.S0022-0302(95)76784-4 PMID:7593855

Petra, A. I., Panagiotidou, S., Hatziagelaki, E., Stewart, J. M., Conti, P., & Theoharides, T. C. (2015). Gut-Microbiota-Brain Axis and Its Effect on Neuropsychiatric Disorders With Suspected Immune Dysregulation. *Clinical Therapeutics*, *37*(5), 984–995. doi:10.1016/j.clinthera.2015.04.002 PMID:26046241

Pham, T. A., & Lawley, T. D. (2014). Emerging insights on intestinal dysbiosis during bacterial infections. *Current Opinion in Microbiology*, *17*, 67–74. doi:10.1016/j.mib.2013.12.002 PMID:24581695

Pimentel, G. D., Micheletti, T. O., Pace, F., Rosa, J. C., Santos, R. V. T., & Lira, F. S. (2012). Gut-central nervous system axis is a target for nutritional therapies. *Nutrition Journal*, *11*(1), 22. doi:10.1186/1475-2891-11-22 PMID:22490672

Pimentel, M. (2004). A link between irritable bowel syndrome and fibromyalgia may be related to findings on lactulose breath testing. *Annals of the Rheumatic Diseases*, *63*(4), 450–452. doi:10.1136/ard.2003.011502 PMID:15020342

Pimentel, M., Soffer, E. E., Chow, E. J., Kong, Y., & Lin, H. C. (2002). Lower frequency of MMC is found in IBS subjects with abnormal lactulose breath test, suggesting bacterial overgrowth. *Digestive Diseases and Sciences*, *47*(12), 2639–2643. doi:10.1023/A:1021039032413 PMID:12498278

Pittman, N., Rawn, S. M., Wang, M., Masetto, A., Beattie, K. A., & Larché, M. (2018). Treatment of small intestinal bacterial overgrowth in systemic sclerosis: A systematic review. *Rheumatology (Oxford, England)*, *57*(10), 1802–1811. doi:10.1093/rheumatology/key175 PMID:29982822

Pituch-Zdanowska, A., Banaszkiewicz, A., & Albrecht, P. (2015). The role of dietary fibre in inflammatory bowel disease. *Przegląd Gastroenterologiczny*, *10*(3), 135–141. doi:10.5114/pg.2015.52753 PMID:26516378

Purchiaroni, F. (2013). The role of intestinal microbiota and the immune system. *European Review for Medical and Pharmacological Sciences*, *17*(3), 323–333. PMID:23426535

Qin, J., Li, R., Raes, J., Arumugam, M., Burgdorf, K. S., Manichanh, C., ... Wang, J. (2010). A human gut microbial gene catalogue established by metagenomic sequencing. *Nature*, *464*(7285), 59–65. doi:10.1038/nature08821 PMID:20203603

Quercia, S., Candela, M., Giuliani, C., Turroni, S., Luiselli, D., Rampelli, S., ... Pirazzini, C. (2014). From lifetime to evolution: Timescales of human gut microbiota adaptation. *Frontiers in Microbiology*, *5*, 587. doi:10.3389/fmicb.2014.00587 PMID:25408692

Rao, S. S. C., & Bhagatwala, J. (2019). Small Intestinal Bacterial Overgrowth: Clinical Features and Therapeutic Management. *Clinical and Translational Gastroenterology*, *10*(10), e00078. doi:10.14309/ctg.0000000000000078 PMID:31584459

Rautava, S., Luoto, R., Salminen, S., & Isolauri, E. (2012). Microbial contact during pregnancy, intestinal colonization and human disease. *Nature Reviews. Gastroenterology & Hepatology*, *9*(10), 565–576. doi:10.1038/nrgastro.2012.144 PMID:22890113

Reitsma, M., Westerhout, J., Wichers, H. J., Wortelboer, H. M., & Verhoeckx, K. C. M. (2014). Protein transport across the small intestine in food allergy. *Molecular Nutrition & Food Research*, *58*(1), 194–205. doi:10.1002/mnfr.201300204 PMID:24395537

Richarte, V., Rosales, K., Corrales, M., Bellina, M., Fadeuilhe, C., Calvo, E., ... Ramos Quiroga, J. A. (2018). El eje intestino-cerebro en el trastorno por déficit de atención/hiperactividad: Papel de la microbiota. *Revista de Neurología*, *66*(S01), S109–S114. doi:10.33588/rn.66S01.2017525 PMID:29516462

Ridker, P. M. (2016). A Test in Context: High-Sensitivity C-Reactive Protein. *Journal of the American College of Cardiology*, *67*(6), 712–723. doi:10.1016/j.jacc.2015.11.037 PMID:26868696

Rinninella, E., Cintoni, Raoul, Lopetuso, Scaldaferri, Pulcini, ... Mele. (2019). Food Components and Dietary Habits: Keys for a Healthy Gut Microbiota Composition. *Nutrients*, *11*(10), 2393. doi:10.3390/nu11102393 PMID:31591348

Rios-Covian, D., Ruas-Madiedo, P., Margolles, A., Gueimonde, M., de los Reyes-Gavilán, C. G., & Salazar, N. (2016). Intestinal Short Chain Fatty Acids and their Link with Diet and Human Health. *Frontiers in Microbiology*, *7*, 185. doi:10.3389/fmicb.2016.00185 PMID:26925050

Roncal, C., Martínez-Aguilar, E., Orbe, J., Ravassa, S., Fernandez-Montero, A., Saenz-Pipaon, G., ... Paramo, J. A. (2019). Trimethylamine-N-Oxide (TMAO) Predicts Cardiovascular Mortality in Peripheral Artery Disease. *Scientific Reports*, *9*(1), 15580. doi:10.103841598-019-52082-z PMID:31666590

Round, J. L., & Mazmanian, S. K. (2009). The gut microbiota shapes intestinal immune responses during health and disease. *Nature Reviews. Immunology*, *9*(5), 313–323. doi:10.1038/nri2515 PMID:19343057

Ruengsomwong, S., La-ongkham, O., Jiang, J., Wannissorn, B., Nakayama, J., & Nitisinprasert, S. (2016). Microbial Community of Healthy Thai Vegetarians and Non-Vegetarians, Their Core Gut Microbiota, and Pathogen Risk. *Journal of Microbiology and Biotechnology*, *26*(10), 1723–1735. doi:10.4014/jmb.1603.03057 PMID:27381339

Scher, J. U., & Abramson, S. B. (2011). The microbiome and rheumatoid arthritis. *Nature Reviews. Rheumatology*, *7*(10), 569–578. doi:10.1038/nrrheum.2011.121 PMID:21862983

Schnorr, S. L., Candela, M., Rampelli, S., Centanni, M., Consolandi, C., Basaglia, G., ... Crittenden, A. N. (2014). Gut microbiome of the Hadza hunter-gatherers. *Nature Communications*, *5*(1), 3654. doi:10.1038/ncomms4654 PMID:24736369

Schwingshackl, L., & Hoffmann, G. (2014). Mediterranean dietary pattern, inflammation and endothelial function: A systematic review and meta-analysis of intervention trials. *Nutrition, Metabolism, and Cardiovascular Diseases*, *24*(9), 929–939. doi:10.1016/j.numecd.2014.03.003 PMID:24787907

Seminario-Amez, M. (2017). Probiotics and oral health: A systematic review. *Medicina Oral, Patologia Oral y Cirugia Bucal*, *22*(3), e282–e288. PMID:28390121

Shah, A., Morrison, M., Burger, D., Martin, N., Rich, J., Jones, M., ... Holtmann, G. J. (2019). Systematic review with meta-analysis: The prevalence of small intestinal bacterial overgrowth in inflammatory bowel disease. *Alimentary Pharmacology & Therapeutics*, *49*(6), 624–635. doi:10.1111/apt.15133 PMID:30735254

Shah, A., Shanahan, E., Macdonald, G., Fletcher, L., Ghasemi, P., Morrison, M., ... Holtmann, G. (2017). Systematic Review and Meta-Analysis: Prevalence of Small Intestinal Bacterial Overgrowth in Chronic Liver Disease. *Seminars in Liver Disease*, *37*(4), 388–400. doi:10.1055-0037-1608832 PMID:29272899

Sheehan, D., Moran, C., & Shanahan, F. (2015). The microbiota in inflammatory bowel disease. *Journal of Gastroenterology*, *50*(5), 495–507. doi:10.100700535-015-1064-1 PMID:25808229

Shen, J., Zuo, Z. X., & Mao, A. P. (2014). Effect of probiotics on inducing remission and maintaining therapy in ulcerative colitis, Crohn's disease, and pouchitis: Meta-analysis of randomized controlled trials. *Inflammatory Bowel Diseases*, *20*(1), 21–35. doi:10.1097/01.MIB.0000437495.30052.be PMID:24280877

Sigthorsson, G., Tibble, J., Hayllar, J., Menzies, I., Macpherson, A., Moots, R., ... Bjarnason, I. (1998). Intestinal permeability and inflammation in patients on NSAIDs. *Gut*, *43*(4), 506–511. doi:10.1136/gut.43.4.506 PMID:9824578

Simopoulos, A. P. (2008). The importance of the omega-6/omega-3 fatty acid ratio in cardiovascular disease and other chronic diseases. *Experimental Biology and Medicine (Maywood, N.J.)*, *233*(6), 674–688. doi:10.3181/0711-MR-311 PMID:18408140

Singh, R. K., Chang, H.-W., Yan, D., Lee, K. M., Ucmak, D., Wong, K., ... Liao, W. (2017). Influence of diet on the gut microbiome and implications for human health. *Journal of Translational Medicine*, *15*(1), 73. doi:10.118612967-017-1175-y PMID:28388917

Skrovanek, S. (2014). Zinc and gastrointestinal disease. *World Journal of Gastrointestinal Pathophysiology*, *5*(4), 496–513. doi:10.4291/wjgp.v5.i4.496 PMID:25400994

Snelson, M., & Coughlan, M. T. (2019). Dietary Advanced Glycation End Products: Digestion, Metabolism and Modulation of Gut Microbial Ecology. *Nutrients*, *11*(2), 215. doi:10.3390/nu11020215 PMID:30678161

Spencer, M., Gupta, A., Dam, L. V., Shannon, C., Menees, S., & Chey, W. D. (2016). Artificial Sweeteners: A Systematic Review and Primer for Gastroenterologists. *Journal of Neurogastroenterology and Motility*, *22*(2), 168–180. doi:10.5056/jnm15206 PMID:26932837

Statovci, D., Aguilera, M., MacSharry, J., & Melgar, S. (2017). The Impact of Western Diet and Nutrients on the Microbiota and Immune Response at Mucosal Interfaces. *Frontiers in Immunology*, *8*, 838. doi:10.3389/fimmu.2017.00838 PMID:28804483

Staudacher, H. M., Lomer, M. C. E., Farquharson, F. M., Louis, P., Fava, F., Franciosi, E., ... Whelan, K. (2017). A Diet Low in FODMAPs Reduces Symptoms in Patients With Irritable Bowel Syndrome and A Probiotic Restores Bifidobacterium Species: A Randomized Controlled Trial. *Gastroenterology*, *153*(4), 936–947. doi:10.1053/j.gastro.2017.06.010 PMID:28625832

Stipanuk, M. H. c. (2013). *Biochemical, Physiological and Molecular Aspects of Human Nutrition* (3rd ed.). Elsevier.

Sturm, R. A., & Duffy, D. L. (2012). Human pigmentation genes under environmental selection. *Genome Biology*, *13*(9), 248. doi:10.1186/gb-2012-13-9-248 PMID:23110848

Suez, J., Korem, T., Zeevi, D., Zilberman-Schapira, G., Thaiss, C. A., Maza, O., ... Elinav, E. (2014). Artificial sweeteners induce glucose intolerance by altering the gut microbiota. *Nature*, *514*(7521), 181–186. doi:10.1038/nature13793 PMID:25231862

Sun, J. (2018). Dietary vitamin D, vitamin D receptor, and microbiome. *Current Opinion in Clinical Nutrition and Metabolic Care*, *21*(6), 471–474. doi:10.1097/MCO.0000000000000516 PMID:30169457

Sun, L., Ma, L., Ma, Y., Zhang, F., Zhao, C., & Nie, Y. (2018). Insights into the role of gut microbiota in obesity: Pathogenesis, mechanisms, and therapeutic perspectives. *Protein & Cell*, *9*(5), 397–403. doi:10.100713238-018-0546-3 PMID:29725936

Swiatecka, D. (2011). The study on the impact of glycated pea proteins on human intestinal bacteria. *International Journal of Food Microbiology*, *145*(1), 267–272. doi:10.1016/j.ijfoodmicro.2011.01.002 PMID:21276631

Szeligowski, T., Yun, A. L., Lennox, B. R., & Burnet, P. W. J. (2020). The Gut Microbiome and Schizophrenia: The Current State of the Field and Clinical Applications. *Frontiers in Psychiatry*, *11*, 156. doi:10.3389/fpsyt.2020.00156 PMID:32226399

Tabatabaeizadeh, S. A. (2018). Vitamin D, the gut microbiome and inflammatory bowel disease. *Journal of Research in Medical Sciences*, *23*(1), 75. doi:10.4103/jrms.JRMS_606_17 PMID:30181757

Tramontano, M., Andrejev, S., Pruteanu, M., Klünemann, M., Kuhn, M., Galardini, M., ... Patil, K. R. (2018). Nutritional preferences of human gut bacteria reveal their metabolic idiosyncrasies. *Nature Microbiology*, *3*(4), 514–522. doi:10.103841564-018-0123-9 PMID:29556107

Ungaro, R., Bernstein, C. N., Gearry, R., Hviid, A., Kolho, K.-L., Kronman, M. P., ... Atreja, A. (2014). Antibiotics associated with increased risk of new-onset Crohn's disease but not ulcerative colitis: A meta-analysis. *The American Journal of Gastroenterology*, *109*(11), 1728–1738. doi:10.1038/ajg.2014.246 PMID:25223575

Van Puyvelde, K., Mets, T., Njemini, R., Beyer, I., & Bautmans, I. (2014). Effect of advanced glycation end product intake on inflammation and aging: A systematic review. *Nutrition Reviews*, *72*(10), 638–650. doi:10.1111/nure.12141 PMID:25231200

Veronese, N., Solmi, M., Caruso, M. G., Giannelli, G., Osella, A. R., Evangelou, E., ... Tzoulaki, I. (2018). Dietary fiber and health outcomes: An umbrella review of systematic reviews and meta-analyses. *The American Journal of Clinical Nutrition*, *107*(3), 436–444. doi:10.1093/ajcn/nqx082 PMID:29566200

Vinolo, M. A., Rodrigues, H. G., Nachbar, R. T., & Curi, R. (2011). Regulation of inflammation by short chain fatty acids. *Nutrients*, *3*(10), 858–876. doi:10.3390/nu3100858 PMID:22254083

Walker, A. W., Ince, J., Duncan, S. H., Webster, L. M., Holtrop, G., Ze, X., ... Flint, H. J. (2011). Dominant and diet-responsive groups of bacteria within the human colonic microbiota. *The ISME Journal*, *5*(2), 220–230. doi:10.1038/ismej.2010.118 PMID:20686513

WHO. (2006). *Probiotics in Food - Health and nutritional properties and guidelines for evaluation*. Available from: http://www.fao.org/tempref/docrep/fao/009/a0512e/a0512e00.pdf

Wijarnpreecha, K. (2019). Obesity and Risk of Small Intestine Bacterial Overgrowth: A Systematic Review and Meta-Analysis. *Digestive Diseases and Sciences*. PMID:31605277

Wolters, M., Ahrens, J., Romaní-Pérez, M., Watkins, C., Sanz, Y., Benítez-Páez, A., ... Günther, K. (2019). Dietary fat, the gut microbiota, and metabolic health - A systematic review conducted within the MyNewGut project. *Clinical Nutrition (Edinburgh, Lothian)*, *38*(6), 2504–2520. doi:10.1016/j.clnu.2018.12.024 PMID:30655101

Wu, G. D., Chen, J., Hoffmann, C., Bittinger, K., Chen, Y.-Y., Keilbaugh, S. A., ... Lewis, J. D. (2011). Linking long-term dietary patterns with gut microbial enterotypes. *Science*, *334*(6052), 105–108. doi:10.1126cience.1208344 PMID:21885731

Yacoub, R., Nugent, M., Cai, W., Nadkarni, G. N., Chaves, L. D., Abyad, S., ... Uribarri, J. (2017). Advanced glycation end products dietary restriction effects on bacterial gut microbiota in peritoneal dialysis patients; a randomized open label controlled trial. *PLoS One*, *12*(9), e0184789. doi:10.1371/journal.pone.0184789 PMID:28931089

Yan, F., & Polk, D. B. (2011). Probiotics and immune health. *Current Opinion in Gastroenterology*, *27*(6), 496–501. doi:10.1097/MOG.0b013e32834baa4d PMID:21897224

Yatsunenko, T., Rey, F. E., Manary, M. J., Trehan, I., Dominguez-Bello, M. G., Contreras, M., ... Gordon, J. I. (2012). Human gut microbiome viewed across age and geography. *Nature*, *486*(7402), 222–227. doi:10.1038/nature11053 PMID:22699611

Zhong, C., Qu, C., Wang, B., Liang, S., & Zeng, B. (2017). Probiotics for Preventing and Treating Small Intestinal Bacterial Overgrowth: A Meta-Analysis and Systematic Review of Current Evidence. *Journal of Clinical Gastroenterology*, *51*(4), 300–311. doi:10.1097/MCG.0000000000000814 PMID:28267052

Zhong, D., Wu, C., Zeng, X., & Wang, Q. (2018). The role of gut microbiota in the pathogenesis of rheumatic diseases. *Clinical Rheumatology*, *37*(1), 25–34. doi:10.100710067-017-3821-4 PMID:28914372

Zmora, N., Suez, J., & Elinav, E. (2019). You are what you eat: Diet, health and the gut microbiota. *Nature Reviews. Gastroenterology & Hepatology*, *16*(1), 35–56. doi:10.103841575-018-0061-2 PMID:30262901

Chapter 16
Safe and Effective Galactogogues From Unani System of Medicine

Aslam Siddiqui
National Research Institute of Unani Medicine for Skin Disorders, India

Mohammad Zakir
https://orcid.org/0000-0003-3003-2292
National Research Institute of Unani Medicine for Skin Disorders, India

Munawwar Husain Kazmi
National Research Institute of Unani Medicine for Skin Disorders, India

ABSTRACT

Malnutrition is one of the major challenges for infants and children throughout the world. Breast feeding is a natural way of providing infants with the essential nutrients and is recommended as a perfect food for newborns. According to the WHO, breast feeding should be initiated within the first hour of birth and should be continued up to six months. Qilla al-Laban is a condition mentioned in Unani medicine in which breast milk production decreases or becomes scanty. It is due to the altered blood quality or quantity, Sū'-i-Mizāj and Ghalaba-i-Akhlat. Muwallid-i-Laban is an agent that promotes the secretion of milk. Synthetic drugs for augmentation of lactation have major safety concerns. Several galactogogues like Satawar, Musli safaid, etc. are being successfully prescribed by Unani physician since ancient times. This chapter describes various galactogogue mentioned in Unani system of medicine for promoting the production and secretion of milk. The dietary recommendations and drugs used to increase milk production are from natural source and chances of adverse effects are minimal.

DOI: 10.4018/978-1-7998-4808-0.ch016

1. INTRODUCTION

Malnutrition refers to deficiencies, excesses, or imbalances in a person's intake of energy and/or nutrients. It includes undernutrition (wasting, stunting and underweight), micronutrient related malnutrition (deficiency or excess of any micronutrient) and overweight, obesity and diet related non communicable diseases (diabetes, cancer etc.) As per latest data 1.9 billion Adults are overweight or obese, while 462 million are underweight all over world. Nearly 47 million children under 5 years of age are wasted, 14.3 million are severely wasted and 144 million are stunted, while 38.3 million are overweight or obese. Around 45% of deaths among children fewer than 5 years of age are linked to undernutrition (WHO, 2020). The World Health Organization (WHO) has recommended exclusive breastfeeding up to six months of age (WHO, 2007; WHO, 2009). Breast milk is complete and balance food for infants and contains antibodies for protection from many childhood ailments. It is the best source of clean and safe food for children. Breast milk provides all nutrients for overall development of the infants and these children are less prone to develop diabetes and other non communicable diseases in later life. Breast milk substitute does not provide required nutrients and energy as well as it is not clean and safe. Globally only 41% of children are exclusively breastfeed for recommended 6 month period and this trend has not changed in two decades (WHO, n.d.).

Breast milk is easy to digest and promotes adequate growth and development in infants. It contains enough water (87%) for the baby's needs of water and nutrients which are well absorbed. Breastfeeding also develops emotional and social bond of the infant with mother (Mother and Child Nutrition, 2020). Suboptimal or non exclusive breastfeeding contributes around 12% mortality in children below 5 years of age (Poshan, 2020). Children who are not breastfed exclusively for initial six months of their life are more prone to gastrointestinal infections, respiratory illness, high mortality (Ip et al., 2009; Jones et al., 2003; Kramer et al., 2003), type II diabetes (Pettitt et al., 1997), and obesity in later life (Kramer, 2010). Several research has provided strong evidence that breast feeding in human decreases the incidence of various infectious diseases (Heinig, 2001) such as bacterial meningitis (Cochi et al., 1986; Istre et al., 1985), diarrhea (Beaudry et al., 1995; Howie et al., 1990; Popkin et al., 1990), respiratory tract infection (Chulada et al., 2003; Lopez-Alarcon et al., 1997; Oddy et al., 2003) and urinary tract infection (Marild et al., 2004; Pisacane et al., 1992). Breast feeding have many beneficial or protective effect such as decreased postpartum bleeding (Chua et al., 1994), decreased menstrual blood loss (Kennedy et al., 1996), decreased risk of breast cancer (Enger et al., 1998; Lee et al., 2003; Newcomb et al., 1994; Tryggvadottir et al., 2001) and ovarian cancer in lactating mother (Rosenblatt & Thomas, 1993).

Several factors play an important role in inhibition of production of breast milk. Preterm labour, illness of mother, endocrine conditions like hypothyroidism, diabetes, and polycystic ovarian syndrome, obesity, anxiety, depression, fear and emotional stress are common causes of suppressed lactation. Galactagogues are food or drugs used to sustain the initiation, continuation, or augmentation of breast milk production. These galactagouges are prescribed to mothers who are not able to feed appropriately due to low production of milk (Abascal & Yarnell, 2008; Mathur & Dhingra, 2009).

According to the Unani system of Medicine milk, semen and blood are different fluids of the body; their composition, texture and other properties differ from each other and produced by different organs but the causes of production of these is common (Arzani, 1924; Jurjani, 2010). The main reason for deficiency of these three body fluids depends upon *Mizāj* (temperament) and *Mādda* (active substance) of whole body or *Mizāj* (temperament) of specific organ for the production of respective fluid (Kabir-al-Din, 2003; Arzani, 1924; Jurjani, 2010). *Akhlat* (humors) are fluids of the body that serve the functions of nutrition, growth and repair of the organs. The body contains four *Akhlat* (humors), *Dam* (sanguine), *Balgham* (phlegm), *Safra'* (yellow bile) and *Sawda'* (black bile). *Khilt-i-Dam* (sanguine) has hot & wet *Mizāj* (temperament), *Khilt-i-Balgham* (phlegm) cold & wet, *Khilt-i-Safra'* (yellow bile) hot & dry while *Khilt-i-Sawda'* (black bile) cold and dry temperament (Ibn Sīnā, 1411).

Sihhat is a state of the body where the *Mizāj* (temperament) of every organ is moderate in all aspects. It is essential that overall effect or combined qualities of the *Akhlat* (humors) are in accordance with the temperament of the individual for the maintenance of health. Dominance or lack of one of the *Khilt* (humor) causes derangement of the *Mizāj* (temperament) of the organ or body and leads to the deficiency or disease in the body. *Mizāj* (temperament) is a quality that is produced by action and reaction of opposite qualities of elements which are broken up in small particles in order to facilitate their mixing. When these components interact among themselves, a condition is produced, which is found in equal proportion in all the particles of the compound, this new formation is known as *Mizāj*. There are four types of *Mizāj* (temperament) i.e. *Damwi al- Mizāj* (sanguineous temperament), *Balghami al- Mizāj* (phlegmatic temperament), *Safrawi al- Mizāj* (bilious temperament) and *Sawdawi al-Mizāj* (bilious temperament). *Damwi al- Mizāj* is caused by the predominance of *Dam* (sanguine) in the body and it is hot and moist. *Balghami al- Mizāj* is caused by the predominance of *Balgham* (phlegm) in the body and it is cold and moist. *Safrawi al- Mizāj* is caused by the predominance of *Safra'* (yellow bile) in the body and it is hot and dry. *Sawdawi al- Mizāj* is caused by the predominance of *Sawda'* (black bile) in the body and it is cold and dry (Ibn Sīnā, 1411). Diet or drugs having qualities opposite to the prevailing one in the diseased organ are used as per the principle of *'Ilāj bi'l Didd* (heteropathy) e.g. while treating the diseases caused by the morbidity of hot humors, diets possessing cold temperament are used and vice versa (Ibn Sīnā, 1411). Ministry of Women and Child Development, Government of India has commenced flagship programme "POSHAN Abhiyan" to improve nutritional effects for lactating mothers along with children, adolescents and pregnant women by influencing tools, a targeted approach and convergence (Poshan, 2020). The aim of this chapter is to explore the role of Unani system of Medicine in the safe and effective management of the suppressed lactation and also to discuss the importance of natural way for the management of *Qilla al-Laban* (suppressed lactation).

2. UNANI SYSTEM OF MEDICINE AND *QILLA AL-LABAN* (SUPPRESSED LACTATION)

Qilla al-Laban (suppressed lactation) is described as the cessation or decreased secretion of milk due to various reasons. The common causes mentioned are malnutrition, anaemia, excessive evacuation of blood, intake of cold and dry food, impaired *Mizāj* (temperament) and weak *Quwwat Jādhiba* (absorptive faculty) of breasts. *Muwallid-i-Laban* (galactopoietics) is an agent which promotes the secretion of milk while *Mudirr-i-Laban* (Galactogogues) is an agent which enhances the output of milk (Al-Kirmani, 1439; Jurjani, 2010; SUMT, 2012). The management of suppressed lactation depends upon the underlying cause of the problem. *Quwwat Mudabbira-i Badan* (the power of body to maintain health) is responsible to preserve health, any reason or factor which is not suitable for body is countered by this power. If it fails it may lead to quantitative or qualitative disturbance or derangement in equilibrium of *Akhlat* (humors) in the body (Ibn Sīnā, 1411). These abnormal humors disturb normal physiology or in some cases changes in anatomy of the organs. This leads to emergence of disease in Human beings. To overcome derangement and to help *Quwwat Mudabbira-i Badan* four types of interventions are used in

Unani Medicine. These are *'Ilāj bi'l Tadbīr* (Regimenal Therapy), *'Ilaj bi'l Ghizā* (Dietotherapy), *'Ilāj bi'd-Dawā* (Drug therapy) and *'Ilāj bi'l Yad* (Surgical treatment) (al-Kirmani, 1439).

3. ETIOPATHOGENESIS OF *QILLA AL-LABAN* (SUPPRESSED LACTATION)

3.1 Qillat-i-Dam (Deficiency of the Blood)

In this condition the quantity of blood decreases in the body due to various reasons like, heavy menstrual bleeding, epistaxis, *fasd* (venesection), and diarrhoea (Kabir-al-Din, 2003; al-Kirmani, 1439; Arzani, 1992; Baghdadi, 2004). It may also be caused by *Sū'-i-Mizāj* (impaired temperament) of the whole body or *Sū'-i-Mizāj* (impaired temperament) of breast alone. Intake of low quantity or low quality (less nutritious) diet produces inadequate quantity of low quality blood (Kabir-al-Din, 2003; Al-Kirmani, 1439; Arzani, 1924; Arzani, 1992; Baghdadi, 2004; Jurjani, 2010). Sometimes lack of milk is due to excess quantity of blood in the body (Kabir-al-Din, 2003; Arzani, 1992). The nutritional requirement of breast impeded due to deficiency of blood and production of milk decreases in quantity.

3.2 Ghalba-i-Akhlat (Humoral Preponderance)

Predominance of *Akhlāt* (humors) is the main cause of any deficiency or disease condition in the body as per Unani concept. One or more *Akhlāt* (humors) like *Safra'* (yellow bile), *Balgham* (phlegm) and *Sawda'* (black bile) exceeds in its normal volume and become dominant or it becomes deranged. This leads to disturbance in homeostasis of the normal constitution of blood (Al-Kirmani, 1439; Arzani, 1924; Arzani, 1992). Some times *Mizāj* (temperament) of the body or breast may be altered due to *Istifrāgh* (temperamental alteration) of other organ or *Waram al-Damwī* (sanguineous inflammation) in an organ of the body (Al-Kirmani, 1439; Arzani, 1992; Jurjani, 2010). Predominance of *Safra'* (yellow bile), *Balgham* (phlegm) and *Sawda'* (black bile) alone or predominance of *Safra'* (yellow bile) and *Balgham* (phlegm) is responsible for suppressed lactation.

3.3 Sign of Ghalba-i-Akhlat

Specific signs appear when a *Khlit* (humor) become predominant in blood and body. These specific signs help physician to find out particular humour involved in this condition. If *Safra'* (yellow bile) is dominant then milk become light orange in colour, its consistency become thin and have sharp smell and taste. In case of dominance of *Balgham* (phlegm), the milk will be whiter; consistency will be thin like water and trashy or acidic in the taste. Dominance of *Sawda'* (black bile) produces very thick milk in small quantity (Al-Kirmani, 1439; Arzani, 1924; Arzani, 1992; Jurjani, 2010).

3.4 General causes

Apart from specific causes mentioned in Unani literature as per fundamental principles some other factors are also responsible for suppressed lactation. Psychological factors affects overall health in general but also affects milk production and secretion specifically. Presence of dolor, bereavement, anxiety, depression and anger are main causes for this condition (Kabir-al-Din, 2003; Al-Kirmani, 1439; Jurjani, 2010). Life style of the person also play important role in this condition. Excessive sexual activities like excessive sexual intercourse during lactation have adverse effect on production of milk. Prolonged sitting near source of heat for long time also affect milk production as well as milk secretion (Al-Kirmani, 1439).

4. MANAGEMENT OF QILLA AL-LABAN (SUPPRESSED LACTATION)

The management of suppressed lactation require comprehensive intervention based on the underlying cause of the problem. Major causes like humoral preponderance or anaemia may be clearly established before starting any treatment or intervention. Sometimes only diet can cure this problem so major emphasis is given to adopt proper diet along with other interventions like exercise and proper counselling for various psychological factors. In most of the cases modification in diet and proper counselling is enough to cure this problem. The management as per Unani concept is inclusive and based on underlying causes; management of whole body by providing proper nutrition and removing other associated factors are the key factors.

As per Unani concept agents which augments production of semen also enhance production of milk e.g. Toodri (seeds of *Cheiranthus cheiri L.*), Tukhm Khashkhas (seeds of *Papaver somniferum* L.) and breast meat of sheep and goat (Kabir-al-Din, 2003; Arzani, 1924; Arzani, 1992; Baghdadi, 2004; Jurjani, 2010). *Ta'dīl-i-Mizāj* (moderation of temperament) by appropriate *Ghizā* (diet) and *Dawā* (drug) has required if *Sū'-i-Mizāj* (impaired temperament) is the cause of the problem. If involvement of *Khilt* (humour) is there then it may be evacuated by proper dugs as per *Mizāj* (temperament) of the *Khilt* (humour) (Kabir-al-Din, 2003; Arzani, 1992; Baghdadi, 2004; Jurjani, 2010). Primary aim of management is to remove or correct the underlying cause of the problem. If incomplete or insufficient diet is the reason then balanced and nutritious diet should be taken to improve production of the healthy blood. In case of *Ghalaba-i-Akhlat* try to remove the excess *Khilt* (humor) from the body and use the diet or drug opposite the *Mizāj* (temperament) of humour (Al-Kirmani, 1439; Jurjani, 2010). Use *Hārr Ratb Ghizā* (Hot and moist diet) like rice with milk, chick meat, hen's egg, milk with honey and fresh fish etc. (Kabir-al-Din, 2003). These intervention not only strengthen breast but overall health of the person improves because the drugs used here also improve other functions by giving nutrition as well as by correcting predominance of certain *Khilt* (humour).

4.1 Common Management

If the underlying cause of the problem is not clear and exact etiology is not established then some common treatment prescription can be adopted as per need. These prescriptions can be chosen as per patient's condition and *Mizāj* (temperament). Some prescriptions are given bellow and can be used as per requirement and condition of the patients taking consideration of her *Mizāj* (temperament). Some important prescriptions mentioned in literature are given here for reference.

Take Nishashta Gandum (starch of *Triticum sativum* L.) 24 gm mix it with 250 ml milk after that add Biranj (*Embelia ribes* Burm. F), Badam (almond), Panbadana (*Gossypium herbaceum* L.), Khaskdana (seeds of *Carthamus tinctorium* L.), Maghz Chilgoza (kernel of *Pinus gerardiana* Wall.) 12 gm each, Badiyan (*Foeniculum vulgare* Gaertn), Heel Khurd (*Elettaria cardamomum* Maton.) 7 gm each, Tukhm Shibbat (*Anethum sowa* L.) 6 gm, Toodri (seeds of *Cheiranthus cheiri* L.) 12 gm and sugar 10 gm, boil it and consume when cooled (Kabir-al-Din, 2003). It will improve overall health by providing nutrition as well as it has some drugs which also increase production of milk.

Another prescription is as follow and contains drugs which have *Mudirr* (diuretic) activities therefore these drugs increases the secretion of milk from the breast. Make a fine powder of drugs i.e. Tukhm Rehan (*Ocimum basilicum* L.), Tukhm Badruj (*Ocimum americanum* L.), Toodri (*Cheiranthus cheiri L.*), Shaqaqul (*Asparagus adscendens* Roxb.), Tukhm Gazar (seeds of *Daucus carota* L.), Maghz Tukhm Kaddu Shireen (kernel of seeds of *Cucurbita maxima* Duch), Maghz Tukhm Hindudana (kernel of seeds of *Citrullus vulgaris* Schrad.) and Tukhm Kharpazah (seeds of *Cucumis melo* L.), 12 gm each, and consume 18 gm daily with milk (Kabir-al-Din, 2003).

Tukhm Halyun (seeds of *Asparagus officinalis* L.) can be used either in powder form or as Joshanda (decoction). For this purpose take 10 gm Tukhm Halyun, boil it in water and add sugar in equal amount and consume It may be used as fine powder after grinding with equal amount of sugar, 7 gm powder may be used with milk (Kabir-al-Din, 2003). *Halwā* (semisolid preparation) is a special nutritious preparation of the Unani system and recommended in weakness of the body or certain organs. It is prepared by nutritious drugs like chickpea, Tukhm Gazar (seeds of *Daucus carota* L. and sugar) etc. and can be used to increase production of milk. *Halwā Bayda-i-Murgh* (semisolid preparation) is made up of eggs and sugar which may be used. Toodri (seeds of *Cheiranthus cheiri L.*) 4 gm with 250 ml milk is very useful to increase milk production (Kabir-al-Din, 2003).

Apart from drugs and diet other associated factors should be dealt with appropriate methods such as life style change, counselling in case of anxiety and depression and other mental conditions. Heavy work or heavy exercise should be avoided during lactation period (Kabir-al-Din, 2003; Jurjani, 2010). Limit sexual activities, avoid frequent intercourse and avoid long sitting near constant heat or source of heat (Al-Kirmani, 1439). Psychological counselling should be done to remove bereavement, anxiety and depression. Some drugs are also mentioned in Unani literature as *Mufarrih-i-Qalb* (exhilarant and mood elevator) and can be used; balance diets & appropriate drugs should be used (Kabir-al-Din, 2003; Al-Kirmani, 1439; Jurjani, 2010).

4.2 Predominance of *Safra'* (Yellow Bile) and its Management

There are four types of *Khilt* (humour) in the body and present in a definite equilibrium state. If a *Khilt* (humour) become predominant then the equilibrium got disturbed and disease process started. *Khilt-i-Safra'* (yellow bile) is one of the four basic humours. It is yellow in colour and has hot and dry temperament. Its predominance is one of the causes of suppressed lactation. It can be corrected by diet and drugs which are described in literature. For the management of predominance of *Safra'* (yellow bile) following intervention may be adopted.

Mā' al-Sha'īr (barley water), baby goat meat or baby sheep meat is recommended to consume as a diet (Al-Kirmani, 1439; Arzani, 1924; Jurjani, 2010). Sour food items like Alu Bukhara (*Prunus domestica* L.), Anar (*Punica granatum* L.) and Lemu (*Citrus aurantifolia* Christm.) may be taken (Al-Kirmani, 1439; Arzani, 1924; Baghdadi, 2004). Maghz Tukhm Khayaren (kernel of seeds of *Cucumis sativus* L. & *Cucumis utilissimus* Roxb.) Maghz Tukhm Kaddu (kernel of seeds of *Cucurbita maxima* Duch.) and goat meat cooked with Palak (*Spinacia oleracea* L.) may be used. *Harira* (curry) prepared with milk, dry fruits and Jao (*Hordeum vulgare* L.) is effective. *Harira* (curry) is a liquid preparation which is recommended in general debility and in convalescent period to improve immunity and health (Arzani, 1924; Jurjani, 2010). The baby goat meat, fish, and curry made up of *Āsh-i-Jav* (barley water) with Khubbazi

(*Malva sylvestris* L.) and Bathwa (*Chenopodium album* L.) may be consumed. Bone marrow of goat or sheep and goat milk in diet is advisable (Arzani, 1924; Baghdadi, 2004). *Mā' al-Sha'īr* (barley water) with *Sharbat Nilofar* (syrup) is suggested. Tukhm Kaddu (kernel of seeds of *Cucurbita maxima* Duch.), Tukhm Khurfa (*Portulaca oleracea* L.), juice from seeds of *Punica granatum* L., *Sikanjabīn sada* (liquid preparation made with water and vinegar) and intake of other sour diet are useful (Kabir-al-Din, 2003). It is advised to consume diet like Chicks cooked with raw grapes water, Kaddu (*Cucurbita maxima* Duch.) and Kahu (*Lactuca serriola* L.) (Kabir-al-Din, 2003; Arzani, 1924). It is advised to refrain from heavy exercise and heavy physical work as well as mental work (Arzani, 1924; Baghdadi, 2004).

4.3 Predominance of *Balgham* (Phlegm) and its Management

Khilt Balgham (phlegm) is another humour which is white in colour and has cold and wet temperament. Its predominance may also causes suppression of lactation. It can be accurated by various diets and drugs described in literature. For the management of predominance of *Balgham* (phlegm) following intervention may be adopted.

Spicy broth/curry containing Tukhm Gazar (seeds of *Daucus carota* L.) and Badiyan (*Foeniculum vulgare* Gaertn.) is effective (Kabir-al-Din, 2003; Arzani, 1924; Baghdadi, 2004; Jurjani, 2010). Broth/ curry with almond oil, chicken meat, breast of sheep is also advised (Al-Kirmani, 1439). Curry prepared with wheat flour, Methi (*Trigonella foenum-graecum* L.) and Badiyan (*Foeniculum vulgare* Gaertn) is also useful. Karafs (*Apium graveolens* L.), Pudina (*Mentha arvensis* L.) and Badiyan (*Foeniculum vulgare* Gaertn) may be used alone or in combination. Roasted diet, meat of Teeter (*Grey Partridge*), Bater (*Grey francolin*) and diet like *Sakbaaz* (curry prepared in vinegar) and *Zerbaaz* (curry prepared in vinegar with meat and cloves) may be taken (Baghdadi, 2004).

4.4 Predominance of *Balgham* (Phlegm) and *Sawda* (Black Bile) and its Management

Khilt-i-Sawda' (black bile) is fourth humour and black in colour and has cold and dry temperament. When predominance of *Balgham* (phlegm) and *Sawda'* (black bile) occurs simultaneously then management become difficult and drugs having corrective qualities for both humours have to be used for rectification of dominance of both. The intervention including diet and drugs used for management of this condition are given here.

The diet should include Tukhm Gazar (*Daucus carota* L.), Badiyan (*Foeniculum vulgare* Gaertn), Soya (*Anethum sowa* L.) and Ajmud (*Apium graveolens* L.). *Harira* (curry) prepared with milk, dry fruits, wheat flour, *Methi* (*Trigonella foenum-graecum* L.), Badiyan (*Foeniculum vulgare* Gaertn.) and honey is recommended (Kabir-al-Din, 2003; Arzani, 1924; Jurjani, 2010). Local application of *Tila* (liniment) made up of Banafsha (*Viola odorata* L.), Khatmi (*Altheae officinalis* L.) and *Jao* (*Hordeum vulgare* L.) on breast and chest is advised (Arzani, 1924; Jurjani, 2010). Take Gandum (*Triticum sativum* L.), 108 gm, Jao (*Hordeum vulgare* L.) 72 gm, Nakhud (*Cicer arietinum* L.) 72 gm, Berg Soya (leaves of *Anethum sowa* L.) 28 gm, Anjeer khushk (dry *Ficus carica* L.) 10 numbers and Toodri (seeds of *Cheiranthus cheiri L.*) 36 gm mix all and make rough powder. Take 72 gm of this rough powder and soak in water overnight, in the morning take decoction of it with 375 ml milk (Jurjani, 2010).

One prescription is Tukhm Gazar (seeds of *Daucus carota* L.), Tukhm Piyaz (seeds of *Allium cepa* L.), Tukhm Shalgham (seeds of *Brassica napus* L.), Tukhm Muli (seeds of *Raphanus sativus* L.), Tukhm

Badiyan (seeds of *Foeniculum vulgare* Gaertn.) one part each, add equal amount of all seeds with roasted flour of Nakhud (*Cicer arietinum* L.) consume 17 gm with milk in the morning daily. Another prescription is Tukhm Kaddu (seeds of *Cucurbita maxima* Duch.), Tukhm Shalgham (seeds of *Brassica napus* L.), Tukhm Soya (seeds of *Anethum sowa* L.), Tukhm Muli (seeds of *Raphanus sativus* L.), Tukhm Badiyan (seeds of *Foeniculum vulgare* Gaertn.) in equal quantity add equal amount of all seeds with roasted flour of Nakhud (*Cicer arietinum* L.) consume 17 gm with milk in the morning daily. One more important prescription includes Tukhm Gandana (*Alium ampeloprasum* L.), Tukhm Soya (seeds of *Anethum sowa* L.), Tukhm Methi (*Trigonella foenum-graecum* L.), Toodri (*Cheiranthus cheiri L.*) and Berg Badiyan (leaves of *Foeniculum vulgare* Gaertn.) 10 gm each, boil in water and filter it add 100 gm honey and 36 gm ghee (clarified butter) and mixed bread in it and consume (Jurjani, 2010).

Take cow ghee (clarified butter) 36 gm and mix it with wine (one cup) and consume. Mix *Roghan Badam* (oil of *Prunus amygdalus* Batsch.) 17 gm and sugar 72 and serve as decoction. Mix flour of Kunjud (*Sesamum indicum* L.) with wine and stir well, decant the wine and drink it while remaining matter may be applied on breast and chest locally. Increase the consumption of liquid diet having more water contents (Jurjani, 2010).

4.5 Predominance of *Sawdā* (Black Bile) and its Management

Predominance of *Khilt-i-Sawda'* (black bile) alone can be the cause of suppressed lactation. It is difficult to treat the conditions where black bile involves. The treatment takes time and not easy to manage. The intervention includes diet and drugs specifically mentioned for management of *Sawda'* (black bile) and some treatment are given bellow.

Harira (curry) prepared with milk, Gandum (*Triticum sativum* L.), Nakhud (*Cicer arietinum* L.) Jao (*Hordeum vulgare* L.) and Anjeer (*Ficus carica* L.) with *Roghan Badam* (almond oil) may be taken (Kabir-al-Din, 2003). *Halwā* (semisolid preparation) by maida flour, chickpea flour and *Baqla flour* (*Vicia faba* L.) equal part and flour of Badam (*Prunus amygdalus* Batsch.) one fourth part, *Badiyan* (*Foeniculum vulgare* Gaertn), Soya (seeds of *Anethum sowa* L.) and Halun (*Eruca sativa* L.) in sufficient quantity and sugar is effective. You may take this prescription also, take Crushed Khurma (*Phoenix dactylifera* L.), crushed wheat, crushed Jao (*Hordeum vulgare* L.), crushed chickpea 100 gm each, crushed Tukhm Ratba (*Trifolium alexandrinum* L.) 70 gm, Anjeer (*Ficus carica* L.) 10 Nos., Til (*Sesamum indicum* L.) 35 gm and Methi (*Trigonella foenum-graecum* L.) and boil it with water and consume 175 gm of it by adding 35 gm sugar and 35 gm almond oil (Baghdadi, 2004).

Some other formulation may be taken i.e. take Tukhm Ratba (*Trifolium alexandrinum* L.), Tukhm Gazar (seeds of *Daucus carota* L.), Halyun (*Asparagus officinalis* L.), Methi (*Trigonella foenum-graecum* L.) and Til (*Sesamum indicum* L.) in equal quantity and boil with juice of fennel and consume with honey and clarified butter. Another prescription is Wheat flour, barley flour, *Baqla flour* (*Vicia faba* L.), chickpea flour 35 gm each, Tukhm Piyaz (seeds of *Allium cepa* L.), Tukhm Shalgham (seeds of *Brassica napus* L.), Halyun (*Asparagus officinalis* L.), Tukhm Ratba (*Trifolium alexandrinum* L.) and Maghz Chilgoza (*Pinus gerardiana* Wall.) 10 gm each, Badiyan (*Foeniculum vulgare* Gaertn), Soya (*Anethum sowa* L.) 12 gm each, Bozidan (*Pyrethrum indicum* L.) 7 gm, make fine powder and consume 17 gm with milk.

Chickpea soaked in milk overnight when used in the morning is useful to increase production of milk. Pulverize wheat and chickpea in milk and cook with goat meat and mix Badiyan (*Foeniculum vulgare* Gaertn) and consume (Baghdadi, 2004). Meat of chick & healthy chicken may be used. Body massage with appropriate oil is effective. *Tila* (liniment) of *Roghan Banafsha* (oil of *Viola odorata* L.) and *Roghan Badam* (oil of *Prunus amygdalus* Batsch) on breast is also recommended (Kabir-al-Din, 2003).

4.6 Deficiency of blood (Anaemia) and its Management

Deficiency of blood is also a very common cause of suppressed lactation usually in under nutrition population. It may be manage by nutritious diet and other drugs if needed. In Unani system the nutrition by diet as well as by some drug is described in detail. Some of the diets and drugs recommended are mentioned here.

Nutritious diet like eggs, butter, etc. may be taken along with some drugs (Al-Kirmani, 1439; Arzani, 1992). Powder of Toodri Surkh (*Cheiranthus cheiri L.*) 12 gm, Satawar (*Asparagus racemosus* Willd.) 10 gm, sugar 10 gm can be used with milk twice daily (Kabir-al-Din, 2003; Al-Kirmani, 1439). Fine powder of Satawar (*Asparagus racemosus* Willd.), Badiyan (*Foeniculum vulgare* Gaertn) and Zeera Safaid (*Cuminum cyminum* L.) in equal quantity may be used in dose of 7gm with sugar. Powder of Satawar (*Asparagus racemosus* Willd.) 10 gm and Zeera Safaid (*Cuminum cyminum* L.) 10 gm with sugar 10 gm can also be used in a dose of 6gm powder twice daily with milk. This prescription can be used, take Tukhm Gazar (seeds of *Daucus carota* L.), Tukhm Shalgham (seeds of *Brassica napus* L.), Tukhm Muli (seeds of *Raphanus sativus* L.), Tukhm Badiyan (*Foeniculum vulgare* Gaertn) in equal quantity add roasted gram equal to all of them and make fine powder. Consume 17 gm in the morning after adding sugar (Popkin et al., 1990). Massage of *Roghan Bed-i-Anjeer* (castor oil obtained from *Ricinus communis* L.) on breast is also useful (Al-Kirmani, 1439).

4.7 Diet and Life Style Changes

Balance diet and healthy life style plays positive effects on health. It is recommended to follow certain instructions to avoid suppressed lactation as well as to treat it. It is advised to remove bereavement, anxiety and depression by using various methods like storytelling, sports and other activities and by *Mufarrih-i-Qalb* (exhilarant and mood elevator) diets & drugs or psychological counselling. Proper rest, adequate sleep should be taken and heavy exercise and heavy physical work should be avoided. *Latīf Zud Hadm Muqawwi Ghidhā'* (easily digestible & high nutritious diet) is recommended (Kabir-al-Din, 2003; Al-Kirmani, 1439; Arzani, 1992). *Muqawwi Ghidhā'* (high nutritious diet) should be taken in under nutrition persons, where deficiency of blood is the cause of the problem (Kabir-al-Din, 2003; Al-Kirmani, 1439; Jurjani, 2010).

4.8 Single Drugs Used for *Qilla Al-Laban* (Suppressed Lactation)

Various single drugs summarizes in Table-1 have been used to treat suppressed lactation and produce their action directly or indirectly. These drugs provide nutrition to the body or induce galactopoietics, spermatogenic, diuretic and adipogenous actions etc. These drugs are obtained from natural sources, mostly from plants; because of this they do not have any severe adverse effects.

Table 1. Single drugs used in Qilla al-Laban (suppressed lactation) and their pharmacological actions as per Unani System of Medicine

Unani name	Botanical Name	Unani pharmacological actions
Anjeer	*Ficus carica* L.	*Mudirr-i-Bawl* (Diuretic), *Kasīr al-Taghdhiya* (high caloric diet) (Kabir-al-Din, 2007; Ghani, 2011; Khare, 2007)
Badam	*Prunus amygdalus* Batsch.	*Muwallid-i-Mani* (spermatogenic), *Muqawwi-i-Bah* (aphrodisiac) (Kabir-al-Din, 2007; Ghani, 2011; Khare, 2007)
Badiyan	*Foeniculum vulgare* Gaertn.	*Muwallid-i-Laban* (galactopoietics), *Mudirr-i-Bawl* (diuretic), *Mudirr-i-Hayd* (emmenogogue) (Kabir-al-Din, 2007; Ghani, 2011; Khare, 2007)
Gandum	*Triticum sativum* L.	*Musammin-i-Badan* (adipogenous) (Kabir-al-Din, 2007; Ghani, 2011; Khare, 2007)
Halun	*Eruca sativa* L.	*Mudirr-i-Bawl* (diuretic), *Mudirr-i-Hayd* (emmenogogue), *Muqawwi-i-Bah* (aphrodisiac) (Ghani, 2011; Khare, 2007)
Khaskdana	*Carthamus tinctorium* L.	*Muqawwi-i-Bah* (aphrodisiac), *Muwallid-i-Mani* (spermatogenic), *Mudirr-i-Hayd* (emmenogogue)(Kabir-al-Din, 2007; Khare, 2007)
Khurma	*Phoenix dactylifera* L.	*Muwallid-i-Mani* (spermatogenic), *Musammin-i-Badan* (adipogenous) (Kabir-al-Din, 2007; Ghani, 2011; Khare, 2007)
Kunjud	*Sesamum indicum* L.	*Muqawwi-i-Bah* (aphrodisiac), *Musammin-i-Badan* (adipogenous) (Ghani, 2011; Khare, 2007)
Maghz Chilgoza	*Pinus gerardiana* Wall.	*Muwallid-i-Mani* (spermatogenic), *Musammin-i-Badan* (adipogenous) (Kabir-al-Din, 2007; Ghani, 2011; Khare, 2007)
Maghz Tukhm Kaddu	*Cucurbita maxima* Duch.	*Mudirr-i-Bawl* (diuretic), *Musammin-i-Badan* (adipogenous) (Kabir-al-Din, 2007; Ghani, 2011; Khare, 2007)
Nakhud/Chana	*Cicer arietinum* L	*Muqawwi-i-Bah* (aphrodisiac), *Mudirr-i-Bawl* (diuretic) (Kabir-al-Din, 2007; Ghani, 2011; Khare, 2007)
Nishashta Gandum	starch of *Triticum sativum* L.	*Musammin-i-Badan* (adipogenous) (Kabir-al-Din, 2007; Ghani, 2011; Khare, 2007)
Panbadana	*Gossypium herbaceum* L.	*Muwallid-i-Mani* (spermatogenic), *Muwallid-i-Laban* (galactopoietics), *Musammin-i-Badan* (adipogenous) (Kabir-al-Din, 2007; Ghani, 2011; Khare, 2007)
Satawar	*Asparagus racemosus* Willd.	*Mughalliz-i-Mani* (increases the viscosity of the semen) (Ghani, 2011; Khare, 2007)
Toodri Surkh	*Cheiranthus cheiri L.*	*Muwallid-i-Laban* (galactopoietics), *Muwallid-i-Mani* (spermatogenic), *Musammin-i-Badan* (adipogenous) (Kabir-al-Din, 2007; Ghani, 2011; Khare, 2007)
Tukhm Gazar	*Daucus carota* L.	*Mudirr-i-Bawl* (diuretic), *Muqawwi-i-Bah* (aphrodisiac) (Kabir-al-Din, 2007; Ghani, 2011; Khare, 2007)
Tukhm Gandana	*Alium ampeloprasum* L.	*Mudirr-i-Bawl* (diuretic), *Mudirr-i-Hayd* (emmenogogue), *Muqawwi-i-Bah* (aphrodisiac) (Kabir-al-Din, 2007; Ghani, 2011; Khare, 2007)
Tukhm Halyun	*Asparagus officinalis* L.	*Mudirr-i-Bawl* (diuretic), *Mudirr-i-Hayd* (emmenogogue) *Muwallid-i-Mani* (spermatogenic), *Muqawwi-i-Bah* (aphrodisiac) (Ghani, 2011; Khare, 2007)
Tukhm Khashkhas Safaid	*Papaver somniferum* L.	*Musammin-i-Badan* (adipogenous), *Musakkin* (neutralizing the heat) (Ghani, 2011; Khare, 2007)
Tukhm Hulba	*Trigonella foenum-graecum* L.	*Muqawwi-i-A'sab (nervine tonic), Mudirr-i-Hayd* (emmenogogue) (Kabir-al-Din, 2007; Ghani, 2011; Khare, 2007)
Tukhm Piyaz	*Allium cepa* L.	*Muqawwi-i-Bah* (aphrodisiac) (Kabir-al-Din, 2007; Ghani, 2011)
Musli Safaid	*Chlorophytum arundinaceum* Baker.	*Muwallid-i-Mani* (spermatogenic),, *Mughalliz-i-Mani* (increases the viscosity of the semen) (Kabir-al-Din, 2007; Ghani, 2011; Khare, 2007)
Musli Siyah	*Curculigo orchioides* Gaertn.	*Muwallid-i-Mani* (spermatogenic),, *Mughalliz-i-Mani* (increases the viscosity of the semen) (Kabir-al-Din, 2007; Ghani, 2011; Khare, 2007)

4.9 Compound Formulations Used for *Qilla Al-Laban* (Suppressed Lactation)

Different compound formulations have also been described in Unani literature that can be used as readymade medicine to improve milk production. These formulation have several other indications and generally used as immunity booster and to improve overall function of the body Table-2.

Table 2. Compound formulations used in Qilla al-Laban (suppressed lactation)

S. No	Name of Compound Formulation	Form/Reference
1.	*Habb-i-Ambar, Habb-i-Jadwar, Habb-i-Jawahir, Habb-i-Qawi, Habb-i-Zahab, Nuqrai and Qurs-e-Luboob.*	Tablet (NFUM, 2006a; NFUM, 2006b; NFUM, 2007; NFUM, 2011)
2.	*Halwa-i-Baiza-i-Murgh, Halwa-i-Gazar, Halwa-i-Badam, Halwa-i-Musammin, Halwa-i-Salab, Halwa-i-Supari Pak, Halwa Gheekwar, Luboob Kabir, Luboob Saghir, Laboob Kabir Khas, Majoon-i-Aarad Khurma, Majoon-i-Sala'b, Majoon-i-Luluvi, Majoon-i-Regmahi, Majun Murawweh ul Arwah, Majun Piyaz, Majun Punba Dana, Jawarish-i-Jalinoos, Shababi* and *Zehbi.*	Semisolid form (NFUM, 2007; NFUM, 2008; NFUM, 2011)
3.	*Jauhar-i-Nuqra, Jawahir Mohra, Kushta-i-Biaza-i-Murgh* and *Kushta Nuqra*	Microfine powder (NFUM, 2006a; NFUM, 2007; NFUM, 2008)
4.	*Ma'ullaham Khaas*	Distillate (NFUM, 2011)

5. CONCLUSION

As per Unani philosophy diet is given prime importance in both health and disease conditions. The management of any disease should be started with diet and most suitable diet for each *Mizāj* (temperament) is defined meticulously in Unani literature. The Unani system of Medicine diagnoses and treats the patients as a whole looking into their overall physical, mental and spiritual aspects. The basic fundamentals, diagnosis and treatment procedures of the system are based on scientific principles and holistic concepts of health and healing. The combination therapy having more than one drug is based on fundamentals and expertise of the physician in accordance with underlying cause of the disease. The *Mizāj* (temperament) have great importance in diagnosis and treatment and played a vital role in selection of suitable diet or drugs for effective management of a particular disease. The management of *Qilla al-Laban* (suppressed lactation) discussed in this chapter has shown that drugs from natural source can be used for effective and safe management. The use of chemical base drugs have safety concerns and should not be used in this condition as the transmission of chemical to the infant can cause adverse effect in breastfed infant and will affect over all development of the child. The use of natural drugs and diet recommended by Unani can overcome the safety concern and will be helpful to manage this condition effectively.

ACKNOWLEDGMENT

Authors are thankful to Director General, Central Council for Research in Unani Medicines (CCRUM), Ministry of AYUSH, Government of India, New Delhi for all facilities and support.

REFERENCES

Abascal, K., & Yarnell, E. (2008). Botanical galactagogues. *Alternative and Complementary Therapies*, *14*(6), 288–294. doi:10.1089/act.2008.14602

al-Din, K., (2003). *Al-Iksir, vol-II*. New Delhi, India: Aijaz Publishing House.

al-Din, K., (2007). *Ilmul Adviya Nafisi*. New Delhi, India: Aijaz Publishing House.

Al-Kirmani. (1439). *Sharh al-Asbab wa'l 'Alamat* (vols. 3-4). New Delhi, India: Aijaz Publishing House.

Arzani, H.M.A. (1924). *Tibb-i Akbar*. Deoband, India: Faisal Publishers.

Arzani, H.M.A. (1992). *Meezan al-Tib*. New Delhi, India: National Council for promotion of Urdu language.

Baghdadi, A.H. (2004). *Kitab al-Mukhtarat fi'l Tibb Vol. III*. New Delhi, India: Central Council for Research in Unani Medicine.

Beaudry, M., Dufour, R., & Marcoux, S. (1995). Relation between infant feeding and infections during the first six months of life. *The Journal of Pediatrics*, *126*(2), 191–197. doi:10.1016/S0022-3476(95)70544-9 PMID:7844664

Chua, S., Arulkumaran, S., Lim, I., Selamat, N., & Ratnam, S. S. (1994). Influence of breastfeeding and nipple stimulation on postpartum uterine activity. *British Journal of Obstetrics and Gynaecology*, *101*(9), 804–805. doi:10.1111/j.1471-0528.1994.tb11950.x PMID:7947531

Chulada, P. C., Arbes, S. J. Jr, Dunson, D., & Zeldin, D. C. (2003). Breast-feeding and the prevalence of asthma and wheeze in children: Analyses from the Third National Health and Nutrition Examination Survey, 1988 –1994. *The Journal of Allergy and Clinical Immunology*, *111*(2), 328–336. doi:10.1067/mai.2003.127 PMID:12589353

Cochi, S. L., Fleming, D. W., Hightower, A. W., Limpakarnjanarat, K., Facklam, R. R., David Smith, J., ... Broome, C. V. (1986). Primary invasive Haemophilus influenzae type b disease: A population-based assessment of risk factors. *The Journal of Pediatrics*, *108*(6), 887–896. doi:10.1016/S0022-3476(86)80922-2 PMID:3712153

Enger, S. M., Ross, R. K., Paganini-Hill, A., & Bernstein, L. (1998). Breastfeeding experience and breast cancer risk among postmenopausal women. *Cancer Epidemiology, Biomarkers & Prevention*, *7*, 365–369. PMID:9610784

Ghani, N. (2011). *Khazainul Advia*. New Delhi, India: Idara Kitabul Shifa.

Heinig, M. J. (2001). Host defense benefits of breastfeeding for the infant. Effect of breastfeeding duration and exclusivity. *Pediatric Clinics of North America*, *48*(1), 105–123. doi:10.1016/S0031-3955(05)70288-1 PMID:11236719

Howie, P. W., Forsyth, J. S., Ogston, S. A., Clark, A., & Florey, C. D. (1990). Protective effect of breast feeding against infection. *BMJ (Clinical Research Ed.)*, *300*(6716), 11–16. doi:10.1136/bmj.300.6716.11 PMID:2105113

Ibn Sīnā. (1990). *Al-Qānūn fi'l Tibb*. New Delhi, India: Idara Kitabul Shifa.

Ip, S., Chung, M., Raman, G., Trikalinos, T.A., & Lau, J. (2009). A summary of the agency for healthcare research and quality's evidence report on breastfeeding in developed countries. *Breastfeeding Medicine*, *4*(S1), S17–30.

Istre, G. R., Conner, J. S., Broome, C. V., Hightower, A., & Hopkins, R. S. (1985). Risk factors for primary invasive Haemophilus influenzae disease: Increased risk from day care attendance and school-aged household members. *The Journal of Pediatrics*, *106*(2), 190–195. doi:10.1016/S0022-3476(85)80285-7 PMID:3871478

Jones, G., Steketee, R. W., Black, R. E., Bhutta, Z. A., & Morris, S. S. (2003). How many child deaths can we prevent this year. *Lancet*, *362*(9377), 65–71. doi:10.1016/S0140-6736(03)13811-1 PMID:12853204

Jurjani, S. (2010). *Zakhira Khawarizm Shahi*. New Delhi, India: Idara Kitabul Shifa.

Kennedy, K. I., Labbok, M. H., & Van Look, P. F. (1996). Lactational amenorrhea method for family planning. *International Journal of Gynaecology and Obstetrics: the Official Organ of the International Federation of Gynaecology and Obstetrics*, *54*(1), 55–57. doi:10.1016/0020-7292(96)02670-7 PMID:8842819

Khare, C. P. (2007). *Indian Medicinal Plants*. New Delhi, India: Springer India Private Limited. doi:10.1007/978-0-387-70638-2

Kramer, M. S. (2010). "Breast is best": The evidence. *Early Human Development*, *86*(11), 729–732. doi:10.1016/j.earlhumdev.2010.08.005 PMID:20846797

Kramer, M. S., Guo, T., Platt, R. W., Sevkovskaya, Z., Dzikovich, I., Collet, J. P., ... Bogdanovich, N. (2003). Infant growth and health outcomes associated with 3 compared with 6 mo of exclusive breastfeeding. *The American Journal of Clinical Nutrition*, *78*(2), 291–295. doi:10.1093/ajcn/78.2.291 PMID:12885711

Lee, S. Y., Kim, M. T., Kim, S. W., Song, M. S., & Yoon, S. J. (2003). Effect of lifetime lactation on breast cancer risk: A Korean women's cohort study. *International Journal of Cancer*, *105*(3), 390–393. doi:10.1002/ijc.11078 PMID:12704674

Lopez-Alarcon, M., Villalpando, S., & Fajardo, A. (1997). Breast-feeding lowers the frequency and duration of acute respiratory infection and diarrhea in infants under six months of age. *The Journal of Nutrition*, *127*(3), 436–443. doi:10.1093/jn/127.3.436 PMID:9082027

Marild, S., Hansson, S., Jodal, U., Oden, A., & Svedberg, K. (2004). Protective effect of breastfeeding against urinary tract infection. *Acta Paediatrica (Oslo, Norway)*, *93*(2), 164–168. doi:10.1111/j.1651-2227.2004.tb00699.x PMID:15046267

Mathur, N. B., & Dhingra, D. (2009). Perceived Breast Milk Insufficiency in Mothers of Neonates Hospitalized in Neonatal Intensive Care Unit. *Indian Journal of Pediatrics*, *76*(10), 1003–1006. doi:10.100712098-009-0204-0 PMID:19907930

Mother and Child Nutrition. (2020). *Benefits of Breastfeeding for the Infant/Young Child.* https://motherchildnutrition.org/healthy-nutrition/about-essential-nutrition-actions/benefits-of-breastfeeding.html.

NFUM, National Formulary of Unani Medicine. (2006a). *Part-I.* New Delhi, India: CCRUM, Department of AYUSH, Ministry of Health & Family Welfare, Government of India.

NFUM, National Formulary of Unani Medicine. (2006b). *Part-IV* (1st ed.). New Delhi, India: Department of AYUSH, Ministry of Health & Family Welfare, Government of India.

NFUM, National Formulary of Unani Medicine. (2007). *Part-II, Vol-I.* New Delhi, India: Department of AYUSH, Ministry of Health & Family Welfare, Government of India.

NFUM, National Formulary of Unani Medicine. (2008). *Part-V.* New Delhi, India: Department of AYUSH, Ministry of Health & Family Welfare, Government of India.

NFUM, National Formulary of Unani Medicine. (2011). *Part-VI.* New Delhi, India: Department of AYUSH, Ministry of Health & Family Welfare, Government of India.

Newcomb, P. A., Storer, B. E., Longnecker, M. P., Mittendorf, R., Greenberg, E. R., Clapp, R. W., ... MacMahon, B. (1994). Lactation and a reduced risk of premenopausal breast cancer. *The New England Journal of Medicine*, *330*(2), 81–87. doi:10.1056/NEJM199401133300201 PMID:8259187

Oddy, W. H., Sly, P. D., & de Klerk, N. H. (2003). Breast feeding and respiratory morbidity in infancy: A birth cohort study. *Archives of Disease in Childhood*, *88*(3), 224–228. doi:10.1136/adc.88.3.224 PMID:12598384

Pettitt, D. J., Forman, M. R., Hanson, R. L., Knowler, W. C., & Bennett, P. H. (1997). Breastfeeding and incidence of non-insulin-dependent diabetes mellitus in pima Indians. *Lancet*, *350*(9072), 166–168. doi:10.1016/S0140-6736(96)12103-6 PMID:9250183

Pisacane, A., Graziano, L., Mazzarella, G., Scarpellino, B., & Zona, G. (1992). Breastfeeding and urinary tract infection. *The Journal of Pediatrics*, *120*(1), 87–89. doi:10.1016/S0022-3476(05)80607-9 PMID:1731031

Popkin, B. M., Adair, L., Akin, J. S., Black, R., Briscoe, J., & Flieger, W. (1990). Breastfeeding and diarrheal morbidity. *Pediatrics*, *86*, 874–882. PMID:2251024

Poshan. (2020). *Exclusive breastfeeding in India: trends and data gaps.* https://poshan.ifpri.info/2017/08/04/exclusive-breastfeeding-in-india-trends-and-data-gaps

Rosenblatt, K. A., & Thomas, D. B. (1993). Lactation and the risk of epithelial ovarian cancer. WHO Collaborative Study of Neoplasia and Steroid contraceptives. *International Journal of Epidemiology*, *22*(2), 192–197. doi:10.1093/ije/22.2.192 PMID:8505173

SUMT Standard Unani Medical Terminology. (2012). New Delhi, India: Central Council for Research in Unani Medicine, Ministry of Ayush, Govt. of India.

Tryggvadottir, L., Tulinius, H., Eyfjord, J. E., & Sigurvinsson, T. (2001). Breastfeeding and reduced risk of breast cancer in an Icelandic cohort study. *American Journal of Epidemiology*, *154*(1), 37–42. doi:10.1093/aje/154.1.37 PMID:11427403

WHO, World Health Organization. (n.d.). *Breastfeeding*. https://www.who.int/health-topics/breastfeeding#tab=tab_1

WHO, World Health Organization. (2007). Indicators for assessing infant and young child feeding practices part 1 definition. Washington, DC: World Health Organization. Dept. of Child and Adolescent Health and Development.

WHO, World Health Organization. (2009). *Infant and young child feeding: model chapter for textbooks for medical students and allied health professionals*. Geneva: World Health Organization.

WHO, World Health Organization. (2020). *Malnutrition*. https://www.who.int/news-room/fact-sheets/detail/malnutrition#:~:text=47%20million%20children%20under%205,%2D%20and%20middle%2Dincome%20countries

Compilation of References

Aarthi, R. (2019). Brusatol-as potent chemotherapeutic regimen and its role on reversing EMT transition. *Journal of Pharmaceutical Sciences and Research*, *11*(5), 1753–1762.

Abascal, K., & Yarnell, E. (2008). Botanical galactagogues. *Alternative and Complementary Therapies*, *14*(6), 288–294. doi:10.1089/act.2008.14602

Abbasi, Z., Tabatabaei, S. R. F., Mazaheri, Y., Barati, F., & Morovvati, H. (2013). Effects of Sesame Oil on the Reproductive Parameters of Diabetes Mellitus-Induced Male Rats. *The World Journal of Men's Health*, *31*(2), 141. doi:10.5534/wjmh.2013.31.2.141 PMID:24044109

Abbott, D. H., Dumesic, D. A., & Franks, S. (2002). Developmental origin of polycystic ovary syndrome - a hypothesis. *The Journal of Endocrinology*, *174*(1), 1–5. doi:10.1677/joe.0.1740001 PMID:12098657

Abdelazim, A., Khater, S., & Ali, H. (2019). Panax ginseng improves glucose metabolism in streptozotocin-induced diabetic rats through 5¢ adenosine monophosphate kinase up-regulation. *Saudi Journal of Biological Sciences, 26*(7), 1436-1441.

Abdel-Magied, E. M., Abdel-Rahman, H. A., & Harraz, F. M. (2001). The effect of aqueous extracts of *Cynomorium coccineum* and *Withania somnifera* on testicular development in immature Wistar rats. *Journal of Ethnopharmacology*, *75*(1), 1–4. doi:10.1016/S0378-8741(00)00348-2 PMID:11282435

Abraham, P., Avenell, A., McGeoch, S. C., Clark, L. F., & Bevan, J. S. (2010). Antithyroid drug regimen for treating Graves' hyperthyroidism. *Cochrane Database of Systematic Reviews*, (1), CD003420. doi:10.1002/14651858.CD003420.pub4 PMID:20091544

Abu-helalah, M., Al-hanaqta, M., Alshraideh, H., & Hijazeen, J. (2014). Quality of life and psychological well-being of breast cancer survivors in Jordan. *Asian Pacific Journal of Cancer Prevention*, *15*(14), 5927–5936. doi:10.7314/APJCP.2014.15.14.5927 PMID:25081724

Ackerknecht, E. H. (1973). *From the primitives to the twentieth century*. Academic Press.

Adaikan, P. G., Gauthaman, K., Prasad, R. N. V., & Ng, S. C. (2000). Proerectile pharmacological effects of *Tribulus terrestris* extract on the rabbit corpus cavernosum. *Annals of the Academy of Medicine, Singapore*, *29*(1), 22–26. PMID:10748960

Adam, Z., Hamid, M., Ismail, A., & Khamis, S. (2009a). Effect of Ficus deltoidea extracts on hepatic basal and insulin-stimulated glucose uptake. *The Journal of Biological Sciences*, *9*(2), 9–16.

Adapa, D., & TK, S. (2020). A Review on Diabetes Mellitus: Complications, Management and Treatment Modalities. *Journal of Medical and Health Sciences*, *4*(3).

Adike, A., & DiBaise, J. K. (2018). Small Intestinal Bacterial Overgrowth: Nutritional Implications, Diagnosis, and Management. *Gastroenterology Clinics of North America*, *47*(1), 193–208. doi:10.1016/j.gtc.2017.09.008 PMID:29413012

Aditya, N. P., Shim, M., Yang, H., Lee, Y. J., & Ko, S. (2014). Antiangiogenic effect of combined treatment with curcumin and genistein on human prostate cancer cell line. *Journal of Functional Foods*, *8*, 204–213. doi:10.1016/j.jff.2014.03.014

Adlercreutz, H. (2007). Lignans and human health. *Critical Reviews in Clinical Laboratory Sciences*, *44*(5-6), 483–525. doi:10.1080/10408360701612942 PMID:17943494

Agarwal, S. (2017). *Nutraceuticals and osteoarthritis. Leading pharmaceutical consultant.* http://www.drsanjayagrawal.com

Agarwal, S., & Rao, A. V. (2000). Tomato lycopene and its role in human health and chronic diseases. *Canadian Medical Association Journal*, *163*(6), 739–744. PMID:11022591

Aggarwal & Kunnumakkara. (2009). Molecular Targets and Therapeutic Uses of Spices: Modern Uses for Ancient Medicine. World Scientific Publishing Co. Pte. Ltd.

Aggarwal, B. B., Sundaram, C., Prasad, S., & Kannappan, R. (2010). Tocotrienols, the vitamin E of the 21st century: Its potential against cancer and other chronic diseases. Biochemical Pharmacology. https://doi.org/ doi:10.1016/j.bcp.2010.07.043

Aggarwal, B. B. (2010). Targeting inflammation-induced obesity and metabolic diseases by curcumin and other nutraceuticals. *Annual Review of Nutrition*, *30*(1), 173–199. doi:10.1146/annurev.nutr.012809.104755 PMID:20420526

Aghajanpour, M., Nazer, M. R., Obeidavi, Z., Akbari, M., Ezati, P., & Kor, N. M. (2017). Functional foods and their role in cancer prevention and health promotion: A comprehensive review. *American Journal of Cancer Research*, *7*(4), 740–769. PMID:28469951

Agrawal, Y. O., Sharma, P. K., Shrivastava, B., Ojha, S., Upadhya, H. M., Arya, D. S., & Goyal, S. N. (2014). Hesperidin produces cardioprotective activity via PPAR-γ pathway in ischemic heart disease model in diabetic rats. *PLoS One*, *9*(11), 1–13. doi:10.1371/journal.pone.0111212 PMID:25369053

Ahmad Ganai, S. (2017). Plant derived inhibitor Sulforaphane in combinatorial therapy against therapeutically challenging Pancreatic Cancer. *Anti-Cancer Agents in Medicinal Chemistry (Formerly Current Medicinal Chemistry-Anti-Cancer Agents)*, *17*(3), 365–373.

Ahmad, B., Tariq, M., Uppal, A. M., & Naveed, A. K. (2009). Effects of *Nigella sativa* oil on some blood parameters in type 2 diabetes mellitus patients. *Asian Journal of Chemistry*, *21*, 5373–5381.

Ahmad, D. S., Jasra, W. A., & Imtiaz, A. (2003). Genetic diversity in Pakistani genotypes of Hypophae rhamnoides L. ssp. Turkestanica. *Int J Agric Biol Sci*, *5*(1), 10–13.

Ahmadi, A., & Mostafavi, M. (2015). Study on the effects of licorice root hydroalcoholiclicorice extract on mice uterus histological structure and level of testosterone improvement with hyperandrogenism following experimental polycystic ovary syndrome. *Majallah-i Pizishki-i Urumiyyah*, *26*, 571–581.

Ahmad, K. (2014). Insulin sources and types: A review of insulin in terms of its mode on diabetes mellitus. *Journal of Traditional Chinese Medicine*, *34*(2), 234–237. doi:10.1016/S0254-6272(14)60084-4 PMID:24783939

Ahmad, M. K., Mahdi, A. A., Shukla, K. K., Islam, N., Rajender, S., Madhukar, D., Shankhwar, S. N., & Ahmad, S. (2010). Withania somnifera improves semen quality by regulating reproductive hormone levels and oxidative stress in seminal plasma of infertile males. *Fertility and Sterility*, *94*(3), 989–996. doi:10.1016/j.fertnstert.2009.04.046 PMID:19501822

Ahmad, M., Mahdi, A., Shukla, K., Islam, N., Jaiswar, S., & Ahmad, S. (2008). Effect of Mucuna pruriens on semen profile and biochemical parameters in seminal plasma of infertile men. *Fertility and Sterility*, *90*(3), 627–635. doi:10.1016/j.fertnstert.2007.07.1314 PMID:18001713

Ahmed, B., & Abubaker, E. (2011). Treatment options for polycystic ovary syndrome. *International Journal of Women's Health*, *3*, 25–35. PMID:21339935

Ahmed, M. K. (2016). Polycystic Ovarian Syndrome: Insights into Pathogenesis, Diagnosis, Prognosis, Pharmacological and Non-Pharmacological Treatment. *Journal of Pharma Research*, *1*, 1.

Ahn, J. H., Kim, E. S., Lee, C., Kim, S., Cho, S. H., Hwang, B. Y., & Lee, M. K. (2013). Chemical constituents from *Nelumbo nucifera* leaves and their anti-obesity effects. *Bioorganic & Medicinal Chemistry Letters*, *23*(12), 3604–3608. doi:10.1016/j.bmcl.2013.04.013 PMID:23642481

Ahn, J., Lee, H., Kima, S., Parka, J., & Taeyoul, H. (2008). The anti-obesity effect of quercetin is mediated by the AMPK and MAPK signaling pathways. *Biochemical and Biophysical Research Communications*, *373*(4), 545–549. doi:10.1016/j.bbrc.2008.06.077 PMID:18586010

Aiello, N. M., Brabletz, T., Kang, Y., Nieto, M. A., Weinberg, R. A., & Stanger, B. Z. (2017). Upholding a role for EMT in pancreatic cancer metastasis. *Nature*, *547*(7661), E7–E8. doi:10.1038/nature22963 PMID:28682339

Ainehchi, N., Khaki, A., Farshbaf-Khalili, A., Hammadeh, M., & Ouladsahebmadarek, E. (2019). The Effectiveness of Herbal Mixture Supplements with and without Clomiphene Citrate in Comparison to Clomiphene Citrate on Serum Antioxidants and Glycemic Biomarkers in Women with Polycystic Ovary Syndrome Willing to be Pregnant: A Randomized Clinical Trial. *Biomolecules*, *9*(6), E215. doi:10.3390/biom9060215 PMID:31163689

Akbas, F., Gasteyger, C., Sjodin, A., Astrup, A., & Larsen, T. M. (2009). A critical review of the cannabinoid receptor as a drug target for obesity management. *Obesity Reviews*, *10*(1), 58–67. doi:10.1111/j.1467-789X.2008.00520.x PMID:18721231

Akhani, S. P., Vishwakarma, S. L., & Goyal, R. K. (2004). Anti-diabetic activity of *Zingiber officinale* in streptozotocin-induced type I diabetic rats. *The Journal of Pharmacy and Pharmacology*, *56*(1), 101–105. doi:10.1211/0022357022403 PMID:14980006

Akiyama, S., Katsumata, S., Suzuki, K., Ishimi, Y., Wu, J., & Uehara, M. (2010). Dietary hesperidin exerts hypoglycemic and hypolipidemic effects in streptozotocin-induced marginal type 1 diabetic rats. *Journal of Clinical Biochemistry and Nutrition*, *46*(1), 87–92. doi:10.3164/jcbn.09-82 PMID:20104270

Al-Aboudi, A., & Afifi, F. U. (2011). Plants used for the treatment of diabetes in Jordan: A review of scientific evidence. *Pharmaceutical Biology*, *49*(3), 221–239. doi:10.3109/13880209.2010.501802 PMID:20979537

Alam, F., Islam, M., Kamal, M., & Gan, S. (2019). Updates on Managing Type 2 Diabetes Mellitus with Natural Products: Towards Antidiabetic Drug Development. *Current Medicinal Chemistry*, *25*(39), 5395–5431. doi:10.2174/0929867323666160813222436 PMID:27528060

Alappat, L., & Awad, A. B. (2010). Curcumin and obesity: Evidence and mechanisms. *Nutrition Reviews*, *68*(12), 729–738. doi:10.1111/j.1753-4887.2010.00341.x PMID:21091916

al-Din, K., (2003). *Al-Iksir, vol-II*. New Delhi, India: Aijaz Publishing House.

al-Din, K., (2007). *Ilmul Adviya Nafisi*. New Delhi, India: Aijaz Publishing House.

Al-Goblan, A. S., Al-Alfi, M. A., & Khan, M. Z. (2014). Mechanism linking diabetes mellitus and obesity. *Diabetes, Metabolic Syndrome and Obesity*, *7*, 587–591. doi:10.2147/DMSO.S67400 PMID:25506234

Ali Khan, M., Kedhari Sundaram, M., Hamza, A., Quraishi, U., Gunasekera, D., Ramesh, L., Goala, P., Al Alami, U., Ansari, M. Z., Rizvi, T. A., Sharma, C., & Hussain, A. (2015). Sulforaphane Reverses the Expression of Various Tumor Suppressor Genes by Targeting DNMT3B and HDAC1 in Human Cervical Cancer Cells. *Evidence-Based Complementary and Alternative Medicine*, *2015*, 2015. doi:10.1155/2015/412149 PMID:26161119

Ali, K. M., Chatterjee, K., De, D., Jana, K., Bera, T. K., & Ghosh, D. (2011). Inhibitory effect of hydro-methanolic extract of seed of Holarrhena antidysenterica on alpha-glucosidase activity and postprandial blood glucose level in normoglycemic rat. *Journal of Ethnopharmacology*, *135*(1), 194–196. doi:10.1016/j.jep.2011.02.034 PMID:21385604

Alissa, E. M., & Ferns, G. A. (2012). Functional foods and nutraceuticals in the primary prevention of cardiovascular diseases. *Journal of Nutrition and Metabolism*, *2012*, 1–16. doi:10.1155/2012/569486 PMID:22570771

Al-Kirmani. (1439). *Sharh al-Asbab wa'l 'Alamat* (vols. 3-4). New Delhi, India: Aijaz Publishing House.

Al-Qarwi, A. A., Abdel-Rehman, H. A., El-Badry, A. A., Harraz, F., Razig, N. A., & Abdel-Magied, E. M. (2000). The effect of extracts of *Cynomorium coccineum* and *Withania somnifera* on gonadotrophins and ovarian follicles of immature Wistar rats. *Phytotherapy Research*, *14*(4), 288–290. doi:10.1002/1099-1573(200006)14:4<288::AID-PTR603>3.0.CO;2-9 PMID:10861976

Al-Sa'aidi, J. A. A., Al-Khuzai, A. L. D., & Al-Zobaydi, N. F. H. (2009). Effect of alcoholic extract of Nigella sativa on fertility in male rats. *Iraqi Journal of Veterinary Sciences*, *23*, 123–128.

Al-Salameh, A., Bucher, S., Bauduceau, B., Benattar-Zibi, L., Berrut, G., Bertin, P., & … . (2018). Sex Differences in the Occurrence of Major Clinical Events in Elderly People with Type 2 Diabetes Mellitus Followed up in the General Practice. *Experimental and Clinical Endocrinology & Diabetes*, (2), 77–132. doi:10.1055/a-0662-5923 PMID:30134475

Al-Tahami, B. A. M., Ab, A. A. S. I., Sanip, Z., Yusoff, Z., Shihabudin, T. M. T., Singh, T. S. P., & Rasool, A. H. G. (2017). Metabolic and Inflammatory Changes with Orlistat and Sibutramine Treatment in Obese Malaysian Subjects. *Journal of Nippon Medical School*, *84*(3), 125–132. doi:10.1272/jnms.84.125 PMID:28724846

Altemimi, A., Lakhssassi, N., Baharlouei, A., Watson, D. G., & Lightfoot, D. A. (2017). Phytochemicals: Extraction, isolation, and identification of bioactive compounds from plant extracts. *Plants (Basel, Switzerland)*, *6*(4), 42.

Altiner, A. (2012). Effect of the antiobesity agent garcinia cambogia extract on serum lipoprotein (a), apolipoproteins a1 and b, and total cholesterol levels in female rats fed atherogenic diet. *The Journal of Animal and Plant Sciences*, *22*, 872–877.

Alves, Q.L., Camardo, S.B., & Silva, D.F. (2019). Role of nutraceuticals in the prevention and treatment of hypertension and cardiovascular diseases. *Journal of Hypertension and Management, 5*, 37.

Amararathna, M., Johnston, M. R., & Vasantha Rupasinghe, H. P. (2016). Plant polyphenols as chemopreventive agents for lung cancer. *International Journal of Molecular Sciences*, *17*(8), 1352. doi:10.3390/ijms17081352 PMID:27548149

Amato, P., & Simpson, J. L. (2004). The genetics of polycystic ovary syndrome. *Best Practice & Research. Clinical Obstetrics & Gynaecology*, *18*(5), 707–718. doi:10.1016/j.bpobgyn.2004.05.002 PMID:15380142

Ambiye, V. R., Langade, D., Dongre, S., Aptikar, P., Kulkarni, M., & Dongre, A. (2013). Clinical Evaluation of the Spermatogenic Activity of the Root Extract of Ashwagandha (Withania somnifera) in Oligospermic Males: A Pilot Study. *Evidence-Based Complementary and Alternative Medicine*, *2013*, 1–6. doi:10.1155/2013/571420 PMID:24371462

American Diabetes Association. (2014). Diagnosis and classification of diabetes mellitus. *Diabetes Care*, *37*(Supplement 1), S81–S90. doi:10.2337/dc14-S081 PMID:24357215

Amin, K. A., & Nagy, M. A. (2009). Effect of Carnitine and herbal mixture extract on obesity induced by high fat diet in rats. *Diabetology & Metabolic Syndrome*, *1*(1), 17. doi:10.1186/1758-5996-1-17 PMID:19835614

Amin, Y. M. N., Rehman, Z. S., & Khan, N. A. (1996). Sexual function improving effect of *M. pruriens* in sexually normal male rats. *Fitoterapial*, *67*, 53–58.

Amjad, S., Jafri, A., Sharma, A., & Serajuddin, M. (2019). A novel strategy of nanotized herbal drugs and their delivery in the treatment of diabetes: Present status and future prospects. *Journal of Herbal Medicine*, *17-18*, 100279. doi:10.1016/j.hermed.2019.100279

Anahita, J., Faezeh, K., Fatemeh, S., Kourosh, S., Zahra, K., & Malihe, A. (2015). Prevalence of polycystic ovary syndrome and its associated complications in Iranian women: A meta-analysis. *Iranian Journal of Reproductive Medicine*, *13*(10), 591–604. PMID:26644787

Anand David, A. V., Arulmoli, R., & Parasuraman, S. (2016). Overviews of biological importance of quercetin: A bioactive flavonoid. Pharmacognosy Reviews, 10(20). https://doi.org/ doi:10.4103/0973-7847.194044

Anawalt, B. D. (2013). Approach to Male Infertility and Induction of Spermatogenesis. *The Journal of Clinical Endocrinology and Metabolism*, *98*(9), 3532–3542. doi:10.1210/jc.2012-2400 PMID:24014811

Anderson, J. W., Baird, P., Davis, R. H., Ferreri, S., Knudtson, M., Koraym, A., Waters, V., & Williams, C. L. (2009). Health benefits of dietary fiber. Nutrition Reviews. https://doi.org/ doi:10.1111/j.1753-4887.2009.00189.x

Andoh, A., Nishida, A., Takahashi, K., Inatomi, O., Imaeda, H., Bamba, S., ... Kobayashi, T. (2016). Comparison of the gut microbial community between obese and lean peoples using 16S gene sequencing in a Japanese population. *Journal of Clinical Biochemistry and Nutrition*, *59*(1), 65–70. doi:10.3164/jcbn.15-152 PMID:27499582

Angeles, L. & Abbvie, P.M. (2015). *Potentiation of growth inhibition and epigenetic modulation by combination of green tea polyphenol and 5-aza-2 ¢ -deoxycytidine i*. Academic Press.

An, S., Han, J. I., Kim, M. J., Park, J. S., Han, J. M., Baek, N. I., Chung, H. G., Choi, M. S., Lee, K. T., & Jeong, T. S. (2010). Ethanolic extracts of *Brassica campestris* spp. rapa roots prevent high-fat diet-induced obesity via beta(3)-adrenergic regulation of white adipocyte lipolytic activity. *Journal of Medicinal Food*, *13*(2), 406–414. doi:10.1089/jmf.2009.1295 PMID:20132043

Anwar, F., Latif, S., Ashraf, M., & Gilani, A. H. (2007). Moringa oleifera: A food plant with multiple medicinal uses. Phytotherapy Research. https://doi.org/ doi:10.1002/ptr.2023

An, Y., Sun, Z., Zhang, Y., Liu, B., Guan, Y., & Lu, M. (2014). The use of berberine for women with polycystic ovary syndrome undergoing IVF treatment. *Horumon To Rinsho*, *80*(3), 425–431. doi:10.1111/cen.12294 PMID:23869585

Aravindan, S., Ramraj, S. K., Somasundaram, S. T., Herman, T. S., & Aravindan, N. (2015). Polyphenols from marine brown algae target radiotherapy-coordinated EMT and stemness-maintenance in residual pancreatic cancer. *Stem Cell Research & Therapy*, *6*(1), 182. doi:10.118613287-015-0173-3 PMID:26395574

Arentz, S., Abbott, J. A., Smith, C. A., & Bensoussan, A. (2014). A survey of the use of complementary medicine by a self- selected community group of Australian women with polycystic ovary syndrome. *BMC Complementary and Alternative Medicine*, *14*(1), 472. doi:10.1186/1472-6882-14-472 PMID:25481654

Arichi, H., Kimura, Y., Okuda, H., Baba, K., Kozawa, M., & Arichi, S. (1982). Effects of stilbene components of the roots of Polygonum cuspidatum Sieb. et Zucc. on lipid metabolism. *Chemical & Pharmaceutical Bulletin*, *30*(5), 1766–1770. doi:10.1248/cpb.30.1766 PMID:7116511

Aronson, J. K. (2017). Defining 'nutraceuticals': neither nutritious nor pharmaceutical. British Journal of Clinical Pharmacology. https://doi.org/ doi:10.1111/bcp.12935

Arora, D., & Jaglan, S. (2016). Nanocarriers based delivery of nutraceuticals for cancer prevention and treatment: A review of recent research developments. *Trends in Food Science & Technology, 54*, 114–126. doi:10.1016/j.tifs.2016.06.003

Arunachalam, G., Yao, H., Sundar, I. K., Caito, S., & Rahman, I. (2010). SIRT1 regulates oxidant-and cigarette smoke-induced eNOS acetylation in endothelial cells: Role of resveratrol. *Biochemical and Biophysical Research Communications, 393*(1), 66–72. doi:10.1016/j.bbrc.2010.01.080 PMID:20102704

Arzani, H.M.A. (1924). *Tibb-i Akbar.* Deoband, India: Faisal Publishers.

Arzani, H.M.A. (1992). *Meezan al-Tib.* New Delhi, India: National Council for promotion of Urdu language.

Asadi, M. H., Zafari, F., Sarveazad, A., Abbasi, M., Safa, M., Koruji, M., ... Miran, R. A. (2013). Saffron Improves Epididymal Sperm Parameters in Rats Exposed to Cadmium. *Nephro-Urology Monthly, 6*(1). Advance online publication. doi:10.5812/numonthly.12125 PMID:24719804

Asadi, M., & Bahrami, S. (2010). The effect of stachys lavandulifolia Vahl. and mespilus germanica L. leaves hydroalcoholic extracts on leishmania major (MRHO/IR/75/ER) in vitro. *Jundishapur Journal of Natural Pharmaceutical Products, 5*(1), 39–43.

Asadi-Samani, M., Bahmani, M., & Rafieian-Kopaei, M. (2014). The chemical composition, botanical characteristic and biological activities of Borago officinalis: A review. *Asian Pacific Journal of Tropical Medicine.* Advance online publication. doi:10.1016/S1995-7645(14)60199-1 PMID:25312125

Ashraf, R., & Shah, N. P. (2014). Immune system stimulation by probiotic microorganisms. *Critical Reviews in Food Science and Nutrition, 54*(7), 938–956. doi:10.1080/10408398.2011.619671 PMID:24499072

Ashwini, S., Bobby, Z., Sridhar, M. G., & Cleetus, C. C. (2017). Insulin Plant (Costus pictus) Extract Restores Thyroid Hormone Levels in Experimental Hypothyroidism. *Pharmacognosy Research, 9*(1), 51–59. doi:10.4103/0974-8490.199766 PMID:28250654

Aslam, M. S., Naveed, S., Ahmed, A., Abbas, Z., Gull, I., & Athar, M. A. (2014). Side Effects of Chemotherapy in Cancer Patients and Evaluation of Patients Opinion about Starvation Based Differential Chemotherapy. *Journal of Cancer Therapy, 5*(8), 817–822. doi:10.4236/jct.2014.58089

Association, A. T., Hyperthyroidism, A. A. C. E. T., Thyrotoxicosis, O. C., Bahn, R. S., Burch, H. B., Cooper, D. S., ... Montori, V. M. (2011). Hyperthyroidism and other causes of thyrotoxicosis: Management guidelines of the American Thyroid Association and American Association of Clinical Endocrinologists. *Thyroid, 21*(6), 593–646. doi:10.1089/thy.2010.0417 PMID:21510801

Astrup, A., Breum, L., & Toubro, S. (1995). Pharmacological and clinical studies of ephedrine and other thermogenic agonists. *Obesity Research, 3*(S4), 537S–540S. doi:10.1002/j.1550-8528.1995.tb00224.x PMID:8697055

Astrup, A., Toubro, S., Christensen, N., & Quade, F. (1992). Pharmacology of thermogenic drugs. *The American Journal of Clinical Nutrition, 55*(1), 246S–248S. doi:10.1093/ajcn/55.1.246s PMID:1345887

Ataabadi, Alaee, Bagheri, & Bahmanpoor. (2017). Role of Essential Oil of Mentha Spicata (Spearmint) in Addressing Reverse Hormonal and Folliculogenesis Disturbances in a Polycystic Ovarian Syndrome in a Rat Model. *Adv Pharm Bull, 7*(4), 651-654.

Atanasov, A. G., Waltenberger, B., Pferschy-Wenzig, E. M., Linder, T., Wawrosch, C., Uhrin, P., Temml, V., Wang, L., Schwaiger, S., Heiss, E. H., Rollinger, J. M., Schuster, D., Breuss, J. M., Bochkov, V., Mihovilovic, M. D., Kopp, B., Bauer, R., Dirsch, V. M., & Stuppner, H. (2015). Discovery and resupply of pharmacologically active plant-derived natural products: A review. *Biotechnology Advances*, *33*(8), 1582–1614. doi:10.1016/j.biotechadv.2015.08.001

Attanayake, A. P., Jayatilaka, K. A., Pathirana, C., & Mudduwa, L. K. (2015). Antihyperglycemic activity of Coccinia grandis (L.) Voigt in streptozotocin induced diabetic rats. *Indian Journal of Traditional Knowledge*, *14*(3), 376–381.

Auyeng, T. W., Chang, K. K. F., To, C. H., Mak, A., & Szeto, M. L. (2002). Three patients with lead poisoning following use of a Chinese herbal pill. *Hong Kong Medical Journal*, *8*, 60–62. PMID:11861997

Avan, A. (2016). 257P Molecular mechanisms involved in the synergistic interaction of novel formulated curcumin with gemcitabine in pancreatic cancer cells. *Annals of Oncology*, 27(suppl_9), p.mdw582.038-mdw582.038. Available at: . doi:10.1093/annonc/mdw582.038

Azab, A. (2017). Carob (Ceratonia siliqua): Health, Medicine And Chemistry. *European Chemical Bulletin*, *6*(10), 456–469. doi:10.17628/ecb.2017.6.456-469

Azaizeh, H., Saad, B., Khaleel, Kh., & Said, O. (2006) The state of the art of traditional Arab herbal medicine in the eastern region of the Mediterranean: a review. *eCAM, 3*, 229–235.

Azeemuddin, Anturlikar, Onkaramurthy, Baig, Ashok, Rao, Rafiq, & Rangesh. (2019). Effect of "DXB-2030," a Poly-herbal Formulation, on Experimental Polycystic Ovary Syndrome Associated with Hyperandrogenism. *Advances in Pharmacological Sciences*. . doi:10.1155/2019/8272850

Azevedo, M. F., Barra, G. B., Naves, L. A., Ribeiro Velasco, L. F., Godoy Garcia Castro, P., de Castro, L. C., Amato, A. A., Miniard, A., Driscoll, D., Schomburg, L., & de Assis Rocha Neves, F. (2010). Selenoprotein-related disease in a young girl caused by nonsense mutations in the SBP2 gene. *The Journal of Clinical Endocrinology and Metabolism*, *95*(8), 4066–4071. doi:10.1210/jc.2009-2611 PMID:20501692

Azzini, E., Giacometti, J., & Russo, G. L. (2017). Antiobesity effects of anthocyanins in preclinical and clinical studies. *Oxidative Medicine and Cellular Longevity*, *2017*(2740364), 1–11. doi:10.1155/2017/2740364 PMID:28785373

Azziz, R., Carmina, E., Dewailly, D., Diamanti-Kandarakis, E., Escobar-Morreale, H. F., Futterweit, W., Janssen, O. E., Legro, R. S., Norman, R. J., Taylor, A. E., & Witchel, S. F. (2006). Position statement: Criteria for defining polycystic ovary syndrome as a predominantly hyperandrogenic syndrome. An Androgen Excess Society guideline. *The Journal of Clinical Endocrinology and Metabolism*, *91*(11), 4237–4245. doi:10.1210/jc.2006-0178 PMID:16940456

Azziz, R., Marin, C., Hoq, L., Badamgarav, E., & Song, P. (2005). Health care-related economic burden of the polycystic ovary syndrome during the reproductive life span. *The Journal of Clinical Endocrinology and Metabolism*, *90*(8), 4650–4658. doi:10.1210/jc.2005-0628 PMID:15944216

Azziz, R., Nestler, J. E., & Dewailly, D. (2006). *Androgen excessdisorders in women: polycystic ovary syndrome and otherdisorders*. Humana Press.

Azziz, R., Woods, K. S., Reyna, R., Key, T. J., Knochenhauer, E. S., & Yildiz, B. O. (2004). The prevalence and features of the polycystic ovary syndrome in an unselected population. *The Journal of Clinical Endocrinology and Metabolism*, *89*(6), 2745–2749. doi:10.1210/jc.2003-032046 PMID:15181052

Babu, P. A., Suneetha, G., Boddepalli, R., Lakshmi, V. V., Rani, T. S., RamBabu, Y., & Srinivas, K. (2006). A database of 389 medicinal plants for diabetes. *Bioinformation*, *1*(4), 130–131. doi:10.6026/97320630001130 PMID:17597872

Baghdadi, A.H. (2004). *Kitab al-Mukhtarat fi'l Tibb Vol. III.* New Delhi, India: Central Council for Research in Unani Medicine.

Baharuddin, P., Satar, N., Fakiruddin, K. S., Zakaria, N., Lim, M. N., Yusoff, N. M., Zakaria, Z., & Yahaya, B. H. (2016). Curcumin improves the efficacy of cisplatin by targeting cancer stem-like cells through p21 and cyclin D1-mediated tumour cell inhibition in non-small cell lung cancer cell lines. *Oncology Reports*, *35*(1), 13–25. doi:10.3892/or.2015.4371 PMID:26531053

Bahceci, M., Aydemir, M., & Tuzcu, A. (2007). Effects of oral fat and glucose Tolerance test on serum lipid profile, apolipoprotein, and CRP concentration, and insulin resistance in patients with polycystic ovary syndrome. *Fertility and Sterility*, *87*(6), 1363–1368. doi:10.1016/j.fertnstert.2006.11.031 PMID:17362944

Baile, C. A., Yang, J. Y., Rayalam, S., Hartzell, D. L., Lai, C. Y., Andersen, C., & Della-Fera, M. A. (2011). Effect of resveratrol on fat mobilization. *Annals of the New York Academy of Sciences*, *1215*(1), 40–47. doi:10.1111/j.1749-6632.2010.05845.x PMID:21261640

Bailey, C. J., & Day, C. (1989). Traditional plant medicines as treatments for diabetes. *Diabetes Care*, *12*(8), 553–564. doi:10.2337/diacare.12.8.553 PMID:2673695

Bak, E. J., Kim, J., Choi, Y. H., Kim, J. H., Lee, D. E., Woo, G. H., Cha, J. H., & Yoo, Y. J. (2014). Wogonin ameliorates hyperglycemia and dyslipidemia via pparα activation in db/db mice. *Clinical Nutrition (Edinburgh, Lothian)*, *33*(1), 156–163. doi:10.1016/j.clnu.2013.03.013 PMID:23623334

Balamurugan, G., & Muralidharan, P. (2010). Antiobesity effect of *Bauhinia variegata* bark extract on female rats fed on hypercaloric diet. *Bangladesh Journal of Pharmacology*, *5*(1), 8–12. doi:10.3329/bjp.v5i1.4310

Balanathan, K., Omar, M. H., Zainul Rashid, M. R., Ong, F. B., Nurshaireen, A., & Jamil, M. A. (2001). A clinical study on the effect of *Tribulus terrestris* (Tribestan) on the semen profile in males with low sperm count and low motility. *Malayasian Journal of Obstetrics Gynecology*, *7*, 69–78.

Bal, D. G., Foerster, S. B., Backman, D. R., & Lyman, D. O. (2001). Dietary change and cancer: Challenges and future direction. *The Journal of Nutrition*, *131*(1), 181S–185S. doi:10.1093/jn/131.1.181S PMID:11208961

Baldwa, V., Bhandari, C., Pangaria, A., & Goyal, R. (1977). Clinical Trial in Patients with Diabetes Mellitus of an Insulin-like Compound Obtained from Plant Source. *Upsala Journal of Medical Sciences*, *82*(1), 39–41. doi:10.3109/03009737709179057 PMID:20078273

Balen, A. H., Morley, L. C., Misso, M., Franks, S., Legro, R. S., Wijeyaratne, C. N., Stener-Victorin, E., Fauser, B. C. J. M., Norman, R. J., & Teede, H. (2016). The management of anovulatory infertility in women with polycystic ovary syndrome: An analysis of the evidence to support the development of global WHO guidance. *Human Reproduction Update*, *22*(6), 687–708. doi:10.1093/humupd/dmw025 PMID:27511809

Bamosa, A. O., Kaatabi, H., Lebdaa, F. M., Elq, A. M., & Al-Sultanb, A. (2010). Effect of *Nigella sativa* seeds on the glycemic control of patients with type 2 diabetes mellitus. *Indian Journal of Physiology and Pharmacology*, *54*, 344–354. PMID:21675032

Bandaranayake, W. M. (2006). Qualitycontrol, screening, toxicity, and regulation of herbal drugs. Modern Phyto medicine Turning Medicinal Plants into Drugs, 25–57.

Bargiota. (2012). The effects of old, new and emerging medicines on metabolic aberrations in PCOS. Therapeutic Advances in Endocrinology and Metabolism, 3(1), 27–47. PubMed

Barnes, J. (2003). Quality, efficacy and safety of complementary medicines: fashions, facts and the future. Part II: Efficacy and safety. 2003 Blackwell Publishing Ltd. *British Journal of Clinical Pharmacology*, *55*(4), 331–340. doi:10.1046/j.1365-2125.2003.01811.x PMID:12680880

Barthélémy, P., Asmane-De la Porte, I., Meyer, N., Duclos, B., Serra, S., Dourthe, L.-M., Amé, S., Litique, V., Giron, C., Goldbarg, V., Fornecker, L., Quoix, E., & Kurtz, J.-E. (2015). Adherence and Patients' Attitudes to Oral Anticancer Drugs: A Prospective Series of 201 Patients Focusing on Targeted Therapies. *Oncology*, *88*(1), 1–8. doi:10.1159/000366226 PMID:25247774

Bashir, L., Shittu, O. K., Sani, S., Busari, M. B., & Adeniyi, K. A. (2015). African Natural Products with Potential Anti-trypanosoma Properties: A Review. *International Journal of Biochemistry Research & Review*, *7*(2), 45–79. doi:10.9734/IJBCRR/2015/16039

Bashtian, H. M., Emami, A. S., & Mousavifar, N. (2013). Evaluation of fenugreek (Trigonella Foenum-graceum L.), effects seeds extract on insulin resistance in women with polycystic ovarian syndrome. *Iranian J. Pharm. Res.: IJPR*, *12*, 475. PMID:24250624

Basisht, G. (2014). Exploring insights towards definition and laws of health in Ayurveda: Global health perspective. *Ayu*, *35*(4), 351–355. doi:10.4103/0974-8520.158975

Basnet, A., Pandita, A., Fullmer, J., & Sivapiragasam, A. (2017). Squamous Cell Carcinoma of the Thyroid as a Result of Anaplastic Transformation from BRAF-Positive Papillary Thyroid Cancer. *Case Reports in Oncological Medicine*, *4276435*, 1–4. Advance online publication. doi:10.1155/2017/4276435 PMID:29158933

Basu, A., Du, M., Sanchez, K., Leyva, M. J., Betts, N. M., Blevins, S., Wu, M., Aston, C. E., & Lyons, T. J. (2011). Green tea minimally affects biomarkers of inflammation obese subjects with metabolic syndrome. *Nutrition (Burbank, Los Angeles County, Calif.)*, *27*(2), 206–213. doi:10.1016/j.nut.2010.01.015 PMID:20605696

Baynest, H. (2015). Classification, Pathophysiology, Diagnosis and Management of Diabetes Mellitus. *Journal of Diabetes & Metabolism*, *06*(05). Advance online publication. doi:10.4172/2155-6156.1000541

Beaudry, M., Dufour, R., & Marcoux, S. (1995). Relation between infant feeding and infections during the first six months of life. *The Journal of Pediatrics*, *126*(2), 191–197. doi:10.1016/S0022-3476(95)70544-9 PMID:7844664

Behloul, N., & Wu, G. (2013). Genistein: A promising therapeutic agent for obesity and diabetes treatment. *European Journal of Pharmacology*, *698*(1-3), 31–38. doi:10.1016/j.ejphar.2012.11.013 PMID:23178528

Bellini, M., Tonarelli, S., Nagy, A. G., Pancetti, A., Costa, F., Ricchiuti, A., ... Rossi, A. (2020). Low FODMAP Diet: Evidence, Doubts, and Hopes. *Nutrients*, *12*(1), 148. doi:10.3390/nu12010148 PMID:31947991

Benhaddou-Andaloussi, A., Martineau, L., Vuong, T., Meddah, B., Madiraju, P., Settaf, A., & Haddad, P. S. (2011). The *in vivo* antidiabetic activity of *Nigella sativa* is mediated through activation of the AMPK Pathway and increased muscle Glut4 Content. *Evidence-Based Complementary and Alternative Medicine*, *2011*, 1–9. doi:10.1155/2011/538671 PMID:21584245

Bensoussan, A., & Lewith, G. T. (2004). Complementary medicine research in Australia: A strategy for the future. *The Medical Journal of Australia*, *181*(6), 331–333. doi:10.5694/j.1326-5377.2004.tb06303.x

Bentzon, J. F., Otsuka, F., Virmani, R., & Falk, E. (2014). Mechanisms of plaque formation and rupture. *Circulation Research*, *114*(12), 1852–1866. doi:10.1161/CIRCRESAHA.114.302721 PMID:24902970

Benzie, I. F., & Wachtel-Galor, S. (Eds.). (2011). *Herbal medicine: biomolecular and clinical aspects*. CRC Press. doi:10.1201/b10787

Beppu, H., Shimpo, K., Chihara, T., Kaneko, T., Tamai, I., Yamaji, S., Ozaki, S., Kuzuya, H., & Sonoda, S. (2006). Antidiabetic effects of dietary administration of Aloe arborescens Miller components on multiple low-dose streptozotocin-induced diabetes in mice: Investigation on hypoglycemic action and systemic absorption dynamics of aloe components. *Journal of Ethnopharmacology*, *103*(3), 468–477. doi:10.1016/j.jep.2005.10.034 PMID:16406411

Bera, T. K., Ali, K. M., Jana, K., Ghosh, A., & Ghosh, D. (2013). Protective effect of aqueous extract of seed of *Psoralea corylifolia* (Somraji) and seed of *Trigonella foenum-graecum* L. (Methi) in streptozotocin-induced diabetic rat: A comparative evaluation. *Pharmacognosy Research*, *5*(4), 277–285. doi:10.4103/0974-8490.118840 PMID:24174822

Berger, K., Winzell, M. S., Mei, J., & Erlanson-Albertsson, C. (2004). Enterostatin and its target mechanisms during regulation of fat intake. *Physiology & Behavior*, *83*(4), 623–630. doi:10.1016/j.physbeh.2004.08.040 PMID:15621068

Bergmann, J., Luft, B., Boehmann, S., Runnebaum, B., & Gerhard, I. (2000). Phyto-Hypophyson_ L for female infertility. Randomized, placebo-controlled, clinical double-blind study. *Forschende Komplementarmedizin und Klassische Naturheilkunde*, *7*(4), 190–199. PMID:11025394

Berliner, J. A., Navab, M., Fogelman, A. M., Frank, J. S., Demer, L. L., Edwards, P. A., ... Lusis, A. J. (1995). Atherosclerosis: basic mechanisms: oxidation, inflammation, and genetics. *Circulation*, *91*(9), 2488–2496. doi:10.1161/01.CIR.91.9.2488 PMID:7729036

Bernardi, J. R., & Escobar, R. S. (2012). Fetal and neonatal levels of omega-3: Effect on neurodevelopment, nutrition and growth. *The Scientific World Journal*.

Berneis, K., Rizzo, M., Hersberger, M., Rini, G. B., DiFede, G., Pepe, I., Spinas, G. A., & Carmina, E. (2009). Atherogenic forms of dyslipidaemia in women with polycystic ovary syndrome. *International Journal of Clinical Practice*, *63*(1), 56–62. doi:10.1111/j.1742-1241.2008.01897.x PMID:19125993

Bhat, F. A., Sharmila, G., Balakrishnan, S., Arunkumar, R., Elumalai, P., Suganya, S., & Arunakaran, J. (2014). Quercetin reverses EGF-induced epithelial to mesenchymal transition and invasiveness in prostate cancer (PC-3) cell line via EGFR/PI3K/Akt pathway. *The Journal of Nutritional Biochemistry*, *25*(11), 1132–1139. doi:10.1016/j.jnutbio.2014.06.008 PMID:25150162

Bhatia, V., & Viswanathan, P. (2006). Insulin resistance and PPAR insulin sensitizers. *Current Opinion in Investigational Drugs (London, England)*, *7*(10), 891–897. PMID:17086933

Bhattacharya, Johnson, Tijani, Hart, Pandey, & Gibreel. (2010). Female Infertility. *BMJ Clin Evid, 819.*

Bhattacharya, S. K., Goel, R. K., Kaur, R., & Ghosal, S. (1987). Anti - stress activity of Sitoindosides VII and VIII. New Acylsterylglucosides from *Withania somnifera. Phytotherapy Research*, *1*(1), 32–37. doi:10.1002/ptr.2650010108

Bhuvaneshwari, S., Poornima, R., & Averal, H. (2015). Management of obesity in polycystic ovary syndrome induced albino rats with Pergularia daemia. *Int. J. Appl. Res*, *1*, 779–783.

Bierie, B., Pierce, S. E., Kroeger, C., Stover, D. G., Pattabiraman, D. R., Thiru, P., & Weinberg, R. A. (2017). Integrin-β4 identifies cancer stem cell-enriched populations of partially mesenchymal carcinoma cells. *Proceedings of the National Academy of Sciences of the United States of America*, *114*(12), E2337–E2346. doi:10.1073/pnas.1618298114 PMID:28270621

Biesalski, H. K. (2016). Nutrition meets the microbiome: Micronutrients and the microbiota. *Annals of the New York Academy of Sciences*, *1372*(1), 53–64. doi:10.1111/nyas.13145 PMID:27362360

Bina, F., & Rahimi, R. (2017). Sweet Marjoram, A Review of Ethnopharmacology, Phytochemistry, and Biological Activities. *Journal of Evidence-Based Complementary & Alternative Medicine*, *22*(1), 175–185. doi:10.1177/2156587216650793 PMID:27231340

Birari, R., Javia, V., & Bhutani, K. K. (2010). Antiobesity and lipid lowering effects of *Murraya koenigii* (L.) Spreng leaves extracts and mahanimbine on high fat diet induced obese rats. *Fitoterapia*, *81*(8), 1129–1133. doi:10.1016/j.fitote.2010.07.013 PMID:20655993

Bischoff, S. C., Barbara, G., Buurman, W., Ockhuizen, T., Schulzke, J.-D., Serino, M., ... Wells, J. M. (2014). Intestinal permeability--a new target for disease prevention and therapy. *BMC Gastroenterology*, *14*(1), 189. doi:10.118612876-014-0189-7 PMID:25407511

Bishayee, A., Barnes, K. F., Bhatia, D., Darvesh, A. S., & Carroll, R. T. (2010). Resveratrol suppresses oxidative stress and inflammatory response in diethylnitrosamine-initiated rat hepatocarcinogenesis. *Cancer Prevention Research (Philadelphia, Pa.)*, *3*(6), 753–763. doi:10.1158/1940-6207.CAPR-09-0171 PMID:20501860

Blaabjerg, S., Artzi, D. M., & Aabenhus, R. (2017). Probiotics for the prevention of antibiotic-associated diarrhea in outpatients—A systematic review and meta-analysis. Antibiotics. https://doi.org/ doi:10.3390/antibiotics6040021

Blair, M. (2016). Diabetes Mellitus Review. *Urologic Nursing*, *36*(1), 27. doi:10.7257/1053-816X.2016.36.1.27 PMID:27093761

Blum, A. (2018). Freestyle Libre Glucose Monitoring System. *Clinical Diabetes*, *36*(2), 203–204. doi:10.2337/cd17-0130 PMID:29686463

Blundell, J. E., & Cooling, J. (2000). Routes to obesity: Phenotypes, food choices and activity. *British Journal of Nutrition*, *83*(S1), S33–S38. doi:10.1017/S0007114500000933 PMID:10889790

Bohlooli, S., Jastan, M., Nakhostin-Roohi, B., Mohammadi, S., & Baghari, Z. (2012). A pilot double-blinded, randomized, clinical trial of topical virgin olive oil versus piroxicam gel in osteoarthritis of the knee. *Journal of Clinical Rheumatology; Practical Reports on Rheumatic & Musculoskeletal Diseases*, *18*(2), 99–101. doi:10.1097/RHU.0b013e31824a47b5 PMID:22334264

Boomsma, C. M., Eijkemans, M. J., Hughes, E. G., Visser, G. H., Fauser, B. C., & Macklon, N. S. (2006, November-December). A meta-analysis of pregnancy outcomes in women with polycystic ovary syndrome. *Human Reproduction Update*, *12*(6), 673–683. doi:10.1093/humupd/dml036 PMID:16891296

Bordbar, H., Esmaeilpour, T., Dehghani, F., & Panjehshahin, M. R. (2013). Stereological study of the effect of ginger's alcoholic extract on the testis in busulfan-induced infertility in rats. *Iranian Journal of Reproductive Medicine*, *11*, 467–472. PMID:24639780

Bordoloi, R., & Dutta, K. N. (2014). A review on herbs used in the treatment of diabetes mellitus. *J Pharm Chem Biol Sci*, *2*(2), 86–92.

Borghi, C., & Cicero, A. F. G. (2017). Nutraceuticals with a clinically detectable blood pressure-lowering effect: a review of available randomized clinical trials and their meta-analyses. British Journal of Clinical Pharmacology. https:// doi.org/ doi:10.1111/bcp.12902

Borgia, F., Cannavo, S., Guarneri, Cannavo, S.P., Vaccaro, M., & Guarneri, B(2004Correlation between endocrinological parameters and acne severity in adult women. *Acta Derm Venereol.*, *84*(3), 201–204.

Borzoei, A., Rafraf, M., Niromanesh, S., Farzadi, L., Narimani, F., & Doostan, F. (2018). Effects of cinnamon supplementation on antioxidant status and serum lipids in women with polycystic ovary syndrome. *Journal of Traditional and Complementary Medicine*, *8*(1), 128–133. doi:10.1016/j.jtcme.2017.04.008 PMID:29322000

Bösenberg, L. H., & Van Zyl, D. G. (2008). The mechanism of action of oral antidiabetic drugs: A review of recent literature. *Journal of Endocrinology. Metabolism and Diabetes of South Africa*, *13*(3), 80–88.

Bosshart, H., & Heinzelmann, M. (2007). Targeting bacterial endotoxin: Two sides of a coin. *Annals of the New York Academy of Sciences*, *1096*(1), 1–17. doi:10.1196/annals.1397.064 PMID:17405910

Bouzakri, K., Roques, M., Gual, P., Espinosa, S., Guebre-Egziabher, F., Riou, J. P., Laville, M., le Marchand-Brustel, Y., Tanti, J. F., & Vidal, H. (2003). Reduced activation of phosphatidylinositol-3 kinase and increased serine 636 phosphorylation of insulin receptor substrate-1 in primary culture of skeletal muscle cells from patients with type 2 diabetes. *Diabetes*, *52*(6), 1319–1325. doi:10.2337/diabetes.52.6.1319 PMID:12765939

Brabletz, T. (2012). To differentiate or not—Routes towards metastasis. *Nature Reviews. Cancer*, *12*(6), 425–436. doi:10.1038/nrc3265 PMID:22576165

Brahmanaidu, P., Uddandrao, V. V. S., Sasikumar, V., Naik, R. R., Pothani, S., Begum, M. S., Rajeshkumar, M. P., Varatharaju, C., Meriga, B., Rameshreddy, P., Kalaivani, A., & Saravanan, G. (2017). Reversal of endothelial dysfunction in aorta of streptozotocin-nicotinamide-induced type-2 diabetic rats by S-Allylcysteine. *Molecular and Cellular Biochemistry*, *432*(1-2), 25–32. doi:10.100711010-017-2994-0 PMID:28258439

Breeher, L., Gerr, F., & Fuortes, L. (2013). A case report of adult lead toxicity following use of Ayurvedic herbal medication. *Journal of Occupational Medicine and Toxicology (London, England)*, *8*(1), 26. doi:10.1186/1745-6673-8-26 PMID:24083830

Brehm, B. J., & D'Alessio, D. A. (2014). Environmental factors influencing obesity. In Endotext. MDText. com, Inc.

Broekmans, F., Knauff, E., Valkenburg, O., Laven, J., Eijkemans, M., & Fauser, B. (2006). PCOS according to the Rotterdam consensus criteria: Change in prevalence among WHO-II anovulation and association with metabolic factors. *BJOG*, *13*(10), 1210–1217. doi:10.1111/j.1471-0528.2006.01008.x PMID:16972863

Brower, V. (1998). Nutraceuticals: Poised for a healthy slice of the healthcare market? *Nature Biotechnology*, *16*(8), 728–731. doi:10.1038/nbt0898-728 PMID:9702769

Brower, V. (2005). A nutraceutical a day may keep the doctor away. *EMBO Reports*. Advance online publication. doi:10.1038j.embor.7400498 PMID:16065061

Brown, G. A., Vukovich, M. D., Martini, E. R., Kohut, M. L., Franke, W. D., Jackson, D. A., & King, D. S. (2001). Endocrine and lipid responses to chronic androstenediol-herbal supplementation in 30 to 58 year old men. *Journal of the American College of Nutrition*, *20*(5), 520–528. doi:10.1080/07315724.2001.10719061 PMID:11601567

Brown, K., DeCoffe, D., Molcan, E., & Gibson, D. L. (2012). Diet-induced dysbiosis of the intestinal microbiota and the effects on immunity and disease. *Nutrients*, *4*(8), 1095–1119. doi:10.3390/nu4081095 PMID:23016134

Brown, P. J. (1991). Culture and the evolution of obesity. *Human Nature (Hawthorne, N.Y.)*, *2*(1), 31–57. doi:10.1007/BF02692180 PMID:24222189

Bruner, B., Chad, K., & Chizen, D. (2006). Effects of exercise and nutritional counseling in women with polycystic ovary syndrome. *Applied Physiology, Nutrition, and Metabolism*, *31*(4), 384–391. doi:10.1139/h06-007 PMID:16900227

Bucher, H. C., Hengstler, P., Schindler, C., & Meier, G. (2002). N-3 polyunsaturated fatty acids in coronary heart disease: A meta-analysis of randomized controlled trials. American Journal of Medicine. https://doi.org/ doi:10.1016/S0002-9343(01)01114-7

Buhrmann, C., Kunnumakkara, A. B., Popper, B., Majeed, M., Aggarwal, B. B., & Shakibaei, M. (2020). Calebin A Potentiates the Effect of 5-FU and TNF-β (Lymphotoxin α) against Human Colorectal Cancer Cells: Potential Role of NF-κB. *International Journal of Molecular Sciences*, *21*(7), 2393. doi:10.3390/ijms21072393 PMID:32244288

Bureau, G., Longpré, F., & Martinoli, M. G. (2008). Resveratrol and quercetin, two natural polyphenols, reduce apoptotic neuronal cell death induced by neuroinflammation. *Journal of Neuroscience Research*, *86*(2), 403–410. doi:10.1002/jnr.21503 PMID:17929310

Bures, J. (2010). Small intestinal bacterial overgrowth syndrome. *World Journal of Gastroenterology*, *16*(24), 2978–2990. doi:10.3748/wjg.v16.i24.2978 PMID:20572300

Bu, T., Liu, M., Zheng, L., Guo, Y., & Lin, X. (2010). α-Glucosidase inhibition and the in vivo hypoglycemic effect of butyl-isobutyl-phthalate derived from the Laminaria japonica rhizoid. *Phytotherapy Research*, *24*(11), 1588–1591. doi:10.1002/ptr.3139 PMID:21031613

Byard, R. W. (2017, February 6). *What risks do herbal products pose to the Australian community?* The Medical Journal of Australia. https://www.mja.com.au/journal/2017/206/2/what-risks-do-herbal-products-pose-australian-community

Cai, L., Wan, D., & Yi, F. (2017). Purification, preliminary characterisation and hepatoprotective effects of polysaccharides from dandelion root. *Molecules (Basel, Switzerland)*, *22*(9), 1409. doi:10.3390/molecules22091409 PMID:28841174

Calvert, J. W., & Lefer, D. J. (2009). Myocardial protection by nitrite. *Cardiovascular Research*, *83*(2), 195–203. doi:10.1093/cvr/cvp079 PMID:19251721

Cano, A., Pérez-Moreno, M. A., Rodrigo, I., Locascio, A., Blanco, M. J., del Barrio, M. G., & Nieto, M. A. (2000). The transcription factor snail controls epithelial–mesenchymal transitions by repressing E-cadherin expression. *Nature Cell Biology*, *2*(2), 76–83. doi:10.1038/35000025 PMID:10655586

Cantorna, M. T., Zhu, Y., Froicu, M., & Wittke, A. (2004). Vitamin D status, 1,25-dihydroxyvitamin D3, and the immune system. *The American Journal of Clinical Nutrition*, *80*(6Suppl), 1717S–1720S. doi:10.1093/ajcn/80.6.1717S PMID:15585793

Capasso, R., Izzo, A. A., Pinto, L., Bifulco, T., Vitobello, C., & Mascolo, N. (2000). Phytotherapy and quality of herbal medicines. *Fitoterapia*, *71*, S58–S65. doi:10.1016/S0367-326X(00)00173-8 PMID:10930714

Capurso, G., Signoretti, M., Archibugi, L., Stigliano, S., & Delle Fave, G. (2016). Systematic review and meta-analysis: Small intestinal bacterial overgrowth in chronic pancreatitis. *United European Gastroenterology Journal*, *4*(5), 697–705. doi:10.1177/2050640616630117 PMID:27733912

Carding, S., Verbeke, K., Vipond, D. T., Corfe, B. M., & Owen, L. J. (2015). Dysbiosis of the gut microbiota in disease. *Microbial Ecology in Health and Disease*, *26*(0), 26191. doi:10.3402/mehd.v26.26191 PMID:25651997

Carmina, E. (2004). Diagnosis of polycystic ovary syndrome: From NIH criteria to ESHRE-ASRM guidelines. *Minerva Ginecologica*, *56*, 1–6. PMID:14973405

Carrizzo, A., Puca, A., Damato, A., Marino, M., Franco, E., Pompeo, F., ... Trimarco, V. (2013). Resveratrol improves vascular function in patients with hypertension and dyslipidemia by modulating NO metabolism. *Hypertension*, *62*(2), 359–366. doi:10.1161/HYPERTENSIONAHA.111.01009 PMID:23753407

Cartea, M. E., & Velasco, P. (2008). Glucosinalates in Brasscia foods: Bioavailability in food and significance for human health. *Phytochemistry Reviews*, *7*(2), 213–229. doi:10.100711101-007-9072-2

Casanova, E., Salvado, J., Crescenti, A., & Gibert-Ramos, A. (2019). Epigallocatechin gallate modulates muscle homeostasis in type 2 diabetes and obesity by targeting energetic and redox pathways: A narrative review. *International Journal of Molecular Sciences*, *20*(3), 532. doi:10.3390/ijms20030532 PMID:30691224

Cassidy-Vu, Joe, & Kirk. (2016). Role of Statin Drugs for Polycystic Ovary Syndrome. *Journal of Family & Reproductive Health*, *10*(4), 165–175. PMID:28546815

Castellarin, S. D., & Di Gaspero, G. (2007). Transcriptional control of anthocyanin biosynthetic genes in extreme phenotypes for berry pigmentation of naturally occurring grapevines. *BMC Plant Biology*, *7*(1), 1–10. doi:10.1186/1471-2229-7-46 PMID:17760970

Castrogiovanni, P., Trovato, F. M., Loreto, C., Nsir, H., Szychlinska, M. A., & Musumeci, G. (2016). Nutraceutical supplements in the management and prevention of osteoarthritis. *International Journal of Molecular Sciences*, *17*(12), 2042. doi:10.3390/ijms17122042 PMID:27929434

CDC. (2004). Lead poisoning associated with Ayurvedic medications – five states, 2000–2003. *MMWR. Morbidity and Mortality Weekly Report*, *53*, 582–584. PMID:15241300

CDC. (2019). *Heart disease facts. Division for heart disease and stroke prevention*. National Center for Chronic Disease prevention and Health Promotion.

Cedars, M., & Jaffe, R. B. (2005). Infertility and women. *The Journal of Clinical Endocrinology and Metabolism*, *90*(4), E2. doi:10.1210/jcem.90.4.9997

Cellular, V., Biology, D. & Gen, H. (2018). *In vitro evaluation of combination of EGCG and Erlotinib with classical chemotherapeutics on JAR cells*. Academic Press.

Cerf-Bensussan, N., & Gaboriau-Routhiau, V. (2010). The immune system and the gut microbiota: Friends or foes? *Nature Reviews. Immunology*, *10*(10), 735–744. doi:10.1038/nri2850 PMID:20865020

Cersosimo, E., & DeFronzo, R. (2006). Insulin resistance and endothelial dysfunction: The road map to cardiovascular diseases. *Diabetes/Metabolism Research and Reviews*, *22*(6), 423–436. doi:10.1002/dmrr.634 PMID:16506274

Chan, C. H., Ngoh, G. C., & Yusoff, R. (2012). A brief review on anti diabetic plants: Global distribution, active ingredients, extraction techniques and acting mechanisms. *Pharmacognosy Reviews*, *6*(11), 22. doi:10.4103/0973-7847.95854 PMID:22654401

Chandra, P. (2017). *Sulforaphane increases the efficacy of anti- androgens by rapidly decreasing androgen receptor levels in prostate cancer cells Sulforaphane increases the efficacy of anti-androgens by rapidly decreasing androgen receptor levels in prostate cancer cells*. Academic Press.

Chandra, A. K., & De, N. (2010). Goitrogenic/antithyroidal potential of green tea extract in relation to catechin in rats. *Food and Chemical Toxicology*, *48*(8-9), 2304–2311. doi:10.1016/j.fct.2010.05.064 PMID:20561943

Chandrasekaran, C. V., Vijayalakshmi, M. A., Prakash, K., Bansal, V. S., Meenakshi, J., & Amit, A. (2012). Herbal Approach for Obesity Management Review Article. *American Journal of Plant Sciences*, *3*(No.7A), 1003–1014. doi:10.4236/ajps.2012.327119

Chang, C.-C., Lin, K.-Y., Peng, K.-Y., Day, Y.-J., & Hung, L.-M. (2015). Resveratrol exerts anti-obesity effects in high-fat diet obese mice and displays differential dosage effects on cytotoxicity, differentiation, and lipolysis in 3T3-L1 cells. *Endocrine Journal*, EJ15–EJ0545. PMID:26698690

Chang, H. Y., Kao, M. C., Way, T. D., Ho, C. T., & Fu, E. (2011). Diosgenin suppresses hepatocyte growth factor (HGF)-induced epithelial–mesenchymal transition by down-regulation of Mdm2 and vimentin. *Journal of Agricultural and Food Chemistry*, *59*(10), 5357–5363. doi:10.1021/jf200598w PMID:21504235

Chang, J. Y., Antonopoulos, D. A., Kalra, A., Tonelli, A., Khalife, W. T., Schmidt, T. M., & Young, V. B. (2008). Decreased diversity of the fecal Microbiome in recurrent Clostridium difficile-associated diarrhea. *The Journal of Infectious Diseases*, *197*(3), 435–438. doi:10.1086/525047 PMID:18199029

Chang, S. H., Liu, C. J., Kuo, C. H., Chen, H., Lin, W.-Y., Teng, K.-Y., Chang, S.-W., Tsai, C.-H., Tsai, F.-J., Huang, C.-Y., Tzang, B.-S., & Kuo, W.-W. (2011). Garlic oil alleviates MAPKs- and IL-6-mediated diabetes-related cardiac hypertrophy in STZ-induced DM rats. *Evidence-Based Complementary and Alternative Medicine*, *950150*, 1–11. Advance online publication. doi:10.1093/ecam/neq075 PMID:21792366

Chan, H.-K., & Ismail, S. (2014). Side Effects of Chemotherapy among Cancer Patients in a Malaysian General Hospital: Experiences, Perceptions and Informational Needs from Clinical Pharmacists. *Asian Pacific Journal of Cancer Prevention*, *15*(13), 5305–5309. doi:10.7314/APJCP.2014.15.13.5305 PMID:25040993

Chan, K. (2003). Some aspects of toxic contaminants in herbal medicines. *Chemosphere*, *52*(9), 1361–1371. doi:10.1016/S0045-6535(03)00471-5 PMID:12867165

Charanraj, N., Venkateswararao, P., Vasudha, B., & Narender, B. (2019). Phytopharmacology of Chloroxylon swietenia: A review. *Journal of Drug Delivery and Therapeutics*, *9*(1), 273–278. doi:10.22270/jddt.v9i1.2188

Chassaing, B., Koren, O., Goodrich, J. K., Poole, A. C., Srinivasan, S., Ley, R. E., & Gewirtz, A. T. (2015). Dietary emulsifiers impact the mouse gut microbiota promoting colitis and metabolic syndrome. *Nature*, *519*(7541), 92–96. doi:10.1038/nature14232 PMID:25731162

Chassaing, B., Van de Wiele, T., De Bodt, J., Marzorati, M., & Gewirtz, A. T. (2017). Dietary emulsifiers directly alter human microbiota composition and gene expression ex vivo potentiating intestinal inflammation. *Gut*, *66*(8), 1414–1427. doi:10.1136/gutjnl-2016-313099 PMID:28325746

Chaturvedi, S., Sharma, P. K., Garg, V. K., & Bansal, M. (2011). Role of nutraceuticals in health promotion. *International Journal of Pharm Tech Research.*

Chaudhari, S. P., Tam, A. Y., & Barr, J. A. (2015). Curcumin: A contact allergen. *The Journal of Clinical and Aesthetic Dermatology*, *8*(11), 43.

Chaudhury, A., Duvoor, C., Reddy Dendi, V. S., Kraleti, S., Chada, A., Ravilla, R., ... Sasapu, A. (2017). Clinical review of antidiabetic drugs: Implications for type 2 diabetes mellitus management. *Frontiers in Endocrinology*, *8*, 6. doi:10.3389/fendo.2017.00006 PMID:28167928

Chauhan, A., Semwal, D. K., Mishra, S. P., & Semwal, R. B. (2017). Ayurvedic concept of Shatkriyakala: Traditional knowledge of cancer pathogenesis and therapy. *Journal of Integrative Medicine*, *15*(2), 88–94. doi:10.1016/S2095-4964(17)60311-X

Chauhan, N. S., & Dixit, V. K. (2008). Spermatogenic activity of rhi-zomes of *Curculigo orchioides* gaertn in male rats. *International Journal of Applied Research in Natural Products*, *1*(2), 26–31.

Chauhan, N. S., Rao, C. V., & Dixit, V. K. (2007). Effect of Curculigo orchioides rhizomes on sexual behaviour of male rats. *Fitoterapia*, *78*(7-8), 530–534. doi:10.1016/j.fitote.2007.06.005 PMID:17643866

Chauhan, N. S., Sharma, V., Dixit, V. K., & Thakur, M. (2014). A Review on Plants Used for Improvement of Sexual Performance and Virility. *BioMed Research International*, *2014*, 1–19. doi:10.1155/2014/868062 PMID:25215296

Cheang, K. I., Nestler, J. E., & Futterweit, W. (2008). Risk of cardiovascular events in mothers of women with polycystic ovary syndrome. *Endocrine Practice*, *14*(9), 1084–1094. doi:10.4158/EP.14.9.1084 PMID:19158047

Chen, B., Kim, J. J.-W., Zhang, Y., Du, L., & Dai, N. (2018). Prevalence and predictors of small intestinal bacterial overgrowth in irritable bowel syndrome: A systematic review and meta-analysis. *Journal of Gastroenterology*, *53*(7), 807–818. doi:10.100700535-018-1476-9 PMID:29761234

Chen, D., Zhong, J., Chen, S., Zhang, Y., Zhang, W., & Wang, G. (2013). Effect of supplemented Wuzi Yanzong decoction on the quality of sperm and secretion of seminal fructose. *Journal of Traditional Chinese Medicine*, *54*, 401–404.

Cheng, T. O. (2006). Obesity is a global challenge. *The American Journal of Medicine*, *119*(6), e11. doi:10.1016/j.amjmed.2006.04.006 PMID:16750947

Cheng, X., Yao, X., Xu, S., Pan, J., Yu, H., Bao, J., Guan, H., Lu, R., & Zhang, L. (2018). Punicalagin induces senescent growth arrest in human papillary thyroid carcinoma BCPAP cells via NF-kappaB signaling pathway. *Biomedicine and Pharmacotherapy*, *103*, 490–498. doi:10.1016/j.biopha.2018.04.074 PMID:29677534

Chen, H. W., Chiang, W. J., & Chen, C. L. (2015). Characteristics and Prescription Patterns of Traditional Chinese Medicine in Polycystic Ovary Syndrome. *Journal of Chengdu University of TCM.*, *38*, 120–123.

Chen, H. Y., Lin, Y. H., Su, I. H., Chen, Y. C., Yang, S. H., & Chen, J. L. (2014). Investigation on Chinese herbal medicine for primary dysmenorrhea: Implication from a nationwide prescription database in Taiwan. *Complementary Therapies in Medicine*, *22*(1), 116–125. doi:10.1016/j.ctim.2013.11.012 PMID:24559826

Chen, J., Duan, Y., Zhang, X., Ye, Y., Ge, B., & Chen, J. (2015). Genistein induces apoptosis by the inactivation of the IGF-1R/p-Akt signaling pathway in MCF-7 human breast cancer cells. *Food & Function*, *6*(3), 995–1000. doi:10.1039/C4FO01141D PMID:25675448

Chen, J.-T., Tominaga, K., Sato, Y., Anzai, H., & Matsuoka, R. (2010). Maitake mushroom (Grifola frondosa) extract induces ovulation in patients with polycystic ovary syndrome: A possible monotherapy and a combination therapy after failure with first-line clomiphene citrate. *Journal of Alternative and Complementary Medicine (New York, N.Y.)*, *16*(12), 1295–1299. doi:10.1089/acm.2009.0696 PMID:21034160

Chen, P. (2013). Genistein reinforces the inhibitory effect of Cisplatin on liver cancer recurrence and metastasis after curative hepatectomy. *Asian Pacific journal of cancer prevention*, *14*(2), 759–764. PMID:23621233

Chen, Q., Wang, E., Ma, L., & Zhai, P. (2012). Dietary resveratrol increases the expression of hepatic 7α-hydroxylase and ameliorates hypercholesterolemia in high-fat fed C57BL/6J mice. *Lipids in Health and Disease*, *11*(1), 56. doi:10.1186/1476-511X-11-56 PMID:22607622

Chen, Y.-R., Yi, F.-F., Li, X.-Y., Wang, C.-Y., Chen, L., Yang, X.-C., ... Cai, J. (2008). Resveratrol attenuates ventricular arrhythmias and improves the long-term survival in rats with myocardial infarction. *Cardiovascular Drugs and Therapy*, *22*(6), 479–485. doi:10.100710557-008-6141-8 PMID:18853243

Chen, Z.-P., Mitchelhill, K. I., Michell, B. J., Stapleton, D., Rodriguez-Crespo, I., Witters, L. A., ... Kemp, B. E. (1999). AMP-activated protein kinase phosphorylation of endothelial NO synthase. *FEBS Letters*, *443*(3), 285–289. doi:10.1016/S0014-5793(98)01705-0 PMID:10025949

Cheon, H., Cho, J. M., Kim, S., Baek, S. H., Lee, M. K., Kim, K. W., Yu, S. W., Solinas, G., Kim, S. S., & Lee, M. S. (2010). Role of JNK activation in pancreatic beta-cell death by streptozotocin. *Molecular and Cellular Endocrinology*, *321*(2), 131–137. doi:10.1016/j.mce.2010.02.016 PMID:20176078

Chittenden, B. G., Fullerton, G., Maheshwari, A., & Bhattacharya, S. (2009). Polycystic ovary syndrome and the risk of gynaecological cancer: A systematic review. *Reproductive Biomedicine Online*, *19*(3), 398–405. doi:10.1016/S1472-6483(10)60175-7 PMID:19778486

Cho, A. S., Jeon, S. M., Kim, M. J., Yeo, J., Seo, K. I., Choi, M. S., & Lee, M. K. (2010). Chlorogenic acid exhibits anti-obesity property and improves lipid metabolism in high-fat diet-induced-obese mice. *Food and Chemical Toxicology*, *48*(3), 937–943. doi:10.1016/j.fct.2010.01.003 PMID:20064576

Choe, S. C., Kim, H. S., Jeong, T. S., Bok, S. H., & Park, Y. B. (2001). Naringin has an antiatherogenic effect with the inhibition of intercellular adhesion molecule-1 in hypercholesterolemic rabbits. *Journal of Cardiovascular Pharmacology*, *38*(6), 947–955. doi:10.1097/00005344-200112000-00017 PMID:11707699

Cho, I. (2012). Effects of Panax ginseng in neurodegenerative diseases. *Journal of Ginseng Research*, *36*(4), 342–353. doi:10.5142/jgr.2012.36.4.342 PMID:23717136

Choi, J. H., Jang, M., Kim, E.-J., Lee, M. J., Park, K. S., Kim, S.-H., In, J.-G., Kwak, Y.-S., Park, D.-H., Cho, S.-S., Nah, S.-Y., Cho, I.-H., & Bae, C.-S. (2019). Korean Red Ginseng alleviates dehydroepiandrosterone-induced polycystic ovarian syndrome in rats via its antiinflammatory and antioxidant activities. *Journal of Ginseng Research*. Advance online publication. doi:10.1016/j.jgr.2019.08.007

Choi, Y. J., Park, S. Y., Kim, J. Y., Won, K. C., Kim, B. R., Son, J. K., Lee, S. H., & Kim, Y. W. (2013). Combined treatment of betulinic acid, a PTP1B inhibitor, with *Orthosiphon stamineus* extract decreases body weight in high-fat-fed mice. *Journal of Medicinal Food*, *16*(1), 2–8. doi:10.1089/jmf.2012.2384 PMID:23256448

Cho, J., Park, W., Lee, S., Ahn, W., & Lee, Y. (2004). Ginsenoside-Rb1 from Panax ginseng C.A. Meyer activates estrogen receptor-alpha and -beta, independent of ligand binding. *The Journal of Clinical Endocrinology and Metabolism*, *89*(7), 3510–3515. doi:10.1210/jc.2003-031823 PMID:15240639

Chojnacka, K., Saeid, A., Witkowska, Z., & Tuhy, L. (2012). Biologically active compounds in seaweed extracts-the prospects for the application. *The Open Conference Proceedings Journal*, *3*(1), 20–28. doi:10.2174/1876326X01203020020

Choo, C. Y., Sulong, N. Y., Man, F., & Wong, T. W. (2012). Vitexin and isovitexin from the Leaves of Ficus deltoidea with in-vivo?? -glucosidase inhibition. *Journal of Ethnopharmacology*, *142*(3), 776–781. doi:10.1016/j.jep.2012.05.062 PMID:22683902

Chopade, V., Phatak, A., Upaganlawar, A., & Tankar, A. (2008). Green tea (Camellia sinensis): Chemistry, traditional, medicinal uses and its pharmacological activities - A review. *Phcog Rev.*, *2*, 157–162.

Chopra, R. N. (2006). *Chopras indigenous drugs of India*. Academic Publishers.

Choudhury, H., Pandey, M., Hua, C., Mun, C., Jing, J., Kong, L., Ern, L. Y., Ashraf, N. A., Kit, S. W., Yee, T. S., Pichika, M. R., Gorain, B., & Kesharwani, P. (2018). An update on natural compounds in the remedy of diabetes mellitus: A systematic review. *Journal of Traditional and Complementary Medicine*, *8*(3), 361–376. doi:10.1016/j.jtcme.2017.08.012 PMID:29992107

Chou, L. F., Chen, C. Y., Yang, W. H., Chen, C. C., Chang, J. L., Leu, Y. L., & Wang, T. H. (2020). Suppression of Hepatocellular Carcinoma Progression through FOXM1 and EMT Inhibition via Hydroxygenkwanin-InducedmiR-320a Expression. *Biomolecules*, *10*(1), 20. doi:10.3390/biom10010020

Chou, T.-C., & Talalay, P. (1984). Quantitative analysis of dose-effect relationships: The combined effects of multiple drugs or enzyme inhibitors. *Advances in Enzyme Regulation*, *22*, 27–55. doi:10.1016/0065-2571(84)90007-4 PMID:6382953

Chua, S., Arulkumaran, S., Lim, I., Selamat, N., & Ratnam, S. S. (1994). Influence of breastfeeding and nipple stimulation on postpartum uterine activity. *British Journal of Obstetrics and Gynaecology*, *101*(9), 804–805. doi:10.1111/j.1471-0528.1994.tb11950.x PMID:7947531

Chueh, W.-H., & Lin, J.-Y. (2011). Berberine, an isoquinoline alkaloid in herbal plants, protects pancreatic islets and serum lipids in nonobese diabetic mice. *Journal of Agricultural and Food Chemistry*, *59*(14), 8021–8027. doi:10.1021/jf201627w PMID:21696141

Chuengsamarn, S., Rattanamongkolgul, S., Luechapudiporn, R., Phisalaphong, C., & Jirawatnotai, S. (2012). Curcumin Extract for Prevention of Type 2 Diabetes. *Diabetes Care*, *35*(11), 2121–2127. doi:10.2337/dc12-0116 PMID:22773702

Chulada, P. C., Arbes, S. J. Jr, Dunson, D., & Zeldin, D. C. (2003). Breast-feeding and the prevalence of asthma and wheeze in children: Analyses from the Third National Health and Nutrition Examination Survey, 1988 –1994. *The Journal of Allergy and Clinical Immunology*, *111*(2), 328–336. doi:10.1067/mai.2003.127 PMID:12589353

Chung, S. H., Choi, C. G., & Park, S. H. (2001). Comparisons between white ginseng radix and rootlet for antidiabetic activity and mechanism in KKAy mice. *Archives of Pharmacal Research*, *24*(3), 214–218. doi:10.1007/BF02978260 PMID:11440080

Chung, S. S., & Vadgama, J. V. (2015). Curcumin and epigallocatechin gallate inhibit the cancer stem cell phenotype via down-regulation of STAT3-NFkappaB signaling. *Anticancer Research*, *35*(1), 39–46. PMID:25550533

Chu, W., & Phang, S. (2016). Marine algae as a potential source for Anti-Obesity Agents. *Marine Drugs*, *14*(12), 222. doi:10.3390/md14120222 PMID:27941599

Cianfrocca, C., Pelliccia, F., Auriti, A., & Santini, M. (2002). Ginkgo biloba-induced frequent ventricular arrhythmia. *Italian Heart Journal*, *3*, 689–691.

Cicero, A. F., & Baggioni, A. (2016). Berberine and its role in chronic disease. *Advances in Experimental Medicine and Biology*, *928*, 27–45. doi:10.1007/978-3-319-41334-1_2 PMID:27671811

Cicero, A. F., & Colletti, A. (2016). Combination of phytomedicines with different lipid lowering activity for dyslipidemia management: The available clinical data. *Phytomedicine*, *23*(11), 1113–1118. doi:10.1016/j.phymed.2015.10.011 PMID:26621556

Ciesielski, T. H., Bartlett, J., & Williams, S. M. (2019). Omega-3 polyunsaturated fatty acid intake norms and preterm birth rate: A cross-sectional analysis of 184 countries. *BMJ Open*, *9*(4), e027249. doi:10.1136/bmjopen-2018-027249 PMID:31005937

Clapp, M., Aurora, N., Herrera, L., Bhatia, M., Wilen, E., & Wakefield, S. (2017). Gut microbiota's effect on mental health: The gut-brain axis. *Clinics and Practice*, *7*(4), 987. doi:10.4081/cp.2017.987 PMID:29071061

Clarke, R. E., Dordevic, A., Tan, S., Ryan, L., & Coughlan, M. (2016). Dietary Advanced Glycation End Products and Risk Factors for Chronic Disease: A Systematic Review of Randomised Controlled Trials. *Nutrients*, *8*(3), 125. doi:10.3390/nu8030125 PMID:26938557

Clauw, D. J. (2009). Fibromyalgia: An overview. *The American Journal of Medicine*, *122*(12Suppl), S3–S13. doi:10.1016/j.amjmed.2009.09.006 PMID:19962494

Clinic, C. (2016). *Insulin Pumps*. Cleveland Clinic. Available at: https://my.clevelandclinic.org/health/articles/9811-insulin-pumps

Cochi, S. L., Fleming, D. W., Hightower, A. W., Limpakarnjanarat, K., Facklam, R. R., David Smith, J., ... Broome, C. V. (1986). Primary invasive Haemophilus influenzae type b disease: A population-based assessment of risk factors. *The Journal of Pediatrics*, *108*(6), 887–896. doi:10.1016/S0022-3476(86)80922-2 PMID:3712153

Collet, T. H., Bauer, D. C., Cappola, A. R., Asvold, B. O., Weiler, S., Vittinghoff, E., ... Thyroid Studies, C. (2014). Thyroid antibody status, subclinical hypothyroidism, and the risk of coronary heart disease: An individual participant data analysis. *The Journal of Clinical Endocrinology and Metabolism*, *99*(9), 3353–3362. doi:10.1210/jc.2014-1250 PMID:24915118

Comijn, J., Berx, G., Vermassen, P., Verschueren, K., van Grunsven, L., Bruyneel, E., & Van Roy, F. (2001). The two-handed E box binding zinc finger protein SIP1 downregulates E-cadherin and induces invasion. *Molecular Cell*, *7*(6), 1267–1278. doi:10.1016/S1097-2765(01)00260-X PMID:11430829

Conlon, M. A., & Bird, A. R. (2014). The impact of diet and lifestyle on gut microbiota and human health. *Nutrients*, *7*(1), 17–44. doi:10.3390/nu7010017 PMID:25545101

Connor, W. E. (2000). Importance of n-3 fatty acids in health and disease. *The American Journal of Clinical Nutrition*, *71*(1Supplement), 171S–175S. doi:10.1093/ajcn/71.1.171S PMID:10617967

Cook, M. R., Luo, J., Ndiaye, M., Chen, H., & Kunnimalaiyaan, M. (2010). Xanthohumol inhibits the neuroendocrine transcription factor achaete-scute complex-like 1, suppresses proliferation, and induces phosphorylated ERK1/2 in medullary thyroid cancer. *American Journal of Surgery*, *199*(3), 315–318. doi:10.1016/j.amjsurg.2009.08.034 PMID:20226902

Cornelison, R., Llaneza, D. C., & Landen, C. N. (2017). Emerging therapeutics to overcome chemoresistance in epithelial ovarian cancer: A mini-review. *International Journal of Molecular Sciences*, *18*(10), 1–20. doi:10.3390/ijms18102171 PMID:29057791

Cory, H., Passarelli, S., Szeto, J., Tamez, M., & Mattei, J. (2018). The role of polyphenols in human health and food systems: A mini-review. *Frontiers in Nutrition*, *5*, 87. doi:10.3389/fnut.2018.00087 PMID:30298133

Costello, M. E., Ciccia, F., Willner, D., Warrington, N., Robinson, P. C., Gardiner, B., ... Brown, M. A. (2015). Brief Report: Intestinal Dysbiosis in Ankylosing Spondylitis. *Arthritis & Rheumatology (Hoboken, N.J.)*, *67*(3), 686–691. doi:10.1002/art.38967 PMID:25417597

Costello, R., & Shivkumar, A. (2019). *Sulfonylureas*. StatPearls Publishing.

Coviello, A. D., Legro, R. S., & Dunaif, A. (2006). Adolescent girls with polycystic ovary syndrome have an increased risk of the metabolic syndrome associated with increasing androgen levels independent of obesity and insulin resistance. *The Journal of Clinical Endocrinology and Metabolism*, *91*(2), 492–497. doi:10.1210/jc.2005-1666 PMID:16249280

Craig, M. E., Hattersley, A., & Donaghue, K. C. (2009). Definition, epidemiology and classification of diabetes in children and adolescents. *Pediatric Diabetes*, *10*, 3–12. doi:10.1111/j.1399-5448.2009.00568.x PMID:19754613

Crosignani, P. (2001). A. Polycystic ovarian disease: Heritability and heterogeneity. *Human Reproduction Update*, *7*(1), 3–7. doi:10.1093/humupd/7.1.3 PMID:11212071

Crozier, A., Jaganath, I. B., & Clifford, M. N. (2009). Dietary phenolics: Chemistry, bioavailability and effects on health. *Natural Product Reports*, *26*(8), 1001–1043. doi:10.1039/b802662a PMID:19636448

Csige, I., Ujvárosy, D., Szabó, Z., Lőrincz, I., Paragh, G., Harangi, M., & Somodi, S. (2018). The impact of obesity on the cardiovascular system. *Journal of Diabetes Research*, *2018*, 2018. doi:10.1155/2018/3407306 PMID:30525052

Csiszar, A., Labinskyy, N., Pinto, J. T., Ballabh, P., Zhang, H., Losonczy, G., ... Zhang, C. (2009). Resveratrol induces mitochondrial biogenesis in endothelial cells. *American Journal of Physiology. Heart and Circulatory Physiology*, *297*(1), H13–H20. doi:10.1152/ajpheart.00368.2009 PMID:19429820

Da Costa, J. P. (2017). A current look at nutraceuticals- Key concepts and future prospects. *Trends in Food Science & Technology*, *62*, 68–78. doi:10.1016/j.tifs.2017.02.010

Dabaghian, F. H., Kamalinejad, M., Shojaei, A., & Fard, M. A. (2012). Presenting anti-diabetic plants in Iranian traditional medicine. *Journal of Diabetes and Endocrinology*, *3*(5), 70–76. doi:10.5897/JDE12.004

Dai, G., Sun, B., Gong, T., Pan, Z., Meng, Q., & Ju, W. (2019). Ginsenoside Rb2 inhibits epithelial-mesenchymal transition of colorectal cancer cells by suppressing TGF-β/Smad signaling. *Phytomedicine*, *56*, 126–135. doi:10.1016/j.phymed.2018.10.025 PMID:30668333

Daliri, E.B.-M., & Lee, B.H. (2015). Current trends and future perspectives on functional foods and nutraceuticals. *Microbiology Monographs*, 221-244.

Dandu, A. M., & Inamdar, N. M. (2009). Evaluation of beneficial effects of antioxidant properties of aqueous leaf extract of *Andrographis paniculata* in STZ-induced diabetes. *Pakistan Journal of Pharmaceutical Sciences*, *22*(1), 49–52. PMID:19168420

Dang, Y.-P., Yuan, X.-Y., Tian, R., Li, D.-G., & Liu, W. (2015). Curcumin improves the paclitaxel-induced apoptosis of HPV-positive human cervical cancer cells via the NF-kappaB-p53-caspase-3 pathway. *Experimental and Therapeutic Medicine*, *9*(4), 1470–1476. doi:10.3892/etm.2015.2240 PMID:25780454

Darbre, P. D. (2017). Endocrine disruptors and obesity. *Current Obesity Reports*, *6*(1), 18–27. doi:10.100713679-017-0240-4 PMID:28205155

Dargham, S. R., Ahmed, L., Kilpatrick, E. S., & Atkin, S. L. (2017). The prevalence and metabolic characteristics of polycystic ovary syndrome in the Qatari population. *PLoS One*, *12*(7), e0181467. doi:10.1371/journal.pone.0181467 PMID:28723965

Das, B., Sarkar, N., Bishayee, A., & Sinha, D. (2019, June). Dietary phytochemicals in the regulation of epithelial to mesenchymal transition and associated enzymes: A promising anticancer therapeutic approach. *Seminars in Cancer Biology*, *56*, 196–218. doi:10.1016/j.semcancer.2018.11.007 PMID:30472212

Das, L., Bhaumik, E., Raychaudhuri, U., & Chakraborty, R. (2012). Role of nutraceuticals in human health. *Journal of Food Science and Technology*, *49*(2), 173–183. doi:10.100713197-011-0269-4 PMID:23572839

Das, L., & Vinayak, M. (2015). Long Term Effect of Curcumin in Restoration of Tumour Suppressor p53 and Phase-II Antioxidant Enzymes via Activation of Nrf2 Signalling and Modulation of Inflammation in Prevention of Cancer. *PLoS One*, *10*(4), e0124000. doi:10.1371/journal.pone.0124000 PMID:25860911

Dattner, A. M. (2003). From medical herbalism to phytotherapy in dermatology: Back to the future. *Dermatologic Therapy*, *16*(2), 106–113. doi:10.1046/j.1529-8019.2003.01618.x PMID:12919112

Daveri, E., Cremonini, E., Mastaloudis, A., Hester, S. N., Wood, S. M., Waterhouse, A. L., Anderson, M., Fraga, C. G., & Oteiza, P. I. (2018). Cyanidin and delphinidin modulate inflammation and altered redox signaling improving insulin resistance in high fat-fed mice. *Redox Biology*, *18*, 16–24. doi:10.1016/j.redox.2018.05.012 PMID:29890336

David, L. A., Maurice, C. F., Carmody, R. N., Gootenberg, D. B., Button, J. E., Wolfe, B. E., ... Turnbaugh, P. J. (2014). Diet rapidly and reproducibly alters the human gut microbiome. *Nature*, *505*(7484), 559–563. doi:10.1038/nature12820 PMID:24336217

Dayani Siriwardene, S. A., Karunathilaka, L. P. A., Kodituwakku, N. D., & Karunarathne, Y. A. U. D. (2010). Clinical efficacy of Ayurveda treatment regimen on Subfertility with Poly Cystic Ovarian Syndrome (PCOS). *Ayu*, *31*(1), 24–27. doi:10.4103/0974-8520.68203 PMID:22131680

De Craene, B., & Berx, G. (2013). Regulatory networks defining EMT during cancer initiation and progression. *Nature Reviews. Cancer*, *13*(2), 97–110. doi:10.1038/nrc3447 PMID:23344542

De Filippis, F., Pellegrini, N., Vannini, L., Jeffery, I. B., La Storia, A., Laghi, L., ... Ercolini, D. (2016). High-level adherence to a Mediterranean diet beneficially impacts the gut microbiota and associated metabolome. *Gut*, *65*(11), 1812–1821. doi:10.1136/gutjnl-2015-309957 PMID:26416813

De Filippo, C., Cavalieri, D., Di Paola, M., Ramazzotti, M., Poullet, J. B., Massart, S., ... Lionetti, P. (2010). Impact of diet in shaping gut microbiota revealed by a comparative study in children from Europe and rural Africa. *Proceedings of the National Academy of Sciences of the United States of America*, *107*(33), 14691–14696. doi:10.1073/pnas.1005963107 PMID:20679230

de Vrese, M., & Schrezenmeir, J. (2008). Probiotics, prebiotics, and synbiotics. *Advances in Biochemical Engineering/Biotechnology*, *111*, 1–66. doi:10.1007/10_2008_097 PMID:18461293

Dehghan, A., Esfandiari, A., & Bigdeli, S. M. (2012). Alternative Treatment of Ovarian Cysts with Tribulus terrestris Extract: A Rat Model. *Reproduction in Domestic Animals*, *47*(1), 12–15. doi:10.1111/j.1439-0531.2011.01877.x PMID:21883512

Deitch, E. A. (1990). Bacterial translocation of the gut flora. *The Journal of Trauma*, *30*(12Suppl), S184–S189. doi:10.1097/00005373-199012001-00037 PMID:2254980

Delzenne, N. M., Neyrinck, A. M., Bäckhed, F., & Cani, P. D. (2011). Targeting gut microbiota in obesity: Effects of prebiotics and probiotics. *Nature Reviews. Endocrinology*, *7*(11), 639–646. doi:10.1038/nrendo.2011.126 PMID:21826100

Delzenne, N. M., Neyrinck, A. M., & Cani, P. D. (2013). Gut microbiota and metabolic disorders: How prebiotic can work? *British Journal of Nutrition*, *109*(S2), S81–S85. doi:10.1017/S0007114512004047 PMID:23360884

Deng, G. F., Shen, C., Xu, X. R., Kuang, R. D., Guo, Y. J., Zeng, L. S., ... Li, H. B. (2012). Potential of fruit wastes as natural resources of bioactive compounds. *International Journal of Molecular Sciences*, *13*(7), 8308–8323. doi:10.3390/ijms13078308 PMID:22942704

Deng, J., Liu, Y., Duan, Z., Zhu, C., Hui, J., Mi, Y., Ma, P., Ma, X., Fan, D., & Yang, H. (2017). Protopanaxadiol and protopanaxatriol-type saponins ameliorate glucose and lipid metabolism in type 2 diabetes mellitus in high-fat Diet/Streptozocin-induced mice. *Frontiers in Pharmacology*, *8*, 506. doi:10.3389/fphar.2017.00506 PMID:28824430

Deng, M., Liu, B., Song, H., Yu, R., Zou, D., Chen, Y., & Lv, Q. (2020). β-Elemene Inhibits the Metastasis of Multidrug-Resistant Gastric Cancer Cells Through miR-1323/Cbl-b/EGFR Pathway. *Phytomedicine*, *69*, 153184. doi:10.1016/j.phymed.2020.153184 PMID:32199253

Deng, R. (2012). A Review of the Hypoglycemic Effects of Five Commonly Used Herbal Food Supplements. *Recent Patents on Food, Nutrition & Agriculture*, *4*(1), 50–60. doi:10.2174/1876142911204010050 PMID:22329631

Deng, X. W., & Xie, N. (2014). Progress of berberine for treatment of type 2 diabetes. *Zhongguo Zhongyao Zazhi*, *39*(8), 1374–1378. PMID:25039167

Deng, Y. X., Zhang, X. J., Shi, Q. Z., Chen, Y. S., Qiu, X. M., & Chen, B. (2012). Anti-hyperglycemic effects and mechanism of traditional Chinese medicine Huanglian Wan in streptozocin-induced diabetic rats. *Journal of Ethnopharmacology*, *144*(2), 425–432. doi:10.1016/j.jep.2012.09.039 PMID:23036812

Deo, P., Hewawasam, E., Karakoulakis, A., Claudie, D. J., Nelson, R., Simpson, B. S., Smith, N. M., & Semple, S. J. (2016). In vitro inhibitory activities of selected Australian medicinal plant extracts against protein glycation, angiotensin converting enzyme (ACE) and digestive enzymes linked to type II diabetes. *BMC Complementary and Alternative Medicine*, *16*(1), 435. doi:10.118612906-016-1421-5 PMID:27809834

Depenbusch, M., Eckardstein, S. V., Simoni, M., & Nieschlag, E. (2002). Maintenance of spermatogenesis in hypogonadotropic hypogonadal men with human chorionic gonadotropin alone. *European Journal of Endocrinology*, *147*(5), 617–624. doi:10.1530/eje.0.1470617 PMID:12444893

Desai, A. G., Qazi, G. N., Ganju, R. K., El-Tamer, M., Singh, J., Saxena, A. K., & Bhat, H. K. (2008). Medicinal plants and cancer chemoprevention. *Current Drug Metabolism*, *9*(7), 581–591. doi:10.2174/138920008785821657 PMID:18781909

Desai, M. Y., Dalal, D., Santos, R. D., Carvalho, J. A., Nasir, K., & Blumenthal, R. S. (2006). Association of body mass index, metabolic syndrome, and leukocyte count. *The American Journal of Cardiology*, *97*(6), 835–838. doi:10.1016/j.amjcard.2005.10.021 PMID:16516585

Desmet, P., Keller, K., Hansel, R., & Chandler, R. (1993). *Adverse effects of herbal drugs 2*. Spriger-Verlag. doi:10.1007/978-3-642-48906-8

Devendra, D., Liu, E., & Eisenbarth, G. S. (2004). Type 1 diabetes: Recent developments. *British Medical Journal*, *328*(7442), 750–754. doi:10.1136/bmj.328.7442.750 PMID:15044291

Devkota, S., & Chang, E. B. (2015). Interactions between Diet, Bile Acid Metabolism, Gut Microbiota, and Inflammatory Bowel Diseases. *Digestive Diseases (Basel, Switzerland)*, *33*(3), 351–356. doi:10.1159/000371687 PMID:26045269

Dghaim, R., Al Khatib, S., Rasool, H., & Khan, M. A. (2015). Determination of Heavy Metals Concentration in Traditional. Herbs Commonly Consumed in the United Arab Emirates. Journal of Environmental and Public Health. Hindawi Publishing Corporation.

Dhuley, J. N. (1998). Effect of ashwagandha on lipid peroxidation in stress induced animals. *Journal of Ethnopharmacology*, *60*(2), 173–178. doi:10.1016/S0378-8741(97)00151-7 PMID:9582008

Di Cosmo, C., McLellan, N., Liao, X. H., Khanna, K. K., Weiss, R. E., Papp, L., & Refetoff, S. (2009). Clinical and molecular characterization of a novel selenocysteine insertion sequence-binding protein 2 (SBP2) gene mutation (R128X). *The Journal of Clinical Endocrinology and Metabolism*, *94*(10), 4003–4009. doi:10.1210/jc.2009-0686 PMID:19602558

Diamanti-Kandarakis, E., Argyrakopoulou, G., Economou, F., Kandaraki, E., & Koutsilieris, M. (2008). Defects in insulin signaling pathways in ovarian steroidogenesis and other tissues in polycystic ovary syndrome (PCOS). *The Journal of Steroid Biochemistry and Molecular Biology*, *109*(3-5), 242–246. doi:10.1016/j.jsbmb.2008.03.014 PMID:18440223

Diamanti-Kandarakis, E., Papavassiliou, A. G., Kandarakis, S. A., & Chrousos, G. P. (2007). Pathophysiology and types of dyslipidemia in PCOS. *Trends in Endocrinology and Metabolism*, *18*(7), 280–285. doi:10.1016/j.tem.2007.07.004 PMID:17692530

Didari, T., Solki, S., Mozaffari, S., Nikfar, S., & Abdollahi, M. (2014). A systematic review of the safety of probiotics. *Expert Opinion on Drug Safety*, *13*(2), 227–239. doi:10.1517/14740338.2014.872627 PMID:24405164

Diejomaoh, M., Jirous, J., Al-Azemi, M., Baig, S., Gupta, M., & Tallat, A. (2003). The relationship of recurrent spontaneous miscarriage with reproductive failure. *Medical Principles and Practice*, *12*(2), 107–111. doi:10.1159/000069122 PMID:12634466

Dillard, C. J., & German, J. B. (2000). Phytochemicals: Nutraceuticals and human health. *Journal of the Science of Food and Agriculture*, *80*(12), 1744–1756. doi:10.1002/1097-0010(20000915)80:12<1744::AID-JSFA725>3.0.CO;2-W

Di-lorenzo, C., Williams, C., Hainal, F., & Valenzuela, J. (1988). Pectin delays gastric emptying and increases satiety in obese subjects. *Gastroenterology*, *95*(5), 1211–1215. doi:10.1016/0016-5085(88)90352-6 PMID:3169489

Ding, H., & Petersen, W. Qu, & Baio. (2017). The prevalence of polycystic ovary syndrome in reproductive aged women of different ethnicity: a systematic review and meta-analysis. Oncotarget, 8(56), 96351–96358. PubMed

Ding, J., Xu, Y., Ma, X., An, J., Yang, X., Liu, Z., & Lin, N. (2015). Estrogenic effect of the extract of Renshen (Radix Ginseng) on reproductive tissues in immature mice. *Journal of Traditional Chinese Medicine*, *35*(4), 460–467. doi:10.1016/S0254-6272(15)30125-4 PMID:26427118

Ding, L., Jin, D., & Chen, X. (2010). Luteolin enhances insulin sensitivity via activation of PPARγ transcriptional activity in adipocytes. *The Journal of Nutritional Biochemistry*, *21*(10), 941–947. doi:10.1016/j.jnutbio.2009.07.009 PMID:19954946

Dinka, P. B., Lana, S., & Roya, O. (2015). Polycystic Ovary Syndrome: Important Underrecognized Cardiometabolic Risk Factor in Reproductive-Age Women. *International Journal of Endocrinology*, 1–17.

Diwakarla, S., Fothergill, L. J., Fakhry, J., Callaghan, B., & Furness, J. B. (2017). Heterogeneity of enterochromaffin cells within the gastrointestinal tract. *Neurogastroenterology and Motility*, *29*(6), e13101. doi:10.1111/nmo.13101 PMID:28485065

Dolinsky, V. W., Chakrabarti, S., Pereira, T. J., Oka, T., Levasseur, J., Beker, D., ... Lopaschuk, G. D. (2013). Resveratrol prevents hypertension and cardiac hypertrophy in hypertensive rats and mice. *Biochimica et Biophysica Acta (BBA)-. Molecular Basis of Disease*, *1832*(10), 1723–1733. doi:10.1016/j.bbadis.2013.05.018 PMID:23707558

Dong, H., Wang, N., Zhao, L., & Lu, F. (2012). Berberine in the treatment of type 2 diabetes mellitus: a systemic review and meta-analysis. *Evidence-based Complementary and Alternative Medicine: eCAM*, 591654. . doi:10.1155/2012/591654

Douchi, T., Oki, T., Yamasaki, H., Kuwahata, R., Nakae, M., & Nagata, Y. (2001). Relationship of androgens to muscle size and bone mineral density in women with polycystic ovary syndrome. *Obstetrics and Gynecology*, *98*(3), 445–449. PubMed

Dragomir, A., & Radulian, G. (2016). Eating habits in normal weight and obese people. *Romanian Journal of Diabetes, Nutrition, & Metabolic Diseases*, *23*(4), 387–395. doi:10.1515/rjdnmd-2016-0045

Draper, L. R., Gyure, L. A., Hall, J. G., & Robertson, D. (1983). Effect of alcohol on the integrity of the intestinal epithelium. *Gut*, *24*(5), 399–404. doi:10.1136/gut.24.5.399 PMID:6840613

Driscoll, D. A. (2000). Polycystic ovary syndrome in adolescence. *Seminars in Reproductive Medicine*, *21*(3), 301–307. PMID:14593553

Düker, E. M., Kopanski, L., Jarry, H., & Wuttke, W. (1991). Effects of extracts from Cimicifuga racemosa on gonadotropin release in menopausal women and ovariectomized rats. *Planta Medica*, *57*(5), 420–424. doi:10.1055-2006-960139 PMID:1798794

Dumitrescu, A. M., & Refetoff, S. (2013). The syndromes of reduced sensitivity to thyroid hormone. *Biochimica et Biophysica Acta*, *1830*(7), 3987–4003. doi:10.1016/j.bbagen.2012.08.005 PMID:22986150

Dunaif, A. (1999). Insulin action in the poly cystic ovary syndrome. *Endocrinology and Metabolism Clinics of North America*, *28*(2), 341–359. doi:10.1016/S0889-8529(05)70073-6 PMID:10352922

Du, Q., Hu, B., an, H.-M., Shen, K.-P., Xu, L., Deng, S., & Wei, M.-M. (2013). Synergistic anticancer effects of curcumin and resveratrol in Hepa1-6 hepatocellular carcinoma cells. *Oncology Reports*, *29*(5), 1851–1858. doi:10.3892/or.2013.2310 PMID:23446753

Du, Q., Wang, Y., Liu, C., Wang, H., Fan, H., Li, Y., Wang, J., Zhang, X., Lu, J., Ji, H., & Hu, R. (2016). Chemopreventive activity of GEN-27, a genistein derivative, in colitis-associated cancer is mediated by p65-CDX2-beta-catenin axis. *Oncotarget*, *7*(14), 17870–17884. doi:10.18632/oncotarget.7554 PMID:26910375

Duthie, G. G., Gardner, P. T., & Kyle, J. A. M. (2003). Plant polyphenols: Are they the new magic bullet? *The Proceedings of the Nutrition Society*, *62*(3), 599–603. doi:10.1079/PNS2003275 PMID:14692595

Dutta, S., Ali, K. M., Dash, S. K., & Giri, B. (2018). Role of nutraceuticals on health promotion and disease prevention: A review. *Journal of Drug Delivery and Therapeutics*, *8*(4), 42–47. doi:10.22270/jddt.v8i4.1759

Edwards, R. L., Lyon, T., Litwin, S. E., Rabovsky, A., Symons, J. D., & Jalili, T. (2007). Quercetin reduces blood pressure in hypertensive subjects. *The Journal of Nutrition*, *137*(11), 2405–2411. doi:10.1093/jn/137.11.2405 PMID:17951477

Ehrmann, D. A., Liljenquist, D. R., Kasza, K., Azziz, R., Legro, R. S., & Ghazzi, M. N. (2006). Prevalence and predictors of the metabolic syndrome in women with polycystic ovary syndrome. *The Journal of Clinical Endocrinology and Metabolism*, *91*(1), 48–53. doi:10.1210/jc.2005-1329 PMID:16249284

Ejaz, A., Wu, D., Kwan, P., & Meydani, M. (2009). Curcumin inhibits adipogenesis in 3T3-L1 adipocytes and angiogenesis and obesity in C57/BL mice. *The Journal of Nutrition*, *139*(5), 919–925. doi:10.3945/jn.108.100966 PMID:19297423

Ekoé, J. M., Punthakee, Z., Ransom, T., Prebtani, A. P., & Goldenberg, R. (2013). Screening for type 1 and type 2 diabetes. *Canadian Journal of Diabetes*, *37*, S12–S15. doi:10.1016/j.jcjd.2013.01.012 PMID:24070932

Ekor, M. (2014). The growing use of herbal medicines: Issues relating to adverse reactions and challenges in monitoring safety. *Frontiers in Pharmacology*, *4*, 177. doi:10.3389/fphar.2013.00177 PMID:24454289

El Hadi, H., Vettor, R., & Rossato, M. (2018). Congenital vitamin E deficiency. In V. R. Preedy & V. B. Patel (Eds.), *Handbook of famine, starvation, and nutrient deprivation* (pp. 1–18). Basel, Switzerland: Springer International Publishing AG. doi:10.1007/978-3-319-40007-5_86-1

El Hayek, Bitar, Hamdar, Mirza, & Daoud. (2016). Poly Cystic Ovarian Syndrome: An Updated Overview. *Frontiers in Physiology, 7.*

El Mgeed, A. A., Bstawi, M., Mohamed, U., & Gabbar, M. A. (2009). Histopathological and biochemical effects of green tea and/or licorice aqueous extracts on thyroid functions in male albino rats intoxicated with dimethylnitrosamine. *Nutrition & Metabolism*, *6*(1), 2. doi:10.1186/1743-7075-6-2 PMID:19138393

El Sohaimy, S. A. (2012). Functional foods and nutraceuticals-modern approach to food science. *World Applied Sciences Journal*, *20*, 691–708.

El-Beshbishy, H., & Bahashwan, S. (2012). Hypoglycemic effect of basil (Ocimum basilicum) aqueous extract is mediated through inhibition of α-glucosidase and α-amylase activities: An in vitro study. *Toxicology and Industrial Health*, *28*(1), 42–50. doi:10.1177/0748233711403193 PMID:21636683

Elham, P. (2018). Lean Women with Polycystic Ovary Syndrome. In Debatable Topics in PCOS Patients. Intech Publishers.

El-Saber Batiha, G., Magdy Beshbishy, A. G., & Wasef, L. (2020). Chemical constituents and pharmacological activities of garlic (*Allium sativum* L.): A review. *Nutrients*, *12*(3), 872. doi:10.3390/nu12030872 PMID:32213941

El-Sharkawy, A. A., Abdelmotaleb, G. S., Aly, M. K., & Kabel, A. M. (2014). Effect of metformin on sleep disorders in adolescent girls with polycystic ovarian syndrome. *Journal of Pediatric and Adolescent Gynecology*, *27*(6), 347–352. doi:10.1016/j.jpag.2014.01.004 PMID:25256878

Elvin-Lewis, M. (2001). Should we be concerned about herbal remedies. *Journal of Ethnopharmacology, 75*(2-3), 141–164. doi:10.1016/S0378-8741(00)00394-9 PMID:11297844

Enger, S. M., Ross, R. K., Paganini-Hill, A., & Bernstein, L. (1998). Breastfeeding experience and breast cancer risk among postmenopausal women. *Cancer Epidemiology, Biomarkers & Prevention, 7*, 365–369. PMID:9610784

Eom, D.-W., Lee, J. H., Kim, Y.-J., Hwang, G. S., Kim, S.-N., Kwak, J. H., Cheon, G. J., Kim, K. H., Jang, H.-J., Ham, J., Kang, K. S., & Yamabe, N. (2015). Synergistic effect of curcumin on epigallocatechin gallate-induced anticancer action in PC3 prostate cancer cells. *BMB Reports, 48*(8), 461–466. doi:10.5483/BMBRep.2015.48.8.216 PMID:25441423

Epstein, L. H., Wing, R. R., Penner, B. C., & Kress, M. J. (1985). Effect of diet and controlled exercise on weight loss in obese children. *The Journal of Pediatrics, 107*(3), 358–361. doi:10.1016/S0022-3476(85)80506-0 PMID:4032130

Erdle, S. C., Chan, E. S., Yang, H., Vallance, B. A., Mill, C., & Wong, T. (2018). First-reported pediatric cases of American ginseng anaphylaxis and allergy. *Allergy, Asthma, and Clinical Immunology: Official Journal of the Canadian Society of Allergy and Clinical Immunology, 14*(1), 1–3.

Escott-Stump, E., & Mahan, L. L. (2000). *Krause's food, nutrition and diet therapy*. Philadelphia: WB Saunders Company.

Esfandiari, A., Dehghan, A., Sharifi, S., Najafi, B., & Vesali, E. (2011). Effect of Tribulus terrestris extract on ovarian activity in immature Wistar rat: A histological evaluation. *Journal of Animal and Veterinary Advances, 10*(7), 883–886. doi:10.3923/javaa.2011.883.886

Etxeberria, U., Arias, N., Boqué, N., Macarulla, M. T., Portillo, M. P., Martínez, J. A., & Milagro, F. I. (2015). Reshaping faecal gut microbiota composition by the intake of trans-resveratrol and quercetin in high-fat sucrose diet-fed rats. *The Journal of Nutritional Biochemistry, 26*(6), 651–660. doi:10.1016/j.jnutbio.2015.01.002 PMID:25762527

Fain, J. N., Madan, A. K., Hiler, M. L., Cheema, P., & Bahouth, S. W. (2004). Comparison of the release of adipokines by adipose tissue, adipose tissue matrix, and adipocytes from visceral and subcutaneous abdominal adipose tissues of obese humans. *Endocrinology, 145*(5), 2273–2282. doi:10.1210/en.2003-1336 PMID:14726444

Falzon, C. C., & Balabanova, A. (2017). Phytotherapy: An introduction to herbal medicine. *Primary Care: Clinics in Office Practice, 44*(2), 217–227. doi:10.1016/j.pop.2017.02.001 PMID:28501226

Fang, L., Xu, W., & Kong, D. (2019). Icariin inhibits cell proliferation, migration and invasion by down-regulation of microRNA-625-3p in thyroid cancer cells. *Biomedicine and Pharmacotherapy, 109*, 2456–2463. doi:10.1016/j.biopha.2018.04.012 PMID:30551506

FAO/WHO. (2001). *Report on joint FAO/WHO expert consultation on evaluation of health and nutritional properties of probiotics in food including powder milk with live lactic acid bacteria*. Author.

Fararh, K. M., Atoji, Y., Shimizu, Y., Shiina, T., Nikami, H., & Takewaki, T. (2004). Mechanisms of the hypoglycaemic and immunopotentiating effects of Nigella sativa L. oil in streptozotocin-induced diabetic hamsters. *Research in Veterinary Science, 77*(2), 123–129. doi:10.1016/j.rvsc.2004.03.002 PMID:15196902

Farhangi, M. A., Dehghan, P., & Tajmiri, S. (2018). Powdered black cumin seeds strongly improves serum lipids, atherogenic index of plasma and modulates anthropometric features in patients with Hashimoto's thyroiditis. *Lipids in Health and Disease, 17*(1), 59. doi:10.118612944-018-0704-x PMID:29587770

Farhangi, M. A., Dehghan, P., Tajmiri, S., & Abbasi, M. M. (2016). The effects of Nigella sativa on thyroid function, serum Vascular Endothelial Growth Factor (VEGF) - 1, Nesfatin-1 and anthropometric features in patients with Hashimoto's thyroiditis: A randomized controlled trial. *BMC Complementary and Alternative Medicine, 16*(1), 471. doi:10.118612906-016-1432-2 PMID:27852303

Farhangi, M. A., & Tajmiri, S. (2020). The effects of powdered black cumin seeds on markers of oxidative stress, intracellular adhesion molecule (ICAM)-1 and vascular cell adhesion molecule (VCAM)-1 in patients with Hashimoto's thyroiditis. *Clinical Nutrition ESPEN*, *37*, 207–212. doi:10.1016/j.clnesp.2020.02.015 PMID:32359745

Farnsworth, N. R., Akerele, O., Bingel, A. S., Soejarto, D. D., & Guo, Z. (1985). Medicinal plants in therapy. *Bulletin of the World Health Organization*, *63*(6), 965. PMID:3879679

Farvid, M. S., Chen, W. Y., Michels, K. B., Cho, E., Willett, W. C., & Eliassen, A. H. (2016). Fruit and vegetable consumption in adolescence and early adulthood and risk of breast cancer: Population based cohort study. *BMJ (Clinical Research Ed.)*, i2343. doi:10.1136/bmj.i2343 PMID:27170029

Fasano, A. (2012a). Zonulin, regulation of tight junctions, and autoimmune diseases. *Annals of the New York Academy of Sciences*, *1258*(1), 25–33. doi:10.1111/j.1749-6632.2012.06538.x PMID:22731712

Fasano, A. (2012b). Intestinal permeability and its regulation by zonulin: Diagnostic and therapeutic implications. *Clinical Gastroenterology and Hepatology*, *10*(10), 1096–1100. doi:10.1016/j.cgh.2012.08.012 PMID:22902773

Fatima, N., Hafizur, R. M., Hameed, A., Ahmed, S., Nisar, M., & Kabir, N. (2015). Ellagic acid in *Emblica officinalis* exerts anti-diabetic activity through the action on β-cells of pancreas. *European Journal of Nutrition*, *56*(2), 591–601. doi:10.100700394-015-1103-y PMID:26593435

Fauser, B. C., Pache, T. D., Lamberts, S. W., Hop, W. C., de Jong, F. H., & Dahl, K. D. (1991). Serum bioactive and immunoreactive luteinizing hormone and follicle-stimulating hormone levels in women with cycle abnormalities, with or without polycystic ovarian disease. *The Journal of Clinical Endocrinology and Metabolism*, *73*(4), 811–817. doi:10.1210/jcem-73-4-811 PMID:1909705

FDA/CFSAN. (1994). *Food and Drug Administration website*. Dietary Supplement Health and Education Act. http://vm.cfsan.fda.gov/~dms/dietsupp.html

Fedorak, R. N., & Madsen, K. L. (2004). Probiotics and the management of inflammatory bowel disease. *Inflammatory Bowel Diseases*, *10*(3), 286–299. doi:10.1097/00054725-200405000-00018 PMID:15290926

Fei, N., & Zhao, L. (2013). An opportunistic pathogen isolated from the gut of obese human causes obesity in germfree mice. *The ISME Journal*, *7*(4), 880–884. doi:10.1038/ismej.2012.153 PMID:23235292

Felizola, S. J. (2015). Ursolic acid in experimental models and human subjects: Potential as an anti-obesity/overweight treatment. *Cancer*, *1*, 2.

Feng, F., Cheng, P., Wang, C., Wang, Y., & Wang, W. (2019). Polyphyllin I and VII potentiate the chemosensitivity of A549/DDP cells to cisplatin by enhancing apoptosis, reversing EMT and suppressing the CIP2A/AKT/mTOR signaling axis. *Oncology Letters*, *18*(5), 5428–5436. doi:10.3892/ol.2019.10895 PMID:31612051

Fernández, C. (2016). *The Future of Diabetes Treatment: Is A Cure Possible?* Available at: https://www.labiotech.eu/in-depth/diabetes-treatment-cure-review/

Fernández, C. (2018). *Needle-Free Diabetes Care: 8 Devices That Painlessly Measure Blood Glucose*. Available at: https://www.labiotech.eu/diabetes/needle-free-glucose-monitoring-for-diabetes-medtech/

Ferreira, C. M., Vieira, A. T., Vinolo, M. A. R., Oliveira, F. A., Curi, R., & Martins, F. S. (2014). The central role of the gut microbiota in chronic inflammatory diseases. *Journal of Immunology Research*, *2014*, 689492. doi:10.1155/2014/689492 PMID:25309932

Ferrero-Miliani, L., Nielsen, O.H., Andersen, P.S., & Girardin, S.E. (2007). Chronic inflammation: Importance of NOD2 and NALP3 in interleukin-1β generation. *Clinical and Experimental Immunology*, *147*(2), 227–235. PMID:17223962

Field, A. E., Coakley, E. H., Must, A., Spadano, J. L., Laird, N., Dietz, W. H., Rimm, E., & Colditz, G. A. (2001). Impact of overweight on the risk of developing common chronic diseases during a 10-year period. *Archives of Internal Medicine*, *161*(13), 1581–1586. doi:10.1001/archinte.161.13.1581 PMID:11434789

Finamore, A., Massimi, M., Conti Devirgiliis, L., & Mengheri, E. (2008). Zinc deficiency induces membrane barrier damage and increases neutrophil transmigration in Caco-2 cells. *The Journal of Nutrition*, *138*(9), 1664–1670. doi:10.1093/jn/138.9.1664 PMID:18716167

Firdous, S. M. (2014). Phytochemicals for treatment of diabetes. *EXCLI Journal*, *13*, 451. PMID:26417272

Firenzuoli, F., & Gori, L. (2007). Herbal medicine today: Clinical and research issues. *Evidence-Based Complementary and Alternative Medicine*, *4*(s1, S1), 37–40. doi:10.1093/ecam/nem096 PMID:18227931

Fischer, K. R., Durrans, A., Lee, S., Sheng, J., Li, F., Wong, S. T., & Schwabe, R. F. (2015). Epithelial-to-mesenchymal transition is not required for lung metastasis but contributes to chemoresistance. *Nature*, *527*(7579), 472–476. doi:10.1038/nature15748 PMID:26560033

Fischer-Posovszky, P., Kukulus, V., Tews, D., Unterkircher, T., Debatin, K. M., Fulda, S., & Wabitsch, M. (2010). Resveratrol regulates human adipocyte number and function in a Sirt1-dependent manner. *The American Journal of Clinical Nutrition*, *92*(1), 5–15. doi:10.3945/ajcn.2009.28435 PMID:20463039

Fokunang, C. N., Ndikum, V., Tabi, O. Y., Jiofack, R. B., Ngameni, B., Guedje, N. M., Tembe-Fokunang, E. A., Tomkins, P., Barkwan, S., Kechia, F., Asongalem, E., Ngoupayou, J., Torimiro, N. J., Gonsu, K. H., Sielinou, V., Ngadjui, B. T., Angwafor, F., 3rd, Nkongmeneck, A., Abena, O. M., Ngogang, J., … Kamsu-Kom. (2011). Traditional medicine: past, present and future research and development prospects and integration in the National Health System of Cameroon. *African Journal of Traditional, Complementary, and Alternative Medicines: AJTCAM*, *8*(3), 284–295.

Ford, E. S., Ajani, U. A., & Mokdad, A. H. (2005). The metabolic syndrome and concentrations of C-reactive protein among US youth. *Diabetes Care*, *28*(4), 878–881. doi:10.2337/diacare.28.4.878

Forni, C., Facchiano, F., Bartoli, M., Pieretti, S., Facchiano, A., D'Arcangelo, D., Norelli, S., Valle, G., Nisini, R., Beninati, S., Tabolacci, C., & Jadeja, R. N. (2019). Beneficial role of phytochemicals on oxidative stress and age-related diseases. BioMed Research International (Vol. 2019). https://doi.org/ doi:10.1155/2019/8748253

Fowler, M. (2008). Microvascular and Macrovascular Complications of Diabetes. *Clinical Diabetes*, *26*(2), 77–82. doi:10.2337/diaclin.26.2.77

Franks, S. (1989). Polycystic ovary syndrome: A changing perspective. *Horumon To Rinsho*, *31*(1), 87–120. doi:10.1111/j.1365-2265.1989.tb00457.x PMID:2513151

Frati-Munari, A., Fernandez, J., Becerril, M., Chavez, A., & Banles, M. (1983). Decrease in serum lipids, glycemia and body weight by *Plantago psyllium* in obese and diabetic patients. *Archivos de Investigacion Medica*, *14*, 259–268. PMID:6322713

Frazier, T. H., DiBaise, J. K., & McClain, C. J. (2011). Gut microbiota, intestinal permeability, obesity-induced inflammation, and liver injury. *JPEN. Journal of Parenteral and Enteral Nutrition*, *35*(5Suppl), 14S–20S. doi:10.1177/0148607111413772 PMID:21807932

Fridlender, M., Kapulnik, Y., & Koltai, H. (2015). Plant derived substances with anti-cancer activity: From folklore to practice. *Frontiers in Plant Science*, *6*, 799. doi:10.3389/fpls.2015.00799 PMID:26483815

Friedl, P., & Mayor, R. (2017). Tuning collective cell migration by cell–cell junction regulation. *Cold Spring Harbor Perspectives in Biology*, *9*(4), a029199. doi:10.1101/cshperspect.a029199 PMID:28096261

Fried, M., Hainer, V., Basdevant, A., Buchwald, H., Deitel, M., Finer, N., ... Steffen, R. (2007). Interdisciplinary European guidelines for surgery for severe (morbid) obesity. *Obesity Surgery*, *17*(2), 260–270. doi:10.100711695-007-9025-2 PMID:17476884

Fujiki, H., & Imai, K. (2015). Innovative strategy of cancer treatment with the combination of green tea catechins and anticancer compounds. Academic Press.

Fujiki, H., Sueoka, E., Watanabe, T., & Suganuma, M. (2015). Primary cancer prevention by green tea, and tertiary cancer prevention by the combination of green tea catechins and anticancer compounds. *Journal of Cancer Prevention*, *20*(1), 1–4. doi:10.15430/JCP.2015.20.1.1 PMID:25853098

Fuke, N., Nagata, N., Suganuma, H., & Ota, T. (2019). Regulation of Gut Microbiota and Metabolic Endotoxemia with Dietary Factors. *Nutrients*, *11*(10), 2277. doi:10.3390/nu11102277 PMID:31547555

Fu, Q., Li, Q., Lin, X., Qiao, R., Yang, R., Li, X., ... Liang, Y. (2017). Antidiabetic effects of tea. *Molecules (Basel, Switzerland)*, *22*(5), 849. doi:10.3390/molecules22050849 PMID:28531120

Futterweit, W. (1999). Polycystic ovary syndrome: Clinical perspectives and management. *Obstetrical & Gynecological Survey*, *54*(6), 403–413. doi:10.1097/00006254-199906000-00024 PMID:10358853

Gallagher, A. M., Flatt, P. R., Duffy, G. A. W. Y., & Abdel-Wahab, Y. H. A. (2003). The effects of traditional antidiabetic plants on in vitro glucose diffusion. *Nutrition Research (New York, N.Y.)*, *23*(3), 413–424. doi:10.1016/S0271-5317(02)00533-X

Galtier, F. (2010). Definition, epidemiology, risk factors. *Diabetes & Metabolism*, *36*(6 Pt 2), 628–651. doi:10.1016/j.diabet.2010.11.014 PMID:21163426

Galvano, F., La Fauci, L., Vitaglione, P., Fogliano, V., Vanella, L., & Felgines, C. (2007). Bioavailability, antioxidant and biological properties of the natural free-radical scavengers cyanidin and related glycosides. *Annali dell'Istituto Superiore di Sanita*, *43*, 382–393. PMID:18209272

Gambineri, A., Pelusi, C., Manicardi, E., Vicennati, V., Cacciari, M., Morselli-Labate, A. M., Pagotto, U., & Pasquali, R. (2004). Glucose intolerance in a large cohort of mediterranean women with polycystic ovary syndrome: Phenotype and associated factors. *Diabetes*, *53*(9), 2353–2358. doi:10.2337/diabetes.53.9.2353 PMID:15331545

Ganesan, A. (2008). The impact of natural products upon modern drug discovery. *Current Opinion in Chemical Biology*, *12*(3), 306–317. doi:10.1016/j.cbpa.2008.03.016 PMID:18423384

Ganji-Arjenaki, M., & Rafieian-Kopaei, M. (2018). Probiotics are a good choice in remission of inflammatory bowel diseases: A meta analysis and systematic review. *Journal of Cellular Physiology*, *233*(3), 2091–2103. doi:10.1002/jcp.25911 PMID:28294322

Garcia-Mantrana, I., Selma-Royo, M., Alcantara, C., & Collado, M. C. (2018). Shifts on Gut Microbiota Associated to Mediterranean Diet Adherence and Specific Dietary Intakes on General Adult Population. *Frontiers in Microbiology*, *9*, 890. doi:10.3389/fmicb.2018.00890 PMID:29867803

Garg, A., Garg, S., Zaneveld, L. J. D., & Singla, A. K. (2001). Chemistry and pharmacology of the Citrus bioflavonoid hesperidin. Phytotherapy Research. https://doi.org/ doi:10.1002/ptr.1074

Gates, M. A., Tworoger, S. S., Hecht, J. L., de Vivo, I., Rosner, B., & Hankinson, S. E. (2007). A prospective study of dietary flavonoid intake and incidence of epithelial ovarian cancer. *International Journal of Cancer*, *121*(10), 2225–2232. doi:10.1002/ijc.22790 PMID:17471564

Gauthaman, K., & Ganesan, A. P. (2008). The hormonal effects of *Tribulus terrestris* and its role in the management of male erectile dysfunction – an evaluation using primates, rabbit and rat. *Phytomedicine*, *15*(1-2), 44–54. doi:10.1016/j.phymed.2007.11.011 PMID:18068966

Geier, M. S., Butler, R. N., & Howarth, G. S. (2006). Probiotics, prebiotics and synbiotics: A role in chemoprevention for colorectal cancer. *Cancer Biology & Therapy*, *5*(10), 1265–1269. doi:10.4161/cbt.5.10.3296 PMID:16969130

Gentile, D., Fornai, M., Pellegrini, C., Colucci, R., Benvenuti, L., Duranti, E., Masi, S., Carpi, S., Nieri, P., Nericcio, A., Garelli, F., Virdis, A., Pistelli, L., Blandizzi, C., & Antonioli, L. (2018). Luteolin prevents cardiometabolic alterations and vascular dysfunction in mice with HFD-induced obesity. *Frontiers in Pharmacology*, *9*, 1094–1107. doi:10.3389/fphar.2018.01094 PMID:30319424

Georgiev, P., Dimitrov, M., & Vitanov, S. (1988). Effect of Tribestan (from *Tribulus terrestris*) on plasma testosterone and spermatogenesis in male lambs and rams. *Veterinarna Sbirka*, *86*(3), 20–22.

Geraldine, M., Herman, D. S. S., & Venkatesh, T. (2006). Lead poisoning as a result of infertility treatment using herbal remedies. *Archives of Gynecology and Obstetrics*, *275*(4), 279–281. doi:10.100700404-006-0227-y PMID:16947057

Gerard, C., Didier, D., & Evanthia, D. (2014). The polycystic ovary syndrome: A position statement from the European Society of Endocrinology. *European Journal of Endocrinology*, *171*(4), 1–29. doi:10.1530/EJE-14-0253 PMID:24849517

Gevers, D., Kugathasan, S., Denson, L. A., Vázquez-Baeza, Y., Van Treuren, W., Ren, B., ... Xavier, R. J. (2014). The treatment-naive microbiome in new-onset Crohn's disease. *Cell Host & Microbe*, *15*(3), 382–392. doi:10.1016/j.chom.2014.02.005 PMID:24629344

Ghaffari, F., Moghadd, M. A. H., & Zare, M. (2018). Neuroprotective effect of quercetin nanocrystal in a 6-hydroxy-dopamine model of Parkinson disease: Biochemical and behavioral evidence. *Basic and Clinical Neuroscience*, *9*(5), 317–324. doi:10.32598/bcn.9.5.317 PMID:30719246

Ghafurniyan, H., Azarnia, M., Nabiuni, M., & Karimzadeh, L. (2015). The effect of green tea extract on reproductive improvement in estradiol valerate-induced polycystic ovarian syndrome in rat, Iran. *J. Pharm. Res: IJPR*, *14*, 1215. PMID:26664389

Ghani, N. (2011). *Khazainul Advia*. New Delhi, India: Idara Kitabul Shifa.

Ghavi, F., Taghizadeh, M., Taebi, M., & Abdolahian, S. (2019). Effect of Foeniculum vulgare essence on symptoms of polycystic ovarian syndrome (PCOS): A randomized double-blind, Placebo-Controlled Trial. *Journal of Herbal Medicine*, *17*, 100277. doi:10.1016/j.hermed.2019.100277

Ghorbani, A. (2017). Mechanisms of antidiabetic effects of flavonoid rutin. *Biomedicine and Pharmacotherapy*, *96*, 305–312. doi:10.1016/j.biopha.2017.10.001 PMID:29017142

Ghosh, D. (2018). Quality issues of herbal medicines: Internal and external factors. *Internationa Journal of Complementary & Alternative Medicine*, *11*(1), 67–69. doi:10.15406/ijcam.2018.11.00350

Ghosh, D., & Konishi, T. (2007). Anthocyanins and anthocyanin-rich extracts: Role in diabetes and eye function. *Asia Pacific Journal of Clinical Nutrition*, *16*(2), 200–208. PMID:17468073

Ghosh, R., Ganapathy, M., Alworth, W. L., Chan, D. C., & Kumar, A. P. (2009). Combination of 2-methoxyestradiol (2-ME2) and eugenol for apoptosis induction synergistically in androgen independent prostate cancer cells. *The Journal of Steroid Biochemistry and Molecular Biology*, *113*(1–2), 25–35. doi:10.1016/j.jsbmb.2008.11.002 PMID:19084597

Giaccari, A., Sorice, G., & Muscogiuri, G. (2009). Glucose toxicity: The leading actor in the pathogenesis and clinical history of type 2 diabetes–mechanisms and potentials for treatment. *Nutrition, Metabolism, and Cardiovascular Diseases*, *19*(5), 365–377. doi:10.1016/j.numecd.2009.03.018 PMID:19428228

Gill, H., & Prasad, J. (2008). Probiotics, immunomodulation, and health benefits. *Advances in Experimental Medicine and Biology*, *606*, 423–454. doi:10.1007/978-0-387-74087-4_17 PMID:18183940

Glaros, T. G. (2013). Causes and consequences of low grade endotoxemia and inflammatory diseases. *Frontiers in Bioscience (Scholar Edition)*, *5*(2), 754–765. doi:10.2741/S405 PMID:23277084

Glenville, M. (2006). Nutritional supplements in pregnancy: Commercial push or evidence based? Current Opinion in Obstetrics and Gynecology. https://doi.org/ doi:10.1097/GCO.0b013e328010214e

Glore, S. R., Van Treeck, D., Knehans, A. W., & Guild, M. (1994). Soluble fiber and serum lipids: A literature review. Journal of the American Dietetic Association. https://doi.org/ doi:10.1016/0002-8223(94)90099-X

Glueck, C. J., Papanna, R., Wang, P., Goldenberg, N., & Sieve-Smith, L. (2003). Incidence and treatment of metabolic syndrome in newly referred women with confirmed polycystic ovarian syndrome. *Metabolism: Clinical and Experimental*, *52*(7), 908–915. doi:10.1016/S0026-0495(03)00104-5 PMID:12870169

Gnoth, C., Godehardt, E., Frank-Herrmann, P., Friol, K., Tigges, J., & Freundl, G. (2005). Definition and prevalence of subfertility and infertility. *Human Reproduction (Oxford, England)*, *20*(5), 1144–1147. doi:10.1093/humrep/deh870 PMID:15802321

Gocmez, S. S., Gacar, N., Utkan, T., Gacar, G., Scarpace, P. J., & Tumer, N. (2016). Protective effects of resveratrol on aging-induced cognitive impairment in rats. *Neurobiology of Learning and Memory*, *131*, 131–136. doi:10.1016/j.nlm.2016.03.022 PMID:27040098

Godinho, R., Mega, C., Teixeira-de-Lemos, E., Carvalho, E., Teixeira, F., Fernandes, R., & Reis, F. (2015). The Place of Dipeptidyl Peptidase-4 Inhibitors in Type 2 Diabetes Therapeutics: A "Me Too" or "the Special One" Antidiabetic Class? *Journal of Diabetes Research*, *2015*, 1–28. doi:10.1155/2015/806979 PMID:26075286

Go, G., Sung, J. S., Jee, S. C., Kim, M., Jang, W. H., Kang, K. Y., Kim, D. Y., Lee, S., & Shin, H. S. (2017). In vitro anti-obesity effects of sesamol mediated by adenosine monophosphate-activated protein kinase and mitogen-activated protein kinase signaling in 3T3-L1 cells. *Food Science and Biotechnology*, *26*(1), 195–200. doi:10.100710068-017-0026-1 PMID:30263528

Gomez-Pinilla, F. (2008). Brain foods: The effects of nutrients on brain function. *Nature Reviews. Neuroscience*, *9*(7), 568–578. doi:10.1038/nrn2421 PMID:18568016

Gonzales, G.F., Cordova, A., Vega, K., Chung, A., Villena, A., & Gonez, C. (2002). *Effect of Lepidium meyenii (MACA) on sexual desire and its absent relationship with serum testosterone levels in adult healthy men.* Academic Press.

González-Rodríguez, Á., Santamaría, B., Mas-Gutierrez, J. A., Rada, P., Fernández-Millán, E., Pardo, V., Álvarez, C., Cuadrado, A., Ros, M., Serrano, M., & Valverde, Á. M. (2015). Resveratrol treatment restores peripheral insulin sensitivity in diabetic mice in a sirt1-independent manner. *Molecular Nutrition & Food Research*, *59*(8), 1431–1442. doi:10.1002/mnfr.201400933 PMID:25808216

Gonzalez-Vallinas, M., Gonzalez-Castejon, M., Rodriguez Casado, A., & Ramírez de Molina, A. (2013). Dietary phytochemicals in cancer prevention and therapy: A complementary approach with promising perspectives. *Nutrition Reviews*, *71*(9), 585–599. doi:10.1111/nure.12051 PMID:24032363

Goodarzi, M. O., Dumesic, D. A., Chazenbalk, G., & Azziz, R. (2011). Polycystic ovary syndrome:etiology, pathogenesis and diagnosis. *Nature Reviews. Endocrinology*, *7*(4), 219–231. doi:10.1038/nrendo.2010.217 PMID:21263450

Gouws, C., Georgousopoulou, E., Mellor, D., McKune, A., & Naumovski, N. (2019). Effects of the Consumption of Prickly Pear Cacti (Opuntia spp.) and its Products on Blood Glucose Levels and Insulin: A Systematic Review. *Medicina*, *55*(5), 138. doi:10.3390/medicina55050138 PMID:31096667

Govender, M., Choonara, Y. E., Kumar, P., Toit, L. C., Vuuren, S. V., & Pillay, V. (2014). A review of the advancements in probiotic delivery: Conventional vs. non-conventional formulations for intestinal flora supplementation. *Journal of the American Association of Pharmaceutical Scientists*, *15*(1), 29–43. PMID:24222267

Governa, P., Baini, G., Borgonetti, V., Cettolin, G., Giachetti, D., Magnano, A. R., Miraldi, E., & Biagi, M. (2018). Phytotherapy in the management of diabetes: A review. *Molecules (Basel, Switzerland)*, *23*(1), 105. doi:10.3390/molecules23010105 PMID:29300317

Grace, E., Shaw, C., Whelan, K., & Andreyev, H. J. N. (2013). Review article: Small intestinal bacterial overgrowth--prevalence, clinical features, current and developing diagnostic tests, and treatment. *Alimentary Pharmacology & Therapeutics*, *38*(7), 674–688. doi:10.1111/apt.12456 PMID:23957651

Grant, P. (2010). Spearmint herbal tea has significant anti-androgen effects in polycystic ovarian syndrome. a randomized controlled trial. *Phytotherapy Research*, *24*(2), 186–188. doi:10.1002/ptr.2900 PMID:19585478

Grant, P., & Ramasamy, S. (2012). An Update on Plant Derived Anti-Androgens. *International Journal of Endocrinology and Metabolism*, *2*(2), 497–502. doi:10.5812/ijem.3644 PMID:23843810

Gregory, J. W. (2019). Prevention of Obesity and Metabolic Syndrome in Children. *Frontiers in Endocrinology*, *10*, 669. doi:10.3389/fendo.2019.00669

Groschwitz, K. R., & Hogan, S. P. (2009). Intestinal barrier function: Molecular regulation and disease pathogenesis. *The Journal of Allergy and Clinical Immunology*, *124*(1), 3–20, quiz 21–22. doi:10.1016/j.jaci.2009.05.038 PMID:19560575

Gruber, L., Kisling, S., Lichti, P., Martin, F.-P., May, S., Klingenspor, M., ... Haller, D. (2013). High fat diet accelerates pathogenesis of murine Crohn's disease-like ileitis independently of obesity. *PLoS One*, *8*(8), e71661. doi:10.1371/journal.pone.0071661 PMID:23977107

Gu, J. (2015). *Protects against doxorubicin-induced cardiotoxicity Resveratrol alleviates cardiomyocytes oxidative stress induced by doxorubicin Resveratrol modulates doxorubicin- induced cardiocyomytes autophagy Resveratrol mitigates cardiomyocytes apoptosis induced by*. Academic Press.

Guariguata, L., Whiting, D., Hambleton, I., Beagley, J., Linnenkamp, U., & Shaw, J. (2014). Global estimates of diabetes prevalence for 2013 and projections for 2035. *Diabetes Research and Clinical Practice*, *103*(2), 137–149. doi:10.1016/j.diabres.2013.11.002 PMID:24630390

Guarner, F. (2005). Inulin and oligofructose: Impact on intestinal disease and disorders. *British Journal of Nutrition*, *93*(S1Supplement), S61–S65. doi:10.1079/BJN20041345 PMID:15877897

Guilherme, A., Virbasius, J. V., Puri, V., & Czech, M. P. (2008). Adipocyte dysfunctions linking obesity to insulin resistance and type 2 diabetes. *Nature Reviews. Molecular Cell Biology*, *9*(5), 367–377. doi:10.1038/nrm2391 PMID:18401346

Gumus, G., & Lee, J. (2011). Alternative Paths To Parenthood: Ivf Or Child Adoption? *Economic Inquiry*, *50*(3), 802–820. doi:10.1111/j.1465-7295.2011.00401.x

Gunawan-Puteri, M. D., Kato, E., & Kawabata, J. (2012). α-Amylase inhibitors from an Indonesian medicinal herb, Phyllanthus urinaria. *Journal of the Science of Food and Agriculture*, *92*(3), 606–609. doi:10.1002/jsfa.4615 PMID:22095704

Guo-Ming, P., Fang-Xu, L., Yong, Y., Yin, Z., Li-Li, K., Pu, Z., & … . (2019). Herbal medicine in the treatment of patients with type 2 diabetes mellitus. *Chinese Medical Journal, 132*(1), 78–85. doi:10.1097/CM9.0000000000000006 PMID:30628962

Gupta, V., Winocour, J., Rodriguez-Feo, C., Bamba, R., Shack, R. B., Grotting, J. C., & Higdon, K. K. (2016). *Safety of aesthetic surgery*. Academic Press.

Gupta, S., Chauhan, D., Mehla, K., Sood, P., & Nair, A. (2010). An overview of nutraceuticals: Current scenario. *Journal of Basic and Clinical Pharmacy*. PMID:24825966

Gupta, V. K., Tuohy, M. G., O'Donovan, A., & Lohani, M. (2015). *Biotechnology of bioactive compounds: Sources and applications*. Wiley-Blackwell. doi:10.1002/9781118733103

Guri, A. J., Hontecillas, R., Si, H., Liu, D., & Bassaganya-Riera, J. (2007). Dietary abscisic acid ameliorates glucose tolerance and obesity-related inflammation in db/db mice fed high-fat diets. *Clinical Nutrition (Edinburgh, Lothian), 26*(1), 107–116. doi:10.1016/j.clnu.2006.07.008 PMID:17000034

Gurib-Fakim, A. (2006). Medicinal plants: Traditions of yesterday and drugs of tomorrow. *Molecular Aspects of Medicine, 27*(1), 1–93. doi:10.1016/j.mam.2005.07.008

Gu, Y., Zhang, X., Sun, D., Zhao, H., Cai, B., & Gao, C. (2015). The Stimulative Effect of Yangjing Capsule on Testosterone Synthesis through Nur77 Pathway in Leydig Cells. *Evidence-Based Complementary and Alternative Medicine*, 1–8. doi:10.1155/2015/408686 PMID:26413123

Hafez, D. A. (2010). Effect of extracts of ginger goots and cinnamon bark on fertility of male diabetic rats. *The Journal of American Science, 6*, 940–947.

Haj-Husein, I. S., Tukan, S., & Alkazaleh, F. (2016). The effect of marjoram (Origanum majorana) tea on the hormonal profile of women with polycystic ovary syndrome: A randomised controlled pilot study. *Journal of Human Nutrition and Dietetics, 29*(1), 105–111. doi:10.1111/jhn.12290 PMID:25662759

Haji Shafiha, M., Zabiri, T., & Salari Lak, S. H. (2007). Investigating validity criteria of vaginal ultrasound (ovarian volume, the ovarian stroma and the stromal surface of the ovary) in the diagnosis of polycystic ovary syndrome. *Majallah-i Pizishki-i Urumiyyah, 3*, 538–543.

Hajian-Tilaki, K., & Heidari, B. (2013). A Comparison between International Obesity Task Force and Center for Disease Control References in Assessment of Overweight and Obesity Among Adolescents in Babol, Northern Iran. *International Journal of Preventive Medicine, 4*(2), 226–232.

Hajimonfarednejad, M., Nimrouzi, M., Heydari, M., Zarshenas, M. M., Raee, M. J., & Jahromi, B. N. (2018). Insulin resistance improvement by cinnamon powder in polycystic ovary syndrome: A randomized double-blind placebo controlled clinical trial. *Phytotherapy Research, 32*(2), 276–283. doi:10.1002/ptr.5970 PMID:29250843

Hajra, K. M., Chen, D. Y., & Fearon, E. R. (2002). The SLUG zinc-finger protein represses E-cadherin in breast cancer. *Cancer Research, 62*(6), 1613–1618. PMID:11912130

Häkkinen, S. H., Kärenlampi, S. O., Heinonen, I. M., Mykkänen, H. M., & Törrönen, A. R. (1999). Content of the flavonols quercetin, myricetin, and kaempferol in 25 edible berries. *Journal of Agricultural and Food Chemistry, 47*(6), 2274–2279. doi:10.1021/jf9811065 PMID:10794622

Halban, P. A., Polonsky, K. S., Bowden, D. W., Hawkins, M. A., Ling, C., Mather, K. J., Powers, A. C., Rhodes, C. J., Sussel, L., & Weir, G. (2014). Beta-cell failure in type 2 diabetes: Postulated mechanisms and prospects for prevention and treatment. *Diabetes Care, 37*(6), 1751–1758. doi:10.2337/dc14-0396 PMID:24812433

Halberstein, R. A. (2005). Medicinal plants: Historical and cross-cultural usage patterns. *Annals of Epidemiology*, *15*(9), 686–699. doi:10.1016/j.annepidem.2005.02.004 PMID:15921929

Hamao, M., Matsuda, H., Nakamura, S., Nakashima, S., Semura, S., Maekubo, S., Wakasugi, S., & Yoshikawa, M. (2011). Anti-obesity effects of the methanolic extract and chakasaponins from the flower buds of *Camellia sinensis* in mice. *Bioorganic & Medicinal Chemistry*, *19*(20), 6033–6041. doi:10.1016/j.bmc.2011.08.042 PMID:21925888

Hamilton, A. C. (2004). Medicinal plants, conservation and livelihoods. *Biodiversity and Conservation*, *13*(8), 1477–1517. doi:10.1023/B:BIOC.0000021333.23413.42

Hamza, A. H., AlBishri, W. M., & Alfaris, M. H. (2019). Effect of Vitex agnus-castus plant extract on polycystic ovary syndrome complications in experimental rat model. *Asian Pacific Journal of Reproduction*, *8*, 63–69.

Hardin, H., Yu, X. M., Harrison, A. D., Larrain, C., Zhang, R., Chen, J., Chen, H., & Lloyd, R. V. (2016). Generation of Novel Thyroid Cancer Stem-Like Cell Clones: Effects of Resveratrol and Valproic Acid. *American Journal of Pathology*, *186*(6), 1662–1673. doi:10.1016/j.ajpath.2016.02.003 PMID:27060227

Hardy, G. (2000). Nutraceuticals and functional foods: Introduction and meaning. *Nutrition (Burbank, Los Angeles County, Calif.)*. Advance online publication. doi:10.1016/S0899-9007(00)00332-4 PMID:10906598

Harmon, A. W., & Patel, Y. M. (2003). Naringenin inhibits phosphoinositide 3-kinase activity and glucose uptake in 3T3-L1 adipocytes. *Biochemical and Biophysical Research Communications*, *305*(3), 229–234. doi:10.1016/S0006-291X(03)00720-4 PMID:12745063

Harrison, C. L., Lombard, C. B., Moran, L. J., & Teede, H. J. (2011). Exercise therapy in polycystic ovary syndrome: A systematic review. *Human Reproduction Update*, *17*(2), 171–183. doi:10.1093/humupd/dmq045 PMID:20833639

Harris, W. S. (2018). The Omega-6:Omega-3 ratio: A critical appraisal and possible successor. *Prostaglandins, Leukotrienes, and Essential Fatty Acids*, *132*, 34–40. doi:10.1016/j.plefa.2018.03.003 PMID:29599053

Harvard, P. (2018). *Type 1 Diabetes Mellitus - Harvard Health*. Retrieved 27 August 2020, from https://www.health.harvard.edu/a_to_z/type-1-diabetes-mellitus-a-to-z

Harvey, A. L. (2008). Natural products in drug discovery. *Drug Discovery Today*, *13*(19-20), 894–901. doi:10.1016/j.drudis.2008.07.004 PMID:18691670

Harvey, J. R., & Ogden, D. E. (2014). Obesity treatment in disadvantaged population groups: Where do we stand and what can we do? *Prev Med (Baltim)*, *68*, 71–75. doi:10.1016/j.ypmed.2014.05.015 PMID:24878585

Hasanein, P., & Fazeli, F. (2014). Role of naringenin in protection against diabetic hyperalgesia and tactile allodynia in male wistar rats. *Journal of Physiology and Biochemistry*, *70*(4), 997–1006. doi:10.100713105-014-0369-5 PMID:25407136

Hasan, T., & Sultana, M. (2018). Antidiabetic potency of Bangladeshi medicinal plants. *J Ayurvedic Herb Med*, *4*(1), 35–42.

Hasanzade, F., Toliat, M., Emami, S. A., & Emamimoghaadam, Z. (2013). The effect of cinnamon on glucose of type II diabetes patients. *Journal of Traditional and Complementary Medicine*, *3*(3), 171–174. doi:10.4103/2225-4110.114900 PMID:24716174

Ha, T. K., Jung, I., Kim, M. E., Bae, S. K., & Lee, J. S. (2017). Anti-cancer activity of myricetin against human papillary thyroid cancer cells involves mitochondrial dysfunction-mediated apoptosis. *Biomedicine and Pharmacotherapy*, *91*, 378–384. doi:10.1016/j.biopha.2017.04.100 PMID:28463801

Haugen, B. R., Alexander, E. K., Bible, K. C., Doherty, G. M., Mandel, S. J., Nikiforov, Y. E., ... Schlumberger, M. (2016). 2015 American Thyroid Association management guidelines for adult patients with thyroid nodules and differentiated thyroid cancer: The American Thyroid Association guidelines task force on thyroid nodules and differentiated thyroid cancer. *Thyroid*, *26*(1), 1–133. doi:10.1089/thy.2015.0020 PMID:26462967

Hawrelak, J. A., & Myers, S. P. (2004). The causes of intestinal dysbiosis: A review. *Alternative Medicine Review*, *9*(2), 180–197. PMID:15253677

Health.gov. (2020). Available at: https://health.gov/sites/default/files/2019-09/paguide.pdf

He, D.-Y., & Dai, S.-M. (2011). Anti-Inflammatory and Immunomodulatory Effects of Paeonia Lactiflora Pall, a Traditional Chinese Herbal Medicine. *Frontiers in Pharmacology*, *2*, 10. doi:10.3389/fphar.2011.00010 PMID:21687505

Hegedus, L., Bonnema, S. J., & Bennedbaek, F. N. (2003). Management of simple nodular goiter: Current status and future perspectives. *Endocrine Reviews*, *24*(1), 102–132. doi:10.1210/er.2002-0016 PMID:12588812

Heidary, M., Vahhabi, S., Reza Nejadi, J., Delfan, B., Birjandi, M., Kaviani, H., & Givrad, S. (2008). Effect of saffron on semen parameters of infertile men. *Urology Journal*, *5*, 255–259. PMID:19101900

Heinig, M. J. (2001). Host defense benefits of breastfeeding for the infant. Effect of breastfeeding duration and exclusivity. *Pediatric Clinics of North America*, *48*(1), 105–123. doi:10.1016/S0031-3955(05)70288-1 PMID:11236719

He, K., Li, X., Chen, X., Ye, X., Huang, J., Jin, Y., Li, P., Deng, Y., Jin, Q., Shi, Q., & Shu, H. (2011). Evaluation of antidiabetic potential of selected traditional Chinese medicines in STZ-induced diabetic mice. *Journal of Ethnopharmacology*, *137*(3), 1135–1142. doi:10.1016/j.jep.2011.07.033 PMID:21798327

Hemaiswarya, S., & Doble, M. (2013). Combination of phenylpropanoids with 5-fluorouracil as anti-cancer agents against human cervical cancer (HeLa) cell line. *Phytomedicine*, *20*(2), 151–158. doi:10.1016/j.phymed.2012.10.009 PMID:23207250

Heppner, K., & Perez-Tilve, D. (2015). GLP-1 based therapeutics: Simultaneously combating T2DM and obesity. *Frontiers in Neuroscience*, *9*. Advance online publication. doi:10.3389/fnins.2015.00092 PMID:25852463

Herman, L. (2015). *Herb and spice companion: the complete guide to over 100 herbs & spices*. Wellfleet Press.

Hertog, M. G. L., Hollman, P. C., & van de Putte, B. (1993). Content of potentially anticarcinogenic flavonoids of tea infusions, wines, and fruit juices. *Journal of Agricultural and Food Chemistry*, *41*(8), 1242–1246. doi:10.1021/jf00032a015

Hevia, A., Delgado, S., Sánchez, B., & Margolles, A. (2015). Molecular Players Involved in the Interaction Between Beneficial Bacteria and the Immune System. *Frontiers in Microbiology*, *6*, 1285. doi:10.3389/fmicb.2015.01285 PMID:26635753

He, X., Wang, Y., Zhu, J., Orloff, M., & Eng, C. (2011). Resveratrol enhances the anti-tumor activity of the mTOR inhibitor rapamycin in multiple breast cancer cell lines mainly by suppressing rapamycin-induced AKT signaling. *Cancer Letters*, *301*(2), 168–176. doi:10.1016/j.canlet.2010.11.012 PMID:21168265

Hickson, M., D'Souza, A. L., Muthu, N., Rogers, T. R., Want, S., Rajkumar, C., & Bulpitt, C. J. (2007). Use of probiotic Lactobacillus preparation to prevent diarrhoea associated with antibiotics: Randomised double blind placebo controlled trial. *British Medical Journal*. Advance online publication. doi:10.1136/bmj.39231.599815.55 PMID:17604300

Hidalgo, M., Oruna-Concha, M. J., Kolida, S., Walton, G. E., Kallithraka, S., Spencer, J. P. E., ... de Pascual-Teresa, S. (2012). Metabolism of anthocyanins by human gut microflora and their influence on gut bacterial growth. *Journal of Agricultural and Food Chemistry*, *60*(15), 3882–3890. doi:10.1021/jf3002153 PMID:22439618

Hiermann, A., Schramm, H., & Laufer, S. (1998). Anti-inflammatory activity of myricetin-3-O-β-d-glucuronide and related compounds. *Inflammation Research*, *47*(11), 421–427. doi:10.1007000110050355 PMID:9865500

Hill, P., Muir, J. G., & Gibson, P. R. (2017). Controversies and Recent Developments of the Low-FODMAP Diet. *Gastroenterology & Hepatology*, *13*(1), 36–45. PMID:28420945

Hinnen, D., Nielsen, L., Waninger, A., & Kushner, P. (2006). Incretin mimetics and DPP-IV inhibitors: New paradigms for the treatment of type 2 diabetes. *Journal of the American Board of Family Medicine*, *19*(6), 612–618. doi:10.3122/jabfm.19.6.612 PMID:17090794

Hoang, J. (2010). Thyroid nodules and evaluation of thyroid cancer risk. *Australasian Journal of Ultrasound in Medicine*, *13*(4), 33–36. doi:10.1002/j.2205-0140.2010.tb00177.x PMID:28191095

Hoermann, R., Quadbeck, B., Roggenbuck, U., Szabolcs, I., Pfeilschifter, J., Meng, W., Reschke, K., Hackenberg, K., Dettmann, J., Prehn, B., Hirche, H., & Mann, K. (2002). Relapse of Graves' disease after successful outcome of antithyroid drug therapy: Results of a prospective randomized study on the use of levothyroxine. *Thyroid*, *12*(12), 1119–1128. doi:10.1089/105072502321085225 PMID:12593726

Ho, L., Chen, L. H., Wang, J., Zhao, W., Talcott, S. T., Ono, K., ... Percival, S. S. (2009). Heterogeneity in red wine polyphenolic contents differentially influences Alzheimer's disease-type neuropathology and cognitive deterioration. *Journal of Alzheimer's Disease*, *16*(1), 59–72. doi:10.3233/JAD-2009-0916 PMID:19158422

Ho, L., Ferruzzi, M. G., Janle, E. M., Wang, J., Gong, B., Chen, T.-Y., ... Talcott, S. T. (2013). Identification of brain-targeted bioactive dietary quercetin-3-O-glucuronide as a novel intervention for Alzheimer's disease. *The FASEB Journal*, *27*(2), 769–781. doi:10.1096/fj.12-212118 PMID:23097297

Holden, K. R., Zuniga, O. F., May, M. M., Su, H., Molinero, M. R., Rogers, R. C., & Schwartz, C. E. (2005). X-linked MCT8 gene mutations: Characterization of the pediatric neurologic phenotype. *Journal of Child Neurology*, *20*(10), 852–857. doi:10.1177/08830738050200101601 PMID:16417886

Hold, G. L. (2014). Role of the gut microbiota in inflammatory bowel disease pathogenesis: What have we learnt in the past 10 years? *World Journal of Gastroenterology*, *20*(5), 1192–1210. doi:10.3748/wjg.v20.i5.1192 PMID:24574795

Hollander, P., Maggs, D.G., Ruggles, J.A., Fineman, M., Shen, L., Koltetman, O.G., & Weyer, C. (2004). Effect of Pramlintide on weight in overweight an obese insulin-treated type2 diabetes patients. *Obese Res.*, *12*, 661-668.

Hollon, J., Puppa, E., Greenwald, B., Goldberg, E., Guerrerio, A., & Fasano, A. (2015). Effect of gliadin on permeability of intestinal biopsy explants from celiac disease patients and patients with non-celiac gluten sensitivity. *Nutrients*, *7*(3), 1565–1576. doi:10.3390/nu7031565 PMID:25734566

Hong, Y. J., Kim, N., Lee, K., Hee Sonn, C., Eun Lee, J., Tae Kim, S., Ho Baeg, I., & Lee, K.-M. (2012). Korean red ginseng (Panax ginseng) ameliorates type 1 diabetes and restores immune cell compartments. *Journal of Ethnopharmacology*, *144*(2), 225–233. doi:10.1016/j.jep.2012.08.009 PMID:22925946

Hong, Y., & Sun, B. (2016). Curative Estimation of Using Modified Cangfu Daotan Pill and Clomiphene in the Treatment of Polycystic Ovarian Syndrome Complicated with Infertility. *Journal of Sichuan of Traditional Chinese Medicine*, *34*, 90–93.

Hoogwerf, B., Doshi, K., & Diab, D. (2008). Pramlintide, the synthetic analogue of amylin: Physiology, pathophysiology, and effects on glycemic control, body weight, and selected biomarkers of vascular risk. *Vascular Health and Risk Management*, *4*(2), 355–362. doi:10.2147/VHRM.S1978 PMID:18561511

Hope, I. (2018). *Diabetes Pathophysiology & Diseases Process (Diagram)*. Retrieved 27 August 2020, from https://rnspeak.com/diabetes-pathophysiology-diseases-process-diagram/

Horakova, O., Kroupova, P., Bardova, K., Buresova, J., Janovska, P., Kopecky, J., & Rossmeisl, M. (2019). Metformin acutely lowers blood glucose levels by inhibition of intestinal glucose transport. *Scientific Reports*, *9*(1), 6156. Advance online publication. doi:10.103841598-019-42531-0 PMID:30992489

Hord, N. G. (2008). Eukaryotic microbiotic crosstalk: Potential mechanism for health benefits of prebiotics and probiotics. *Annual Review of Nutrition*, *28*(1), 215–231. doi:10.1146/annurev.nutr.28.061807.155402 PMID:18489258

Hormann, V., Kumi-Diaka, J., Durity, M., & Rathinavelu, A. (2012). Anticancer activities of genistein-topotecan combination in prostate cancer cells. *Journal of Cellular and Molecular Medicine*, *16*(11), 2631–2636. doi:10.1111/j.1582-4934.2012.01576.x PMID:22452992

Horne, B. D., Muhlestein, J. B., & Anderson, J. L. (2015). Health effects of intermittent fasting: Hormesis or harm? A systematic review. *The American Journal of Clinical Nutrition*, *102*(2), 464–470. doi:10.3945/ajcn.115.109553 PMID:26135345

Hossain, M. K., Dayem, A. A., Han, J., Yin, Y., Kim, K., Saha, S. K., Yang, G. M., Choi, H. Y., & Cho, S. G. (2016). Molecular mechanisms of the anti-obesity and anti-diabetic properties of flavonoids. *International Journal of Molecular Sciences*, *17*(4), 569–601. doi:10.3390/ijms17040569 PMID:27092490

Hossein, K. J., Leila, K. J., Ebrahim, T., Nazanin, S., Farzad, P., Elham, R., Mohammad, P., & Zahra, H. (2015). The effect of pomegranate juice extract on hormonal changes of female wistar rats caused by polycystic ovarian syndrome. *Biomedical & Pharmacology Journal*, *8*(2), 971–977. doi:10.13005/bpj/849

Hosseinzadeh, H., Ziaee, T., & Sadeghi, A. (2008). The effect of saffron, Crocus sativus stigma, extract and its constituents, safranal and crocin on sexual behaviors in normal male rats. *Phytomedicine*, *15*(6-7), 491–495. doi:10.1016/j.phymed.2007.09.020 PMID:17962007

Howells, L. M., Berry, D. P., Elliott, P. J., Jacobson, E. W., Hoffmann, E., Hegarty, B., ... Gescher, A. J. (2011). Phase I randomized, double-blind pilot study of micronized resveratrol (SRT501) in patients with hepatic metastases—Safety, pharmacokinetics, and pharmacodynamics. *Cancer Prevention Research (Philadelphia, Pa.)*, *4*(9), 1419–1425. doi:10.1158/1940-6207.CAPR-11-0148 PMID:21680702

Howie, P. W., Forsyth, J. S., Ogston, S. A., Clark, A., & Florey, C. D. (1990). Protective effect of breast feeding against infection. *BMJ (Clinical Research Ed.)*, *300*(6716), 11–16. doi:10.1136/bmj.300.6716.11 PMID:2105113

Howkins & Shaw. (1999). *Textbook of Gynaecology* (12th ed.). B.I. Churchill Livingstone Pvt. Ltd.

Hseu, Y. C., Huang, Y. C., Thiyagarajan, V., Mathew, D. C., Lin, K. Y., Chen, S. C., Liu, J.-Y., Hsu, L.-S., Li, M.-L., & Yang, H. L. (2019). Anticancer activities of chalcone flavokawain B from Alpinia pricei Hayata in human lung adenocarcinoma (A549) cells via induction of reactive oxygen species-mediated apoptotic and autophagic cell death. *Journal of Cellular Physiology*, *234*(10), 17514–17526. doi:10.1002/jcp.28375 PMID:30847898

Hsia, D., Grove, O., & Cefalu, W. (2017). An Update on SGLT2 Inhibitors for the Treatment of Diabetes Mellitus. *Current Opinion in Endocrinology, Diabetes, and Obesity*, *24*(1), 73–79. PMID:27898586

Hsu, C. L., Wu, C. H., Huang, S. L., & Yen, G. C. (2009). Phenolic compounds rutin and o-coumaric acid ameliorate obesity induced by high-fat diet in rats. *Journal of Agricultural and Food Chemistry*, *57*(2), 425–431. doi:10.1021/jf802715t PMID:19119847

Hu, S. (2016). *The synergistic effect of resveratrol in combination with cisplatin on apoptosis via modulating autophagy in A549 cells*. Academic Press.

Huang, H., Xin, H., Liu, X., Xu, Y., Wen, D., Zhang, Y., & Zhu, Y. Z. (2012). Novel anti-diabetic effect of SCM-198 via inhibiting the hepatic NF-kappaB pathway in db/db mice. *Bioscience Reports*, *32*(2), 185–195. doi:10.1042/BSR20110017 PMID:21859425

Huang, R. Y., Wong, M. K., Tan, T. Z., Kuay, K. T., Ng, A. H. C., Chung, V. Y., & Sim, W. J. (2013). An EMT spectrum defines an anoikis-resistant and spheroidogenic intermediate mesenchymal state that is sensitive to E-cadherin restoration by a src-kinase inhibitor, saracatinib (AZD0530). *Cell Death & Disease*, *4*(11), e915–e915. doi:10.1038/cddis.2013.442 PMID:24201814

Huang, R., Wang, K., & Hu, J. (2016). Effect of Probiotics on Depression: A Systematic Review and Meta-Analysis of Randomized Controlled Trials. *Nutrients*, *8*(8), 483. doi:10.3390/nu8080483 PMID:27509521

Huang, W. Y., Zhang, H. C., Liu, W. X., & Li, C. Y. (2012). Survey of antioxidant capacity and phenolic composition of blueberry, blackberry, and strawberry in nanjing. *Journal of Zhejiang University. Science. B.*, *13*(2), 94–102. doi:10.1631/jzus.B1100137 PMID:22302422

Huang, W.-C., Chen, C.-Y., Lin, S.-J., & Chang, C.-S. (2016). Medication adherence to oral anticancer drugs: Systematic review. *Expert Review of Anticancer Therapy*, *16*(4), 423–432. doi:10.1586/14737140.2016.1159515 PMID:26935964

Hueda, M. C. (2020). *Introductory chapter: Nutraceuticals as an alternative to maintain a healthy lifestyle, nutraceuticals- past, present and future*. IntechOpen. doi:10.5772/intechopen.89875

Hu, F. B., & Willett, W. C. (2002). Optimal diets for prevention of coronary heart disease. *Journal of the American Medical Association*, *288*(20), 25692578. doi:10.1001/jama.288.20.2569 PMID:12444864

Hui, H., Tang, G., & Go, V. L. (2009). Hypoglycemic herbs and their action mechanisms. *Chinese Medicine*, *4*(1), 11. doi:10.1186/1749-8546-4-11 PMID:19523223

Hussain, A., Brahmbhatt, K., Priyani, A., Ahmed, M., Rizvi, T. A., & Sharma, C. (2011). Eugenol enhances the chemotherapeutic potential of gemcitabine and induces anticarcinogenic and anti-inflammatory activity in human cervical cancer cells. *Cancer Biotherapy & Radiopharmaceuticals*, *26*(5), 519–527. doi:10.1089/cbr.2010.0925 PMID:21939359

Hussain, A., Harish, G., Prabhu, S. A., Mohsin, J., Khan, M. A., Rizvi, T. A., & Sharma, C. (2012). Inhibitory effect of genistein on the invasive potential of human cervical cancer cells via modulation of matrix metalloproteinase-9 and tissue inhibitiors of matrix metalloproteinase-1 expression. *Cancer Epidemiology*, *36*(6), e387–e393. doi:10.1016/j.canep.2012.07.005 PMID:22884883

Hussain, A., Mohsin, J., Prabhu, S. A., Begum, S., Nusri, Q. E.-A., Harish, G., Javed, E., Khan, M. A., & Sharma, C. (2013). Sulforaphane inhibits growth of human breast cancer cells and augments the therapeutic index of the chemotherapeutic drug, gemcitabine. *Asian Pacific Journal of Cancer Prevention*, *14*(10), 5855–5860. doi:10.7314/APJCP.2013.14.10.5855 PMID:24289589

Hussain, K., Majeed, M. T., Ismail, Z., Sadikun, A., & Ibrahim, P. (2009). Traditional and complementary medicines: Quality assessment strategies and safe usage. *Southern Med Review*, *2*(1), 19–23.

Hussain, S., Ahmed, A. A., Mahwi, T. O., & Aziz, T. A. (2012). Postprandial hyperglycemia in type 2 diabetic patients challenged with carbohydrates load. *International Journal of Experimental Diabetes Research*, *1*(3), 32–35. doi:10.5923/j.diabetes.20120103.01

Hwang, J. H., Jung, H. W., Kang, S. Y., Kang, A. N., Ma, J. N., Meng, X. L., Hwang, M., & Park, Y. K. (2018). Therapeutic effects of acupuncture with MOK, a polyherbal medicine, on PTU-induced hypothyroidism in rats. *Experimental and Therapeutic Medicine, 16*(1), 310–320. doi:10.3892/etm.2018.6190 PMID:29896255

Hyun-Jin, C., Mi Ja, C., & Seung-Shi, H. (2010). Antiobese and hypocholesterolaemic effects of an *Adenophora triphylla* extract in HepG2 cells and high fat diet-induced obese mice. *Food Chemistry, 119*(2), 437–444. doi:10.1016/j.foodchem.2009.06.039

Ibn Sīnā. (1990). *Al-Qānūn fi'l Tibb*. New Delhi, India: Idara Kitabul Shifa.

Imparl-Radosevich, J., Deas, S., Polansky, M. M., Baedke, D. A., Ingebritsen, T. S., Anderson, R. A., & Graves, D. J. (1998). Regulation of PTP-1 and insulin receptor kinase by fractions from cinnamon: Implications for cinnamon regulation of insulin signalling. *Hormone Research, 50*(3), 177–182. doi:10.1159/000023270 PMID:9762007

International Diabetes Federation. (2017). *IDF Diabetes Atlas* (Eighth edition 2017). doi:10.1016/S0140-6736(16)31679-8

International Diabetes Foundation. (2019). *Diabetes: facts and figures*. Available from: https://www.idf.org/WDD15-guide/facts-and-figures.html

IOM. (2000). Selenium. In Dietary reference intakes for vitamin C, vitamin E, selenium and carotenoids. Food and Nutrition Board, Institute of Medicine. National Academy Press.

IOM. (2002). *Dietary reference intakes for energy, carbohydrate, fiber, fat, fatty acids, cholesterol, protein and amino acids*. Institute of Medicine.

Ip, S., Chung, M., Raman, G., Trikalinos, T.A., & Lau, J. (2009). A summary of the agency for healthcare research and quality's evidence report on breastfeeding in developed countries. *Breastfeeding Medicine, 4*(S1), S17–30.

Iriti, M., & Faoro, F. (2006). Grape phytochemicals: A bouquet of old and new nutraceuticals for human health. *Medical Hypotheses*. Advance online publication. doi:10.1016/j.mehy.2006.03.049 PMID:16759816

Irudayaraj, S. S., Stalin, A., Sunil, C., Duraipandiyan, V., Al-Dhabi, N. A., & Ignacimuthu, S. (2016). Antioxidant, antilipidemic and antidiabetic effects of ficusin with their effects on GLUT4 translocation and PPARγ expression in type 2 diabetic rats. *Chemico-Biological Interactions, 256*, 85–93. doi:10.1016/j.cbi.2016.06.023 PMID:27350165

Islam, S., Mokhtari, R. B., Akbari, P., Hatina, J., Yeger, H., & Farhat, W. A. (2017). Simultaneous Targeting of Bladder Tumor Growth, Survival, and Epithelial-to-Mesenchymal Transition with a Novel Therapeutic Combination of Acetazolamide (AZ) and Sulforaphane (SFN). *Targeted Oncology, 11*(2), 209–227. doi:10.100711523-015-0386-5 PMID:26453055

Isomaa, B., Almgren, P., Tuomi, T., Forsen, B., Lahti, K., Nissen, M., Taskinen, M.-R., & Groop, L. (2001). Cardiovascular morbidity and mortality associated with the metabolic syndrome. *Diabetes Care, 24*(4), 683–689. doi:10.2337/diacare.24.4.683 PMID:11315831

Istre, G. R., Conner, J. S., Broome, C. V., Hightower, A., & Hopkins, R. S. (1985). Risk factors for primary invasive Haemophilus influenzae disease: Increased risk from day care attendance and school-aged household members. *The Journal of Pediatrics, 106*(2), 190–195. doi:10.1016/S0022-3476(85)80285-7 PMID:3871478

Iuvone, T., Esposito, G., Capasso, F., & Izzo, A. A. (2003). Induction of nitric oxide synthase expression by Withania somnifera in macrophages. *Life Sciences, 72*(14), 1617–1625. doi:10.1016/S0024-3205(02)02472-4 PMID:12551750

Izar, M. C., Tegani, D. M., Kasmas, S. H., & Fonseca, F. A. (2011). Phytosterols and phytosterolemia: Gene-diet interactions. *Genes & Nutrition, 6*(1), 17–26. doi:10.100712263-010-0182-x PMID:21437027

Jachak, S. M., & Saklani, A. (2007). Challenges and opportunities in drug discovery from plants. *Current Science*, 1251–1257.

Jahanafrooz, Z., Motamed, N., Rinner, B., Mokhtarzadeh, A., & Baradaran, B. (2018). Silibinin to improve cancer therapeutic, as an apoptotic inducer, autophagy modulator, cell cycle inhibitor, and microRNAs regulator. *Life Sciences*, *213*, 236–247. doi:10.1016/j.lfs.2018.10.009 PMID:30308184

Jakicic, J. M., & Otto, A. D. (2005). Physical activity considerations for the treatment and prevention of obesity. *The American Journal of Clinical Nutrition*, *82*(1), 226–229. doi:10.1093/ajcn/82.1.226S PMID:16002826

Jalilian, N., Modarresi, M., Rezaie, M., Ghaderi, L., & Bozorgmanesh, M. (2013). Phytotherapeutic management of polycystic ovary syndrome: Role of aerial parts of wood betony (Stachys lavandulifolia). *Phytotherapy Research*, *27*(11), 1708–1713. doi:10.1002/ptr.4921 PMID:23307315

James, M. I., Iwuji, C., Irving, G., Karmokar, A., Higgins, J. A., Griffin-Teal, N., Thomas, A., Greaves, P., Cai, H., Patel, S. R., Morgan, B., Dennison, A., Metcalfe, M., Garcea, G., Lloyd, D. M., Berry, D. P., Steward, W. P., Howells, L. M., & Brown, K. (2015). Curcumin inhibits cancer stem cell phenotypes in <em>ex vivo</em> models of colorectal liver metastases, and is clinically safe and tolerable in combination with FOLFOX chemotherapy. *Cancer Letters*, *364*(2), 135–141. doi:10.1016/j.canlet.2015.05.005 PMID:25979230

Janczarek, M., Bachanek, T., Mazur, E., & Chalas, R. (2016). The role of probiotics in prevention of oral diseases. Postepy Higiency I. *Medycyna Doswiadczalna*, *70*(0), 850–885. PMID:27594560

Jang, W. S., & Choung, S. Y. (2013). Antiobesity effects of the ethanol extract of *Laminaria japonica* Areshoung in high-fat-diet-induced obese rat. *Evidence-Based Complementary and Alternative Medicine*, *2013*, 492807. doi:10.1155/2013/492807 PMID:23365609

Jang, Y., Kim, M., & Hwang, S. W. (2020). Molecular mechanisms underlying the actions of arachidonic acid-derived prostaglandins on peripheral nociception. *Journal of Neuroinflammation*, *17*(1), 30. doi:10.118612974-020-1703-1 PMID:31969159

Janovskà, P., Flachs, P., Kazdova, L., & Kopecký, J. (2013). Anti-obesity effect of n-3 polyunsaturated fatty acids in mice fed high-fat diet is independent of cold-induced thermogenesis. *Physiological Research*, *62*, 153–161. doi:10.33549/physiolres.932464 PMID:23234412

Jaradat, N., & Zaid, A. N. (2019). Herbal remedies used for the treatment of infertility in males and females by traditional healers in the rural areas of the West Bank/Palestine. *BMC Complementary and Alternative Medicine*, *19*(1), 194. doi:10.118612906-019-2617-2 PMID:31366346

Jatwa, R., & Kar, A. (2009). Amelioration of metformin-induced hypothyroidism by Withania somnifera and Bauhinia purpurea extracts in Type 2 diabetic mice. *Phytotherapy Research*, *23*(8), 1140–1145. doi:10.1002/ptr.2765 PMID:19170137

Javir, G., Joshi, K., Khedkar, V., & Rojatkar, S. (2020). 6 α-Hydroxy-4 [14], 10 [15]-guainadien-8β, 12-olide induced cell cycle arrest via modulation of EMT and Wnt/β-catenin pathway in HER-2 positive breast cancer cells. *The Journal of Steroid Biochemistry and Molecular Biology*, *197*, 105514. doi:10.1016/j.jsbmb.2019.105514 PMID:31678110

Jayaprasad, B., Sharavanan, P. S., & Sivaraj, R. (2016). Antidiabetic effect of *Chloroxylon swietenia* bark extracts on streptozotocin induced diabetic rats. *Beni-Suef Univ. Journal of Basic and Applied Sciences*, *5*(1), 1–9.

Jazani, Hamdi, Tansaz, Nazemiyeh, Bazargani, Fazljou, & Azgomi. (2018). *Herbal Medicine for Oligomenorrhea and Amenorrhea: A Systematic Review of Ancient and Conventional Medicine*. Hindawi BioMed Research International. doi:10.1155/2018/3052768

Jedel, E., Waern, M., Gustafson, D., Landén, M., Eriksson, E., Holm, G., Nilsson, L., Lind, A.-K., Janson, P. O., & Stener-Victorin, E. (2010). Anxiety and depression symptoms in women with polycystic ovary Syndrome compared with controls matched for body mass index. *Human Reproduction (Oxford, England)*, *25*(2), 450–456. doi:10.1093/humrep/dep384 PMID:19933236

Jelodar, K. A. (2012). Effect of Vitex agnus-castus fruits hydroalcoholic extract on sex hormones in rat with induced polycystic ovary syndrome (PCOS). *Physiol. Pharmacol.*, *16*, 62–69.

Jensen, E. X., Fusch, C., Jaeger, P., Peheim, E., & Horber, F. F. (1995). Impact of chronic cigarette smoking on body composition and fuel metabolism. *The Journal of Clinical Endocrinology and Metabolism*, *80*(7), 2181–2185. PMID:7608276

Jeong, S., Min Cho, J., Kwon, Y., Kim, S., Yeob Shin, D., & Ho Lee, J. (2019). Chitosan oligosaccharide (GO2KA1) improves postprandial glycemic response in subjects with impaired glucose tolerance and impaired fasting glucose and in healthy subjects: A crossover, randomized controlled trial. *Nutrition & Diabetes*, *9*(1), 31. Advance online publication. doi:10.103841387-019-0099-4 PMID:31685797

Jernberg, C., Löfmark, S., Edlund, C., & Jansson, J. K. (2007). Long-term ecological impacts of antibiotic administration on the human intestinal microbiota. *The ISME Journal*, *1*(1), 56–66. doi:10.1038/ismej.2007.3 PMID:18043614

Jernberg, C., Löfmark, S., Edlund, C., & Jansson, J. K. (2010). Long-term impacts of antibiotic exposure on the human intestinal microbiota. *Microbiology*, *156*(Pt 11), 3216–3223. doi:10.1099/mic.0.040618-0 PMID:20705661

Jia, K., Tong, X., Wang, R., & Song, X. (2018). The clinical effects of probiotics for inflammatory bowel disease: A meta-analysis. *Medicine; Analytical Reviews of General Medicine, Neurology, Psychiatry, Dermatology, and Pediatries*, *97*(51), e13792. doi:10.1097/MD.0000000000013792 PMID:30572537

Jiang, J., & Dutta, S. (2017). *PDB101: Global Health: Diabetes Mellitus: Monitoring: Complications.* Retrieved 24 August 2020, from https://pdb101.rcsb.org/global-health/diabetes-mellitus/monitoring/complications

Jiang, D. (2017). TCM Treatment of Polycystic Ovary and PCOS. *J Complement Med Alt Healthcare J*, *2*(1), 1–5. doi:10.19080/JCMAH.2017.02.555578

Jiang, M., Huang, O., Zhang, X., Xie, Z., Shen, A., Liu, H., Geng, M., & Shen, K. (2013). Curcumin Induces Cell Death and Restores Tamoxifen Sensitivity in the Antiestrogen-Resistant Breast Cancer Cell Lines MCF-7/LCC2 and MCF-7/LCC9. *Molecules (Basel, Switzerland)*, *18*(1), 701–720. doi:10.3390/molecules18010701 PMID:23299550

Jiang, Z., Cao, Q., Dai, G., Wang, J., Liu, C., Lv, L., & Pan, J. (2019). Celastrol inhibits colorectal cancer through TGF-β1/Smad signaling. *OncoTargets and Therapy*, *12*, 509–518. doi:10.2147/OTT.S187817 PMID:30666129

Jiang, Z., Wang, J., Li, X., & Zhang, X. (2016). Echinacoside and Cistanche tubulosa (Schenk) R. wight ameliorate bisphenol A-induced testicular and sperm damage in rats through gonad axis regulated steroidogenic enzymes. *Journal of Ethnopharmacology*, *193*, 321–328. doi:10.1016/j.jep.2016.07.033 PMID:27422164

Jianping, J.Y., & Jiaa, Y. W. (2012). Effects and mechanisms of berberine in diabetes treatment. *Acta Pharmaceutica Sinica B*, *2*(4), 327-334.

Ji, H., & Zhang, H. (2008). Multipotent natural agents to combat Alzheimer's disease. Functional spectrum and structural features. *Acta Pharmacologica Sinica*, *29*(2), 143–151. doi:10.1111/j.1745-7254.2008.00752.x PMID:18215342

Jolly, M. K., Tripathi, S. C., Jia, D., Mooney, S. M., Celiktas, M., Hanash, S. M., & Levine, H. (2016). Stability of the hybrid epithelial/mesenchymal phenotype. *Oncotarget*, *7*(19), 27067–27084. doi:10.18632/oncotarget.8166 PMID:27008704

Jones, G., Steketee, R. W., Black, R. E., Bhutta, Z. A., & Morris, S. S. (2003). How many child deaths can we prevent this year. *Lancet*, *362*(9377), 65–71. doi:10.1016/S0140-6736(03)13811-1 PMID:12853204

Jong-Anurakkun, N., Bhandari, M. R., Hong, G., & Kawabata, J. (2008). α-Glucosidase inhibitor from Chinese aloes. *Fitoterapia*, *79*(6), 456–457. doi:10.1016/j.fitote.2008.02.010 PMID:18508205

Jonsson, A. L., & Backhed, F. (2017). Role of gut microbiota in atherosclerosis. *Nature Reviews. Cardiology*, *14*(2), 79–87. doi:10.1038/nrcardio.2016.183 PMID:27905479

Jordan, N. V., Johnson, G. L., & Abell, A. N. (2011). Tracking the intermediate stages of epithelial-mesenchymal transition in epithelial stem cells and cancer. *Cell Cycle (Georgetown, Tex.)*, *10*(17), 2865–2873. doi:10.4161/cc.10.17.17188 PMID:21862874

Jorge, A. P., Horst, H., de Sousa, E., Pizzolatti, M. G., & Silva, F. R. (2004). Insulinomimetic effects of kaempferitrin on glycaemia and on 14C-glucose uptake in rat soleus muscle. *Chemico-Biological Interactions*, *49*(2-3), 89–96. doi:10.1016/j.cbi.2004.07.001 PMID:15501431

Joslin, D. (2020). *Advantages and disadvantages of insulin pump*. Retrieved 24 August 2020, from https://onlineclasses.joslin.org/info/the_advantages_and_disadvantages_of_an_insulin_pump.html

Juengel, E., Euler, S., Maxeiner, S., Rutz, J., Justin, S., Roos, F., Khoder, W., Nelson, K., Bechstein, W. O., & Blaheta, R. A. (2017). Sulforaphane as an adjunctive to everolimus counteracts everolimus resistance in renal cancer cell lines. *Phytomedicine*, *27*, 1–7. doi:10.1016/j.phymed.2017.01.016 PMID:28314474

Jungbauer, A., & Medjakovic, S. (2014). Phytoestrogens and the metabolic syndrome. *The Journal of Steroid Biochemistry and Molecular Biology*, *139*, 277–289. doi:10.1016/j.jsbmb.2012.12.009 PMID:23318879

Jung, U. J., Lee, M. K., Jeong, K. S., & Choi, M. S. (2004). The hypoglycemic effects of hesperidin and naringin are partly mediated by hepatic glucose-regulating enzymes in C57BL/KsJ-*db/db* mice. *The Journal of Nutrition*, *134*(10), 2499–2503. doi:10.1093/jn/134.10.2499 PMID:15465737

Jung, U. J., Lee, M. K., Park, Y. B., Kang, M. A., & Choi, M. S. (2006). Effect of citrus flavonoids on lipid metabolism and glucose-regulating enzyme mRNA levels in type-2 diabetic mice. *The International Journal of Biochemistry & Cell Biology*, *38*(7), 1134–1145. doi:10.1016/j.biocel.2005.12.002 PMID:16427799

Jungwirth, A., Giwercman, A., Tournaye, H., Diemer, T., Kopa, Z., Dohle, G., & Krausz, C. (2012). European Association of Urology Guidelines on Male Infertility: The 2012 update. *European Urology*, *62*(2), 324–332. doi:10.1016/j.eururo.2012.04.048 PMID:22591628

Jurjani, S. (2010). *Zakhira Khawarizm Shahi*. New Delhi, India: Idara Kitabul Shifa.

Kaatabi, H., Bamosa, A. O., Badar, A., Al-Elq, A., Abou-Hozaifa, B., Lebda, F., Al-Khadra, A., & Al-Almaie, S. (2015). *Nigella sativa* improves glycemic control and ameliorates oxidative stress in patients with type 2 diabetes mellitus: Placebo controlled participant blinded clinical trial. *PLoS One*, *10*(2), e0113486. doi:10.1371/journal.pone.0113486 PMID:25706772

Kaczmarczyk, M. M., Miller, M. J., & Freund, G. G. (2012). The health benefits of dietary fiber: Beyond the usual suspects of type 2 diabetes mellitus, cardiovascular disease and colon cancer. *Metabolism: Clinical and Experimental*, *61*(8), 1058–1066. doi:10.1016/j.metabol.2012.01.017 PMID:22401879

Kadooka, Y., Sato, M., Imaizumi, K., Ogawa, A., Ikuyama, K., Akai, Y., Okano, M., Kagoshima, M., & Tsuchida, T. (2010). Regulation of abdominal adiposity by probiotics (*Lactobacillus gasseri* SBT2055) in adults with obese tendencies in a randomized controlled trial. *European Journal of Clinical Nutrition*, *64*(6), 636–643. doi:10.1038/ejcn.2010.19 PMID:20216555

Kaguelidou, F., Alberti, C., Castanet, M., Guitteny, M. A., Czernichow, P., & Leger, J. (2008). Predictors of autoimmune hyperthyroidism relapse in children after discontinuation of antithyroid drug treatment. *The Journal of Clinical Endocrinology and Metabolism*, *93*(10), 3817–3826. doi:10.1210/jc.2008-0842 PMID:18628515

Kalhotra, P., Chittepu, V.C.S.R., Osorio-Revilla, G. & Gallardo-Velazquez, T. (2020). Phytochemicals in garlic extract inhibit therapeutic enzyme DPP-4 and induce skeletal muscle cell proliferation: A possible mechanism of action to benefit the treatment of diabetes mellitus. *Biomolecules*, *10*(2), 305.

Kalia, A. N. (2005). *Textbook of industrial pharmacognocy*. New Delhi: CBS Publisher and Distributor.

Kaliannan, K., Wang, B., Li, X.-Y., Kim, K.-J., & Kang, J. X. (2015). A host-microbiome interaction mediates the opposing effects of omega-6 and omega-3 fatty acids on metabolic endotoxemia. *Scientific Reports*, *5*(1), 11276. doi:10.1038rep11276 PMID:26062993

Kalra, E. K. (2003). Nutraceuticals-Definition and introduction. *American Association of Pharmaceutical Scientists*, *5*(3), 27–28.

Kalsi, T., Babic-Illman, G., Ross, P. J., Maisey, N. R., Hughes, S., Fields, P., Martin, F. C., Wang, Y., & Harari, D. (2015). The impact of comprehensive geriatric assessment interventions on tolerance to chemotherapy in older people. *British Journal of Cancer*, *112*(9), 1435–1444. doi:10.1038/bjc.2015.120 PMID:25871332

Kamel, H. H. (2013). Role of phyto-oestrogens in ovulation induction in women with polycystic ovarian syndrome. *European Journal of Obstetrics, Gynecology, and Reproductive Biology*, *168*(1), 60–63. doi:10.1016/j.ejogrb.2012.12.025 PMID:23347605

Kanai, M., Yoshimura, K., Asada, M., Imaizumi, A., Suzuki, C., Matsumoto, S., Nishimura, T., Mori, Y., Masui, T., Kawaguchi, Y., Yanagihara, K., Yazumi, S., Chiba, T., Guha, S., & Aggarwal, B. B. (2011). A phase I/II study of gemcitabine-based chemotherapy plus curcumin for patients with gemcitabine-resistant pancreatic cancer. *Cancer Chemotherapy and Pharmacology*, *68*(1), 157–164. doi:10.100700280-010-1470-2 PMID:20859741

Kandasamy, N., & Ashokkumar, N. (2014). Protective effect of bioflavonoid myricetin enhances carbohydrate metabolic enzymes and insulin signaling molecules in streptozotocin-cadmium induced diabetic nephrotoxic rats. *Toxicology and Applied Pharmacology*, *279*(2), 173–185. doi:10.1016/j.taap.2014.05.014 PMID:24923654

Kang, H. J., Youn, Y. K., Hong, M. K., & Kim, L. S. (2011). Antiproliferation and redifferentiation in thyroid cancer cell lines by polyphenol phytochemicals. *Journal of Korean Medical Science*, *26*(7), 893–899. doi:10.3346/jkms.2011.26.7.893 PMID:21738342

Kang, J. H., Kang, H. S., Kim, I. K., Lee, H. Y., Ha, J. H., Yeo, C. D., Kang, H. H., Moon, H. S., & Lee, S. H. (2015). Curcumin sensitizes human lung cancer cells to apoptosis and metastasis synergistically combined with carboplatin. *Experimental Biology and Medicine*, *240*(11), 1416–1425. doi:10.1177/1535370215571881 PMID:25716014

Kang, J. H., Tsuyoshi, G., Han, I. S., Kawada, T., Kim, Y. M., & Yu, R. (2010). Dietary capsaicin reduces obesity-induced insulin resistance and hepatic steatosis in obese mice fed a high-fat diet. *Obesity (Silver Spring, Md.)*, *18*(4), 780–787. doi:10.1038/oby.2009.301 PMID:19798065

Kang, O. H., Shon, M. Y., Kong, R., Seo, Y. S., Zhou, T., Kim, D. Y., Kim, Y. S., & Kwon, D. Y. (2017). Anti-diabetic effect of black ginseng extract by augmentation of AMPK protein activity and upregulation of GLUT2 and GLUT4 expression in db/db mice. *BMC Complementary and Alternative Medicine*, *17*(1), 341–352. doi:10.118612906-017-1839-4 PMID:28662663

Kanitsoraphan, C., Rattanawong, P., Charoensri, S., & Senthong, V. (2018). Trimethylamine N-Oxide and Risk of Cardiovascular Disease and Mortality. *Current Nutrition Reports*, *7*(4), 207–213. doi:10.100713668-018-0252-z PMID:30362023

Kanter, R., & Caballero, B. (2012). Global gender disparities in obesity: A review. *Advances in Nutrition*, *3*(4), 491–498. doi:10.3945/an.112.002063 PMID:22797984

Kao, Y. H., Hiipakka, R. A., & Liao, S. (2000). Modulation of endocrine systems and food intake by green tea epigallocatechin gallate. *Endocrinology*, *141*(3), 980–987. doi:10.1210/endo.141.3.7368 PMID:10698173

Kar, A., Panda, S., & Bharti, S. (2002). Relative efficacy of three medicinal plant extracts in the alteration of thyroid hormone concentrations in male mice. *Journal of Ethnopharmacology*, *81*(2), 281–285. doi:10.1016/S0378-8741(02)00048-X PMID:12065164

Karlsson, F. H., Fåk, F., Nookaew, I., Tremaroli, V., Fagerberg, B., Petranovic, D., ... Nielsen, J. (2012). Symptomatic atherosclerosis is associated with an altered gut metagenome. *Nature Communications*, *3*(1), 1245. doi:10.1038/ncomms2266 PMID:23212374

Karmase, A., Birari, R., & Bhutani, K. K. (2013). Evaluation of anti-obesity effect of *Aegle marmelos* leaves. *Phytomedicine*, *20*(10), 805–812. doi:10.1016/j.phymed.2013.03.014 PMID:23632084

Karmisholt, J., Andersen, S. L., Bulow-Pedersen, I., Carle, A., Krejbjerg, A., & Nygaard, B. (2019). Predictors of Initial and Sustained Remission in Patients Treated with Antithyroid Drugs for Graves' Hyperthyroidism: The RISG Study. *Journal of Thyroid Research*, *5945178*, 1–9. Advance online publication. doi:10.1155/2019/5945178 PMID:30719273

Karri, S., Sharma, S., Hatware, K., & Patil, K. (2019). Natural anti-obesity agents and their therapeutic role in management of obesity: A future trend perspective. *Biomedicine and Pharmacotherapy*, *110*, 224–238. doi:10.1016/j.biopha.2018.11.076 PMID:30481727

Karthick, C., Periyasamy, S., Jayachandran, K. S., & Anusuyadevi, M. (2016). Intrahippocampal administration of ibotenic acid induced cholinergic dysfunction via NR2A/NR2B expression: Implications of resveratrol against Alzheimer disease pathophysiology. *Frontiers in Molecular Neuroscience*, *9*, 28. doi:10.3389/fnmol.2016.00028 PMID:27199654

Karthik, M., & Gayathri, C. (2013). Effect of ethanolic extract of *Hibiscus cannabinus* leaf on high cholesterol diet induced obesity in female albino rats. *Asian Journal of Pharmaceutical and Clinical Research*, *6*(4), 65–67.

Karuppagounder, S. S., Pinto, J. T., Xu, H., Chen, H.-L., Beal, M. F., & Gibson, G. E. (2009). Dietary supplementation with resveratrol reduces plaque pathology in a transgenic model of Alzheimer's disease. *Neurochemistry International*, *54*(2), 111–118. doi:10.1016/j.neuint.2008.10.008 PMID:19041676

Kashani,, L., & Akhondzadeh, S. (2016). Herbal Medicine in the Treatment of Polycystic Ovary Syndrome. *Faslnamah-i Giyahan-i Daruyi*, *15*, 59.

Kasiotis, K. M., Pratsinis, H., Kletsas, D., & Haroutounian, S. A. (2013). Resveratrol and related stilbenes: Their anti-aging and anti-angiogenic properties. *Food and Chemical Toxicology*, *61*, 112–120. doi:10.1016/j.fct.2013.03.038 PMID:23567244

Kasubuchi, M., Hasegawa, S., Hiramatsu, T., Ichimura, A., & Kimura, I. (2015). Dietary gut microbial metabolites, short-chain fatty acids, and host metabolic regulation. *Nutrients*, *7*(4), 2839–2849. doi:10.3390/nu7042839 PMID:25875123

Kaufinan, P., Cseke, L., Warber, S., Duke, J., & Brielmann, H. (1999). *Natural products from plants*. CRC Press.

Kaul, K., Apostolopoulou, M., & Roden, M. (2015). Insulin resistance in type 1 diabetes mellitus. *Metabolism, 64*(12), 1629-1639.

Kaul, K., Tarr, J., Ahmad, S., Kohner, E., & Chibber, R. (2012). Introduction to diabetes mellitus. *Advances in Experimental Medicine and Biology*, *771*, 1–11. PMID:23393665

Kaur, G., Mukundan, S., Wani, V., & Kumar, M. S. (2015). Nutraceuticals in the management and prevention of metabolic syndrome. *Austin Journal of Pharmacology and Therapeutics*, *3*, 1–6.

Kaur, J. (2014). A comprehensive review of metabolic syndrome. *Cardiology Research and Practice*, *2014*, 943162. doi:10.1155/2014/943162

Kaur, J., Kaur, S., & Mahajan, A. (2013). Herbal medicines: Possible risks and benefits. *Am J Phytomed Clin Ther*, *1*(2), 226–239.

Kaur, R., Mahajan, P., & Goswami, M. (2018). Diabetes mellitus: An emerging risk factor to public health. *World Journal of Pharmaceutical Research*, *7*(12), 257–281.

Kavanagh, K. T., Hafer, L. J., Kim, D. W., Mann, K. K., Sherr, D. H., Rogers, A. E., & Sonenshein, G. E. (2001). Green tea extracts decrease carcinogen-induced mammary tumor burden in rats and rate of breast cancer cell proliferation in culture. *Journal of Cellular Biochemistry*, *82*(3), 387–398. doi:10.1002/jcb.1164 PMID:11500915

Kawser Hossain, M., Abdal Dayem, A., Han, J., Kumar Saha, S., Yang, G. M., Choi, H. Y., & Cho, S. G. (2016). Recent advances in disease modeling and drug discovery for diabetes mellitus using induced pluripotent stem cells. *International Journal of Molecular Sciences*, *17*(2), 256–273. doi:10.3390/ijms17020256 PMID:26907255

Kazeem, M. I., Adamson, J. O., & Ogunwande, I. A. (2013). Modes of inhibition of α-amylase and α-glucosidase by aqueous extract of Morinda lucida Benth leaf. *BioMed Research International*. PMID:24455701

Kellow, N. J., & Savige, G. S. (2013). Dietary advanced glycation end-product restriction for the attenuation of insulin resistance, oxidative stress and endothelial dysfunction: A systematic review. *European Journal of Clinical Nutrition*, *67*(3), 239–248. doi:10.1038/ejcn.2012.220 PMID:23361161

Kelly, J. R., Kennedy, P. J., Cryan, J. F., Dinan, T. G., Clarke, G., & Hyland, N. P. (2015). Breaking down the barriers: The gut microbiome, intestinal permeability and stress-related psychiatric disorders. *Frontiers in Cellular Neuroscience*, *9*, 392. doi:10.3389/fncel.2015.00392 PMID:26528128

Kenjale, R., Shah, R., & Sathaye, S. (2008). Effects of *Chlorophytum borivil- ianum* on sexual behaviour and sperm count in male rats. *Phytotherapy Research*, *22*(6), 796–801. doi:10.1002/ptr.2369 PMID:18412148

Kennedy, D. O. (2016). B vitamins and the brain: Mechanism, dose and efficacy- A review. *Nutrients*, *8*(2), 68. doi:10.3390/nu8020068 PMID:26828517

Kennedy, D. O., & Wightman, E. L. (2011). Herbal extracts and phytochemicals: Plant secondary metabolites and the enhancement of human brain function. *Advances in Nutrition (Bethesda, Md.)*, *2*(1), 32–50. doi:10.3945/an.110.000117 PMID:22211188

Kennedy, K. I., Labbok, M. H., & Van Look, P. F. (1996). Lactational amenorrhea method for family planning. *International Journal of Gynaecology and Obstetrics: the Official Organ of the International Federation of Gynaecology and Obstetrics*, *54*(1), 55–57. doi:10.1016/0020-7292(96)02670-7 PMID:8842819

Kernan, W. N., Inzucchi, S. E., Sawan, C., Macko, R. F., & Furie, K. L. (2013). Obesity: A stubbornly obvious target for stroke prevention. *Stroke*, *44*(1), 278–286. doi:10.1161/STROKEAHA.111.639922 PMID:23111440

Kerr, C. (2018). Combination cisplatin and sulforaphane treatment reduces proliferation, invasion, and tumor formation in epidermal squamous cell carcinoma. Academic Press.

Khaki, A. A. (2012). Pp-1 The Effects Of Ginger On Spermatogenesis And Sperm Parameters Of Rat. *Reproductive Biomedicine Online*, *24*, S5. Advance online publication. doi:10.1016/S1472-6483(12)60133-3

Khan, A., Safdar, M., Khan, M. A., Khattak, K. N., & Anderson, R. A. (2003). Cinnamon improves glucose and lipids of people with type 2 diabetes. *Diabetes Care*, *26*(12), 3215–3218. doi:10.2337/diacare.26.12.3215 PMID:14633804

Khanage, S. G., Subhash, T. Y., & Bhaiyyasaheb, I. R. (2019). Herbal drugs for the treatment of Polycystic ovary syndrome (PCOS) and its complications. *Pharmaceutical Research*, *2*(1), 5–13. PMID:31823112

Khani, B., Rabbani Bidgoli, S., Moattar, F., & Hassani, H. (2013). Effect of sesame on sperm quality of infertile men. *Journal of Research in Medical Sciences*, *18*(3), 184–187. PMID:23930112

Khan, M. A. B., Hashim, J. M., King, J. K., Govender, R. D., Mustafa, H., & Kaabi, J. A. (2020). Epidemiology of type 2 diabetes-global burden of disease and forecasted trends. *Journal of Epidemiology and Global Health*, *10*(1), 107–111. doi:10.2991/jegh.k.191028.001 PMID:32175717

Khan, M. J., Gerasimidis, K., Edwards, C. A., & Shaikh, M. G. (2016). Role of Gut Microbiota in the Aetiology of Obesity: Proposed Mechanisms and Review of the Literature. *Journal of Obesity*, *2016*, 7353642. doi:10.1155/2016/7353642 PMID:27703805

Khan, M., Hussain, A., Sundaram, M. K., Alalami, U., Gunasekera, D., Ramesh, L., Hamza, A., & Quraishi, U. (2015). (-)-Epigallocatechin-3-gallate reverses the expression of various tumor-suppressor genes by inhibiting DNA methyltransferases and histone deacetylases in human cervical cancer cells. *Oncology Reports*, *33*(4), 1–9. doi:10.3892/or.2015.3802 PMID:25682960

Khare, C. P. (2007). *Indian Medicinal Plants*. New Delhi, India: Springer India Private Limited. doi:10.1007/978-0-387-70638-2

Kharroubi, A., & Darwish, H. (2015). Diabetes mellitus: The epidemic of the century. *World Journal of Diabetes*, *6*(6), 850–867. doi:10.4239/wjd.v6.i6.850 PMID:26131326

Khatoon, A., Rashid, I., Shaikh, S., Rizvi, S. M. D., Shakil, S., Pathak, N., ... Srivastava, P. (2018). ADNCD: a compendious database on anti-diabetic natural compounds focusing on mechanism of action. *3 Biotech, 8*(8), 361.

Khomami, M. B., Tehrani, F. R., Hashemi, S., Farahmand, M., & Azizi, F. (2015). Of PCOS symptoms, hirsutism has the most significant impact on the quality of life of Iranian women. *PLoS One*, *10*(4), e0123608. doi:10.1371/journal.pone.0123608 PMID:25874409

Khorami, S. A. H., Movahedi, A., Khaza'ai, H., Mutalib, A., & Sokhini, M. (2015). PI3K/AKT pathway in modulating glucose homeostasis and its alteration in diabetes. *Annals of Medical and Biomedical Sciences*, *1*(2), 46–55.

Khot, Lad, Patil, & Kakad. (2013). Clinical Efficacy Of Ayurveda Treatment On Polycystic Ovarian Syndrome. *IOSR Journal of Pharmacy, 3*(4), 21-25.

Kianbakht, S., Khalighi-Sigaroodi, F., & Dabaghian, F. (2013). Improved Glycemic Control in Patients with Advanced Type 2 Diabetes Mellitus Taking Urticadioica Leaf Extract: A Randomized Double-Blind Placebo-Controlled Clinical Trial. *Clinical Laboratory*, *59*(09+10/2013). Advance online publication. doi:10.7754/Clin.Lab.2012.121019 PMID:24273930

Kim, E. K., Choi, E. J., & Debnath, T. (2016). Role of phytochemicals in the inhibition of epithelial–mesenchymal transition in cancer metastasis. *Food & Function*, *7*(9), 3677–3685. doi:10.1039/C6FO00901H PMID:27507108

Kim, H. J., Oh, G. T., Park, Y. B., Lee, M. K., Seo, H. J., & Choi, M. S. (2004). Naringin alters the cholesterol biosynthesis and antioxidant enzyme activities in ldl receptor-knockout mice under cholesterol fed condition. *Life Sciences*, *74*(13), 1621–1634. doi:10.1016/j.lfs.2003.08.026 PMID:14738906

Kim, K. H., Lee, D., Lee, H. L., Kim, C. E., Jung, K., & Kang, K. S. (2018). Beneficial effects of Panax ginseng for the treatment and prevention of neurodegenerative diseases: Past findings and future directions. *Journal of Ginseng Research*, *42*(3), 239–247. doi:10.1016/j.jgr.2017.03.011 PMID:29989012

Kim, S. H., Han, J., Seog, D. H., Chung, J. Y., Kim, N., Hong Park, Y., & Lee, S. K. (2015). Antidepressant effect of Chaihu-Shugan-San extract and its constituents in rat models of depression. *Life Sciences*, *76*(11), 1297–1306. doi:10.1016/j.lfs.2004.10.022 PMID:15642599

Kim, S. R., Lee, E. Y., Kim, D. J., Kim, H. J., & Park, H. R. (2020). Quercetin Inhibits Cell Survival and Metastatic Ability via the EMT-Mediated Pathway in Oral Squamous Cell Carcinoma. *Molecules (Basel, Switzerland)*, *25*(3), 757. doi:10.3390/molecules25030757 PMID:32050534

Kim, S., Jin, Y., Choi, Y., & Park, T. (2011). Resveratrol exerts anti-obesity effects via mechanisms involving down-regulation of adipogenic and inflammatory processes in mice. *Biochemical Pharmacology*, *81*(11), 1343–1351. doi:10.1016/j.bcp.2011.03.012 PMID:21439945

Kimura, M., Waki, I., Chujo, T., Kikuchi, T., Hiyama, C., Yamazaki, K., & Tanaka, O. (1981). Effects of hypoglycemic components in ginseng radix on blood insulin level in alloxan diabetic mice and on insulin release from perfused rat pancreas. *Journal of Pharmacobio-Dynamics*, *4*(6), 410–417. doi:10.1248/bpb1978.4.410 PMID:7026762

Kin, R., Kato, S., Kaneto, N., Sakurai, H., Hayakawa, Y., Li, F., & Yokoyama, S. (2013). Procyanidin C1 from Cinnamomi Cortex inhibits TGF-β-induced epithelial-to-mesenchymal transition in the A549 lung cancer cell line. *International Journal of Oncology*, *43*(6), 1901–1906. doi:10.3892/ijo.2013.2139 PMID:24141365

Kiseleva, I. A., Teplaia, E. V., & Kaminskii, A. V. (2012). Application of herbal medicine alba in treatment of patients with the pathology of thyroid. *Likars'Ka Sprava*, (8), 116–119. PMID:23786024

Kitabchi, A. E., Umpierrez, G. E., Miles, J. M., & Fisher, J. N. (2009). Hyperglycemic crises in adult patients with diabetes. *Diabetes Care*, *32*(7), 1335–1343. doi:10.2337/dc09-9032 PMID:19564476

Klatte, E. T., Scharre, D. W., Nagaraja, H. N., Davis, R. A., & Beversdorf, D. Q. (2003). Combination therapy of donepezil and vitamin E in Alzheimer disease. *Alzheimer Disease and Associated Disorders*. Advance online publication. doi:10.1097/00002093-200304000-00010 PMID:12794389

Kleerebezem, M., Boels, I. C., Groot, M. N., Mierau, I., Sybesma, W., & Hugenholtz, J. (2002). Metabolic engineering of Lactococcus lactis: The impact of genomics and metabolic modelling. *Journal of Biotechnology*. Advance online publication. doi:10.1016/S0168-1656(02)00132-3 PMID:12141987

Knochenhauer, E. S., Key, T. J., Kahsar-Miller, M., Waggoner, W., Boots, L. R., & Azziz, R. (1998). Prevalence of the polycystic ovary syndrome in unselected black and white women of the Southeastern United States: A prospective study. *The Journal of Clinical Endocrinology and Metabolism*, *83*(9), 3078–3082. doi:10.1210/jc.83.9.3078 PMID:9745406

Knutson, K. L. (2012). Does inadequate sleep play a role in vulnerability to obesity? *American Journal of Human Biology*, *24*(3), 361–371. doi:10.1002/ajhb.22219 PMID:22275135

Ko, B.-S., Choi, S. B., Park, S. K., Jang, J. S., Kim, Y. E., & Park, S. (2005). Insulin sensitizing and insulinotropic action of berberine from Cortidis rhizoma. *Biological & Pharmaceutical Bulletin*, *28*(8), 1431–1437. doi:10.1248/bpb.28.1431 PMID:16079488

Koch, C. E., Ganjam, G. K., Steger, J., Legler, K., Stohr, S., Schumacher, D., Hoggard, N., Heldmaier, G., & Tups, A. (2013). The dietary flavonoids naringenin and quercetin acutely impair glucose metabolism in rodents possibly via inhibition of hypothalamic insulin signalling. *British Journal of Nutrition*, *109*(6), 1040–1051. doi:10.1017/S0007114512003005 PMID:22850125

Kodali, M., Parihar, V. K., Hattiangady, B., Mishra, V., Shuai, B., & Shetty, A. K. (2015). Resveratrol prevents age-related memory and mood dysfunction with increased hippocampal neurogenesis and microvasculature, and reduced glial activation. *Scientific Reports*, *5*(1), 8075. doi:10.1038rep08075 PMID:25627672

Kokate, C. K., Purohit, A. P., & Gokhale, S. B. (2002). *Nutraceutical and cosmaceutical* (21st ed.). Pune, India: Pharmacognosy, Nirali Prakashan.

Kolahdooz, M., Nasri, S., Modarres, S. Z., Kianbakht, S., & Huseini, H. F. (2014). Effects of Nigella sativa L. seed oil on abnormal semen quality in infertile men: A randomized, double-blind, placebo-controlled clinical trial. *Phytomedicine*, *21*(6), 901–905. doi:10.1016/j.phymed.2014.02.006 PMID:24680621

Kong, J., Zhang, Z., Musch, M. W., Ning, G., Sun, J., Hart, J., ... Li, Y. C. (2008). Novel role of the vitamin D receptor in maintaining the integrity of the intestinal mucosal barrier. *American Journal of Physiology. Gastrointestinal and Liver Physiology*, *294*(1), G208–G216. doi:10.1152/ajpgi.00398.2007 PMID:17962355

Kong, W.-J., Zhang, H., Song, D.-Q., Xue, R., Zhao, W., Wei, J., Wang, Y.-M., Shan, N., Zhou, Z.-X., Yang, P., You, X.-F., Li, Z.-R., Si, S.-Y., Zhao, L.-X., Pan, H.-N., & Jiang, J.-D. (2009). Berberine reduces insulin resistance through protein kinase C-dependent up-regulation of insulin receptor expression. *Metabolism: Clinical and Experimental*, *58*(1), 109–119. doi:10.1016/j.metabol.2008.08.013 PMID:19059538

Kooti, W., Farokhipour, M., Asadzadeh, Z., Ashtary-Larky, D., & Asadi-Samani, M. (2016). The role of medicinal plants in the treatment of diabetes: A systematic review. *Electronic Physician*, *8*(1), 1832–1842. doi:10.19082/1832 PMID:26955456

Kort, D. H., & Lobo, R. A. (2014). Preliminary evidence that cinnamon improves menstrual cyclicity in women with polycystic ovary syndrome: A randomized controlled trial. *American Journal of Obstetrics and Gynecology*, *211*(5), 487.e481–487.e486. doi:10.1016/j.ajog.2014.05.009 PMID:24813595

Kousaxidis, A., Petrou, A., Lavrentaki, V., Fesatidou, M., Nicolaou, I., & Geronikaki, A. (2020). Aldose reductase and protein tyrosine phosphatase 1B inhibitors as a promising therapeutic approach for diabetes mellitus. *European Journal of Medicinal Chemistry*, *112742*. Advance online publication. doi:10.1016/j.ejmech.2020.112742 PMID:32871344

Ko, Y. S., Lee, W. S., Panchanathan, R., Joo, Y. N., Choi, Y. H., Kim, G. S., & Kim, H. J. (2016). Polyphenols from artemisia annua L inhibit adhesion and EMT of highly metastatic breast cancer cells MDA-MB-231. *Phytotherapy Research*, *30*(7), 1180–1188. doi:10.1002/ptr.5626 PMID:27151203

Kposowa, A. (2013). Mortality from Diabetes by Hispanic Groups: Evidence from the US National Longitudinal Mortality Study. *International Journal of Population Research*, *2013*, 1–12. doi:10.1155/2013/571306

Kramer, M. S. (2010). "Breast is best": The evidence. *Early Human Development*, *86*(11), 729–732. doi:10.1016/j.earlhumdev.2010.08.005 PMID:20846797

Kramer, M. S., Guo, T., Platt, R. W., Sevkovskaya, Z., Dzikovich, I., Collet, J. P., ... Bogdanovich, N. (2003). Infant growth and health outcomes associated with 3 compared with 6 mo of exclusive breastfeeding. *The American Journal of Clinical Nutrition*, *78*(2), 291–295. doi:10.1093/ajcn/78.2.291 PMID:12885711

Krebs, A. M., Mitschke, J., Losada, M. L., Schmalhofer, O., Boerries, M., Busch, H., & Brunton, V. G. (2017). The EMT-activator Zeb1 is a key factor for cell plasticity and promotes metastasis in pancreatic cancer. *Nature Cell Biology*, *19*(5), 518–529. doi:10.1038/ncb3513 PMID:28414315

Kreft, S., Knapp, M., & Kreft, I. (1999). Extraction of rutin from buckwheat (*Fagopyrum esculentummoench*) seeds and determination by capillary electrophoresis. *Journal of Agricultural and Food Chemistry*, *47*(11), 4649–4652. doi:10.1021/jf990186p PMID:10552865

Krentz, A. J., & Bailey, C. J. (2005). Oral antidiabetic agents: Current role in type 2 diabetes mellitus. *Drugs*, *65*(3), 385–411. doi:10.2165/00003495-200565030-00005 PMID:15669880

Kris-Etherton, P. M., Hecker, K. D., Bonanome, A., Coval, S. M., Binkoski, A. E., Hilpert, K. F., ... Etherton, T. D. (2003). Bioactive compounds in foods: Their role in the prevention of cardiovascular disease and cancer. *The American Journal of Medicine*, *113*(Supplement 9B), 71S–88S. doi:10.1016/S0002-9343(01)00995-0 PMID:12566142

Krzewska, A., & Ben-Skowronek, I. (2016). Effect of Associated Autoimmune Diseases on Type 1 Diabetes Mellitus Incidence and Metabolic Control in Children and Adolescents. *BioMed Research International*, *2016*, 1–12. doi:10.1155/2016/6219730 PMID:27525273

Kumar, S., Nasim, B., & Abraham, E. (2018). *Nanorobots a Future Device for Diagnosis and Treatment.* Retrieved 29 February 2020, from https://www.ommegaonline.org/article-details/NANOROBOTS-A-FUTURE-DEVICE-FOR-DIAGNOSIS-AND-TREATMENT/1815

Kumar, A., Woods, K. S., Bartolucci, A. A., & Azziz, R. (2005). Prevalence of adrenal androgen excess in patients with the polycystic ovary syndrome (PCOS). *Horumon To Rinsho*, *62*(6), 644–649. doi:10.1111/j.1365-2265.2005.02256.x PMID:15943823

Kumari, M., & Kozyrskyj, A. L. (2017). Gut microbial metabolism defines host metabolism: An emerging perspective in obesity and allergic inflammation. *Obesity Reviews*, *18*(1), 18–31. doi:10.1111/obr.12484 PMID:27862824

Kumar, K. K., Jayaprakash, A. P., & Srinivasan, K. K. (2015). Antidiabetic evaluation of Hemionitis arifolia leaves by in vitro methods. *Manipal Journal of Pharmaceutical Sciences*, *1*(1), 13–20.

Kumar, K., Fateh, V., Verma, B., & Pandey, S. (2014). Some herbal drugs used for treatment of diabetes. *International Journal of Research and Development in Pharmacy & Life Sciences*, *3*, 1116–1120.

Kumar, R., Singh, G., Krishan, P., Kumari, P., Rizwi, S. I., & Gautam, S. P. (2013). Nutraceuticals: A boom to medical industry. *Pharmaceutical Sciences*, *2*, 1–8.

Kumar, V., Bhandari, U., Tripathi, C. D., & Khanna, G. (2012). Evaluation of antiobesity and cardioprotective effect of *Gymnema sylvestre* extract in murine model. *Indian Journal of Pharmacology*, *44*(5), 607–613. doi:10.4103/0253-7613.100387 PMID:23112423

Kuo, S. M. (2013). The interplay between fiber and the intestinal microbiome in the inflammatory response. *Advances in Nutrition*, *4*(1), 16–28. doi:10.3945/an.112.003046 PMID:23319119

Kuruvilla, A. (2002). Herbal Formulations as Pharmacotherapeutic Agents. *Indian Journal of Experimental Biology*, *40*, 7–11. PMID:12561961

Ku, S. K., & Bae, J. S. (2015). Baicalin, baicalein and wogonin inhibits high glucose-induced vascular inflammation *in vitro* and *in vivo*. *BMB Reports*, *48*(9), 519–524. doi:10.5483/BMBRep.2015.48.9.017 PMID:25739393

Kwon, Y.-I., Apostolidis, E., & Shetty, K. (2007). Evaluation of pepper (Capsicum annuum) for management of diabetes and hypertension. *Journal of Food Biochemistry*, *31*(3), 370–385. doi:10.1111/j.1745-4514.2007.00120.x

Labban, L., Mustafa, U. E.-S., & Ibrahim, Y. M. (2014). The effects of Rosemary (Rosmarinus officinalis) leaves powder on glucose level, lipid profile and lipid perodoxation. *International Journal of Clinical Medicine*, *5*(06), 297–304. doi:10.4236/ijcm.2014.56044

Lama, A., Pirozzi, C., Avagliano, C., Annunziata, C., Mollica, M.P., Calignano, A., Meli, R., & Raso, G.M. (2020). Nutraceuticals: An integrative approach to starve Parkinson's disease. *Brain, Behavior and Immunity- Health, 2*, 100037.

Lamouille, S., Xu, J., & Derynck, R. (2014). Molecular mechanisms of epithelial–mesenchymal transition. *Nature Reviews. Molecular Cell Biology*, *15*(3), 178–196. doi:10.1038/nrm3758 PMID:24556840

Landsberg, L., Aronne, L. J., Beilin, L. J., Burke, V., Igel, L. I., Lloyd-Jones, D., & Sowers, J. (2013). Obesity- related hypertension: Pathogenesis, cardiovascular risk, and treatment—a position paper of the obesity society and the American society of hypertension. *Obesity (Silver Spring, Md.)*, *21*(1), 8–24. doi:10.1002/oby.20181 PMID:23401272

Lankarani, M., Valizadeh, N., Heshmat, R., Shafaee, A.R., Amini, M.R., & Ardeshir Larijani, M.B. (2005). Evaluation of dyslipidemia in polycystic ovary syndrome. *J Diabetes Metab Disord, 4*, E11+E11i-E11x.

Larion, S., & Khurana, S. (2018). Clinical studies investigating the effect of vitamin E therapy in patients with NASH. *Clinics in Liver Disease*, *11*(1), 16–21. doi:10.1002/cld.687 PMID:30992781

Lattrich, C., Lubig, J., Springwald, A., Goerse, R., Ortmann, O., & Treeck, O. (2011). Additive effects of trastuzumab and genistein on human breast cancer cells. *Anti-Cancer Drugs*, *22*(3), 253–261. doi:10.1097/CAD.0b013e3283427bb5 PMID:21160418

Laurberg, P. (1984). Forskolin stimulation of thyroid secretion of T4 and T3. *FEBS Letters*, *170*(2), 273–276. doi:10.1016/0014-5793(84)81327-7 PMID:6327383

Lavle, C. J., & Milani, R. V. (2005). Cardiac rehabilitation and exercise training pogrammes in metabolic syndrome and diabetes. *Journal of Cardiopulmonary Rehabilitation*, *25*(2), 59–66. doi:10.1097/00008483-200503000-00001 PMID:15818190

Lazzer, S., Bedogni, G., Lafortuna, C. L., Marazzi, N., Busti, C., Galli, R., de Col, A., Agosti, F., & Sartorio, A. (2010). Relationship between basal metabolic rate, gender, age, and body composition in 8,780 white obese subjects. *Obesity (Silver Spring, Md.)*, *18*(1), 71–78. doi:10.1038/oby.2009.162 PMID:19478787

Leclercq, S., Matamoros, S., Cani, P. D., Neyrinck, A. M., Jamar, F., Stärkel, P., ... Delzenne, N. M. (2014). Intestinal permeability, gut-bacterial dysbiosis, and behavioral markers of alcohol-dependence severity. *Proceedings of the National Academy of Sciences of the United States of America*, *111*(42), E4485–E4493. doi:10.1073/pnas.1415174111 PMID:25288760

Lee, S. O. L. H. W. A. (2015). Anti - angiogenic effects of resveratrol in combination with 5 - fluorouracil on B16 murine melanoma cells. Academic Press.

Leea, J. H., & Jo, J. (2017). Successful treatment with Korean herbal medicine and lifestyle management in an obese woman with polycystic ovarian syndrome. *Integrative Medicine Research*, *6*(3), 325–328. doi:10.1016/j.imr.2017.06.002 PMID:28951847

Lee, C. H. (2019). Reversal of Epithelial–Mesenchymal Transition by Natural Anti-Inflammatory and Pro-Resolving Lipids. *Cancers (Basel)*, *11*(12), 1841. doi:10.3390/cancers11121841 PMID:31766574

Lee, I. C., & Choi, B. Y. (2016). Withaferin-A—A natural anticancer agent with pleitropic mechanisms of action. *International Journal of Molecular Sciences*, *17*(3), 290. doi:10.3390/ijms17030290 PMID:26959007

Lee, S. Y., Kim, M. T., Kim, S. W., Song, M. S., & Yoon, S. J. (2003). Effect of lifetime lactation on breast cancer risk: A Korean women's cohort study. *International Journal of Cancer*, *105*(3), 390–393. doi:10.1002/ijc.11078 PMID:12704674

Lee, T. T., & Rausch, M. E. (2012). Polycystic ovarian syndrome: Role of imaging in diagnosis. *Radiographics*, *32*(6), 1643–1657. doi:10.1148/rg.326125503 PMID:23065162

Lee, Y. M., Yoon, Y., Yoon, H., Park, H. M., Song, S., & Yeum, K. J. (2017). Dietary anthocyanins against obesity and inflammation. *Nutrients*, *9*(10), 1089–1104. doi:10.3390/nu9101089 PMID:28974032

Lee, Y. S., Kim, W. S., Kim, K. H., Yoon, M. J., Cho, H. J., Shen, Y., Ye, J.-M., Lee, C. H., Oh, W. K., Kim, C. T., Hohnen-Behrens, C., Gosby, A., Kraegen, E. W., James, D. E., & Kim, J. B. (2006). Berberine, a natural plant product, activates AMP-activated protein kinase with beneficial metabolic effects in diabetic and insulin-resistant states. *Diabetes*, *55*(8), 2256–2264. doi:10.2337/db06-0006 PMID:16873688

Lee, Y. S., Lee, S., Lee, H. S., Kim, B. K., Ohuchi, K., & Shin, K. H. (2005). Inhibitory effects of isorhamnetin-3-O-β-d-glucoside from *Salicornia herbacea* on rat lens aldose reductase and sorbitol accumulation in streptozotocin-induced diabetic rat tissues. *Biological & Pharmaceutical Bulletin*, *28*(5), 916–918. doi:10.1248/bpb.28.916 PMID:15863906

Leger, J., & Carel, J. C. (2018). Diagnosis and management of hyperthyroidism from prenatal life to adolescence. *Best Practice & Research. Clinical Endocrinology & Metabolism*, *32*(4), 373–386. doi:10.1016/j.beem.2018.03.014 PMID:30086864

Legro, R. S. (1998). Polycystic ovary syndrome: Current and future treatment paradigms. *American Journal of Obstetrics and Gynecology*, *179*(6 Pt 2), S101–S8. doi:10.1016/S0002-9378(98)70240-6 PMID:9855616

Legro, R. S., Kunselman, A. R., Dodson, W. C., & Dunaif, A. (1999). Prevalence and predictors of risk for type 2 diabetes mellitus and impaired glucose tolerance in polycystic ovary syndrome: A prospective, controlled study in 254 affected women. *The Journal of Clinical Endocrinology and Metabolism*, *84*(1), 165–169. PMID:9920077

Leibel, R. L., Rosenbaum, M., & Hirsch, J. (1995). Changes in energy expenditure resulting from altered body weight. *The New England Journal of Medicine*, *332*(10), 621–628. doi:10.1056/NEJM199503093321001 PMID:7632212

Leikert, J. F., Räthel, T. R., Wohlfart, P., Cheynier, V., Vollmar, A. M., & Dirsch, V. M. (2002). Red wine polyphenols enhance endothelial nitric oxide synthase expression and subsequent nitric oxide release from endothelial cells. *Circulation*, *106*(13), 1614–1617. doi:10.1161/01.CIR.0000034445.31543.43 PMID:12270851

Leite-Silva, C., Gusmão, C. L. S., & Takahashi, C. S. (2007). Genotoxic and antigenotoxic effects of *Fucus vesiculosus* extract on cultured human lymphocytes using the chromosome aberration and Comet assays. *Genetics and Molecular Biology*, *30*(1), 105–111. doi:10.1590/S1415-47572007000100019

Lemaure, B., Touché, A., Zbinden, I., Moulin, J., Courtois, D., Macé, K., & Darimont, C. (2007). Administration of Cyperus rotundus tubers extract prevents weight gain in obese Zucker rats. *Phytotherapy Research*, *21*(8), 724–730. doi:10.1002/ptr.2147 PMID:17444573

Leng, S. H., Lu, F. E., & Xu, L. J. (2004). Therapeutic effects of berberine in impaired glucose tolerance rats and its influence on insulin secretion. *Acta Pharmacologica Sinica*, *25*(4), 496–502. PMID:15066220

Lenoir-Wijnkoop, I., Sanders, M. E., Cabana, M. D., Caglar, E., Corthier, G., Rayes, N., ... Timmerman, H. M. (2007). Probiotic and prebiotic influence beyond the intestinal tract. *Nutrition Reviews*, *65*(11), 469–489. doi:10.1111/j.1753-4887.2007.tb00272.x PMID:18038940

Lepage, P., Häsler, R., Spehlmann, M. E., Rehman, A., Zvirbliene, A., Begun, A., ... Schreiber, S. (2011). Twin study indicates loss of interaction between microbiota and mucosa of patients with ulcerative colitis. *Gastroenterology*, *141*(1), 227–236. doi:10.1053/j.gastro.2011.04.011 PMID:21621540

Leray, C., Wiesel, M. L., Freund, M., Cazenave, J. P., & Gachet, C. (2001). Long-chain n-3 fatty acids specifically affect rat coagulation factors dependent on vitamin K relation to peroxidative stress. *Arteriosclerosis, Thrombosis, and Vascular Biology*. Advance online publication. doi:10.1161/01.ATV.21.3.459 PMID:11231929

Lesbros-Pantoflickova, D., Corthesy-Theulaz, I., & Blum, A. L. (2007). Helicobacter pylori and probiotics. *The Journal of Nutrition*, *137*(3), 812S–818S. doi:10.1093/jn/137.3.812S PMID:17311980

Leung, L., Birtwhistle, R., Kotecha, J., Hannah, S., & Cuthbertson, S. (2009). Anti-diabetic and hypoglycaemic effects of Momordicacharantia (bitter melon): A mini review. *British Journal of Nutrition, 102*(12), 1703–1708. doi:10.1017/S0007114509992054 PMID:19825210

Li, H., Wang, Z., & Liu, Y. (2003). Review in the studies on tannins activity of cancer prevention and anticancer. Zhong yao cai = Zhongyaocai = Journal of Chinese Medicinal Materials.

Liang, C., Li, H., Shen, C., Lai, J., Shi, Z., Liu, B., & Tao, H. (2012). Genistein potentiates the anti-cancer effects of gemcitabine in human osteosarcoma via the downregulation of Akt and nuclear factor-kappaB pathway. *Anti-cancer Agents in Medicinal Chemistry, 12*(5), 554–563. doi:10.2174/187152012800617867 PMID:22263786

Liao, Hu, & Hung. (2018). *Complementary Therapy with Traditional Chinese Medicine for Polycystic Ovarian Syndrome*. Intech Open Science. doi:10.5772/intechopen.71654

Liao, W.-T., Chiang, J.-H., Li, C.-J., Lee, M.-T., Su, C.-C., & Yen, H.-R. (2018). Investigation on the Use of Traditional Chinese Medicine for Polycystic Ovary Syndrome in a Nationwide Prescription Database in Taiwan. *Journal of Clinical Medicine, 7*(7), 179. doi:10.3390/jcm7070179 PMID:30037150

Li, C., He, J. Z., Zhou, X. D., & Xu, X. (2017). Berberine regulates type 2 diabetes mellitus related with insulin resistance. *Zhongguo Zhongyao Zazhi, 42*(12), 2254–2260. PMID:28822177

Liew, R., Stagg, M. A., MacLeod, K. T., & Collins, P. (2005). The red wine polyphenol, resveratrol, exerts acute direct actions on guinea-pig ventricular myocytes. *European Journal of Pharmacology, 519*(1-2), 1–8. doi:10.1016/j.ejphar.2005.06.017 PMID:16102748

Li, G. Q., Kam, A., Wong, K. H., Zhou, X., Omar, E. A., Alqahtani, A., Li, K. M., Razmovski-Naumovski, V., & Chan, K. (2012). Herbal medicines for the management of diabetes. *Advances in Experimental Medicine and Biology, 771*, 396–413. doi:10.1007/978-1-4614-5441-0_28 PMID:23393692

Li, J., Xiang, S. T., Zhang, Q. H., Wu, J. J., Tang, Q., Zhou, J. F., Yang, L. J., Chen, Z. Q., & Hann, S. S. (2015). Combination of curcumin and bicalutamide enhanced the growth inhibition of androgen-independent prostate cancer cells through SAPK/JNK and MEK/ERK1/2-mediated targeting NF-κB/p65 and MUC1-C. *Journal of Experimental & Clinical Cancer Research, 34*(1), 46. doi:10.118613046-015-0168-z PMID:25971429

Li, L., & Somerset, S. (2014). The clinical significance of the gut microbiota in cystic fibrosis and the potential for dietary therapies. *Clinical Nutrition (Edinburgh, Lothian), 33*(4), 571–580. doi:10.1016/j.clnu.2014.04.004 PMID:24767984

Li, L., Wang, X., Sharvan, R., Gao, J., & Qu, S. (2017). Berberine could inhibit thyroid carcinoma cells by inducing mitochondrial apoptosis, G0/G1 cell cycle arrest and suppressing migration via PI3K-AKT and MAPK signaling pathways. *Biomedicine and Pharmacotherapy, 95*, 1225–1231. doi:10.1016/j.biopha.2017.09.010 PMID:28931215

Limer, J. L., & Speirs, V. (2004). Phyto-oestrogens and breast cancer chemoprevention. Breast Cancer Research. https://doi.org/ doi:10.1186/bcr781

Lim, S. S., Norman, R. J., Davies, M. J., & Moran, L. J. (2013). The effect of obesity on polycystic ovary syndrome: A systematic review and meta-analysis. *Obesity Reviews, 14*(2), 95–109. doi:10.1111/j.1467-789X.2012.01053.x PMID:23114091

Lim, S., Yoon, J. W., Choi, S. H., Cho, B. J., Kim, J. T., Chang, H. S., Park, H. S., Park, K. S., Lee, H. K., Kim, Y. B., & Jang, H. C. (2009). Effect of ginsam, a vinegar extract from *Panax ginseng*, on body weight and glucose homeostasis in an obese insulin-resistant rat model. *Metabolism: Clinical and Experimental, 58*(1), 8–15. doi:10.1016/j.metabol.2008.07.027 PMID:19059525

Lin, H., Hao, Y., Wan, X., He, J., & Tong, Y. (2020). Baicalein inhibits cell development, metastasis and EMT and induces apoptosis by regulating ERK signaling pathway in osteosarcoma. *Journal of Receptors and Signal Transduction, 40*(1), 49–57. doi:10.1080/10799893.2020.1713807 PMID:31948366

Lin, L., & Zhang, J. (2017). Role of intestinal microbiota and metabolites on gut homeostasis and human diseases. *BMC Immunology, 18*(1), 2. doi:10.118612865-016-0187-3 PMID:28061847

Lin, X., Li, K., Yang, Z., Chen, B., & Zhang, T. (2020). Dulcitol suppresses proliferation and migration of hepatocellular carcinoma via regulating SIRT1/p53 pathway. *Phytomedicine, 66*, 153112. doi:10.1016/j.phymed.2019.153112 PMID:31786318

Li, Q., Han, Y., Dy, A. B. C., & Hagerman, R. J. (2017). The Gut Microbiota and Autism Spectrum Disorders. *Frontiers in Cellular Neuroscience, 11*, 120. doi:10.3389/fncel.2017.00120 PMID:28503135

Liskova, A., Kubatka, P., Samec, M., Zubor, P., Mlyncek, M., Bielik, T., & Büsselberg, D. (2019). Dietary phytochemicals targeting cancer stem cells. *Molecules (Basel, Switzerland), 24*(5), 899. doi:10.3390/molecules24050899 PMID:30836718

Little, T. J., Horowitz, M., & Feinle-Bisset, C. (2005). Role of cholecystokinin in appetite control and body weight regulation. *Obesity Reviews, 6*(4), 297–306. doi:10.1111/j.1467-789X.2005.00212.x PMID:16246215

Liu, D. (2014). Genistein enhances the effect of cisplatin on the inhibition of non-small cell lung cancer A549 cell growth in vitro and in vivo. *Oncology Letters, 8*(6), 2806–2810. Available at: https://www.ncbi.nlm.nih.gov/pmc/articles/PMC4214458/

Liu, W. J. (Ed.). (2011). Traditional herbal medicine research methods: identification, analysis, bioassay, and pharmaceutical and clinical studies. John Wiley & Sons. doi:10.1002/9780470921340

Liu, Y., Zhong, G., & Liu, H. (2015). Therapeutic effect of HaizaoYuhu decoction with/without seaweed and liquorice anti-drug combination on goiter rats in preferred dosage conditions. *Science and Technology Review, 33*, 87-91.

Liu, C.-T., Hsu, T.-W., Chen, K.-M., Tan, Y.-P., Lii, C.-K., & Sheen, L.-Y. (2012). The antidiabetic effect of garlic oil is associated with ameliorated oxidative stress but not ameliorated level of pro-inflammatory cytokines in skeletal muscle of streptozotocin-induced diabetic rats. *Journal of Traditional and Complementary Medicine, 2*(2), 135–144. doi:10.1016/S2225-4110(16)30087-6 PMID:24716126

Liu, D., & Chen, Z. (2013). The effect of curcumin on breast cancer cells. *Journal of Breast Cancer, 16*(2), 133–137. doi:10.4048/jbc.2013.16.2.133 PMID:23843843

Liu, I. M., Tzeng, T. F., Liou, S. S., & Lan, T. W. (2007). Myricetin, a naturally occurring flavonol, ameliorates insulin resistance induced by a high-fructose diet in rats. *Life Sciences, 81*(21-22), 1479–1488. doi:10.1016/j.lfs.2007.08.045 PMID:17976658

Liu, L., Yu, Y. L., Yang, J. S., Li, Y., Liu, Y.-W., Liang, Y., Liu, X.-D., Xie, L., & Wang, G.-J. (2010). Berberine suppresses intestinal disaccharidases with beneficial metabolic effects in diabetic states, evidences from in vivo and in vitro study. *Naunyn-Schmiedeberg's Archives of Pharmacology, 381*(4), 371–381. doi:10.100700210-010-0502-0 PMID:20229011

Liu, R., Wang, Q., Ding, Z., Zhang, X., Li, Y., Zang, Y., & Zhang, G. (2020). Silibinin Augments the Antifibrotic Effect of Valsartan Through Inactivation of TGF-β1 Signaling in Kidney. *Drug Design, Development and Therapy, 14*, 603–611. doi:10.2147/DDDT.S224308 PMID:32103902

Liu, S. C., Huang, C. M., Bamodu, O. A., Lin, C. S., Liu, B. L., Tzeng, Y. M., & Chen, T. M. (2019). Ovatodiolide suppresses nasopharyngeal cancer by targeting stem cell-like population, inducing apoptosis, inhibiting EMT and dysregulating JAK/STAT signaling pathway. *Phytomedicine, 56*, 269–278. doi:10.1016/j.phymed.2018.05.007 PMID:30668347

Liu, S., Li, D., Huang, B., Chen, Y., Lu, X., & Wang, Y. (2013). Inhibition of pancreatic lipase, α-glucosidase, α-amylase, and hypolipidemic effects of the total flavonoids from Nelumbo nucifera leaves. *Journal of Ethnopharmacology*, *149*(1), 263–269. doi:10.1016/j.jep.2013.06.034 PMID:23811214

Liu, Y., Fu, X., Lan, N., Li, S., Zhang, J., Wang, S., Li, C., Shang, Y., Huang, T., & Zhang, L. (2014). Luteolin protects against high fat diet-induced cognitive deficits in obesity mice. *Behavioural Brain Research*, *267*, 178–188. doi:10.1016/j.bbr.2014.02.040 PMID:24667364

Liu, Y., & Mao, L. H. (2013). Effect of danzhi xiaoyao pill on ovulation induction of polycystic ovarian syndrome patients of pathogenic fire derived from stagnation of gan-qi. Zhongguo. *Zhong Xi Yi Jie He Za Zhi.*, *33*, 1191–1195. PMID:24273971

Liu, Y., Sun, M., Yao, H., Liu, Y., & Gao, R. (2017). Herbal medicine for the treatment of obesity: An overview of scientific evidence from 2007 to 2017. *Evidence-Based Complementary and Alternative Medicine*. doi:10.1155/2017/8943059 PMID:29234439

Liu, Y., & Wang, M. W. (2008). Botanical drugs: challenges and opportunities: contribution to Linnaeus Memorial Symposium 2007. *Life Sciences*, *82*(9-10), 445–449. doi:10.1016/j.lfs.2007.11.007

Liu, Y., Weng, W., Gao, R., & Liu, Y. (2019). New Insights for Cellular and Molecular Mechanisms of Aging and Aging-Related Diseases: Herbal Medicine as Potential Therapeutic Approach. *Oxidative Medicine and Cellular Longevity*, *2019*, 1–25. doi:10.1155/2019/4598167

Liu, Z., Zhu, Y.-Y., Li, Z.-Y., & Ning, S.-Q. (2016). Evaluation of the efficacy of paclitaxel with curcumin combination in ovarian cancer cells. *Oncology Letters*, *12*(5), 3944–3948. doi:10.3892/ol.2016.5192 PMID:27895754

Li, W. L., Dai, Y., Xu, D., & Ji, Y. B. (2007). Effects of different polar fractions from Jinkuishenqiwan on testosterone and oxidative stress in rats with kidney-yang deficiency induced by hydrocortisone. *Zhongguo Xin Yao Zazhi*, *16*, 1944–1946.

Li, Y., Meeran, S. M., Patel, S. N., Chen, H., Hardy, T. M., & Tollefsbol, T. O. (2013). Epigenetic reactivation of estrogen receptor-α (ERα) by genistein enhances hormonal therapy sensitivity in ERα-negative breast cancer. *Molecular Cancer*, *12*(1), 9. doi:10.1186/1476-4598-12-9 PMID:24063558

Lohiya, N. K., Balasubramanian, K., & Ansari, A. S. (2016). Indian folklore medicine in managing mens health and wellness. *Andrologia*, *48*(8), 894–907. doi:10.1111/and.12680 PMID:27681646

Lohr, J.-M. (2016). A phase I dose escalation trial of AXP107-11, a novel multi-component crystalline form of genistein, in combination with gemcitabine in chemotherapy-naive patients with unresectable pancreatic cancer. *Pancreatology*, *16*(4), 640–645.

Loman, B. R., Hernández-Saavedra, D., An, R., & Rector, R. S. (2018). Prebiotic and probiotic treatment of nonalcoholic fatty liver disease: A systematic review and meta-analysis. *Nutrition Reviews*, *76*(11), 822–839. doi:10.1093/nutrit/nuy031 PMID:30113661

Lomax, A. R., & Calder, P. C. (2009). Probiotics, immune function, infection and inflammation: A review of the evidence from studies conducted in humans. *Current Pharmaceutical Design*, *15*(13), 1428–1518. doi:10.2174/138161209788168155 PMID:19442167

Lopez-Alarcon, M., Villalpando, S., & Fajardo, A. (1997). Breast-feeding lowers the frequency and duration of acute respiratory infection and diarrhea in infants under six months of age. *The Journal of Nutrition*, *127*(3), 436–443. doi:10.1093/jn/127.3.436 PMID:9082027

Lorenzati, B., Zucco, C., Miglietta, S., Lamberti, F., & Bruno, G. (2010). Oral hypoglycemic drugs: pathophysiological basis of their mechanism of actionoral hypoglycemic drugs: pathophysiological basis of their mechanism of action. *Pharmaceuticals*, *3*(9), 3005–3020. doi:10.3390/ph3093005 PMID:27713388

Losso, J. N. (2003). Targeting excessive angiogenesis with functional foods and nutraceuticals. *Trends in Food Science & Technology*. Advance online publication. doi:10.1016/S0924-2244(03)00156-0

Losurdo, G., Cubisino, R., Barone, M., Principi, M., Leandro, G., Ierardi, E., & Leo, A. D. (2018). Probiotic monotherapy and Helicobacter pylori eradication: A systematic review with pooled-data analysis. *World Journal of Gastroenterology*, *24*(1), 139–149. doi:10.3748/wjg.v24.i1.139 PMID:29358890

Lubecka, K., Kaufman-Szymczyk, A., & Fabianowska-Majewska, K. (2018). Inhibition of breast cancer cell growth by the combination of clofarabine and sulforaphane involves epigenetically mediated CDKN2A upregulation. *Nucleosides, Nucleotides & Nucleic Acids*, *37*(5), 1–10. doi:10.1080/15257770.2018.1453075 PMID:29634384

Lubecka-Pietruszewska, K. (2015). Sulforaphane Alone and in Combination with Clofarabine Epigenetically Regulates the Expression of DNA Methylation-Silenced Tumour Suppressor Genes in Human Breast Cancer Cells. *Lifestyle Genomics*, *8*(2), 91–101. https://www.karger.com/DOI/10.1159/000439111 PMID:26372775

Luhach, S., Goel, A., Taj, G., Goyal, P., & Kumar, A. (2013). Phyto diab care: Phytoremedial database for antidiabetics. *Bioinformation*, *9*(7), 375–377. doi:10.6026/97320630009375 PMID:23750083

Lu, J. J., Bao, J. L., Chen, X. P., Huang, M., & Wang, Y. T. (2012). Alkaloids isolated from natural herbs as the anticancer agents. *Evidence-Based Complementary and Alternative Medicine*, *2012*, 2012. doi:10.1155/2012/485042 PMID:22988474

Lujan, M. E., Jarrett, B. Y., Brooks, E. D., Reines, J. K., Peppin, A. K., Muhn, N., Haider, E., Pierson, R. A., & Chizen, D. R. (2013). Updated ultrasound criteria for polycystic ovary syndrome: Reliable thresholds for elevated follicle population and ovarian volume. *Human Reproduction (Oxford, England)*, *28*(5), 1361–1368. doi:10.1093/humrep/det062 PMID:23503943

Luna, B., & Feinglos, M. (2001). Oral Agents in the Management of Type 2 Diabetes Mellitus. *American Family Physician*, *63*(9), 1747–1757. PMID:11352285

Luo, H.A.O. (2016). *Resveratrol Overcomes Cellular Resistance to Vemurafenib Through Dephosphorylation of AKT in BRAF -mutated Melanoma Cells*. Academic Press.

Luo, J. Z., & Luo, L. (2009). Ginseng on hyperglycemia: Effects and mechanisms. *Evidence-Based Complementary and Alternative Medicine*, *6*(4), 423–427. doi:10.1093/ecam/nem178 PMID:18955300

Luo, Q., Li, Z., Huang, X., Yan, J., Zhang, S., & Cai, Y.-Z. (2006). Lycium barbarum polysaccharides: Protective effects against heat-induced damage of rat testes and H2O2-induced DNA damage in mouse testicular cells and beneficial effect on sexual behavior and reproductive function of hemicastrated rats. *Life Sciences*, *79*(7), 613–621. doi:10.1016/j.lfs.2006.02.012 PMID:16563441

Lutgarda, B., Giuseppina, C., Giuseppe, D. P., Paola, C., Claudia, V., Marilena, V., Angela, A. R., & Giovanni, A. (2018). Dietary Fibre as a Unifying Remedy for the Whole Spectrum of Obesity-Associated Cardiovascular Risk. *Nutrients*, *10*(7), 943. doi:10.3390/nu10070943 PMID:30037123

Lv, L., Huang, W., Yu, X., Ren, H., & Sun, R. (2009). Comparative research of different Bupleurum chinense composition to influence of hepatotoxicity of rats and oxidative damage mechanism. *Zhongguo Zhongyao Zazhi*, *34*(18), 2364–2368. PMID:20030090

Macfarlane, S., Macfarlane, G. T., & Cummings, J. H. (2006). Review article: Prebiotics in the gastrointestinal tract. *Alimentary Pharmacology & Therapeutics*, *24*(5), 701–714. doi:10.1111/j.1365-2036.2006.03042.x PMID:16918875

Madrid, A. M., Poniachik, J., Quera, R., & Defilippi, C. (2011). Small intestinal clustered contractions and bacterial overgrowth: A frequent finding in obese patients. *Digestive Diseases and Sciences*, *56*(1), 155–160. doi:10.100710620-010-1239-9 PMID:20431947

Madsen, H. L., & Bertelsen, G. (1995). Spices as antioxidants. *Trends in Food Science & Technology*, *6*(8), 271–277. doi:10.1016/S0924-2244(00)89112-8

Maeda, H., Hosokawa, M., Sashima, T., Funayama, K., & Miyashita, K. (2005). Fucoxanthin from edible seaweed, *Undaria pinnatifida*, shows antiobesity effect through UCP1 expression in white adipose tissues. *Biochemical and Biophysical Research Communications*, *332*(2), 392–397. doi:10.1016/j.bbrc.2005.05.002 PMID:15896707

Mahabadi, J. A., Bafrani, H. H., Nikzad, H., Taherian, A., & Salehi, M. (2013). Effect of Diet Contains Sesame Seed on Adult Wistar Rat Testis. *International Journal of Morphology*, *31*(1), 197–202. doi:10.4067/S0717-95022013000100033

Makheswari, M. U., & Sudarsanam, D. (2012). Database on antidiabetic indigenous plants of Tamil Nadhu, India. *International Journal of Pharmaceutical Sciences and Research*, *3*(2), 287–293.

Makris, A., & Foster, G. D. (2011). Dietary approaches to the treatment of obesity. *Psychiatria Clinica*, *34*(4), 813–827. PMID:22098806

Ma, L., Jia, M., Nan, Y. Y., Liu, M. L., Wang, Z. R., & Ma, J. (2011). Effects of Jin- gui Shenqi pills on sperm quality and contents of hormones in adenine-induced infertility rats. *J Shandong Univ Tradit Chin Med*, *35*, 431–433.

Malatji, B. G., Meyer, H., Mason, S., Engelke, U. F. H., Wevers, R. A., van Reenen, M., & Reinecke, C. J. (2017). A diagnostic biomarker profile for fibromyalgia syndrome based on an NMR metabolomics study of selected patients and controls. *BMC Neurology*, *17*(1), 88. doi:10.118612883-017-0863-9 PMID:28490352

Malekshahi, H., Bahrami, G., Miraghaee, S., Ahmadi, S. A., Sajadimajd, S., Hatami, R., Mohammadi, B., & Keshavarzi, S. (2019). *Momordica charantia* reverses type II diabetes in rat. *Journal of Food Biochemistry*, *43*(11), e13021. doi:10.1111/jfbc.13021 PMID:31441956

Malhotra, A., Nair, P., & Dhawan, D. K. (2014). Study to evaluate molecular mechanics behind synergistic chemo-preventive effects of curcumin and resveratrol during lung carcinogenesis. *PLoS One*, *9*(4), e93820. doi:10.1371/journal.pone.0093820 PMID:24705375

Mali, P. Y., Bigoniya, P., Panchal, S. S., & Muchhandi, I. S. (2013). Anti-obesity activity of chloroform-methanol extract of *Premna integrifolia* in mice fed with cafeteria diet. *Journal of Pharmacy & Bioallied Sciences*, *5*(3), 229–236. doi:10.4103/0975-7406.116825 PMID:24082700

Malviya, N., Jain, S., & Malviya, S. (2010). Antidiabetic potential of medicinal plants Acta Pol Pharmaceutical. *Drug Research*, *67*, 113–118.

Malviya, N., Jain, S., & Malviya, S. A. P. N. A. (2010). Antidiabetic potential of medicinal plants. *Acta Poloniae Pharmaceutica*, *67*(2), 113–118. PMID:20369787

Manda, G., Rojo, A. I., Martínez-Klimova, E., Pedraza-Chaverri, J., & Cuadrado, A. (2020). Nordihydroguaiaretic Acid: From Herbal Medicine to Clinical Development for Cancer and Chronic Diseases. *Frontiers in Pharmacology*, *11*, 151. doi:10.3389/fphar.2020.00151

Manganaris, G. A., Goulas, V., Vicente, A. R., & Terry, L. A. (2014). Berry antioxidants: Small fruits providing large benfits. *Journal of the Science of Food and Agriculture*, *94*(5), 825–833. doi:10.1002/jsfa.6432 PMID:24122646

Manichanh, C. (2006). Reduced diversity of faecal microbiota in Crohn's disease revealed by a metagenomic approach. *Gut*, *55*(2), 205–211. doi:10.1136/gut.2005.073817 PMID:16188921

Mannerås-Holm, L., Baghaei, F., Holm, G., Janson, P. O., Ohlsson, C., Lonn, M., & Stener-Victorin, E. (2011). Coagulation and fibrinolytic disturbances in women with polycystic ovary syndrome. *The Journal of Clinical Endocrinology and Metabolism*, *96*(4), 1068–1076. doi:10.1210/jc.2010-2279 PMID:21252248

Ma, R. J., Zhou, J., Fang, J. Q., Yang, D. H., & Qu, F. (2011). Combination of acupuncture and chinese medicinal herbs in treating model rats with polycystic ovary syndrome. *Afr. J. Tradit. Complement. Altern. Med. AJTCAM.*, *8*(4), 353–361. doi:10.4314/ajtcam.v8i4.3 PMID:22654211

March, W. A., Moore, V. M., Willson, K. J., Phillips, D. I., Norman, R. J., & Davies, M. J. (2010). The prevalence of polycystic ovary syndrome in a community sample assessed under contrasting diagnostic criteria. *Human Reproduction (Oxford, England)*, *25*(2), 544–551. doi:10.1093/humrep/dep399 PMID:19910321

Mardani, M., Vaez, A., & Razavi, S. (2014). Effect of saffron on rat sperm chromatin integrity. *Iranian Journal of Reproductive Medicine*, *12*, 343–350. PMID:25031579

Marild, S., Hansson, S., Jodal, U., Oden, A., & Svedberg, K. (2004). Protective effect of breastfeeding against urinary tract infection. *Acta Paediatrica (Oslo, Norway)*, *93*(2), 164–168. doi:10.1111/j.1651-2227.2004.tb00699.x PMID:15046267

Markowiak, P., & Slizewska, K. (2017). Effects of probiotics, prebiotics and synbiotics on human health. *Nutrients*, *9*(9), 1021. doi:10.3390/nu9091021 PMID:28914794

Marques da Fonseca, L., Jacques da Silva, L. R., Santos dos Reis, J., Rodrigues da Costa Santos, M. A., de Sousa Chaves, V., Monteiro da Costa, K., & de Alcântara-Pinto, D. C. (2020). Piperine Inhibits TGF-β Signaling Pathways and Disrupts EMT-Related Events in Human Lung Adenocarcinoma Cells. *Medicines (Basel, Switzerland)*, *7*(4), 19. doi:10.3390/medicines7040019 PMID:32276474

Marre, M., & Penfornis, A. (2011). GLP-1 receptor agonists today. *Diabetes Research and Clinical Practice*, *93*(3), 317–327. doi:10.1016/j.diabres.2011.01.004 PMID:21767888

Marsh, A., Eslick, E. M., & Eslick, G. D. (2016). Does a diet low in FODMAPs reduce symptoms associated with functional gastrointestinal disorders? A comprehensive systematic review and meta-analysis. *European Journal of Nutrition*, *55*(3), 897–906. doi:10.100700394-015-0922-1 PMID:25982757

Marum, A. P., Moreira, C., Saraiva, F., Tomas-Carus, P., & Sousa-Guerreiro, C. (2016). A low fermentable oligo-di-mono saccharides and polyols (FODMAP) diet reduced pain and improved daily life in fibromyalgia patients. *Scandinavian Journal of Pain*, *13*(1), 166–172. doi:10.1016/j.sjpain.2016.07.004 PMID:28850525

Mata, R., Cristians, S., Escandón-Rivera, S., Juárez-Reyes, K., & Rivero-Cruz, I. (2013). Mexican antidiabetic herbs: Valuable sources of inhibitors of α-glucosidases. *Journal of Natural Products*, *76*(3), 468–483. doi:10.1021/np300869g PMID:23398496

Mathur, N. B., & Dhingra, D. (2009). Perceived Breast Milk Insufficiency in Mothers of Neonates Hospitalized in Neonatal Intensive Care Unit. *Indian Journal of Pediatrics*, *76*(10), 1003–1006. doi:10.100712098-009-0204-0 PMID:19907930

Matijasic, B. B., Obermajer, T., Lipoglavšek, L., Grabnar, I., Avguštin, G., & Rogelj, I. (2014). Association of dietary type with fecal microbiota in vegetarians and omnivores in Slovenia. *European Journal of Nutrition*, *53*(4), 1051–1064. doi:10.100700394-013-0607-6 PMID:24173964

Matos, R. S., Baroncini, L.A., Précoma, L. B., Winter, G., Lambach, P.H., Caron, E.Y., . . . Précoma, D.B. (2012). Resveratrol causes antiatherogenic effects in an animal model of atherosclerosis. *Arquivos Brasileiros de Cardiologia*, *98*(2), 136–142. doi:10.1590/S0066-782X2012005000006 PMID:22231915

Matsuda, H., Morikawa, T., & Yoshikawa, M. (2002). Antidiabetogenic constituents from several natural medicines. *Pure and Applied Chemistry*, *74*(7), 1301–1308. doi:10.1351/pac200274071301

Matsui, T., Ogunwande, I. A., Abesundara, K. J., & Matsumoto, K. (2006). Anti-hyperglycemic Potential of Natural Products. *Mini-Reviews in Medicinal Chemistry*, *6*(3), 349–356. doi:10.2174/138955706776073484 PMID:16515474

Maury, E., Ehala-Aleksejev, K., Guiot, Y., Detry, R., Vandenhooft, A., & Brichard, S. M. (2007). Adipokines oversecreted by omental adipose tissue in human obesity. *American Journal of Physiology. Endocrinology and Metabolism*, *293*(3), E656–E665. doi:10.1152/ajpendo.00127.2007 PMID:17578888

Mayo Clinic. (2020). *The Best Ways To Cut Calories From Your Diet*. Available at: https://www.mayoclinic.org/healthy-lifestyle/weight-loss/in-depth/calories/art-20048065

Mayoclinic.org. (2020a). *Blood Pressure Test - Mayo Clinic*. Available at: https://www.mayoclinic.org/tests-procedures/blood-pressure-test/about/pac-20393098

Mayoclinic.org. (2020b). *Cholesterol Test - Mayo Clinic*. Available at: https://www.mayoclinic.org/tests-procedures/cholesterol-test/about/pac-20384601

Mayoclinic.org. (2020c). *Liposuction - Mayo Clinic*. Available at: https://www.mayoclinic.org/tests-procedures/liposuction/about/pac-20384586

Ma, Z., Yang, J., Yang, Y., Wang, X., Chen, G., Shi, A., Lu, L., Jia, S., Kang, X., & Lu, L. (2020). Rosmarinic acid exerts an anticancer effect on osteosarcoma cells by inhibiting DJ-1 via regulation of the PTEN-PI3K-Akt signaling pathway. *Phytomedicine*, *68*, 153186. doi:10.1016/j.phymed.2020.153186 PMID:32088353

McEwen, L., Casagrande, S., Kuo, S., & Herman, W. (2017). Why Are Diabetes Medications So Expensive and What Can Be Done to Control Their Cost? *Current Diabetes Reports*, *17*(9), 17. doi:10.100711892-017-0893-0 PMID:28741264

Mclachlan, R. I. (2000). The endocrine control of spermatogenesis. *Best Practice & Research. Clinical Endocrinology & Metabolism*, *14*(3), 345–362. doi:10.1053/beem.2000.0084 PMID:11097780

Medagama, A. (2015). The glycaemic outcomes of Cinnamon, a review of the experimental evidence and clinical trials. *Nutrition Journal*, *14*(1), 108. Advance online publication. doi:10.118612937-015-0098-9 PMID:26475130

Meddah, B., Ducroc, R., El Abbes Faouzi, M., Eto, B., Mahraoui, L., Benhaddou-Andaloussi, A., Martineau, L. C., Cherrah, Y., & Haddad, P. S. (2009). Nigella sativa inhibits intestinal glucose absorption and improves glucose tolerance in rats. *Journal of Ethnopharmacology*, *121*(3), 419–424. doi:10.1016/j.jep.2008.10.040 PMID:19061948

Meenatchi, P., Purushothaman, A., & Maneemegalai, S. (2017). Antioxidant, antiglycation and insulinotrophic properties of Coccinia grandis (L.) in vitro: Possible role in prevention of diabetic complications. *Journal of Traditional and Complementary Medicine*, *7*(1), 54–64. doi:10.1016/j.jtcme.2016.01.002 PMID:28053889

Metchinkoff, E. (1907). *The prolongation of life*. New York: Putmans Sons.

Metro, D., Cernaro, V., Papa, M., & Benvenga, S. (2018). Marked improvement of thyroid function and autoimmunity by Aloe barbadensis miller juice in patients with subclinical hypothyroidism. *Journal of Clinical & Translational Endocrinology*, *11*, 18–25. doi:10.1016/j.jcte.2018.01.003 PMID:29527506

Meydani, M. (2000). Effect of functional food ingredients: Vitamin E modulation of cardiovascular diseases and immune status in the elderly. *The American Journal of Clinical Nutrition*, *71*(6), 1665S–1668S. doi:10.1093/ajcn/71.6.1665S PMID:10837312

Miean, K. H., & Mohamed, S. (2001). Flavonoid (myricetin, quercetin, kaempferol, luteolin, and apigenin) content of edible tropical plants. *Journal of Agricultural and Food Chemistry*, *49*(6), 3106–3112. doi:10.1021/jf000892m PMID:11410016

Mi, J., He, W., Lv, J., Zhuang, K., Huang, H., & Quan, S. (2019). Effect of berberine on the HPA-axis pathway and skeletal muscle GLUT4 in type 2 diabetes mellitus rats. *Diabetes, Metabolic Syndrome and Obesity*, *12*, 1717–1725. doi:10.2147/DMSO.S211188 PMID:31564939

Mikaili, Mojaverrostami, & Moloudizargari, & Aghajanshakeri. (2013). Pharmacological and therapeutic effects of Mentha Longifolia L. and its main constituent, menthol. *Ancient Science of Life*, *33*(2), 131–138. PMID:25284948

Miksits, M., Wlcek, K., Svoboda, M., Kunert, O., Haslinger, E., Thalhammer, T., ... Jäger, W. (2009). Antitumor activity of resveratrol and its sulfated metabolites against human breast cancer cells. *Planta Medica*, *75*(11), 1227–1230. doi:10.1055-0029-1185533 PMID:19350482

Mikulskia, M. A., Wichmanb, M. D., Simmonsc, D. L., Phama, A. N., Clotteya, V., & Fuortesa, L. J. (2017). Toxic metals in ayurvedic preparations from a public health lead poisoning cluster investigation. *International Journal of Occupational and Environmental Health*, *23*(3), 187–192. doi:10.1080/10773525.2018.1447880 PMID:29528276

Milanov, S., Maleeva, A., & Tashkov, M. T. (1981). Effect on the concentration of some hormones in the serum of healthy subjects. Sofia, Bulgaria: Company Documentation, Chemical Pharmaceutical Research Institute.

Mills & Bone. (2013). *The Principles and Practices of Phytotherapy*. Churchill.

Minami, J. I., Kondo, S., Yanagisawa, N., Odamaki, T., Xiao, J. Z., Abe, F., Nakajima, S., Hamamoto, Y., Saitoh, S., & Shimoda, T. (2015). Oral administration of Bifidobacterium breve B-3 modifies metabolic functions in adults with obese tendencies in a randomised controlled trial. *Journal of Nutritional Science*, *4*, e1–e7. doi:10.1017/jns.2015.5 PMID:26090097

Miner, S. A., Robins, S., Zhu, Y. J., Keeren, K., Gu, V., Read, S. C., & Zelkowitz, P. (2018). Evidence for the use of complementary and alternative medicines during fertility treatment: A scoping review. *BMC Complementary and Alternative Medicine*, *18*(1), 158. Advance online publication. doi:10.118612906-018-2224-7 PMID:29764413

Mirfeizi, M., Tourzani, Z. M., Mirfeizi, S. Z., Jafarabadi, M. A., Rezvani, H. R., & Afzali, M. (2015). Controlling type 2 diabetes mellitus with herbal medicines: A triple-blind randomized clinical trial of efficacy and safety. *Journal of Diabetes*, *8*(5), 647–656. doi:10.1111/1753-0407.12342 PMID:26362826

Mishra, L. C., Singh, B. B., & Dagenais, S. (2000). Scientific basis for the therapeutic use of Withania somnifera (ashwagandha): A Review. *Alternative Medicine Review*, *5*(4), 334–346. PMID:10956379

Mishra, R. K., Verma, H. P., Singh, N., & Singh, S. K. (2012). Male infertility: Lifestyle and oriental remedies. *Journal of Science Research*, *56*, 93–101.

Misra, L., & Wagner, H. (2007). Extraction of bioactive principle from *Mucuna pruriens* seeds. *Indian Journal of Biochemistry & Biophysics*, *44*, 56–60. PMID:17385342

Mitra, K., Afsaneh, K., & Ahmad, K. (2017). The Effect of Herbal Teas on Management of Polycystic Ovary Syndrome: A Systematic Review. *Journal of Midwifery and Reproductive Health*, *5*(4), 1098–1106.

Mitsou, E. K., Kakali, A., Antonopoulou, S., Mountzouris, K. C., Yannakoulia, M., Panagiotakos, D. B., & Kyriacou, A. (2017). Adherence to the Mediterranean diet is associated with the gut microbiota pattern and gastrointestinal characteristics in an adult population. *British Journal of Nutrition*, *117*(12), 1645–1655. doi:10.1017/S0007114517001593 PMID:28789729

Mizutani, T., Suzuki, K., Kondo, N., & Yamagata, Z. (2007). Association of maternallife style including smoking during pregnancy with childhood obesity. *Obesity (Silver Spring, Md.)*, *15*(12), 33133–31399. doi:10.1038/oby.2007.373 PMID:18198324

Mohamed Sham Shihabudeen, H., Hansi Priscilla, D., & Thirumurugan, K. (2011). Cinnamon extract inhibits α-glucosidase activity and dampens postprandial glucose excursion in diabetic rats. *Nutrition & Metabolism*, *8*(1), 46. doi:10.1186/1743-7075-8-46 PMID:21711570

Mohammed, S. I., Chopda, M. Z., Patil, R. H., Vishwakarma, K. S., & Maheshwari, V. L. (2016). In vivo antidiabetic and antioxidant activities of Coccinia grandis leaf extract against streptozotocin induced diabetes in experimental rats. *Asian Pacific Journal of Tropical Disease*, *6*(4), 298–304. doi:10.1016/S2222-1808(15)61034-9

Mohanraj, K., Karthikeyan, B. S., Vivek-Ananth, R. P., Chand, R. B., Aparna, S. R., Mangalapandi, P., & Samal, A. (2018). IMPPAT: A curated database of Indian Medicinal Plants, Phytochemistry And Therapeutics. *Scientific Reports*, *8*(1), 1–17. doi:10.103841598-018-22631-z PMID:29311619

Mohd Bukhari, D. A., Siddiqui, M. J., Shamsudin, S. H., Rahman, M. M., & So'ad, S. Z. M. (2017). α-Glucosidase inhibitory activity of selected Malaysian plants. *Journal of Pharmacy & Bioallied Sciences*, *9*(3), 164–170. doi:10.4103/jpbs.JPBS_35_17 PMID:28979070

Mohebbi-Kian, E., Mohammad-Alizadeh-Charandabi, S., & Bekhradi, R. (2014). Efficacy of fennel and combined oral contraceptive on depot medroxyprogesterone acetate-induced amenorrhea: A randomized placebo-controlled trial. *Contraception*, *90*(4), 440–446. doi:10.1016/j.contraception.2014.05.001 PMID:24981150

Mohseni, R., ArabSadeghabadi, Z., Ziamajidi, N., Abbasalipourkabir, R., & RezaeiFarimani, A. (2019). Oral administration of resveratrol-loaded solid lipid nanoparticle improves insulin resistance through targeting expression of SNARE Proteins in adipose and muscle tissue in rats with type 2 diabetes. *Nanoscale Research Letters*, *14*(1), 227. doi:10.118611671-019-3042-7 PMID:31290033

Mokaberinejad, R., Akhtari, E., Tansaz, M., Bioos, S., Kamalinejad, M., Zafarghandi, N., Ghobadi, A., Sohrabvand, F., & Akhbari, A. (2014). Effect of Mentha longifolia on FSH Serum Level in Premature Ovarian Failure. *Open Journal of Obstetrics and Gynecology*, *4*(7), 356–360. doi:10.4236/ojog.2014.47053

Mokaberinejad, R., Zafarghandi, N., Bioos, S., Dabaghian, F. H., Naseri, M., Kamalinejad, M., Amin, G., Ghobadi, A., Tansaz, M., Akhbari, A., & Hamiditabar, M. (2012). Mentha longifolia syrup in secondary amenorrhea: A double-blind, placebo-controlled, randomized trials. *Daru: Journal of Faculty of Pharmacy, Tehran University of Medical Sciences*, *20*(1), 97. doi:10.1186/2008-2231-20-97 PMID:23351184

Mokdad, A. H., Bowman, B. A., Ford, E. S., Vinicor, F., Marks, J. S., & Koplan, J. P. (2001). The continuing epidemics of obesity and diabetes in the United States. *Journal of the American Medical Association*, *286*(10), 1195–1200. doi:10.1001/jama.286.10.1195 PMID:11559264

Molan, A. L., Liu, Z., & Plimmer, G. (2014). Evaluation of the effect of blackcurrant products on gut microbiota and on markers of risk for colon cancer in humans. *Phytotherapy Research*, *28*(3), 416–422. doi:10.1002/ptr.5009 PMID:23674271

Molloy, S. A., Rowan, E. N., Brien, J. T. O., McKeith, I. G., Wesnes, K., & Burn, D. J. (2006). Effect of levodopa on cognitive function in Parkinson's disease with and without dementia with Lewy bodies. *Journal of Neurology, Neurosurgery, and Psychiatry*, *77*(12), 1323–1328. doi:10.1136/jnnp.2006.098079 PMID:16952917

Monday, O. M., & Uzoma, A. I. (2013). Histological changes and antidiabetic activities of Icacina trichantha tuber extract in beta–cells of alloxan induced diabetic rats. *Asian Pacific Journal of Tropical Biomedicine*, *3*(8), 628–633. doi:10.1016/S2221-1691(13)60127-6 PMID:23905020

Monteith, G. R., Davis, F. M., & Roberts-Thomson, S. J. (2012). Calcium channels and pumps in cancer: Changes and consequences. *The Journal of Biological Chemistry*, *287*(38), 31666–31673. doi:10.1074/jbc.R112.343061 PMID:22822055

Moradi, B., Abbaszadeh, S., Shahsavari, S., Alizadeh, M., & Beyranvand, F. (2018). The most useful medicinal herbs to treat diabetes. *Biomedical Research and Therapy*, *5*(8), 2538–2551. doi:10.15419/bmrat.v5i8.463

Mora, J. C., Przkora, R., & Cruz-Almeida, Y. (2018). Knee osteoarthritis: Pathophysiology and current treatment modalities. *Journal of Pain Research*, *11*, 2189–2196. doi:10.2147/JPR.S154002 PMID:30323653

Moran, L. J., Brinkworth, G. D., & Norman, R. J. (2008). Dietary therapy in polycystic ovary syndrome. *Seminars in Reproductive Medicine*, *26*(1), 85–92. doi:10.1055-2007-992928 PMID:18181086

Moran, L. J., Pasquali, R., Teede, H. J., Hoeger, K. M., & Norman, R. J. (2009). Treatment of obesity in polycystic ovary syndrome: A position statement of the Androgen Excess and Polycystic Ovary Syndrome Society. *Fertility and Sterility*, *92*(6), 1966–1982. doi:10.1016/j.fertnstert.2008.09.018 PMID:19062007

Moreira, D. L., Teixeira, S. S., Monteiro, M. H. D., De-Oliveira, A. C. A. X., & Paumgartten, F. J. R. (2014). Traditional use and safety of herbal medicines. *Revista Brasileira de Farmacognosia*, *24*(2), 248–257. doi:10.1016/j.bjp.2014.03.006

Mother and Child Nutrition. (2020). *Benefits of Breastfeeding for the Infant/Young Child.* https://motherchildnutrition.org/healthy-nutrition/about-essential-nutrition-actions/benefits-of-breastfeeding.html.

Mukherjee, P. K., Venkatesh, P., & Ponnusankar, S. (2010). Ethnopharmacology and integrative medicine - Let the history tell the future. *Journal of Ayurveda and Integrative Medicine*, *1*(2), 100–109. doi:10.4103/0975-9476.65077

Musmar, S., Afaneh, A., & Mo'alla, H. (2013). Epidemiology of polycystic ovary syndrome: A cross sectional study of university students at An-Najah national university-Palestine. *Reproductive Biology and Endocrinology*, *11*(1), 47. doi:10.1186/1477-7827-11-47 PMID:23688000

Mutlu Altundag, E., Mine Yilmaz, A., Kasaci, T., Corek, C., Taga, Y., & Suha Yalcin, A. (2014). The role of HSP90 in Quercetin-induced apoptosis in human papillary thyroid (B-CPAP) cancer cells. *Free Radical Biology & Medicine*, *75*(Suppl 1), S43. doi:10.1016/j.freeradbiomed.2014.10.797 PMID:26461378

Nabilatul, H. M., Ismail, W. I. W., Zainah, A., Siti, S. J., & Aishah, A. (2013). Potential roles of *Stevia rebaudiana* Bertoni in arogating insulin resistance and diabetes: A review. *Evidence-Based Complementary and Alternative Medicine*, *2013*, 718049. PMID:24324517

Nagappa, A. N., Thakurdesai, P. A., Venkat Rao, N., & Singh, J. (2003). Antidiabetic activity of *Terminalia catappa* Linn fruits. *Journal of Ethnopharmacology*, *88*(1), 45–50. doi:10.1016/S0378-8741(03)00208-3 PMID:12902049

Nagendran, J., Waller, T. J., & Dyck, J. R. B. (2013). AMPK signalling and the control of substrate use in the heart. *Molecular and Cellular Endocrinology*, *366*(2), 180–193. doi:10.1016/j.mce.2012.06.015 PMID:22750050

Nahid, M. A., Satoh, M., & Chan, E. K. (2015). Interleukin 1beta-Responsive MicroRNA-146a Is Critical for the Cytokine-Induced Tolerance and Cross-Tolerance to Toll-Like Receptor Ligands. *Journal of Innate Immunity*, *7*(4), 428–440. doi:10.1159/000371517 PMID:25896300

Naimi, M., Vlavcheski, F., Shamshoum, H., & Tsiani, E. (2017). Rosemary extract as a potential anti-hyperglycemic agent: Current evidence and future perspectives. *Nutrients*, *9*(9), 968. doi:10.3390/nu9090968 PMID:28862678

Nair, G. R., Naidu, G. S., Jain, S., Nagi, R., Makkad, R. S., & Jha, A. (2016). Clinical effectiveness of aloe vera in the management of oral mucosal diseases- A systematic review. *Journal of Clinical and Diagnostic Research: JCDR*, *10*(8), ZE01–ZE07. PMID:27656587

Najafian, J., Abdar-Esfahani, M., Arab-Momeni, M., & Akhavan-Tabib, A. (2014). Safety of herbal medicine in treatment of weight loss. *ARYA Atherosclerosis*, *10*(1), 55. PMID:24963315

Nakagawa, T., Goto, H., Hussein, G., Hikiami, H., Shibahara, N., & Shimada, Y. (2008). Keishibukuryogan ameliorates glucose intolerance and hyperlipidemia in Otsuka Long-Evans Tokushima Fatty (OLETF) rats. *Diabetes Research (Edinburgh, Lothian)*, *80*(1), 40–47. doi:10.1016/j.diabres.2007.11.019 PMID:18242756

Nakamura, H., Noh, J. Y., Itoh, K., Fukata, S., Miyauchi, A., & Hamada, N. (2007). Comparison of methimazole and propylthiouracil in patients with hyperthyroidism caused by Graves' disease. *The Journal of Clinical Endocrinology and Metabolism*, *92*(6), 2157–2162. doi:10.1210/jc.2006-2135 PMID:17389704

Nambiar, D. K., Rajamani, P., & Singh, R. P. (2015). Silibinin attenuates ionizing radiation-induced pro-angiogenic response and EMT in prostate cancer cells. *Biochemical and Biophysical Research Communications*, *456*(1), 262–268. doi:10.1016/j.bbrc.2014.11.069 PMID:25446081

Nardo, L. G., Patchava, S., & Laing, I. (2008). Polycystic ovary syndrome: Pathophysiology, molecular aspects and clinical implications. *Panminerva Medica*, *50*(4), 267–278. PMID:19078868

Nasri, H., Baradaran, A., Shirzad, H., & Kopaei, M. R. (2014). New concepts in nutraceuticals as alternative for pharmaceuticals. *International Journal of Preventive Medicine*. PMID:25709784

National Institutes of Health, Department of Health and Human Services. (2008). *Beyond Infertility: Polycystic Ovary Syndrome (PCOS)*. NIH Pub, No. 08-5863.

Nava, A., Azizeh, F. K., Aliyeh, G., Kobra, H., Arash, K., Elaheh, O., Abbas, D., Fahimeh, B., & Masoumeh, M. (2019). The Effect of Herbal Medicine Supplementation on Clinical and Para-clinical Outcomes in Women With PCOS: A Systematic Review and Meta-analysis. *International Journal of Women's Health and Reproduction Sciences*, *7*(4), 423–433. doi:10.15296/ijwhr.2019.72

Ndarubu, T. A., Chiamaka, O. S., Alfa, S., Aishatu, M., Chinedu, O. E., Wenawo, D. L., ... Eustace, B. B. (2019). Phytochemicals, hypoglycemic and hypolipidemic effects of methanol leaf extract of Hibiscus sabdariffa in alloxan induced diabetic rats. *GSC Biological and Pharmaceutical Sciences, 8*(3), 070-078.

Nejatbakhsh, F., Nazem, E., Goushegir, A., & Isfahani, M. M., Nikbakht Nasrabadi, A., & Baygom Siahpoosh, M. (2012). Recommended foods for male infertility in Iranian traditional medicine. *Iranian Journal of Reproductive Medicine*, *10*, 511–516. PMID:25246919

Nejatbakhsh, F., Shirbeigi, L., Rahimi, R., & Abolhassani, H. (2016). Review of local herbal compounds found in the Iranian traditional medicine known to optimise male fertility. *Andrologia*, *48*(8), 850–859. doi:10.1111/and.12675 PMID:27681643

Nelson-Dooley, C., Della-Fera, M. A., Hamrick, M., & Baile, C. A. (2005). Novel treatments for obesity and osteoporosis: Targeting apoptotic pathways in adipocytes. *Current Medicinal Chemistry*, *12*(19), 2215–2225. doi:10.2174/0929867054864886 PMID:16178781

Nelson, J. C., & Papakostas, G. I. (2009). A Typical antipsychotic augmentation in major depressive disorder: A meta-analysis of placebo-controlled randomized trials. *The American Journal of Psychiatry*, *166*(9), 980–991. doi:10.1176/appi.ajp.2009.09030312 PMID:19687129

Ness-Abramof, R., & Apovian, C. M. (2006). Diet modification for treatment and prevention of obesity. *Endocrine*, *29*(1), 5–9. doi:10.1385/ENDO:29:1:5 PMID:16622287

Nestler, J. E., Powers, L. P., Matt, D. W., Steingold, K. A., Plymate, S. R., Rittmaster, R. S., Clore, J. N., & Blackard, W. G. (1991). A direct effect of hyperinsulinemia on serum sex hormone-binding globulin levels in obese women with the polycystic ovary syndrome. *The Journal of Clinical Endocrinology and Metabolism*, *72*(1), 83–89. doi:10.1210/jcem-72-1-83 PMID:1898744

Neuhouser, M. L. (2004). Dietary flavonoids and cancer risk: Evidence from human population studies. *Nutrition and Cancer*, *50*(1), 1–7. doi:10.120715327914nc5001_1 PMID:15572291

Newcomb, P. A., Storer, B. E., Longnecker, M. P., Mittendorf, R., Greenberg, E. R., Clapp, R. W., ... MacMahon, B. (1994). Lactation and a reduced risk of premenopausal breast cancer. *The New England Journal of Medicine*, *330*(2), 81–87. doi:10.1056/NEJM199401133300201 PMID:8259187

Newman, D. J., & Cragg, G. M. (2016). Natural products as sources of new drugs from 1981 to 2014. *Journal of Natural Products*, *79*(3), 629–661. doi:10.1021/acs.jnatprod.5b01055

NFUM, National Formulary of Unani Medicine. (2006a). *Part-I*. New Delhi, India: CCRUM, Department of AYUSH, Ministry of Health & Family Welfare, Government of India.

NFUM, National Formulary of Unani Medicine. (2006b). *Part-IV* (1st ed.). New Delhi, India: Department of AYUSH, Ministry of Health & Family Welfare, Government of India.

NFUM, National Formulary of Unani Medicine. (2007). *Part-II, Vol-I*. New Delhi, India: Department of AYUSH, Ministry of Health & Family Welfare, Government of India.

NFUM, National Formulary of Unani Medicine. (2008). *Part-V*. New Delhi, India: Department of AYUSH, Ministry of Health & Family Welfare, Government of India.

NFUM, National Formulary of Unani Medicine. (2011). *Part-VI*. New Delhi, India: Department of AYUSH, Ministry of Health & Family Welfare, Government of India.

Ng, F., Yun, H., Lei, X., Danishefsky, S. J., Fahey, J., Stephenson, K., Flexner, C., & Lee, L. (2008). (3R,9R,10R)-Panaxytriol: A molecular-based nutraceutical with possible application to cancer prevention and treatment. *Tetrahedron Letters*. Advance online publication. doi:10.1016/j.tetlet.2008.09.169 PMID:20011028

Ng, M., Fleming, T., Robinson, M., Thomson, B., Graetz, N., Margono, C., Mullany, E. C., Biryukov, S., Abbafati, C., Abera, S. F., Abraham, J. P., Abu-Rmeileh, N. M. E., Achoki, T., AlBuhairan, F. S., Alemu, Z. A., Alfonso, R., Ali, M. K., Ali, R., Guzman, N. A., ... Gakidou, E. (2014). Global, regional, and national prevalence of overweight and obesity in children and adults during 1980- 2013: A systematic analysis for the Global Burden of Disease Study 2013. *Lancet*, *384*(9945), 766–781. doi:10.1016/S0140-6736(14)60460-8 PMID:24880830

Nieto, M. A., Huang, R. Y. J., Jackson, R. A., & Thiery, J. P. (2016). EMT: 2016. *Cell*, *166*(1), 21–45. doi:10.1016/j.cell.2016.06.028 PMID:27368099

NIH. (2020). *Selenium, Health professional fact sheet*. National Institute of Healths, Office of Dietary Supplements.

Nimesh, S., Tomar, R., & Dhiman, S. (2019). Medicinal Herbal Plants and Allopathic Drugs to Treat Diabetes Mellitus: A glance. *Advances In Pharmacology And Clinical Trials*, *4*(1), 1–13.

Nirav, R. S. (2017). Current Management on PCOS (Polycystic Ovary Syndrome)/Stein-Leventhal Syndrome. *Invest Gynecol Res Women's Health*, *1*(3), 46–48.

Nirmala, P., & Ramanathan, M. (2011). Effect of kaempferol on lipid peroxidation and antioxidant status in 1,2-dimethyl hydrazine induced colorectal carcinoma in rats. *European Journal of Pharmacology*, *654*(1), 75–79. doi:10.1016/j.ejphar.2010.11.034 PMID:21172346

Niu, Y., Na, L., Feng, R., Gong, L., Zhao, Y., Li, Q., Li, Y., & Sun, C. (2013). The phytochemical, EGCG, extends lifespan by reducing liver and kidney function damage and improving age-associated inflammation and oxidative stress in healthy rats. *Aging Cell*, *12*(6). Advance online publication. doi:10.1111/acel.12133 PMID:23834676

Noriega, B. S., Sanchez-Gonzalez, M. A., Salyakina, D., & Coffman, J. (2016). Understanding the Impact of Omega-3 Rich Diet on the Gut Microbiota. *Case Reports in Medicine*, *2016*, 3089303. doi:10.1155/2016/3089303 PMID:27065349

Norman, R. J., Davies, M. J., Lord, J., & Moran, L. J. (2002). The role of lifestyle modification in polycystic ovary syndrome. *Trends in Endocrinology and Metabolism*, *13*(6), 251–257. doi:10.1016/S1043-2760(02)00612-4 PMID:12128286

Norman, R. J., Dewailly, D., Legro, R. S., & Hickey, T. E. (2007). Polycystic ovary syndrome. *Lancet*, *370*(9588), 685–697. doi:10.1016/S0140-6736(07)61345-2 PMID:17720020

Nowak, D. A., Snyder, D. C., Brown, A. J., & Wahnefried, W. D. (2007). The Effect of Flaxseed Supplementation on Hormonal Levels Associated with Polycystic Ovarian Syndrome: A Case Study. *Current Topics in Nutraceutical Research*, *5*(4), 177–181. PMID:19789727

O'Hara, A. M., & Shanahan, F. (2006). The gut flora as a forgotten organ. *EMBO Reports*, *7*(7), 688–693. doi:10.1038j.embor.7400731 PMID:16819463

O'Keeffe, M., Jansen, C., Martin, L., Williams, M., Seamark, L., Staudacher, H. M., ... Lomer, M. C. (2018). Long-term impact of the low-FODMAP diet on gastrointestinal symptoms, dietary intake, patient acceptability, and healthcare utilization in irritable bowel syndrome. *Neurogastroenterology and Motility*, *30*(1), e13154. doi:10.1111/nmo.13154 PMID:28707437

O'Malley, B., & Strott, C. (1999). Steroid hormones: Metabolism and mechanism of action. In Reproductive Endocrinology- Physiology, pathophysiology and clinical management. Philadelphia: WB Saunders Company.

Obata, S., Okauchi, S., Kimura, T., Hirukawa, H., Tanabe, A., Kinoshita, T., Kohara, K., Tatsumi, F., Shimoda, M., Kamei, S., Nakanishi, S., Mune, T., Kaku, K., & Kaneto, H. (2017). Advanced breast cancer in a relatively young man with severe obesity and type 2 diabetes mellitus. *Journal of Diabetes Investigation*, *8*(3), 395–396. doi:10.1111/jdi.12570 PMID:28470916

Oboh, G., Ademiluyi, A. O., Akinyemi, A. J., Henle, T., Saliu, J. A., & Schwarzenbolz, U. (2012). Inhibitory effect of polyphenol-rich extracts of jute leaf (Corchorus olitorius) on key enzyme linked to type 2 diabetes (α-amylase and α-glucosidase) and hypertension (angiotensin I converting) in vitro. *Journal of Functional Foods*, *4*(2), 450–458. doi:10.1016/j.jff.2012.02.003

Ocaña, O. H., Córcoles, R., Fabra, Á., Moreno-Bueno, G., Acloque, H., Vega, S., & Nieto, M. A. (2012). Metastatic colonization requires the repression of the epithelial-mesenchymal transition inducer Prrx1. *Cancer Cell*, *22*(6), 709–724. doi:10.1016/j.ccr.2012.10.012 PMID:23201163

Oddy, W. H., Sly, P. D., & de Klerk, N. H. (2003). Breast feeding and respiratory morbidity in infancy: A birth cohort study. *Archives of Disease in Childhood*, *88*(3), 224–228. doi:10.1136/adc.88.3.224 PMID:12598384

Oelker, L. (2005). Quality control in herbal supplements. *Annali dell'Istituto Superiore di Sanita, 41*(1), 43–48. PMID:16037649

Ogden, C. L., Carroll, M. D., Curtin, L. R., McDowell, M. A., Tabak, C. J., & Flegal, K. M. (2006). Prevalence of overweight and obesity in the United States, 1999-2004. *Journal of the American Medical Association, 295*(13), 1549–1555. doi:10.1001/jama.295.13.1549 PMID:16595758

Ogunwande, I. A., Matsui, T., Fujise, T., & Matsumoto, K. (2007). α-Glucosidase inhibitory profile of Nigerian medicinal plants in immobilized assay system. *Food Science and Technology Research, 13*(2), 169–172. doi:10.3136/fstr.13.169

Oh, M. R., Park, S. H., Kim, S. Y., Back, H.-I., Kim, M.-G., Jeon, J.-Y., Ha, K.-C., Na, W.-T., Cha, Y.-S., Park, B.-H., Park, T., & Chae, S.-W. (2014). Postprandial glucose-lowering effects of fermented red ginseng in subjects with impaired fasting glucose or type 2 diabetes: A randomized, double-blind, placebo-controlled clinical trial. *BMC Complementary and Alternative Medicine, 14*(1), 237. doi:10.1186/1472-6882-14-237 PMID:25015735

Oh, S. D., Kim, M., Min, B. I., Choi, G. S., Kim, S. K., Bae, H., Kang, C., Kim, D. G., Park, B. J., & Kim, C. K. (2014). Effect of *Achyranthes bidentata* blume on 3T3-L1 adipogenesis and rats fed with a high-fat diet. *Evidence-Based Complementary and Alternative Medicine, 2014*(158018), 1–8. PMID:24963319

Okoroh, E. M., Hooper, W. C., Atrash, H. K., Yusuf, H. R., & Boulet, S. L. (2012). Prevalence of polycystic ovary syndrome among the privately insured, United States, 2003–2008. *Obstetrics and Gynecology, 207*, 299.e1–299.e7. PMID:22921097

Oldroyd, J., Unwin, N., White, M., Mathers, J., & Alberti, K. (2006). Randomised controlled trial evaluating lifestyle interventions in people with impaired glucose tolerance. *Diabetes Research and Clinical Practice, 72*(2), 117–127. doi:10.1016/j.diabres.2005.09.018 PMID:16297488

Olokoba, A., Obateru, O., & Olokoba, L. (2012). Type 2 Diabetes Mellitus: A Review of Current Trends. *Oman Medical Journal, 27*(4), 269–273. doi:10.5001/omj.2012.68 PMID:23071876

Ong, K. J., Theodoru, E., & Ledger, W. (2006). Long-term consequence of polycystic ovarian syndrome. *Current Obstetrics & Gynaecology, 16*(6), 333–336. doi:10.1016/j.curobgyn.2006.09.002

Ong, M., Peng, J., Jin, X., & Qu, X. (2017). Chinese Herbal Medicine for the Optimal Management of Polycystic Ovary Syndrome. *The American Journal of Chinese Medicine, 45*(03), 405–422. doi:10.1142/S0192415X17500252 PMID:28359195

Orel, R., & Kamhi Trop, T. (2014). Intestinal microbiota, probiotics and prebiotics in inflammatory bowel disease. *World Journal of Gastroenterology, 20*(33), 11505–11524. doi:10.3748/wjg.v20.i33.11505 PMID:25206258

Ortiz-Andrade, R. R., Garcia-Jimenez, S., Castillo-Espana, P., Ramirez-Avila, G., Villalobos-Molina, R., & Estrada-Soto, S. (2007). α-Glucosidase inhibitory activity of the methanolic extract from Tournefortia hartwegiana: An antihyperglycemic agent. *Journal of Ethnopharmacology, 109*(1), 48–53. doi:10.1016/j.jep.2006.07.002 PMID:16920301

Osada, K., Takahashi, M., Hoshina, S., Nakamura, M., Nakamura, S., & Sugano, M. (2001). Tea catechins inhibit cholesterol oxidation accompanying oxidation of low density lipoprotein *in vitro*. *Comparative Biochemistry and Physiology-Part C, 128*(2), 153–164. doi:10.1016/S1532-0456(00)00192-7 PMID:11239828

Othman, M., Aguero, R., & Lin, H. C. (2008). Alterations in intestinal microbial flora and human disease. *Current Opinion in Gastroenterology, 24*(1), 11–16. doi:10.1097/MOG.0b013e3282f2b0d7 PMID:18043226

Owolabi, O. J., Inninh, S. O., Anaka, O. N., & Iyamu, O. A. (2014). Antidiabetic and Hypolipidemic Effects of Methanol Leaf Extract of *Napoleona vogelii* (Lecythidaceae). *Hook and Planch on Alloxan–Induced Diabetes Mellitus in Rats Tropical Journal of Pharmaceutical Research, 13*(11), 1903–1909.

Ozdal, T., Sela, D. A., Xiao, J., Boyacioglu, D., Chen, F., & Capanoglu, E. (2016). The Reciprocal Interactions between Polyphenols and Gut Microbiota and Effects on Bioaccessibility. *Nutrients, 8*(2), 78. doi:10.3390/nu8020078 PMID:26861391

Pacana, T., & Sanyal, A. J. (2012). Vitamin E and non-alcoholic fatty liver disease. *Current Opinion in Clinical Nutrition and Metabolic Care, 15*(6), 641–648. doi:10.1097/MCO.0b013e328357f747 PMID:23075940

Pachiappan, Matheswaran, Pushkalai, Saravanan, & Muthusamy. (2017). Medicinal plants for polycystic ovary syndrome: A review of phytomedicine research. *International Journal of Herbal Medicine, 5*(2), 78-80.

Padiya, R., & Banerjee, S. K. (2013). Garlic as an anti-diabetic agent: Recent progress and patent reviews. *Recent Patents on Food, Nutrition & Agriculture, 5*(2), 105–127. doi:10.2174/18761429113059990002 PMID:23270395

Padwal, R. S., & Majumdur, S. R. (2007). Drug treatments for obesity: Olistat, Sibutramine, rimonabant. *Lancet, 369*(9555), 371–377. doi:10.1016/S0140-6736(07)60033-6 PMID:17208644

Pal, H. C., Sharma, S., Strickland, L. R., Katiyar, S. K., Ballestas, M. E., Athar, M., Elmets, C. A., & Afaq, F. (2014). Fisetin inhibits human melanoma cell invasion through promotion of mesenchymal to epithelial transition and by targeting MAPK and NFκB signaling pathways. *PLoS One, 9*(1), e86338. doi:10.1371/journal.pone.0086338 PMID:24466036

Palsamy, P., & Subramanian, S. (2008). Resveratrol, a natural phytoalexin, normalizes hyperglycemia in streptozotocin-nicotinamide induced experimental diabetic rats. *Biomedicine and Pharmacotherapy, 62*(9), 598–605. doi:10.1016/j.biopha.2008.06.037 PMID:18675532

Panche, A. N., Diwan, A. D., & Chandra, S. R. (2016). Flavonoids: An overview. *Journal of Nutritional Science, 5*, e47. doi:10.1017/jns.2016.41 PMID:28620474

Panda, A. K., Chakraborty, D., Sarkar, I., Khan, T., & Sa, G. (2017). New insights into therapeutic activity and anticancer properties of curcumin. *Journal of Experimental Pharmacology, 9*, 31–45. doi:10.2147/JEP.S70568 PMID:28435333

Panda, S., & Kar, A. (1999). Withania somnifera and Bauhinia purpurea in the regulation of circulating thyroid hormone concentrations in female mice. *Journal of Ethnopharmacology, 67*(2), 233–239. doi:10.1016/S0378-8741(99)00018-5 PMID:10619390

Panda, S., & Kar, A. (2005). Guggulu (Commiphora mukul) potentially ameliorates hypothyroidism in female mice. *Phytotherapy Research, 19*(1), 78–80. doi:10.1002/ptr.1602 PMID:15798994

Panda, S., & Kar, A. (2006). Evaluation of the antithyroid, antioxidative and antihyperglycemic activity of scopoletin from Aegle marmelos leaves in hyperthyroid rats. *Phytotherapy Research, 20*(12), 1103–1105. doi:10.1002/ptr.2014 PMID:17078113

Panda, S., & Kar, A. (2007). Annona squamosa seed extract in the regulation of hyperthyroidism and lipid-peroxidation in mice: Possible involvement of quercetin. *Phytomedicine, 14*(12), 799–805. doi:10.1016/j.phymed.2006.12.001 PMID:17291737

Panda, S., & Kar, A. (2007). Apigenin (4¢,5,7-trihydroxyflavone) regulates hyperglycaemia, thyroid dysfunction and lipid peroxidation in alloxan-induced diabetic mice. *The Journal of Pharmacy and Pharmacology, 59*(11), 1543–1548. doi:10.1211/jpp.59.11.0012 PMID:17976266

Panda, S., Sharma, R., & Kar, A. (2019). Chavibetol corrects thyrotoxicosis through alterations in thyroid peroxidase. *Naunyn-Schmiedeberg's Archives of Pharmacology*, *392*(5), 541–550. doi:10.100700210-018-01606-x PMID:30610248

Panda, S., Sharma, R., Khan, A., & Kar, A. (2020). Ameliorative effect of Aloe gel against L-T4-induced hyperthyroidism via suppression of thyrotropin receptors, inflammation and oxidative stress. *Molecular Biology Reports*, *47*(4), 2801–2810. doi:10.100711033-020-05405-7 PMID:32242301

Pandey, K. R., Naik, S. R., & Vaki, B. V. (2015). Probiotics, prebiotics and synbiotics- A review. *Journal of Food Science and Technology*, *52*(12), 7577–7587. doi:10.100713197-015-1921-1 PMID:26604335

Pandey, M. M., Rastogi, S., & Rawat, A. K. S. (2013). Indian traditional ayurvedic system of medicine and nutritional supplementation. *Evidence-Based Complementary and Alternative Medicine*, *2013*, 2013. doi:10.1155/2013/376327

Pandey, M., Verma, R. K., & Saraf, S. A. (2010). Nutraceuticals: New era of medicine and health. *Asian Journal of Pharmaceutical and Clinical Research*, *3*, 11–15.

Pang, B., Zhao, L.-H., Zhou, Q., Zhao, T.-Y., Wang, H., Gu, C.-H., & Tong, X.-L. (2015). Application of berberine on treating type 2 diabetes mellitus. *International Journal of Endocrinology*, *905749*, 1–12. Advance online publication. doi:10.1155/2015/905749 PMID:25861268

Pan, M.-H., Lai, C.-S., Tsai, M.-L., Wu, J.-C., & Ho, C.-T. (2012). Molecular mechanisms for anti-aging by natural dietary compounds. *Molecular Nutrition & Food Research*, *56*(1), 88–115. doi:10.1002/mnfr.201100509 PMID:22083941

Pan, S. T., Li, Z.-L., He, Z.-X., Qiu, J.-X., & Zhou, S.-F. (2016). Molecular mechanisms for tumour resistance to chemotherapy. *Clinical and Experimental Pharmacology & Physiology*, *43*(8), 723–737. doi:10.1111/1440-1681.12581 PMID:27097837

Papathanasopoulos, A., & Camilleri, M. (2010). Dietary fiber supplements: Effects in obesity and metabolic syndrome and relationship to gastrointestinal functions. *Gastroenterology*, *138*(1), 65–72. doi:10.1053/j.gastro.2009.11.045 PMID:19931537

Papi, A., Govoni, M., Ciavarella, C., Spisni, E., Orlandi, M., & Farabegoli, F. (2016). Epigallocatechin-3-gallate increases RXRγ-mediated pro-apoptotic and anti-invasive effects in gastrointestinal cancer cell lines. *Current Cancer Drug Targets*, *16*(4), 373–385. doi:10.2174/1568009615666150817120931 PMID:26278714

Park, H. S., Cho, J. H., Kim, K. W., Chung, W. S., & Song, M. Y. (2018). Effects of Panax ginseng on obesity in animal models: A Systematic review and meta-analysis. *Evidence-based Complementary and Alternative Medicine: eCAM*, 2719794.

Park, E. Y., Kim, H. J., Kim, Y. K., Park, S. U., Choi, J. E., Cha, J. Y., & Jun, H. S. (2012). Increase in insulin secretion induced by Panax ginseng berry extracts contributes to the amelioration of hyperglycemia in streptozotocin-induced diabetic mice. *Journal of Ginseng Research*, *36*(2), 153–160. doi:10.5142/jgr.2012.36.2.153 PMID:23717115

Parker, J., McCullough, K., Field, B., Minnion, J. S., Martin, N. M., Ghatei, M. A., & Bloom, S. R. (2013). Glucagon and GLP-1 inhibit food intake and increase c-fos expression in similar appetite regulating centres in the brainstem and amygdala. *International Journal of Obesity*, *37*(10), 1391–1398. doi:10.1038/ijo.2012.227 PMID:23337772

Park, H. J., Cho, J.-Y., Kim, M. K., Koh, P.-O., Cho, K.-W., Kim, C. H., Lee, K.-S., Chung, B. Y., Kim, G.-S., & Cho, J.-H. (2012). Anti-obesity effect of *Schisandra chinensis* in 3T3-L1 cells and high fat diet-induced obese rats. *Food Chemistry*, *134*(1), 227–234. doi:10.1016/j.foodchem.2012.02.101 PMID:23265481

Park, H. Y., Kim, M., & Han, J. (2011). Stereospecific microbial production of isoflavanones from isoflavones and isoflavone glucosides. *Applied Microbiology and Biotechnology*, *91*(4), 1173–1181. doi:10.100700253-011-3310-7 PMID:21562980

Park, S. J., Nam, J., Ahn, C. W., & Kim, Y. (2019). Anti-diabetic properties of different fractions of Korean red ginseng. *Journal of Ethnopharmacology*, *236*, 220–230. doi:10.1016/j.jep.2019.01.044 PMID:30849506

Park, S. Y., Kim, G., Bae, S.-J., Yoo, Y., & Choi, Y. (2007). Induction of apoptosis by isothiocyanate sulforaphane in human cervical carcinoma HeLa and hepatocarcinoma HepG2 cells through activation of caspase-3. *Oncology Reports*, *18*(1), 181–187. doi:10.3892/or.18.1.181 PMID:17549366

Parvez, M. K. (2017). Natural or Plant Products for the Treatment of Neurological Disorders: Current Knowledge. *Current Drug Metabolism*. Advance online publication. doi:10.2174/1389200218666170710190249 PMID:28699506

Pasqualotto, F. F., Lucon, A. M., Sobreiro, B. P., Pasqualotto, E. B., & Arap, S. (2004). Effects of medicaltherapy, alcohol, smoking, and endocrine disruptors on male infertility. *Revista do Hospital das Clínicas*, *59*(6), 375–382. doi:10.1590/S0041-87812004000600011 PMID:15654492

Pastushenko, I., Brisebarre, A., Sifrim, A., Fioramonti, M., Revenco, T., Boumahdi, S., & De Clercq, S. (2018). Identification of the tumour transition states occurring during EMT. *Nature*, *556*(7702), 463–468. doi:10.103841586-018-0040-3 PMID:29670281

Patade, G. R., & Marita, A. R. (2014). Metformin: A Journey from countryside to the bedside. *Journal of Obesity and Metabolic Research*, *1*(2), 127. doi:10.4103/2347-9906.134435

Patel, D. K., Kumar, R., Laloo, D., & Hemalatha, S. (2012). Diabetes mellitus: An overview on its pharmacological aspects and reported medicinal plants having antidiabetic activity. *Asian Pacific Journal of Tropical Biomedicine*, *2*(5), 411–420. doi:10.1016/S2221-1691(12)60067-7 PMID:23569941

Patel, D. K., Prasad, S. K., Kumar, R., & Hemalatha, S. (2012). An overview on antidiabetic medicinal plants having insulin mimetic property. *Asian Pacific Journal of Tropical Biomedicine*, *2*(4), 320–330. doi:10.1016/S2221-1691(12)60032-X PMID:23569923

Patel, P. N., Yu, X. M., Jaskula-Sztul, R., & Chen, H. (2014). Hesperetin activates the Notch1 signaling cascade, causes apoptosis, and induces cellular differentiation in anaplastic thyroid cancer. *Annals of Surgical Oncology*, *21*(S4, Suppl 4), S497–S504. doi:10.124510434-013-3459-7 PMID:24419754

Patel, S. (2018). Polycystic ovary syndrome, an inflammatory, systemic, lifestyle endocrinopathy. *The Journal of Steroid Biochemistry and Molecular Biology*, *182*, 27–36. doi:10.1016/j.jsbmb.2018.04.008 PMID:29678491

Pathania, S., Ramakrishnan, S. M., & Bagler, G. (2015). Phytochemica: A platform to explore phytochemicals of medicinal plants. *Database (Oxford)*, *2015*, 2015. doi:10.1093/database/bav075 PMID:26255307

Patil, C. S. (2011). Current Trends and Future Prospective of Nutraceuticals in Health Promotion. *BIOINFO Pharmaceutical Biotechnology*, *1*(1), 1–7. https://bioinfopublication.org/viewhtml.php?artid=BIA0000894

Patil, A., Jadhav, V., & Arvindekar Aand More, T. (2014). Antidiabetic Activity of Maesa indica (Roxb.) Stem Bark in Streptozotocin Induced Diabetic Rats. *American Journal of Phytomedicine and Clinical Therapeutics*, *2*(8), 957–962.

Patil, C. S. (2011). Current trends and future prospective of nutraceuticals in health promotion. *BIOINFO Pharmaceutical Biotechnology*, *1*(1), 1–7.

Patil, S. B., Takalikar, S. S., Joglekar, M. M., Haldavnekar, V. S., & Arvindekar, A. U. (2013). Insulinotropic and β-cell protective action of cuminaldehyde, cuminol and an inhibitor isolated from Cuminum cyminum in streptozotocin-induced diabetic rats. *British Journal of Nutrition*, *110*(8), 1434–1443. doi:10.1017/S0007114513000627 PMID:23507295

Patwardhan, B., Vaidya, A., Chorghade, M., & Joshi, S. (2008). Reverse Pharmacology and Systems Approaches for Drug Discovery and Development. *Current Bioactive Compounds*. Advance online publication. doi:10.2174/157340708786847870

Patwardhan, B., Warude, D., Pushpangadan, P., & Bhatt, N. (2005). Ayurveda and traditional Chinese medicine: A comparative overview. *Evidence-Based Complementary and Alternative Medicine*, *2*(4), 465–473. doi:10.1093/ecam/neh140

Payab, M., Hasani-Ranjbar, S., Shahbal, N., Qorbani, M., Aletaha, A., Haghi-Aminjan, H., & Abdollahi, M. (2020). Effect of the herbal medicines in obesity and metabolic syndrome: A systematic review and meta-analysis of clinical trials. *Phytotherapy Research*, *34*(3), 526–545. doi:10.1002/ptr.6547

Pearson, K. J., Baur, J. A., Lewis, K. N., Peshkin, L., Price, N. L., Labinskyy, N., ... Perez, E. (2008). Resveratrol delays age-related deterioration and mimics transcriptional aspects of dietary restriction without extending life span. *Cell Metabolism*, *8*(2), 157–168. doi:10.1016/j.cmet.2008.06.011 PMID:18599363

Pearson, T. A., Mensah, G. A., Alexander, R. W., Anderson, J. L., Cannon, R. O. III, Criqui, M., ... Vinicor, F. (2003). Markers of inflammation and cardiovascular disease: application to clinical and public health practice: A statement for healthcare professionals from the Centers for Disease Control and Prevention and the American Heart Association. *Circulation*, *107*(3), 499–511. doi:10.1161/01.CIR.0000052939.59093.45 PMID:12551878

Pendyala, Walker, & Holt. (2012). A high-fat diet is associated with endotoxemia that originates from the gut. *Gastroenterology*, *142*(5), 1100-1101.

Peng, Y., & Hu, K. (2018). Effect of garlic on rats with chronic intermittent hypoxia combined with diabetes mellitus. *Molecular Medicine Reports*, *17*(4), 6174–6184. doi:10.3892/mmr.2018.8568 PMID:29436658

Perdigon, G., Alvarez, S., Rachid, M., Agüero, G., & Gobbato, N. (1995). Immune system stimulation by probiotics. *Journal of Dairy Science*, *78*(7), 1597–1606. doi:10.3168/jds.S0022-0302(95)76784-4 PMID:7593855

Pereira, A. S., den Haan, H., Peña-García, J., Moreno, M. M., Pérez-Sánchez, H., & Apostolides, Z. (2019). Exploring african medicinal plants for potential anti-diabetic compounds with the DIA-DB inverse virtual screening web server. *Molecules (Basel, Switzerland)*, *24*(10), 2002. doi:10.3390/molecules24102002 PMID:31137754

Pérez-Moreno, M. A., Locascio, A., Rodrigo, I., Dhondt, G., Portillo, F., Nieto, M. A., & Cano, A. (2001). A new role for E12/E47 in the repression ofe-cadherin expression and epithelial-mesenchymal transitions. *The Journal of Biological Chemistry*, *276*(29), 27424–27431. doi:10.1074/jbc.M100827200 PMID:11309385

Perrone, D., Fuggetta, M. P., Ardito, F., Cottarelli, A., De Filippis, A., Ravagnan, G., De Maria, S., & Lo Muzio, L. (2017). Resveratrol (3,5,4¢-trihydroxystilbene) and its properties in oral diseases. *Experimental and Therapeutic Medicine*, *14*(1), 3–9. doi:10.3892/etm.2017.4472 PMID:28672886

Petra, A. I., Panagiotidou, S., Hatziagelaki, E., Stewart, J. M., Conti, P., & Theoharides, T. C. (2015). Gut-Microbiota-Brain Axis and Its Effect on Neuropsychiatric Disorders With Suspected Immune Dysregulation. *Clinical Therapeutics*, *37*(5), 984–995. doi:10.1016/j.clinthera.2015.04.002 PMID:26046241

Petrovska, B. B. (2012). Historical review of medicinal plants' usage. *Pharmacognosy Reviews*, *6*(11), 1. doi:10.4103/0973-7847.95849

Pettitt, D. J., Forman, M. R., Hanson, R. L., Knowler, W. C., & Bennett, P. H. (1997). Breastfeeding and incidence of non-insulin-dependent diabetes mellitus in pima Indians. *Lancet*, *350*(9072), 166–168. doi:10.1016/S0140-6736(96)12103-6 PMID:9250183

Pham, T. A., & Lawley, T. D. (2014). Emerging insights on intestinal dysbiosis during bacterial infections. *Current Opinion in Microbiology*, *17*, 67–74. doi:10.1016/j.mib.2013.12.002 PMID:24581695

Philipson, L. (2017). *Monogenic Diabetes (Neonatal Diabetes Mellitus & MODY) | NIDDK*. Retrieved 22 August 2020, from https://www.niddk.nih.gov/health-information/diabetes/overview/what-is-diabetes/monogenic-neonatal-mellitus-mody

Phillipson, J. D. (2001). Phytochemistry and medicinal plants. *Phytochemistry*, *56*(3), 237–243. doi:10.1016/S0031-9422(00)00456-8 PMID:11243450

Pilch, S. M. (1987). Physiologic effects and health consequences of dietary fiber. Life Science Research Office, Federation of American Societies for Experimental Biology.

Pimentel, G. D., Micheletti, T. O., Pace, F., Rosa, J. C., Santos, R. V. T., & Lira, F. S. (2012). Gut-central nervous system axis is a target for nutritional therapies. *Nutrition Journal*, *11*(1), 22. doi:10.1186/1475-2891-11-22 PMID:22490672

Pimentel, M. (2004). A link between irritable bowel syndrome and fibromyalgia may be related to findings on lactulose breath testing. *Annals of the Rheumatic Diseases*, *63*(4), 450–452. doi:10.1136/ard.2003.011502 PMID:15020342

Pimentel, M., Soffer, E. E., Chow, E. J., Kong, Y., & Lin, H. C. (2002). Lower frequency of MMC is found in IBS subjects with abnormal lactulose breath test, suggesting bacterial overgrowth. *Digestive Diseases and Sciences*, *47*(12), 2639–2643. doi:10.1023/A:1021039032413 PMID:12498278

Pinhas-Hamiel, O., & Zeitler, P. (2005). The global spread of type 2 diabetes mellitus in children and adolescents. *The Journal of Pediatrics*, *146*(5), 693–700. doi:10.1016/j.jpeds.2004.12.042 PMID:15870677

Pirbalouti, A. G., & Mohammadi, M. (2013). Phytochemical composition of the essential oil of different populations of Stachys lavandulifolia Vahl. *Asian Pacific Journal of Tropical Biomedicine*, *3*(2), 123–128. doi:10.1016/S2221-1691(13)60036-2 PMID:23593591

Pirzada, A. M., Ali, H. H., Naeem, M., Latif, M., Bukhari, A. H., & Tanveer, A. (2015). Traditional uses, phytochemistry, and pharmacological activities. *Journal of Ethnopharmacology*, *174*, 540–560. doi:10.1016/j.jep.2015.08.012 PMID:26297840

Pisacane, A., Graziano, L., Mazzarella, G., Scarpellino, B., & Zona, G. (1992). Breastfeeding and urinary tract infection. *The Journal of Pediatrics*, *120*(1), 87–89. doi:10.1016/S0022-3476(05)80607-9 PMID:1731031

Pittman, N., Rawn, S. M., Wang, M., Masetto, A., Beattie, K. A., & Larché, M. (2018). Treatment of small intestinal bacterial overgrowth in systemic sclerosis: A systematic review. *Rheumatology (Oxford, England)*, *57*(10), 1802–1811. doi:10.1093/rheumatology/key175 PMID:29982822

Pituch-Zdanowska, A., Banaszkiewicz, A., & Albrecht, P. (2015). The role of dietary fibre in inflammatory bowel disease. *Przegląd Gastroenterologiczny*, *10*(3), 135–141. doi:10.5114/pg.2015.52753 PMID:26516378

Pivari, F., Mingione, A., Brasacchio, C., & Soldati, L. (2019). Curcumin and Type 2 Diabetes Mellitus: Prevention and Treatment. *Nutrients*, *11*(8), 1837. doi:10.3390/nu11081837 PMID:31398884

Poirier, P., Giles, T. D., Bray, G. A., Hong, Y., Stern, J. S., Pi-Sunyer, F. X., & Eckel, R. H. (2006). Obesity and cardiovascular diseases: Pathophysiology, evaluation, and effect of weight loss: an update of 1997 American Heart Association Scientific statement on obesity and heart disease from the obesity committee of the council on nutrition, physical activity, and metabolism. *Circulation*, *113*(6), 898–918. doi:10.1161/CIRCULATIONAHA.106.171016 PMID:16380542

Polson, D. W., Franks, S., Reed, M. J., Cheng, R. W., Adams, J., & James, V. H. (1987). The distribution of oestradiol in plasma in relation to uterine cross-sectional area in women with polycystic or multifollicular ovaries. *Horumon To Rinsho, 26*(5), 581–588. doi:10.1111/j.1365-2265.1987.tb00813.x PMID:3665120

Poncin, S., Gerard, A. C., Boucquey, M., Senou, M., Calderon, P. B., Knoops, B., Lengelé, B., Many, M.-C., & Colin, I. M. (2008). Oxidative stress in the thyroid gland: From harmlessness to hazard depending on the iodine content. *Endocrinology, 149*(1), 424–433. doi:10.1210/en.2007-0951 PMID:17884933

Pongchaidecha, A., Lailerd, N., Boonprasert, W., & Chattipakorn, N. (2009). Effects of curcuminoid supplement on cardiac autonomic status in high-fat-induced obese rats. *Nutrition (Burbank, Los Angeles County, Calif.), 25*(7-8), 870–878. doi:10.1016/j.nut.2009.02.001 PMID:19398300

Popkin, B. M., Adair, L., Akin, J. S., Black, R., Briscoe, J., & Flieger, W. (1990). Breastfeeding and diarrheal morbidity. *Pediatrics, 86*, 874–882. PMID:2251024

Poshan. (2020). *Exclusive breast feeding in India: trends and data gaps*. https://poshan.ifpri.info/2017/08/04/exclusive-breastfeeding-in-india-trends-and-data-gaps

Poudyala, H., Panchald, S. K., Waandersb, J., Wardc, L., & Browna, L. (2012). Lipid redistribution by α-linolenic acid-rich chia seed inhibits stearoyl-CoA desaturase-1 and induces cardiac and hepatic protection in diet-induced obese rats. *The Journal of Nutritional Biochemistry, 23*(2), 153–162. doi:10.1016/j.jnutbio.2010.11.011 PMID:21429727

Prabhakar, P. K., & Doble, M. (2011). Mechanism of action of natural products used in the treatment of diabetes mellitus. *Chinese Journal of Integrative Medicine, 17*(8), 563–574. doi:10.100711655-011-0810-3 PMID:21826590

Prakash, D., & Gupta, K. R. (2009). The Antioxidant Phytochemicals of Nutraceutical Importance. *The Open Nutraceuticals Journal*. Advance online publication. doi:10.2174/1876396000902010020

Prakash, D., Niranjan, A., & Tewari, S. K. (2001). Some nutritional properties of the seeds of three *Mucuna species. International Journal of Food Sciences and Nutrition, 52*, 79–82. doi:10.1080/09637480020027264 PMID:11225181

Prasad, S., Phromnoi, K., Yadav, V. R., Chaturvedi, M. M., & Aggarwal, B. B. (2010). Targeting inflammatory pathways by flavonoids for prevention and treatment of cancer. *Planta Medica, 76*(11), 1044–1063. doi:10.1055-0030-1250111 PMID:20635307

Prasannaraja, C., Kamalanathan, A. S., Vijayalakshmi, M. A., & Venkataraman, K. A. (2020). A dipyrrole derivative from *Aloe vera* inhibits an anti-diabetic drug target dipeptidyl peptidase (DPP)-IV *in vitro. Preparative Biochemistry & Biotechnology, 8*(5), 1–10. doi:10.1080/10826068.2019.1710712 PMID:31910723

Pratap, S. A., & Rajender, S. (2012). Potent natural aphrodisiacs for the management of erectile dysfunction and male sexual debilities. *Frontiers in Bioscience (Scholar Edition), 4*(1), 167–180. doi:10.2741259 PMID:22202051

Prevarskaya, N., Skryma, R., & Shuba, Y. (2011). Calcium in tumour metastasis: New roles for known actors. *Nature Reviews. Cancer, 11*(8), 609–618. doi:10.1038/nrc3105 PMID:21779011

Prietl, B., Treiber, G., Pieber, T. R., & Amrein, K. (2013). Vitamin D and immune function. Nutrients. https://doi.org/ doi:10.3390/nu5072502

Prince, P., & Kamalakkannan, N. (2006). Rutin improves glucose homeostasis in streptozotocin diabetic tissues by altering glycolytic and gluconeogenic enzymes. *Journal of Biochemical and Molecular Toxicology, 20*(2), 96–102. doi:10.1002/jbt.20117 PMID:16615078

Pugsley, M. K., Authier, S., & Curtis, M. J. (2008). Principles of safety pharmacology. *British Journal of Pharmacology, 154*(7), 1382–1399. doi:10.1038/bjp.2008.280

Puisieux, A., Brabletz, T., & Caramel, J. (2014). Oncogenic roles of EMT-inducing transcription factors. *Nature Cell Biology*, *16*(6), 488–494. doi:10.1038/ncb2976 PMID:24875735

Punthakee, Z., Goldenberg, R., & Katz, P. (2018). Definition, Classification and Diagnosis of Diabetes, Prediabetes and Metabolic Syndrome. *Canadian Journal of Diabetes*, *42*, S10–S15. doi:10.1016/j.jcjd.2017.10.003 PMID:29650080

Puranik, N., Kammar, K. F., & Devi, S. (2010). Anti-diabetic activity of *Tinospora cordifolia* (Willd.) in streptozotocin diabetic rats; does it act like sulfonylureas? *Turkish Journal of Medical Sciences*, *40*(2), 265–270.

Purchiaroni, F. (2013). The role of intestinal microbiota and the immune system. *European Review for Medical and Pharmacological Sciences*, *17*(3), 323–333. PMID:23426535

Pyzik, A., Grywalska, E., Matyjaszek-Matuszek, B., & Rolinski, J. (2015). Immune disorders in Hashimoto's thyroiditis: What do we know so far? *Journal of Immunology Research*, *979167*, 1–8. Advance online publication. doi:10.1155/2015/979167 PMID:26000316

Qin, B., Panickar, K. S., & Anderson, R. A. (2010). Cinnamon: Potential role in the prevention of insulin resistance, metabolic syndrome, and type 2 diabetes. *Journal of Diabetes Science and Technology*, *4*(3), 685–693. doi:10.1177/193229681000400324 PMID:20513336

Qin, J., Li, R., Raes, J., Arumugam, M., Burgdorf, K. S., Manichanh, C., ... Wang, J. (2010). A human gut microbial gene catalogue established by metagenomic sequencing. *Nature*, *464*(7285), 59–65. doi:10.1038/nature08821 PMID:20203603

Qiu, J. (2007). Traditional medicine: A culture in the balance. *Nature*, *448*(7150), 126–128. doi:10.1038/448126a PMID:17625539

Quercia, S., Candela, M., Giuliani, C., Turroni, S., Luiselli, D., Rampelli, S., ... Pirazzini, C. (2014). From lifetime to evolution: Timescales of human gut microbiota adaptation. *Frontiers in Microbiology*, *5*, 587. doi:10.3389/fmicb.2014.00587 PMID:25408692

Radha, M., & Laxmipriya, N. (2016). Efficacy of non-polar extract (NPE) of aloe barbadensis mill. In polycystic ovarian syndrome (PCOS) rodent model-an 'in vivo' study. *International Journal of Pharmaceutical Sciences and Research*, *7*, 4933.

Rafehi, H., Ververis, K., & Karagiannis, T. C. (2012). Controversies surrounding the clinical potential of cinnamon for the management of diabetes. *Diabetes, Obesity & Metabolism*, *14*(6), 493–499. doi:10.1111/j.1463-1326.2011.01538.x PMID:22093965

Rafieian-kopaei, M. (2012). Medicinal plants and the human needs. Journal of HerbMed Pharmacology. https://doi.org/doi:10.1016/S2222-1808(14)60708-8

Rafieian-Kopaei, M., Nasri, H., Sahinfard, N., Rafieian, M., Rafieian, S., & Shirzad, M. (2014). Turmeric: A spice with multifunctional medicinal properties. *Journal of HerbMed Pharmacology*.

Ragavan, B., & Krishnakumari, S. (2006). Antidiabetic effect of *T. arjuna* bark extract in alloxan induced diabetic rats. *Indian Journal of Clinical Biochemistry*, *21*(2), 123–128. doi:10.1007/BF02912926 PMID:23105628

Rahmani, A.H., Al shabrmi, F.M., Aly, S.M. (2014). Active ingredients of ginger as potential candidates in the prevention and treatment of diseases via modulation of biological activities. *International Journal of Physiology, Pathophysiology and Pharmacology*, *6*, 125–136. PMID:25057339

Rajaa, K. (2013). The Effect Of Aqueous Extract Of Anastatica Hierochuntica On Some Hormones In Mouse Females. *Ibn Al-Haitham Jour. for Pure & Appl. Sci.*

Ramaa, C. S., Shirode, A. R., Mundada, A. S., & Kadam, V. J. (2006). Nutraceuticals- An emerging era in the treatment and prevention of cardiovascular diseases. *Current Pharmaceutical Biotechnology*, *7*(1), 15–23. doi:10.2174/138920106775789647 PMID:16472130

Ramadan, M. F. (2007). Nutritional value, functional properties and nutraceutical applications of black cumin (*Nigella sativa* L.): An overview. *International Journal of Food Science & Technology*, *42*(10), 1208–1218. doi:10.1111/j.1365-2621.2006.01417.x

Ramaswamy, S., & Weinbauer, G. F. (2014). Endocrine control of spermatogenesis: Role of FSH and LH/ testosterone. *Spermatogenesis*, *4*(2), e996025. Advance online publication. doi:10.1080/21565562.2014.996025 PMID:26413400

Rani Javalkar, S. (2019). The economic burden of health expenditure on diabetes mellitus among urban poor: A cross sectional study. *International Journal of Community Medicine And Public Health*, *6*(3), 1162. doi:10.18203/2394-6040.ijcmph20190604

Ranilla, L. G., Kwon, Y. I., Apostolidis, E., & Shetty, K. (2010). Phenolic compounds, antioxidant activity and in vitro inhibitory potential against key enzymes relevant for hyperglycemia and hypertension of commonly used medicinal plants, herbs and spices in Latin America. *Bioresource Technology*, *101*(12), 4676–4689. doi:10.1016/j.biortech.2010.01.093 PMID:20185303

Rani, N., Sharma, S. K., & Vasudeva, N. (2012). Assessment of antiobesity potential of *Achyranthes aspera* Linn. seed. *Evidence-Based Complementary and Alternative Medicine*, *2012*(715912), 1–7. doi:10.1155/2012/715912 PMID:22919417

Ranjana, & Tripathi, Y.B. (2014). Insulin secreting and alpha-glucosidase inhibitory activity of hexane extract of *Annona squamosa* Linn. in streptozotocin (STZ) induced diabetic rats. *Indian Journal of Experimental Biology, 52*, 623-629.

Ranjbar, H. S., Jouyandeh, Z., & Abdollahi, M. (2013). *A Systematic Review Of Anti-Obesity Medicinal Plants - An Update*. J Diabetes Met Dis.

Rao, S. S. C., & Bhagatwala, J. (2019). Small Intestinal Bacterial Overgrowth: Clinical Features and Therapeutic Management. *Clinical and Translational Gastroenterology*, *10*(10), e00078. doi:10.14309/ctg.0000000000000078 PMID:31584459

Rashidi, A. A., Mirhashemi, S. M., Taghizadeh, M., & Sarkhail, P. (2013). Iranian medicinal plants for diabetes mellitus: A systematic review. *Pakistan journal of biological sciences. PJBS*, *16*(9), 401. PMID:24498803

Rasool Hassan, B. (2012). Medicinal plants (importance and uses). *Pharmaceutica Analytica Acta*, *3*(10), e139. doi:10.4172/2153-2435.1000e139

Rathera, M. A., Dara, B. A., Sofia, S. N., Bhata, B. A., & Qurishi, M. A. (2016). Foeniculum vulgare: A comprehensive review of its traditional use, phytochemistry, pharmacology, and safety. *Arabian Journal of Chemistry*, *9*(2), S1574–S1583. doi:10.1016/j.arabjc.2012.04.011

Rau, O., Wurglics, M., Dingermann, T., Abdel-Tawab, M., & Schubert-Zsilavecz, M. (2006). Screening of herbal extracts for activation of the human peroxisome proliferator-activated receptor. *Die Pharmazie-An International Journal of Pharmaceutical Sciences.*, *61*(11), 952–956. PMID:17152989

Raut, A., Bichile, L., Chopra, A., Patwardhan, B., & Vaidya, A. (2013). Comparative study of amrutbhallataka and glucosamine sulphate in osteoarthritis: Six months open label randomized controlled clinical trial. *Journal of Ayurveda and Integrative Medicine*, *4*(4), 229–236. doi:10.4103/0975-9476.123708 PMID:24459390

Rautava, S., Luoto, R., Salminen, S., & Isolauri, E. (2012). Microbial contact during pregnancy, intestinal colonization and human disease. *Nature Reviews. Gastroenterology & Hepatology*, *9*(10), 565–576. doi:10.1038/nrgastro.2012.144 PMID:22890113

Ravi, R., & Krishnamurthy, V. (2019). Beneficial Effects of Medicinal Plants Used For the Management of Obesity-A Review. *International Journal of Health Sciences and Research*, *9*(12), 174–194.

Rebar, R., Judd, H. L., Yen, S. S., Rakoff, J., Vandenberg, G., & Naftolin, F. (1976). Characterization of the inappropriate gonadotropin secretion in polycystic ovary syndrome. *The Journal of Clinical Investigation*, *7*(5), 1320–1329. doi:10.1172/JCI108400 PMID:770505

Reeds, D. N., Patterson, B. W., Okunade, A., Holloszy, J. O., Polonsky, K. S., & Klein, S. (2011). Ginseng and ginsenoside Re do not improve beta-cell function or insulin sensitivity in overweight and obese subjects with impaired glucose tolerance or diabetes. *Diabetes Care*, *34*(5), 1071–1076. doi:10.2337/dc10-2299 PMID:21411505

Reitsma, M., Westerhout, J., Wichers, H. J., Wortelboer, H. M., & Verhoeckx, K. C. M. (2014). Protein transport across the small intestine in food allergy. *Molecular Nutrition & Food Research*, *58*(1), 194–205. doi:10.1002/mnfr.201300204 PMID:24395537

Remacle, J. E., Kraft, H., Lerchner, W., Wuytens, G., Collart, C., Verschueren, K., & Huylebroeck, D. (1999). New mode of DNA binding of multi-zinc finger transcription factors: δEF1 family members bind with two hands to two target sites. *The EMBO Journal*, *18*(18), 5073–5084. doi:10.1093/emboj/18.18.5073 PMID:10487759

Ren, M. Q., Kuhn, G., Wegner, J., & Chen, J. (2001). Isoflavones, substances with multibiological and clinical properties. *European Journal of Nutrition*, *40*(4), 135–146. doi:10.1007/PL00007388 PMID:11905954

Reyes-Escogido, M. L., Gonzalez-Mondragon, E. G., & Vazquez-Tzompantzi, E. (2011). Chemical and pharmacological aspects of capsaicin. *Molecules (Basel, Switzerland)*, *16*(2), 1253–1270. doi:10.3390/molecules16021253 PMID:21278678

Rezaei Farimani, A., Saidijam, M., Goodarzi, M. T., Yadegar Azari, R., Asadi, S., Zarei, S., & Shabab, N. (2015). Effect of resveratrol supplementation on the SNARE Proteins expression in adipose tissue of streptozotocin-nicotinamide induced type 2 diabetic rats. *Iranian Journal of Medical Sciences*, *40*(3), 248–255. PMID:25999625

RH, R. U. (2015). Traditional herbal medicine, pharmacognosy, and pharmacopoeial standards: a discussion at the crossroads. In Evidence-Based Validation of Herbal Medicine (pp. 45-85). Academic Press.

Ricardo Azziz, M. P. H., & Daniel, A. (2011). Polycystic ovary syndrome: An ancient disorder? *Fertility and Sterility*, *95*(5), 1544–1548. doi:10.1016/j.fertnstert.2010.09.032 PMID:20979996

Richard, S. L., Silva, A. A., David, A. E., & Kathleen, M. H. (2013). Diagnosis and Treatment of Polycystic Ovary Syndrome: An Endocrine Society Clinical Practice Guideline. *The Journal of Clinical Endocrinology and Metabolism*, *98*(12), 4565–4592. doi:10.1210/jc.2013-2350 PMID:24151290

Richarte, V., Rosales, K., Corrales, M., Bellina, M., Fadeuilhe, C., Calvo, E., ... Ramos Quiroga, J. A. (2018). El eje intestino-cerebro en el trastorno por déficit de atención/hiperactividad: Papel de la microbiota. *Revista de Neurología*, *66*(S01), S109–S114. doi:10.33588/rn.66S01.2017525 PMID:29516462

Richette, P., & Bardin, T. (2010). Gout. *Lancet*, *375*(9711), 318–328. doi:10.1016/S0140-6736(09)60883-7 PMID:19692116

Rideout, T. C., Harding, S. V., & Jones, P. J. H. (2010). Consumption of plant sterols reduces plasma and hepatic triglycerides and modulates the expression of lipid regulatory genes and de novo lipogenesis in C57BL/6J mice. *Molecular Nutrition & Food Research*, *54*(S1), S7–S13. doi:10.1002/mnfr.201000027 PMID:20333723

Ridker, P. M. (2016). A Test in Context: High-Sensitivity C-Reactive Protein. *Journal of the American College of Cardiology*, *67*(6), 712–723. doi:10.1016/j.jacc.2015.11.037 PMID:26868696

Ried, K. (2015). Chinese herbal medicine for female infertility: An updated meta-analysis. *Complementary Therapies in Medicine*, *23*(1), 116–128. doi:10.1016/j.ctim.2014.12.004 PMID:25637159

Ring, J., Lwin, A., & Köhler, T. (2016). Current medical management of endocrine-related male infertility. *Asian Journal of Andrology, 18*(3), 357. doi:10.4103/1008-682X.179252 PMID:27098657

Rinninella, E., Cintoni, Raoul, Lopetuso, Scaldaferri, Pulcini, ... Mele. (2019). Food Components and Dietary Habits: Keys for a Healthy Gut Microbiota Composition. *Nutrients, 11*(10), 2393. doi:10.3390/nu11102393 PMID:31591348

Rios-Covian, D., Ruas-Madiedo, P., Margolles, A., Gueimonde, M., de los Reyes-Gavilán, C. G., & Salazar, N. (2016). Intestinal Short Chain Fatty Acids and their Link with Diet and Human Health. *Frontiers in Microbiology, 7*, 185. doi:10.3389/fmicb.2016.00185 PMID:26925050

Rios, J. L., & Recio, M. C. (2005). Medicinal plants and antimicrobial activity. *Journal of Ethnopharmacology, 100*(1-2), 80–84. doi:10.1016/j.jep.2005.04.025 PMID:15964727

Rissanen, T. H., Voutilainen, S., Virtanen, J. K., Venho, B., Vanharanta, M., Mursu, J., & Salonen, J. T. (2003). Low intake of fruits, berries and vegetables in associated with excess mortality in men: The Kuopio ischaemic heart disease risk factor (KIHD) study. *The Journal of Nutrition, 133*(1), 199–204. doi:10.1093/jn/133.1.199 PMID:12514290

Rivera, Loya, & Ceballo. (2013). Use of Herbal Medicines and Implications for Conventional Drug Therapy Medical Sciences. *Altern Integ, 2*(6).

Rivkees, S. A., & Mattison, D. R. (2009). Ending propylthiouracil-induced liver failure in children. *The New England Journal of Medicine, 360*(15), 1574–1575. doi:10.1056/NEJMc0809750 PMID:19357418

Rizzo, M., Berneis, K., Hersberger, M., Pepe, I., DiFede, G., Rini, G. B., Spinas, G. A., & Carmina, E. (2009). Milder forms of atherogenic dyslipidemia inovulatory versus anovulatory Polycystic ovary syndrome phenotype. *Human Reproduction (Oxford, England), 24*(9), 2286–2292. doi:10.1093/humrep/dep121 PMID:19454589

Robert, L. R., & David, A. E. (2016). The Pathogenesis of Polycystic Ovary Syndrome (PCOS): The Hypothesis of PCOS as Functional Ovarian Hyperandrogenism Revisited. *Endocrine Reviews, 37*(5), 467–520. doi:10.1210/er.2015-1104 PMID:27459230

Rocha-González, H. I., Ambriz-Tututi, M., & Granados-Soto, V. (2008). Resveratrol: A natural compound with pharmacological potential in neurodegenerative diseases. *CNS Neuroscience & Therapeutics, 14*(3), 234–247. doi:10.1111/j.1755-5949.2008.00045.x PMID:18684235

Rocha, K. K. R., Souza, G. A., Ebaid, G. X., Seiva, F. R. F., Cataneo, A. C., & Novelli, E. L. B. (2009). Resveratrol toxicity: Effects on risk factors for atherosclerosis and hepatic oxidative stress in standard and high-fat diets. *Food and Chemical Toxicology, 47*(6), 1362–1367. doi:10.1016/j.fct.2009.03.010 PMID:19298841

Roche, A., Florkowski, C., & Walmsley, T. (2005). Lead poisoning due to ingestion of Indian herbal remedies. *The New Zealand Medical Journal, 118*(1219), U1589. PMID:16059407

Rodriguez-Casado, A. (2016). The Health Potential of Fruits and Vegetables Phytochemicals: Notable Examples. *Critical Reviews in Food Science and Nutrition, 56*(7), 1097–1107. doi:10.1080/10408398.2012.755149 PMID:25225771

Rogal, J., Zbinden, A., Schenke-Layland, K., & Loskill, P. (2019). Stem-cell based organ-on-a-chip models for diabetes research. *Advanced Drug Delivery Reviews, 140*, 101–128. doi:10.1016/j.addr.2018.10.010 PMID:30359630

Roldan, B., San Millan, J. L., & Escobar-Morreale, H. F. (2004). Genetic basis of metabolic abnormalities in polycystic ovary syndrome: Implications for therapy. *American Journal of Pharmacogenomics, 4*(2), 93–107. doi:10.2165/00129785-200404020-00004 PMID:15059032

Roman-Ramos, R., Flores-Saenz, J. L., & Alarcon-Aguilar, F. J. (1995). Anti-hyperglycemic effect of some edible plants. *Journal of Ethnopharmacology, 48*(1), 25–32. doi:10.1016/0378-8741(95)01279-M PMID:8569244

Romm, A. (2010). *Botanical Medicine for Women's Health*. Churchill Livingstone.

Roncal, C., Martínez-Aguilar, E., Orbe, J., Ravassa, S., Fernandez-Montero, A., Saenz-Pipaon, G., ... Paramo, J. A. (2019). Trimethylamine-N-Oxide (TMAO) Predicts Cardiovascular Mortality in Peripheral Artery Disease. *Scientific Reports*, *9*(1), 15580. doi:10.103841598-019-52082-z PMID:31666590

Rosenblatt, K. A., & Thomas, D. B. (1993). Lactation and the risk of epithelial ovarian cancer. WHO Collaborative Study of Neoplasia and Steroid contraceptives. *International Journal of Epidemiology*, *22*(2), 192–197. doi:10.1093/ije/22.2.192 PMID:8505173

Rosencrantz, M. A., Coffler, M. S., Haggan, A., Duke, K. B., Donohue, M. C., Shayya, R. F., Su, H. I., & Chang, R. J. (2011). Clinical evidence for predominance of delta-5 steroid production in women with polycystic ovary syndrome. *The Journal of Clinical Endocrinology and Metabolism*, *96*(4), 1106–1113. doi:10.1210/jc.2010-2200 PMID:21270326

Roth, L. W., Ryan, A. R., & Meacham, R. B. (2013). Clomiphene citrate in the management of male infertility. *Seminars in Reproductive Medicine*, *31*(04), 245–250. doi:10.1055-0033-1345271 PMID:23775379

Round, J. L., & Mazmanian, S. K. (2009). The gut microbiota shapes intestinal immune responses during health and disease. *Nature Reviews. Immunology*, *9*(5), 313–323. doi:10.1038/nri2515 PMID:19343057

Ruengsomwong, S., La-ongkham, O., Jiang, J., Wannissorn, B., Nakayama, J., & Nitisinprasert, S. (2016). Microbial Community of Healthy Thai Vegetarians and Non-Vegetarians, Their Core Gut Microbiota, and Pathogen Risk. *Journal of Microbiology and Biotechnology*, *26*(10), 1723–1735. doi:10.4014/jmb.1603.03057 PMID:27381339

Rush, J. W. E., Quadrilatero, J., Levy, A. S., & Ford, R. J. (2007). Chronic resveratrol enhances endothelium-dependent relaxation but does not alter eNOS levels in aorta of spontaneously hypertensive rats. *Experimental Biology and Medicine, 232*(6), 814-822.

Rusinek, D., Chmielik, E., Krajewska, J., Jarzab, M., Oczko-Wojciechowska, M., Czarniecka, A., & Jarzab, B. (2017). Current Advances in Thyroid Cancer Management. Are We Ready for the Epidemic Rise of Diagnoses? *International Journal of Molecular Sciences*, *18*(8), 1817. Advance online publication. doi:10.3390/ijms18081817 PMID:28829399

Saad, B., Azaizeh, H., & Said, O. (2008). Arab herbal medicines. In Botanical Medicine in Clinical Practice (pp.31–39). CABI. doi:10.1079/9781845934132.0031

Sabita, N. S., & Trygve, O. T. (2012). The role of nutraceuticals in chemoprevention and chemotheraphy and their clinical outcomes. *Journal of Oncology*, *64*, 1–23.

Sabra, M. M., & Di Cristofano, A. (2019). *89th Annual Meeting of the American Thyroid Association*. Mary Ann Liebert, Inc.

Sacco, S. M., Horcajada, M. N., & Offord, E. (2013). Pytonutrients for bone health during ageing. *British Journal of Clinical Pharmacology*, *75*(3), 697–707. doi:10.1111/bcp.12033 PMID:23384080

Sahu, S. C. (2002). Dual role of organosulfur compounds in foods: A review. *Journal of Environmental Science and Health. Part C, Environmental Carcinogenesis & Ecotoxicology Reviews*. Advance online publication. doi:10.1081/GNC-120005388 PMID:12734054

Saibil, F. (1989). Diarrhea due to fiber overload. *The New England Journal of Medicine*, *320*(9), 599. doi:10.1056/NEJM198903023200920 PMID:2536897

Said, O., Khalil, K., Fulder, S., & Azaizeh, H. (2002). Ethnopharmacological survey of medicinal herbs in Israel, the Golan Heights and the West Bank region. *Journal of Ethnopharmacology*, *83*(3), 251–265. doi:10.1016/S0378-8741(02)00253-2 PMID:12426094

Saini, R. K., Chouhan, R., Bagri, L. P., & Bajpai, A. K. (2012). Strategies of targeting tumors and cancers. *Journal of Cancer Research Updates*, *1*(1), 129–152.

Saiyed, Jahan, Makbul, Ansari, Bano, & Habib. (2016). Effect of combination of Withania somnifera Dunal and Tribulus terrestris Linn on letrozole induced polycystic ovarian syndrome in rats. *Integr Med Res, 5*, 293–300.

Sakamoto, Y., Mikuriya, H., Tayama, K., Takahashi, H., Nagasawa, A., Yano, N., ... Aoki, N. (2001). Goitrogenic effects of green tea extract catechins by dietary administration in rats. *Archives of Toxicology*, *75*(10), 591–596. doi:10.100700204-001-0286-6 PMID:11808919

Sakr, S. A., Zowail, M. E., & Marzouk, A. M. (2014). Effect of saffron (Crocus sativusL.) on sodium valporate induced cytogenetic and testicular alterations in albino rats. *Anatomy & Cell Biology*, *47*(3), 171. doi:10.5115/acb.2014.47.3.171 PMID:25276476

Saksena, S., & Dixit, V. K. (1987). Role of total alkaloids of *Mucuna pruriens* Baker in spermatogenesis in Albino rats. *Indian Journal of Natural Products*, *3*, 3–7.

Sakurai, A., Takeda, K., Ain, K., Ceccarelli, P., Nakai, A., Seino, S., Bell, G. I., Refetoff, S., & DeGroot, L. J. (1989). Generalized resistance to thyroid hormone associated with a mutation in the ligand-binding domain of the human thyroid hormone receptor beta. *Proceedings of the National Academy of Sciences of the United States of America*, *86*(22), 8977–8981. doi:10.1073/pnas.86.22.8977 PMID:2510172

Salehi, B., Ata, A., Anil, V., Kumar, N., Sharopov, F., Ramírez-Alarcón, K., Ruiz-Ortega, A., & ... . (2019). Antidiabetic Potential of Medicinal Plants and Their Active Components. *Biomolecules*, *9*(10), 551. doi:10.3390/biom9100551 PMID:31575072

Salehi, B., Varoni, E. M., Sharifi-Rad, M., Rajabi, S., Zucca, P., Iriti, M., & Sharifi-Rad, J. (2019). Epithelial-mesenchymal transition as a target for botanicals in cancer metastasis. *Phytomedicine*, *55*, 125–136. doi:10.1016/j.phymed.2018.07.001 PMID:30668422

Salman, R., AlSayyad, A., & Ludwig, C. (2019). Type 2 diabetes and healthcare resource utilisation in the Kingdom of Bahrain. *BMC Health Services Research*, *19*(1), 939. Advance online publication. doi:10.118612913-019-4795-5 PMID:31805932

Saminathan, M., Rai, R. B., Dhama, K., Tiwari, R., & Chakraborty, S. (2013). Systematic review on anticancer potential and other health beneficial pharmacological activities of novel medicinal plant *Morinda citrifolia* (Noni). *International Journal of Pharmacology*, *9*(8), 462–492. doi:10.3923/ijp.2013.462.492

Sandborn, W. J., & Faubion, W. A. (2000). Clinical pharmacology of inflammatory bowel disease therapies. *Current Gastroenterology Reports*, *2*(6), 440–445. doi:10.100711894-000-0005-0 PMID:11079044

Sanders, M. E. (1994). Lactic Acid Bacteria as Promoters of Human Health. Functional Foods. https://doi.org/doi:10.1007/978-1-4615-2073-3_14

Sanni, O., Erukainure, O. L., Chukwuma, C. I., Koorbanally, N. A., Ibeji, C. U., & Islam, M. S. (2019). *Azadirachta indica* inhibits key enzyme linked to type 2 diabetes *in vitro*, abates oxidative hepatic injury and enhances muscle glucose uptake *ex vivo. Biomedicine and Pharmacotherapy*, *109*, 734–743. doi:10.1016/j.biopha.2018.10.171 PMID:30551526

Santosh, K. (2008). Mehla RK, Dang AK. (2008). Use of shatavari (Asparagus Racemosus) as a galactopoietic and therapeutic herb-A review. *Agricultural Reviews (Karnal)*, *29*(2), 132–138.

Sarkar, S., Das, D., Dutta, P., Kalita, J., Wann, S., & Manna, P. (2020). Chitosan: A promising therapeutic agent and effective drug delivery system in managing diabetes mellitus. *Carbohydrate Polymers*, *247*, 116594. doi:10.1016/j.carbpol.2020.116594 PMID:32829787

Sartippour, M. R., Shao, Z. M., Heber, D., Beatty, P., Zhang, L., Liu, C., Ellis, L., Liu, W., Go, V. L., & Brooks, M. N. (2002). Green tea inhibits vascular endothelial growth factor (VEGF) induction in human breast cancer cells. *The Journal of Nutrition*, *132*(8), 2307–2311. doi:10.1093/jn/132.8.2307 PMID:12163680

Satapathy, S., Das, N., Bandyopadhyay, D., Mahapatra, S. C., Sundar Sahu, D., & Meda, M. (2017). Effect of Tulsi (Ocimum sanctum Linn.) Supplementation on Metabolic Parameters and Liver Enzymes in Young Overweight and Obese Subjects. *Indian Journal of Clinical Biochemistry*, *32*(3), 357–363. doi:10.100712291-016-0615-4 PMID:28811698

Sattanathan, K. C., Dhanapal, R., & Umarani, R. (2011). ManavalanBeneficial health effects of rutin supplementation in patients with diabetes mellitus. *Journal of Applied Pharmaceutical Science*, *1*(8), 227–231.

Savagner, P. (2015). Epithelial–mesenchymal transitions: from cell plasticity to concept elasticity. Current Topics in Developmental Biology, (112), 273-300.

Saxena, A., & Vikram, N. K. (2004). Role of selected Indian plants in management of type 2 diabetes: A review. *Journal of Alternative and Complementary Medicine (New York, N.Y.)*, *10*(2), 369–378. doi:10.1089/107555304323062365 PMID:15165418

Scarlatti, F., Maffei, R., Beau, I., Codogno, P., & Ghidoni, R. (2008). Role of non-canonical Beclin 1-independent autophagy in cell death induced by resveratrol in human breast cancer cells. *Cell Death and Differentiation*, *15*(8), 1318–1329. doi:10.1038/cdd.2008.51 PMID:18421301

Scheidt, P., Dellarco, M., & Dearry, A. A. (2009). Major milestone for the National Children's Study. *Environmental Health Perspectives*, *117*(1), A13. doi:10.1289/ehp.12416 PMID:19165365

Scher, J. U., & Abramson, S. B. (2011). The microbiome and rheumatoid arthritis. *Nature Reviews. Rheumatology*, *7*(10), 569–578. doi:10.1038/nrrheum.2011.121 PMID:21862983

Schippmann, U. W. E., Leaman, D., & Cunningham, A. B. (2006). A comparison of cultivation and wild collection of medicinal and aromatic plants under sustainability aspects. *Frontis*, (17), 75-95.

Schmatz, R., Mazzanti, C. M., Spanevello, R., Stefanello, N., Gutierres, J., Maldonado, A., Correa, M., da Rosa, C. S., Becker, L., Bagatini, M., Gonçalves, J. F., Jaques, J. D. S., Schetinger, M. R., & Morsch, V. M. (2010). Ectonucleotidase and acetylcholinesterase activities in synaptosomes from the cerebral cortex of streptozotocin-induced diabetic rats and treated with resveratrol. *Brain Research Bulletin*, *80*(6), 371–376. doi:10.1016/j.brainresbull.2009.08.019 PMID:19723569

Schmatz, R., Schetinger, M. R., Spanevello, R. M., Mazzanti, C. M., Stefanello, N., Maldonado, P. A., Gutierres, J., Corrêa, M. C., Girotto, E., Moretto, M. B., & Morsch, V. M. (2009). Effects of resveratrol on nucleotide degrading enzymes in streptozotocin-induced diabetic rats. *Life Sciences*, *84*(11-12), 345–350. doi:10.1016/j.lfs.2008.12.019 PMID:19166862

Schmid, P., Adams, S., Rugo, H. S., Schneeweiss, A., Barrios, C. H., Iwata, H., & Henschel, V. (2018). Atezolizumab and nab-paclitaxel in advanced triple-negative breast cancer. *The New England Journal of Medicine*, *379*(22), 2108–2121. doi:10.1056/NEJMoa1809615 PMID:30345906

Schmidt, J. (2011). *Polycystic ovary syndrome Ovarian pathophysiology and consequences after the menopause* (Thesis). Geson Hylte Tryck.

Schnorr, S. L., Candela, M., Rampelli, S., Centanni, M., Consolandi, C., Basaglia, G., ... Crittenden, A. N. (2014). Gut microbiome of the Hadza hunter-gatherers. *Nature Communications*, *5*(1), 3654. doi:10.1038/ncomms4654 PMID:24736369

Schomburg, L., Dumitrescu, A. M., Liao, X. H., Bin-Abbas, B., Hoeflich, J., Kohrle, J., & Refetoff, S. (2009). Selenium supplementation fails to correct the selenoprotein synthesis defect in subjects with SBP2 gene mutations. *Thyroid, 19*(3), 277–281. doi:10.1089/thy.2008.0397 PMID:19265499

Schonfeld, G. (2010). Plant sterols in atherosclerosis prevention. *The American Journal of Clinical Nutrition, 92*(1), 3–4. doi:10.3945/ajcn.2010.29828 PMID:20519556

Schroder-van der Elst, J. P., van der Heide, D., Romijn, J. A., & Smit, J. W. (2004). Differential effects of natural flavonoids on growth and iodide content in a human Na*/I- symporter-transfected follicular thyroid carcinoma cell line. *European Journal of Endocrinology, 150*(4), 557–564. doi:10.1530/eje.0.1500557 PMID:15080787

Schulz, V., Hänsel, R., & Tyler, V. E. (2001). *Rational phytotherapy: a physician's guide to herbal medicine*. Psychology Press. doi:10.1007/978-3-642-98093-0

Schuster, R., Holzer, W., Doerfler, H., Weckwerth, W., Viernstein, H., Okonogi, S., & Mueller, M. (2016). *Cajanus cajan* - A source of PPARγ activators leading to anti-inflammatory and cytotoxic effects. *Food & Function, 7*(9), 3798–3806. doi:10.1039/C6FO00689B PMID:27603115

Schwingshackl, L., & Hoffmann, G. (2014). Mediterranean dietary pattern, inflammation and endothelial function: A systematic review and meta-analysis of intervention trials. *Nutrition, Metabolism, and Cardiovascular Diseases, 24*(9), 929–939. doi:10.1016/j.numecd.2014.03.003 PMID:24787907

Seib, C. D., & Sosa, J. A. (2019). Evolving Understanding of the Epidemiology of Thyroid Cancer. *Endocrinology and Metabolism Clinics of North America, 48*(1), 23–35. doi:10.1016/j.ecl.2018.10.002 PMID:30717905

Seidlova-Wuttke, D., Hesse, O., Jarry, H., Christoffel, V., Spengler, B., Becker, T., & Wuttke, W. (2003). Evidence for selective estrogen receptor modulator activity in a Black Cohosh (Cimicifuga racemosa) extract: Comparison with estradiol-17beta. *European Journal of Endocrinology, 149*(4), 351–362. doi:10.1530/eje.0.1490351 PMID:14514351

Sellandi, T. M., Thakar, A. B., & Baghel, M. S. (2012). Clinical study of *Trib- ulus terrestris* Linn. in Oligozoospermia: A double blind study. *Ayu, 33*(3), 356–364. doi:10.4103/0974-8520.108822 PMID:23723641

Selvaraj, B., & Periyasamy, S. (2016). *Indian medicinal plants for diabetes: text data mining the literature of different electronic databases for future therapeutics*. Academic Press.

Selvaraj, S., Sun, Y., Sukumaran, P., & Singh, B. B. (2016). Resveratrol activates autophagic cell death in prostate cancer cells via downregulation of STIM1 and the mTOR pathway. *Molecular Carcinogenesis, 55*(5), 818–831. doi:10.1002/mc.22324 PMID:25917875

Seminario-Amez, M. (2017). Probiotics and oral health: A systematic review. *Medicina Oral, Patologia Oral y Cirugia Bucal, 22*(3), e282–e288. PMID:28390121

Semwal, B. C., Gupta, J., Singh, S., Kumar, Y., & Giri, M. (2009). Antihyperglycemic activity of root of *Berberis aristata* DC in alloxan-induced diabetic rats. *International Journal of Green Pharmacy, 3*(3), 259–262. doi:10.4103/0973-8258.56288

Semwal, B., Shah, K., Chauhan, N., Badhe, R., & Divakar, K. (2008). Anti-diabetic activity of stem bark of *Berberis aristata* D.C. in alloxan induced diabetic rats. *International Journal of Pharmacology, 6*(1), 1–8.

Sen, S., Chakraborty, R., & De, B. (2011). Challenges and opportunities in the advancement of herbal medicine: India's position and role in a global context. *Journal of Herbal Medicine, 1*(3-4), 67–75. doi:10.1016/j.hermed.2011.11.001

Sen, S., Querques, M. A., & Chakrabarti, S. (2013). North American Ginseng (Panax quinquefolius) prevents hyperglycemia and associated pancreatic abnormalities in diabetes. *Journal of Medicinal Food, 16*(7), 587–592. doi:10.1089/jmf.2012.0192 PMID:23875898

Serretti, A., & Mandelli, L. (2010). Antidepressants and body weight: A comprehensive review and meta-analysis. *The Journal of Clinical Psychiatry*, *71*(10), 1259–1272. doi:10.4088/JCP.09r05346blu PMID:21062615

Shah, A., Morrison, M., Burger, D., Martin, N., Rich, J., Jones, M., ... Holtmann, G. J. (2019). Systematic review with meta-analysis: The prevalence of small intestinal bacterial overgrowth in inflammatory bowel disease. *Alimentary Pharmacology & Therapeutics*, *49*(6), 624–635. doi:10.1111/apt.15133 PMID:30735254

Shah, A., Shanahan, E., Macdonald, G., Fletcher, L., Ghasemi, P., Morrison, M., ... Holtmann, G. (2017). Systematic Review and Meta-Analysis: Prevalence of Small Intestinal Bacterial Overgrowth in Chronic Liver Disease. *Seminars in Liver Disease*, *37*(4), 388–400. doi:10.1055-0037-1608832 PMID:29272899

Shahnazi, M., Khalili, A. F., Hamdi, K., & Ghahremaninasab, P. (2016). The effects of combined low-dose oral contraceptives and Vitex agnus on the improvement of clinical and paraclinical parameters of polycystic ovarian syndrome: A triple-blind, randomized, controlled clinical trial. *Iranian Red Crescent Medical Journal*, *18*(12). doi:10.5812/ircmj.37510

Shakibaei, M., Mobasheri, A., Lueders, C., Busch, F., Shayan, P., & Goel, A. (2013). Curcumin Enhances the Effect of Chemotherapy against Colorectal Cancer Cells by Inhibition of NF-κB and Src Protein Kinase Signaling Pathways. *PLoS One*, *8*(2), e57218. doi:10.1371/journal.pone.0057218 PMID:23451189

Shakya, A. K. (2016). Medicinal plants: Future source of new drugs. *Int. J. Herb. Med.*, *4*(4), 59–64.

Shang, A., Cao, S., Xu, X., Gan, R., Tang, G., Corke, H., ... Li, H. (2019). Bioactive compounds and biological functions of garlic (*Allium sativum* L.). *Foods*, *8*(7), 246. doi:10.3390/foods8070246 PMID:31284512

Shang, X. J., Guo, J., Chen, L., Deng, C. H., Sun, X. Z., & Geng, Q. (2011). Qilin pills for oligoasthenospermia: A multi-centered clinical trial. *Natl J Androl*, *17*, 1139–1142. PMID:22235686

Sharma, S., Khinchi, M. P., Sharma, N., Agrawal, D., & Gupta, M. K. (2011). Female Infertility: An Overview. *IJPSR*, *2*(1). https://ijpsr.com/bft-article/female-infertility-an-overview/?view=fulltext

Sharma. (1938). *Ashwagandharishta - Rastantra Sar Evam Sidhyaprayog Sangrah-Krishna-Gopal Ayurveda Bhawan*. Dharmarth Trust.

Sharma, A. K., Basu, I., & Singh, S. (2018). Efficacy and Safety of Ashwagandha Root Extract in Subclinical Hypothyroid Patients: A Double-Blind, Randomized Placebo-Controlled Trial. *Journal of Alternative and Complementary Medicine (New York, N.Y.)*, *24*(3), 243–248. doi:10.1089/acm.2017.0183 PMID:28829155

Sharma, C., Nusri, Q. E.-A., Begum, S., Javed, E., Rizvi, T. A., & Hussain, A. (2012). (-)-Epigallocatechin-3-gallate induces apoptosis and inhibits invasion and migration of human cervical cancer cells. *Asian Pacific Journal of Cancer Prevention*, *13*(9), 4815–4822. doi:10.7314/APJCP.2012.13.9.4815 PMID:23167425

Sharma, C., Sadrieh, L., Priyani, A., Ahmed, M., Hassan, A. H., & Hussain, A. (2011). Anti-carcinogenic effects of sulforaphane in association with its apoptosis-inducing and anti-inflammatory properties in human cervical cancer cells. *Cancer Epidemiology*, *35*(3), 272–278. doi:10.1016/j.canep.2010.09.008 PMID:20956097

Sharma, N. K., Ahirwar, D., Jhade, D., & Jain, V. K. (2012). *In-vitro* anti-obesity assay of alcoholic and aqueous extracts of *Camellia sinensis* leaves. *International Journal of Pharmaceutical Sciences and Research*, *3*(1), 863–1866.

Sharma, R., Amin, H., & Prajapati, P. K. (2016). Comparative lipid profile of type 2 obese diabetics and obese non-diabetics: A hospital based study from hilly terrains of Mandi, Himachal Pradesh. *International Journal of Health & Allied Sciences*, *5*(1), 63–64. doi:10.4103/2278-344X.173876

Sharma, S., & Tripathi, P. (2019). Gut microbiome and type 2 diabetes: Where we are and where to go? *The Journal of Nutritional Biochemistry*, *63*, 101–108. doi:10.1016/j.jnutbio.2018.10.003 PMID:30366260

Sharpe, R. M. (1986). Paracrine control of the testis. *Clinics in Endocrinology and Metabolism, 15*(1), 185–207. doi:10.1016/S0300-595X(86)80049-4 PMID:3514003

Sheehan, D., Moran, C., & Shanahan, F. (2015). The microbiota in inflammatory bowel disease. *Journal of Gastroenterology, 50*(5), 495–507. doi:10.100700535-015-1064-1 PMID:25808229

Sheng-Ji, P. (2001). Ethnobotanical approaches of traditional medicine studies: some experiences from Asia. *Pharmaceutical Biology, 39*(sup1), 74-79.

Shen, J., Zuo, Z. X., & Mao, A. P. (2014). Effect of probiotics on inducing remission and maintaining therapy in ulcerative colitis, Crohn's disease, and pouchitis: Meta-analysis of randomized controlled trials. *Inflammatory Bowel Diseases, 20*(1), 21–35. doi:10.1097/01.MIB.0000437495.30052.be PMID:24280877

Sherwani, S., Khan, H., Ekhzaimy, A., Masood, A., & Sakharkar, M. (2016). Significance of HbA1c Test in Diagnosis and Prognosis of Diabetic Patients. *Biomarker Insights, 11. BMI, S38440.* Advance online publication. doi:10.4137/bmi.s38440 PMID:27398023

Shetti, S., Kumar, C. D., Sriwastava, N. K., & Sharma, I. P. (2011). Pharmacovigilance of herbal medicines: Current state and future directions. *Pharmacognosy Magazine, 7*(25), 69. doi:10.4103/0973-1296.75905

Shilo, S., & Hirsch, H. J. (1986). Iodine-induced hyperthyroidism in a patient with a normal thyroid gland. *Postgraduate Medical Journal, 62*(729), 661–662. doi:10.1136/pgmj.62.729.661 PMID:3748931

Shinde, N., Bangar, B., Deshmukh, S., & Kumbhar, P. (2014). Nutraceuticals: A review on current status. Research Journal of Pharmacy and Technology.

Shirazi, A. (2009). The Storehouse of Medicaments. Tehran University of Medical Sciences: Institute for Islamic and Complementary Medicine, Tehran, Iran.

Shi, Y., & Hu, F. B. (2014). The global implications of diabetes and cancer. *Lancet, 383*(9933), 1947–1948. doi:10.1016/S0140-6736(14)60886-2 PMID:24910221

Shubhashree, M. N. (2012). Female Infertility: An Overview (12th ed.). Academic Press.

Shukla, K. K., Mahdi, A. A., Ahmad, M. K., Jaiswar, S. P., Shankwar, S. N., & Tiwari, S. C. (2010). *Mucuna pruriens* reduces stress and improves the quality of semen in infertile men. *Evidence-Based Complementary and Alternative Medicine: eCAM, 7*, 137–144.

Shukla, V., Chandra, V., Sankhwar, P., Popli, P., Kaushal, J. B., Sirohi, V. K., & Dwivedi, A. (2015). Phytoestrogen genistein inhibits EGFR/PI3K/NF-kB activation and induces apoptosis in human endometrial hyperplasial cells. *RSC Advances, 5*(69), 56075–56085. doi:10.1039/C5RA06167A

Sidhu, M. C., & Tanu, S. (2013). A database of antidiabetic plant species of family Asteraceae, Euphorbiaceae, Fabaceae, Lamiaceae and Moraceae. *International Journal of Herbal Medicine, 1*(2), 187–199.

Siezen, R. J., Kok, J., Abee, T., & Schaafsma, G. (2002). Lactic acid bacteria: Genetics, metabolism and applications. *International Journal of General and Molecular Microbiology.* doi:10.1023/A:1020685028897

Sigman, M., & Jarow, J. P. (1997). Endocrine evaluation of infertile men. *Urology, 50*(5), 659–664. doi:10.1016/S0090-4295(97)00340-3 PMID:9372871

Sigthorsson, G., Tibble, J., Hayllar, J., Menzies, I., Macpherson, A., Moots, R., ... Bjarnason, I. (1998). Intestinal permeability and inflammation in patients on NSAIDs. *Gut, 43*(4), 506–511. doi:10.1136/gut.43.4.506 PMID:9824578

Sikka, S. C., Kendirci, M., & Naz, R. (2004). Endocrine Disruptors and Male Infertility. *Endocrine Disruptors (Austin, Tex.)*, 291–312. doi:10.1201/9781420038866-9

Silanikove, N., Leitner, G., & Merin, U. (2015). The interrelationships between lactose intolerance and the modern dairy industry: Global perspectives in evolutional and historical backgrounds. Nutrients. https://doi.org/ doi:10.3390/nu7095340

Simopoulos, A. P. (2008). The importance of the omega-6/omega-3 fatty acid ratio in cardiovascular disease and other chronic diseases. *Experimental Biology and Medicine (Maywood, N.J.)*, *233*(6), 674–688. doi:10.3181/0711-MR-311 PMID:18408140

Singh, A. P., Sarkar, S., Tripathi, M., & Rajender, S. (2013). *Mucuna pruriens* and its major constituent L-DOPA recover spermatogenic loss by com- bating ROS, loss of mitochondrial membrane potential and apoptosis. *PLoS One*, *8*(1), e54655. doi:10.1371/journal.pone.0054655 PMID:23349947

Singh, A., Holvoet, S., & Mercenier, A. (2011). Dietary polyphenols in the prevention and treatment of allergic diseases. *Clinical and Experimental Allergy*, *41*(10), 1346–1359. doi:10.1111/j.1365-2222.2011.03773.x PMID:21623967

Singh, J., Cumming, E., Manoharan, G., Kalasz, H., & Adeghate, E. (2011). Medicinal chemistry of the anti-diabetic effects of momordica charantia: Active constituents and modes of actions. *The Open Medicinal Chemistry Journal*, *5*(supplement 2), 70–77. doi:10.2174/1874104501105010070 PMID:21966327

Singh, J., & Sinha, S. (2012). Classification, Regulatory Acts and Applications of Nutraceuticals for Health. *International Journal of Pharma and Bio Sciences*, *2*(1), 177–187.

Singh, K., & Thakar, A. B. (2018). A clinical study to evaluate the role of Triphaladya Guggulu along with Punarnavadi Kashaya in the management of hypothyroidism. *Ayu*, *39*(1), 50–55. doi:10.4103/ayu.AYU_62_17 PMID:30595635

Singh, R. K., Chang, H.-W., Yan, D., Lee, K. M., Ucmak, D., Wong, K., ... Liao, W. (2017). Influence of diet on the gut microbiome and implications for human health. *Journal of Translational Medicine*, *15*(1), 73. doi:10.118612967-017-1175-y PMID:28388917

Singh, S., Gupta, S. K., Sabir, G., Gupta, M. K., & Seth, P. K. (2009). A database for anti-diabetic plants with clinical/experimental trials. *Bioinformation*, *4*(6), 263–268. doi:10.6026/97320630004263 PMID:20975921

Sirmans, S., & Pate, K. (2014). Epidemiology, diagnosis, and management of polycystic ovary syndrome. *Clinical Epidemiology*, *6*, 1–13. PubMed

Skinner, M. K. (1991). Cell-cell interaction in the testis. *Endocrine Reviews*, *12*(1), 45–77. doi:10.1210/edrv-12-1-45 PMID:2026122

Skrovanek, S. (2014). Zinc and gastrointestinal disease. *World Journal of Gastrointestinal Pathophysiology*, *5*(4), 496–513. doi:10.4291/wjgp.v5.i4.496 PMID:25400994

Skyler, J., Bakris, G., Bonifacio, E., Darsow, T., Eckel, R., Groop, L., Groop, P.-H., Handelsman, Y., Insel, R. A., Mathieu, C., McElvaine, A. T., Palmer, J. P., Pugliese, A., Schatz, D. A., Sosenko, J. M., Wilding, J. P. H., & Ratner, R. E. (2016). Differentiation of Diabetes by Pathophysiology, Natural History, and Prognosis. *Diabetes*, *66*(2), 241–255. doi:10.2337/db16-0806 PMID:27980006

Slavin, J. L. (2005). Dietary fiber and body weight. *Nutrition (Burbank, Los Angeles County, Calif.)*, *21*(3), 411–418. doi:10.1016/j.nut.2004.08.018 PMID:15797686

Slavin, J. L., & Lloyd, B. (2012). Health benefits of fruits and vegetables. *Advances in Nutrition*, *3*(4), 506–516. doi:10.3945/an.112.002154 PMID:22797986

Snelson, M., & Coughlan, M. T. (2019). Dietary Advanced Glycation End Products: Digestion, Metabolism and Modulation of Gut Microbial Ecology. *Nutrients*, *11*(2), 215. doi:10.3390/nu11020215 PMID:30678161

Snow, V., Barry, P., Fitterman, N., Qaseem, A., & Weiss, K. (2005). Pharmacologic and surgical management of obesityin primary care: A clinical practice guideline from theAmerican College of Physicians. *Annals of Internal Medicine*, *142*(7), 525–531. doi:10.7326/0003-4819-142-7-200504050-00011 PMID:15809464

Sobolev, V. S., & Cole, R. J. (1999). trans-Resveratrol content in commercial peanuts and peanut products. *Journal of Agricultural and Food Chemistry*, *47*(4), 1435–1439. doi:10.1021/jf9809885 PMID:10563995

Soetaert, W., Schwengers, D., Buchholz, K., & Vandamme, E. J. (1995). A wide range of carbohydrate modifications by a single micro-organism: Leuconostoc mesenteroides. Progress in Biotechnology. https://doi.org/ doi:10.1016/S0921-0423(06)80116-4

Solecki, R. S. (1975). Shanidar IV, a Neanderthal flower burial in northern Iraq. *Sci*, *190*(4217), 880–881. doi:10.1126cience.190.4217.880

Song, M. Y., Lv, N., Kim, E. K., Kwon, K. S., Yoo, Y. B., Kim, J. H., Lee, S. W., Song, J. H., Lee, J. H., Lee, S. K., Shin, B. C., Ryu, D. G., Park, B. H., & Kwon, K. B. (2009). Antiobesity activity of aqueous extracts of rhizoma *Dioscoreae tokoronis* on high-fat diet-induced obesity in mice. *Journal of Medicinal Food*, *12*(2), 304–309. doi:10.1089/jmf.2008.1010 PMID:19459730

Sonkamble, V. V., & Kamble, L. H. (2015). Antidiabetic potential and identification of phytochemicals from Tinospora cordifolia. *American Journal of Phytomedicine and Clinical Therapeutics*, *3*(1), 97-110.

Son, M. J., Rico, C. W., Nam, S. H., & Kang, M. Y. (2010). Influence of oryzanol and ferulic acid on the lipid metabolism and antioxidative status in high fat-fed mice. *Journal of Clinical Biochemistry and Nutrition*, *46*(2), 150–156. doi:10.3164/jcbn.09-98 PMID:20216948

Soumya, V., Muzib, Y. I., Venkatesh, P., & Hariprasath, K. (2014). GC-MS analysis of Cocus nucifera flower extract and its effects on heterogeneous symptoms of polycystic ovarian disease in female Wistar rats. *Chinese Journal of Natural Medicines*, *12*(9), 677–684. doi:10.1016/S1875-5364(14)60103-5 PMID:25263979

Soylemez, S., Sepici, A., & Akar, F. (2009). Resveratrol supplementation gender independently improves endothelial reactivity and suppresses superoxide production in healthy rats. *Cardiovascular Drugs and Therapy*, *23*(6), 449–458. doi:10.100710557-009-6198-z PMID:19809869

Spencer, M., Gupta, A., Dam, L. V., Shannon, C., Menees, S., & Chey, W. D. (2016). Artificial Sweeteners: A Systematic Review and Primer for Gastroenterologists. *Journal of Neurogastroenterology and Motility*, *22*(2), 168–180. doi:10.5056/jnm15206 PMID:26932837

Spiteri-Grech, J., & Nieschlag, E. (1993). Paracrine factors relevant to the regulation of spermatogenesis-a review. *Journal of Reproduction and Fertility*, *98*(1), 1–14. doi:10.1530/jrf.0.0980001 PMID:8345452

Sreejayan, & Rao, M. N. A. (1994). Curcuminoids as Potent Inhibitors of Lipid Peroxidation. *The Journal of Pharmacy and Pharmacology*, *46*(12), 1013–1016. doi:10.1111/j.2042-7158.1994.tb03258.x PMID:7714712

Sreekanth, C. N., Bava, S. V., Sreekumar, E., & Anto, R. J. (2011). Molecular evidences for the chemosensitizing efficacy of liposomal curcumin in paclitaxel chemotherapy in mouse models of cervical cancer. *Oncogene*, *30*(28), 3139–3152. doi:10.1038/onc.2011.23 PMID:21317920

Stancioiu, F., Mihai, D., Papadakis, G. Z., Tsatsakis, A., Spandidos, D. A., & Badiu, C. (2019). Treatment for benign thyroid nodules with a combination of natural extracts. *Molecular Medicine Reports*, *20*(3), 2332–2338. doi:10.3892/mmr.2019.10453 PMID:31322200

Statovci, D., Aguilera, M., MacSharry, J., & Melgar, S. (2017). The Impact of Western Diet and Nutrients on the Microbiota and Immune Response at Mucosal Interfaces. *Frontiers in Immunology*, *8*, 838. doi:10.3389/fimmu.2017.00838 PMID:28804483

Staudacher, H. M., Lomer, M. C. E., Farquharson, F. M., Louis, P., Fava, F., Franciosi, E., ... Whelan, K. (2017). A Diet Low in FODMAPs Reduces Symptoms in Patients With Irritable Bowel Syndrome and A Probiotic Restores Bifidobacterium Species: A Randomized Controlled Trial. *Gastroenterology*, *153*(4), 936–947. doi:10.1053/j.gastro.2017.06.010 PMID:28625832

Stein, I., & Leventhal, M. (1935). Amenorrhea associated with bilateral polycystic ovaries. *American Journal of Obstetrics and Gynecology*, *29*(2), 181–191. doi:10.1016/S0002-9378(15)30642-6

Stephen, J. M., & Gary, D. H. (2014). *Pathophysiology of disease-an introduction to clinical medicine: Medical*. Academic Press.

Stephen, D. (2012). A report of national nutraceutical center. Nutaceuticals India. *Webinar*, *2012*, 1–22.

Stepto, N. K., Cassar, S., Joham, A. E., Hutchison, S. K., Harrison, C. L., Goldstein, R. F., & Teede, H. J. (2013). Women with polycystic ovary syndrome have intrinsic insulin resistance on euglycaemic-hyperinsulaemic clamp. *Human Reproduction (Oxford, England)*, *28*(3), 777–784. doi:10.1093/humrep/des463 PMID:23315061

Stipanuk, M. H. c. (2013). *Biochemical, Physiological and Molecular Aspects of Human Nutrition* (3rd ed.). Elsevier.

Stoll, A. L., Severus, W. E., Freeman, M. P., Rueter, S., Zboyan, H. A., Diamond, E., Cress, K. K., & Marangell, L. B. (1999). Omega 3 fatty acids in bipolar disorder: A preliminary double-blind, placebo-controlled trial. *Archives of General Psychiatry*. Advance online publication. doi:10.1001/archpsyc.56.5.407 PMID:10232294

Strauss, J.F. (2003). Some new thoughts on the pathophysiology and genetics of polycystic ovary syndrome. *Ann 1N Y Acad Sci, 997*, 42-48.

Struja, T., Fehlberg, H., Kutz, A., Guebelin, L., Degen, C., Mueller, B., & Schuetz, P. (2017). Can we predict relapse in Graves' disease? Results from a systematic review and meta-analysis. *European Journal of Endocrinology*, *176*(1), 87–97. doi:10.1530/EJE-16-0725 PMID:27780830

Sturm, R. A., & Duffy, D. L. (2012). Human pigmentation genes under environmental selection. *Genome Biology*, *13*(9), 248. doi:10.1186/gb-2012-13-9-248 PMID:23110848

Suanarunsawat, T., Anantasomboon, G., & Piewbang, C. (2016). Anti-diabetic and anti-oxidative activity of fixed oil extracted from *Ocimum sanctum* L. leaves in diabetic rats. *Experimental and Therapeutic Medicine*, *11*(3), 832–840. doi:10.3892/etm.2016.2991 PMID:26998000

Suez, J., Korem, T., Zeevi, D., Zilberman-Schapira, G., Thaiss, C. A., Maza, O., ... Elinav, E. (2014). Artificial sweeteners induce glucose intolerance by altering the gut microbiota. *Nature*, *514*(7521), 181–186. doi:10.1038/nature13793 PMID:25231862

Suke, S. G., Kosta, P., & Negi, H. (2015). Role of Pharmacovigilance in India: An overview. *Online Journal of Public Health Informatics*, *7*(2), e223. doi:10.5210/ojphi.v7i2.5595

Sulaiman, M. R., Hussain, M. K., Zakaria, Z. A., Somchit, M. N., Moin, S., Mohamad, A. S., & Israf, D. A. (2008). Evaluation of the antinociceptive activity of Ficus deltoidea aqueous extract. *Fitoterapia*, *79*(7-8), 557–561. doi:10.1016/j.fitote.2008.06.005 PMID:18672036

SUMT Standard Unani Medical Terminology. (2012). New Delhi, India: Central Council for Research in Unani Medicine, Ministry of Ayush, Govt. of India.

Sun, N. (2014). *Pathophysiology | Diabetes Mellitus Type 2*. Retrieved 27 August 2020, from https://u.osu.edu/diabetestype2/diagnosis/

Sunde, R. A. (2006). Selenium. In B. Bowman & R. Russell (Eds.), *Present knowledge in nutrition* (9th ed., pp. 480–497). Washington, DC: International Life Science Institute.

Sunde, R. A. (2010). Selenium. In *Encyclopedia of Dietary Supplements* (2nd ed., pp. 711–718). London: Informa Healthcare. doi:10.1201/b14669-82

Suneetha, D. S., Divya, T. B., & Ali, F. (2013). Antiobesity values of methanolic extract of *Sapindus emariganatus* on monosodium glutamate induced model in rats. *International Journal of Pharmacognosy and Phytochemical Research*, *5*(4), 267–270.

Sun, J. (2018). Dietary vitamin D, vitamin D receptor, and microbiome. *Current Opinion in Clinical Nutrition and Metabolic Care*, *21*(6), 471–474. doi:10.1097/MCO.0000000000000516 PMID:30169457

Sun, L., Ma, L., Ma, Y., Zhang, F., Zhao, C., & Nie, Y. (2018). Insights into the role of gut microbiota in obesity: Pathogenesis, mechanisms, and therapeutic perspectives. *Protein & Cell*, *9*(5), 397–403. doi:10.100713238-018-0546-3 PMID:29725936

Sun, N.-N., Wu, T.-Y., & Chau, C.-F. (2016). Natural dietary and herbal products in anti- obesity treatment. *Molecules (Basel, Switzerland)*, *21*(10), 1351. doi:10.3390/molecules21101351 PMID:27727194

Sun, W. S., Imai, A., Tagami, K., Sugiyama, M., Furui, T., & Tamaya, T. (2004). In vitro stimulation of granulosa cells by a combination of different active ingredients of unkei-to. *The American Journal of Chinese Medicine*, *32*(4), 569–578. doi:10.1142/S0192415X0400220X PMID:15481646

Sun, X., Chang, X., Wang, Y., Xu, B., & Cao, X. (2019). Oroxylin A Suppresses the Cell Proliferation, Migration, and EMT via NF-κB Signaling Pathway in Human Breast Cancer Cells. *BioMed Research International*, *2019*, 2019. doi:10.1155/2019/9241769

Sun, X., Yu, W., & Hu, C. (2014). Genetics of Type 2 Diabetes: Insights into the Pathogenesis and Its Clinical Application. *BioMed Research International*, *2014*, 1–15. doi:10.1155/2014/926713 PMID:24864266

Sun, Z. G., Lian, F., Jiang, K. P., Zhang, J. W., Ma, F. M., & Zhang, N. (2012). Shengjing prescription improves semen parameters of oligo-asthenozoospermia patients: Efficacy and mechanism. *Natl J Androl*, *18*, 764–767. PMID:22934526

Surks, M. I., Ortiz, E., Daniels, G. H., Sawin, C. T., Col, N. F., Cobin, R. H., ... Denke, M. A. (2004). Subclinical thyroid disease: Scientific review and guidelines for diagnosis and management. *Journal of the American Medical Association*, *291*(2), 228–238. doi:10.1001/jama.291.2.228 PMID:14722150

Susan, A., Jason, A. A., Caroline, A. S., & Alan, B. (2014). Herbal medicine for the management of polycystic ovary syndrome (PCOS) and associated oligo/amenorrhoea and hyperandrogenism; a review of the laboratory evidence for effects with corroborative clinical findings. *BMC Complementary and Alternative Medicine*, *14*(1), 511. doi:10.1186/1472-6882-14-511 PMID:25524718

Suvarna, V. C., & Boby, V. U. (2005). Probiotics in human health: A current assessment. *Current Science*, *88*, 1744–1748.

Suzuki, R. (2014). Genistein potentiates the antitumor effect of 5-fluorouracil by inducing apoptosis and autophagy in human pancreatic cancer cells. *Anticancer Research, 34*(9), 4685–4692. https://www.ncbi.nlm.nih.gov/pmc/articles/PMC4240628/ PMID:25202045

Swiatecka, D. (2011). The study on the impact of glycated pea proteins on human intestinal bacteria. *International Journal of Food Microbiology, 145*(1), 267–272. doi:10.1016/j.ijfoodmicro.2011.01.002 PMID:21276631

Szeligowski, T., Yun, A. L., Lennox, B. R., & Burnet, P. W. J. (2020). The Gut Microbiome and Schizophrenia: The Current State of the Field and Clinical Applications. *Frontiers in Psychiatry, 11*, 156. doi:10.3389/fpsyt.2020.00156 PMID:32226399

Szkudelska, K., Nogowski, L., & Szkudelski, T. (2000). Genistein affects lipogenesis and lipolysis in isolated rat adipocytes. *The Journal of Steroid Biochemistry and Molecular Biology, 75*(4-5), 265–271. doi:10.1016/S0960-0760(00)00172-2 PMID:11282281

Szkudelska, K., Szkudelski, T., & Nogowski, L. (2002). Daidzein, coumestrol and zearalenone affect lipogenesis and lipolysis in rat adipocytes. *Phytomedicine, 9*(4), 338–345. doi:10.1078/0944-7113-00148 PMID:12120815

Tabakova, P., Dimitrov, M., & Tashkov, B. (1984). *Clinical studies on the preparation Tribestan in women with endocrine infertility or menopausal syndrome.* Sofia, Bulgaria: 1st Obstetrical and Gynecological Hospital.

Tabatabaeizadeh, S. A. (2018). Vitamin D, the gut microbiome and inflammatory bowel disease. *Journal of Research in Medical Sciences, 23*(1), 75. doi:10.4103/jrms.JRMS_606_17 PMID:30181757

Takahashi, K., & Kitao, M. (1994). Effect of TJ-68 (shakuyaku-kanzo-to) on polycystic ovarian disease. *International Journal of Fertility and Menopausal Studies, 39*(2), 69. PMID:8012442

Takahashi, T. (2011). Mechanism of acupuncture on neuromodulation in the gut—A review. *Neuromodulation, 14*(1), 8–12. doi:10.1111/j.1525-1403.2010.00295.x PMID:21992155

Takahashi, T., & Miyazawa, M. (2012). Potent α-glucosidase inhibitors from safflower (Carthamus tinctorius L.) seed. *Phytotherapy Research, 26*(5), 722–726. doi:10.1002/ptr.3622 PMID:22021176

Takano, S., Reichert, M., Bakir, B., Das, K. K., Nishida, T., Miyazaki, M., & Maitra, A. (2016). Prrx1 isoform switching regulates pancreatic cancer invasion and metastatic colonization. *Genes & Development, 30*(2), 233–247. doi:10.1101/gad.263327.115 PMID:26773005

Takeuchi, T., Nishii, O., Okamura, T., & Yaginuma, T. (1989). Effect of traditional herbal medicine, shakuyaku-kanzo-to on total and free serum testosterone levels. *The American Journal of Chinese Medicine, 17*(1-2), 35–44. doi:10.1142/S0192415X89000073 PMID:2511749

Takikawa, M., Inoue, S., Horio, F., & Tsuda, T. (2010). Dietary anthocyanin-rich bilberry extract ameliorates hyperglycemia and insulin sensitivity via activation of AMP-activated protein kinase in diabetic mice. *The Journal of Nutrition, 140*(3), 527–533. doi:10.3945/jn.109.118216 PMID:20089785

Talbott, E. O., Guzick, D. S., Sutton-Tyrrell, K., McHugh-Pemu, K. P., Zborowski, J. V., Remsberg, K. E., & Kuller, L. H. (2000). Evidence for association between polycystic ovary syndrome and premature carotid atherosclerosis in middle-aged women. *Arteriosclerosis, Thrombosis, and Vascular Biology, 20*(11), 2414–2421. doi:10.1161/01.ATV.20.11.2414 PMID:11073846

Talbott, E., Clerici, A., Berga, S. L., Kuller, L., Guzick, D., Detre, K., Daniels, T., & Engberg, R. A. (1998). Adverse lipid and coronary heart disease risk profiles in young women with polycystic ovary syndrome: Results of a case-control study. *Journal of Clinical Epidemiology, 51*(5), 415–422. doi:10.1016/S0895-4356(98)00010-9 PMID:9619969

Tamadon, M. R., Baradaran, A., & Rafieian-Kopaei, M. (2013). Antioxidant and kidney protection; differential impacts of single and whole natural antioxidants. *Journal of Renal Injury Prevention*. Advance online publication. doi:10.12861/jrip.2014.14 PMID:25340165

Tang, H. (2017). *Reversal of 5-fluorouracil resistance by EGCG is mediate by inactivation of TFAP2A / VEGF signaling pathway and down- regulation of MDR-1 and P-gp expression in gastric cancer*. Academic Press.

Tan, G. H., & Gharib, H. (1997). Thyroid incidentalomas: Management approaches to nonpalpable nodules discovered incidentally on thyroid imaging. *Annals of Internal Medicine*, *126*(3), 226–231. doi:10.7326/0003-4819-126-3-199702010-00009 PMID:9027275

Tang, D., Liu, L., Ajiakber, D., Ye, J., Xu, J., Xin, X., & Aisa, H. A. (2018). Anti-diabetic effect of *Punica granatum* flower polyphenols extract in type 2 diabetic rats: Activation of Akt/GSK-3β and inhibition of IRE1α-XBP1 pathways. *Frontiers in Endocrinology*, *9*(586), 1–11. doi:10.3389/fendo.2018.00586

Tang, T., Glanville, J., Hayden, C. J., White, D., Barth, J. H., & Balen, A. H. (2006). Combined lifestyle modification and metformin in obese patients with polycystic ovary syndrome. A randomized, placebo-controlled, double-blind multicentre study. *Human Reproduction (Oxford, England)*, *21*(1), 80–89. doi:10.1093/humrep/dei311 PMID:16199429

Tao, J. J., Visvanathan, K., & Wolff, A. C. (2016). Long term side effects of adjuvant chemotherapy in patients with early breast cancer. *The Breast*, *24*(2), 1–12. PMID:26299406

Tapas, P., Suraj, V., & Dr.Deepak, D. (2017). A herbal approach to obesity management: A review. *Asian Journal of Pharmaceutical Education and Research*, *6*(3), 1–15.

Taranto, M. P., Vera, J. L., Hugenholtz, J., De Valdez, G. F., & Sesma, F. (2003). Lactobacillus reuteri CRL1098 produces cobalamin. *Journal of Bacteriology*. Advance online publication. doi:10.1128/JB.185.18.5643-5647.2003 PMID:12949118

Tawfeek, F. K. (2006). Effect of nigella sativa oil treatment on the sex organs and sperm characters in rats exposed to hydrogen peroxide. *Mesopotamia Journal of Agriculture*, *34*(1), 2–8. doi:10.33899/magrj.2006.38488

Taylor, P. (2014). *Digestive System Effects of Dietary Components on Cancer of the Digestive System*. Academic Press.

Teede, H., Hutchinson, S.K., & Zoungas, S. (2007). The management of insulin in polycystic ovary syndrome. *Trends in Endocrinology and Metabolism*(18273-279.

Teede, H. J., Misso, M. L., Costello, M. F., Dokras, A., Laven, J., Moran, L., Piltonen, T., & Norman, R. J. (2018). The International PCOS Network. Recommendations from the international evidence-based guideline for the assessment and management of polycystic ovary syndrome. *Horumon To Rinsho*, *89*(3), 251–268. doi:10.1111/cen.13795 PMID:30024653

Teede, H. J., Misso, M. L., Deeks, A. A., Moran, L. J., Stuckey, B. G., Wong, J. L., Norman, R. J., & Costello, M. F. (2011). Assessmentandmanagementofpolycysticovarysyndrome: Summary of an evidence-based guideline. *The Medical Journal of Australia*, *195*(S6), S65–S112. doi:10.5694/mja11.10915 PMID:21929505

Teoh, S. L., & Das, S. (2018). Phytochemicals and their effective role in the treatment of diabetes mellitus: A short review. *Phytochemistry Reviews*, *17*(5), 1111–1128. doi:10.100711101-018-9575-z

Thaker, V. V. (2017). Genetic and epigenetic causes of obesity. *Adolescent Medicine: State of the Art Reviews*, *28*(2), 379. PMID:30416642

Thakur, M., Chauhan, N. S., Bhargava, S., & Dixit, V. K. (2009). A Comparative Study on Aphrodisiac Activity of Some Ayurvedic Herbs in Male Albino Rats. *Archives of Sexual Behavior*, *38*(6), 1009–1015. doi:10.100710508-008-9444-8 PMID:19139984

Thakur, M., Loeppert, R., Praznik, W., & Dixit, V. K. (2008). Effect of Some Ayurvedic Vajikaran Rasayana Herbs on Heat Induced Testicular Damage in Male Albino Rats. *Journal of Complementary & Integrative Medicine*, *5*(1). Advance online publication. doi:10.2202/1553-3840.1112

Thatte, U., & Bhalerao, S. (2008). Pharmacovigilance of ayurvedic medicines in India. *Indian Journal of Pharmacology*, *40*(Suppl 1), S10–S12.

Thessaloniki ESHRE/ASRM-Sponsored PCOS Consensus Workshop Group. (2008). Consensus on infertility treatment related to polycystic ovary syndrome. *Human Reproduction, 23*, 462–477.

Thiery, J. P., Acloque, H., Huang, R. Y., & Nieto, M. A. (2009). Epithelial-mesenchymal transitions in development and disease. *Cell, 139*(5), 871-890.

Thirumalai, T., Therasa, S. V., Elumalai, E. K., & David, E. (2011). Hypoglycemic effect of *Brassica juncea* (seeds) on streptozotocin induced diabetic male albino rat. *Asian Pacific Journal of Tropical Biomedicine*, *1*(4), 323–325. doi:10.1016/S2221-1691(11)60052-X PMID:23569784

Thomford, N. E., Dzobo, K., Chopera, D., Wonkam, A., Skelton, M., Blackhurst, D., Chirikure, S., & Dandara, C. (2015). Pharmacogenomics implications of using herbal medicinal plants on African populations in health transition. *Pharmaceuticals (Basel, Switzerland)*, *8*(3), 637–663. doi:10.3390/ph8030637 PMID:26402689

Thompson, E. W., & Newgreen, D. F. (2005). Carcinoma invasion and metastasis: A role for epithelial-mesenchymal transition? *Cancer Research*, *65*(14), 5991–5995. doi:10.1158/0008-5472.CAN-05-0616 PMID:16024595

Tian, T., Li, J., Li, B., Wang, Y., Li, M., Ma, D., & Wang, X. (2014). Genistein exhibits anti-cancer effects via down-regulating FoxM1 in H446 small-cell lung cancer cells. *Tumour Biology*, *35*(5), 4137–4145. doi:10.100713277-013-1542-0 PMID:24379139

Tilburt, J. C., & Kaptchuk, T. J. (2008). Herbal medicine research and global health: An ethical analysis. *Bulletin of the World Health Organization*, *86*(8), 594–599. doi:10.2471/BLT.07.042820 PMID:18797616

Toden, S., Okugawa, Y., Jascur, T., Wodarz, D., Komarova, N. L., Buhrmann, C., Shakibaei, M., Boland, C. R., & Goel, A. (2015). Curcumin mediates chemosensitization to 5-fluorouracil through miRNA-induced suppression of epithelial-to-mesenchymal transition in chemoresistant colorectal cancer. *Carcinogenesis*, *36*(3), 355–367. doi:10.1093/carcin/bgv006 PMID:25653233

Toklu, H. Z., Şehirli, Ö., Erşahin, M., Süleymanoğlu, S., Yiğiner, Ö., Emekli-Alturfan, E., ... Şener, G. (2010). Resveratrol improves cardiovascular function and reduces oxidative organ damage in the renal, cardiovascular and cerebral tissues of two-kidney, one-clip hypertensive rats. *The Journal of Pharmacy and Pharmacology*, *62*(12), 1784–1793. doi:10.1111/j.2042-7158.2010.01197.x PMID:21054406

Tomé-Carneiro, J., Gonzálvez, M., Larrosa, M., Yáñez-Gascón, M. J., García-Almagro, F. J., Ruiz-Ros, J. A., ... Espín, J. C. (2013). Grape resveratrol increases serum adiponectin and downregulates inflammatory genes in peripheral blood mononuclear cells: A triple-blind, placebo-controlled, one-year clinical trial in patients with stable coronary artery disease. *Cardiovascular Drugs and Therapy*, *27*(1), 37–48. doi:10.100710557-012-6427-8 PMID:23224687

Torresan, M. M., Garrino, L., Borraccino, A., Macchi, G., De Luca, A., & Dimonte, V. (2015). Adherence to treatment in patient with severe cancer pain: A qualitative enquiry through illness narratives. *European Journal of Oncology Nursing*, *19*(4), 397–404. doi:10.1016/j.ejon.2015.01.001 PMID:25691299

Tota, K., Rayabarapu, N., Moosa, S., Talla, V., Bhyravbhatla, B., & Rao, S. (2013). InDiaMed: A comprehensive database of Indian medicinal plants for diabetes. *Bioinformation*, *9*(7), 378–380. doi:10.6026/97320630009378 PMID:23750084

Tracy, W., Rami, M., & Samuel, P. (2016). Diagnosis and Treatment of Polycystic Ovary Syndrome. *American Family Physician, 94*(2), 106–113. PMID:27419327

Tramontano, M., Andrejev, S., Pruteanu, M., Klünemann, M., Kuhn, M., Galardini, M., ... Patil, K. R. (2018). Nutritional preferences of human gut bacteria reveal their metabolic idiosyncrasies. *Nature Microbiology, 3*(4), 514–522. doi:10.103841564-018-0123-9 PMID:29556107

Tran, H. D., Luitel, K., Kim, M., Zhang, K., Longmore, G. D., & Tran, D. D. (2014). Transient SNAIL1 expression is necessary for metastatic competence in breast cancer. *Cancer Research, 74*(21), 6330–6340. doi:10.1158/0008-5472.CAN-14-0923 PMID:25164016

Trevisan, M., Liu, J., Bahsas, F.B., & Menotti, A. (1998). Syndrome X and mortality: a population based study. Risk Factor and Life Expectancy Research Group. *Am J Epidemiol, 148*(10), 958-66.

Trigueros, L., Peña, S., Ugidos, A., Sayas-Barberá, E., Pérez-Álvarez, J., & Sendra, E. (2013). Food ingredients as anti-obesity agents: A review. *Critical Reviews in Food Science and Nutrition, 53*(9), 929–942. doi:10.1080/10408398.2011.574215 PMID:23768185

Trollo, P. J., & Rogers, R. M. (1996). Obstructive sleep apnea. *The New England Journal of Medicine, 334*(2), 99–104. doi:10.1056/NEJM199601113340207 PMID:8531966

Trottier, G., Bostrom, P. J., Lawrentschul, N., & Fleshner, N. E. (2010). Nutraceuticals and prostate cancer prevention: A current review. *Nature Reviews. Urology, 7*(1), 21–30. doi:10.1038/nrurol.2009.234 PMID:19997071

Tryggvadottir, L., Tulinius, H., Eyfjord, J. E., & Sigurvinsson, T. (2001). Breastfeeding and reduced risk of breast cancer in an Icelandic cohort study. *American Journal of Epidemiology, 154*(1), 37–42. doi:10.1093/aje/154.1.37 PMID:11427403

Tsai, J. H., Donaher, J. L., Murphy, D. A., Chau, S., & Yang, J. (2012). Spatiotemporal regulation of epithelial- mesenchymal transition is essential for squamous cell carcinoma metastasis. *Cancer Cell, 22*(6), 725–736. doi:10.1016/j.ccr.2012.09.022 PMID:23201165

Tsuda, T., Ueno, Y., Aoki, H., Koda, T., Horio, F., Takahashi, N., Kawada, T., & Osawa, T. (2004). Anthocyanin enhances adipocytokine secretion and adipocyte-specific gene expression in isolated rat adipocytes. *Biochemical and Biophysical Research Communications, 316*(1), 149–157. doi:10.1016/j.bbrc.2004.02.031 PMID:15003523

Tucci, S. A. (2010). Phytochemicals in the control of human appetite and body weight. *Pharmaceuticals, 3*(3), 748–763. doi:10.3390/ph3030748 PMID:27713277

Tu, P. F., Guo, H. Z., & Guo, D. A. (2002). Researches on active constituents of natural and traditional medicine and development of new drugs. *J. Peking Univ. Health Sci., 34*, 513–518.

Turan, E., Sozmen, B., Eltutan, M., & Sozmen, E. (2017). Serum chitotriosidase enzyme activity is closely related to HbA1c levels and the complications in patients with diabetes mellitus type 2. *Diabetes & Metabolic Syndrome, 11*, S503–S506. doi:10.1016/j.dsx.2017.03.044 PMID:28392356

Turati, F., Rossi, M., Pelucchi, C., Levi, F., & La Vecchia, C. (2015). Fruit and vegetables and cancer risk: A review of southern European studies. *British Journal of Nutrition, 113*(S2), S102–S110. doi:10.1017/S0007114515000148 PMID:26148912

Tzeng, T. F., Liou, S. S., & Liu, I. M. (2011). Myricetin ameliorates defective post-receptor insulin signaling via beta-endorphin signaling in the skeletal muscles of fructose-fed rats. *Evidence-Based Complementary and Alternative Medicine, 2011*(150752), 1–19. doi:10.1093/ecam/neq017 PMID:21785619

Tzotzas, T., Papazisis, K., Perros, P., & Krassas, G. E. (2008). Use of somatostatin analogues in obesity. *Drugs, 68*(14), 1963–1973. doi:10.2165/00003495-200868140-00003 PMID:18778119

Uche, A. N., Angie, E., & Monica, R. G. (2013). Polycystic Ovary Syndrome A Review of Treatment Options With a Focus on Pharmacological Approaches. *P&T, 38*(6), 336–355. PMID:23946629

Uchiyama, Jikyo, Takeda, & Ogata. (2013). Lepidium Meyenii (Maca) Enhances the Serum Levels of Luteinising Hormone in Female Rats. *J Ethnopharmacol., 151*(2), 897-902.

Uemura, T., Goto, T., Kang, M. S., Mizoguchi, N., Hirai, S., Lee, J. Y., Nakano, Y., Shono, J., Hoshino, S., Taketani, K., Tsuge, N., Narukami, T., Makishima, M., Takahashi, N., & Kawada, T. (2011). Diosgenin, the main aglycon of fenugreek, inhibits LXRα activity in HepG2 cells and decreases plasma and hepatic triglycerides in obese diabetic mice. *The Journal of Nutrition, 141*(1), 17–23. doi:10.3945/jn.110.125591 PMID:21106928

Ulrich, K. (2011). Dietary Proteins in Obesity and in Diabetes. *Int. J. Vitam. Nutr. Res., 81*(2 – 3), 125 – 133.

Ungaro, R., Bernstein, C. N., Gearry, R., Hviid, A., Kolho, K.-L., Kronman, M. P., ... Atreja, A. (2014). Antibiotics associated with increased risk of new-onset Crohn's disease but not ulcerative colitis: A meta-analysis. *The American Journal of Gastroenterology, 109*(11), 1728–1738. doi:10.1038/ajg.2014.246 PMID:25223575

Unites State Pharmacopeia (USP). (2006). *The regulation of dietary supplements.* http://www.usp.org/pdf/EN/USPVerified/dietarySupplementRegulation.pdf

Unnikrishnan, A. G., & Menon, U. V. (2011). Thyroid disorders in India: An epidemiological perspective. *Indian Journal of Endocrinology and Metabolism, 15*(6, Suppl 2), S78–S81. doi:10.4103/2230-8210.83329 PMID:21966658

Urbanek, M. (2007). The genetics of the polycystic ovary syndrome. *Nature Clinical Practice. Endocrinology & Metabolism, 3*(2), 103–111. doi:10.1038/ncpendmet0400 PMID:17237837

US FDA. (2014). *Summary of qualified health claims subject to enforcement discretion.* Author.

Ushiroyama, T., Hosotani, T., Mori, K., Yamashita, Y., Ikeda, A., & Ueki, M. (2006). Effects of switching to wen-jing-tang (unkei-to) from preceding herbal preparations selected by eight-principle pattern identification on endocrinological status and ovulatory induction in women with polycystic ovary syndrome. *The American Journal of Chinese Medicine, 34*(02), 177–187. doi:10.1142/S0192415X06003746 PMID:16552830

Ushiroyama, T., Ikeda, A., Sakai, M., Hosotani, T., Suzuki, Y., Tsubokura, S., & Ueki, M. (2001). Effects of unkei-to, an herbal medicine, on endocrine function and ovulation in women with high basal levels of luteinizing hormone secretion. *The Journal of Reproductive Medicine, 46*(5), 451–456. PMID:11396371

Vaidya, A. D., & Devasagayam, T. P. (2007). Current status of herbal drugs in India: An overview. *Journal of Clinical Biochemistry and Nutrition, 41*(1), 1–11. doi:10.3164/jcbn.2007001

Valizadeh, E., Ghalichi, F., & Ostadrahimi, A. (2016). Traditional herbal medicine for weight management: A review. *International Journal of Medical Research & Health Sciences, 5*(11), 393–399.

Valkenburg, O., Steegers-Theunissen, R. P., Smedts, H. P., Dallinga-Thie, G. M., Fauser, B. C., Westerveld, E. H., & Laven, J. S. E. (2008). A more atherogenic serum lipoprotein profile is present in women with polycystic ovary syndrome: A case-control study. *The Journal of Clinical Endocrinology and Metabolism, 93*(2), 470–476. doi:10.1210/jc.2007-1756 PMID:18056772

Vallianou, N. G., Evangelopoulos, A., & Kazazis, C. (2013). Resveratrol and diabetes. *The Review of Diabetic Studies; RDS, 10*(4), 236–242. doi:10.1900/RDS.2013.10.236 PMID:24841877 van Berleere, M., & Dauchet, L. (2017). Fruits, Vegetables, and Health: Evidence From Meta-analyses of Prospective Epidemiological Studies. In *Vegetarian and Plant-Based Diets in Health and Disease Prevention* (pp. 215–248). Elsevier. doi:10.1016/B978-0-12-803968-7.00013-7

Van der Klaauw, A., Keogh, J., Henning, E., Trowse, V., Dhillo, W., Ghatei, M., & Farooqi, I. S. (2013). High protein intake stimulates postprandial GLP1 and PYY release. *Obesity (Silver Spring, Md.), 2013*(21), 1602–1607. doi:10.1002/oby.20154 PMID:23666746

Van Puyvelde, K., Mets, T., Njemini, R., Beyer, I., & Bautmans, I. (2014). Effect of advanced glycation end product intake on inflammation and aging: A systematic review. *Nutrition Reviews, 72*(10), 638–650. doi:10.1111/nure.12141 PMID:25231200

Van Rooijen, R. J., Van Schalkwijk, S., & De Vos, W. M. (1991). Molecular cloning, characterization, and nucleotide sequence of the tagatose 6-phosphate pathway gene cluster of the lactose operon of Lactococcus lactis. *Journal of Biological Chemistry.*

van Santbrink, E. J., Hop, W. C., & Fauser, B. C. (1997). Classification of normogonadotropic infertility: Polycystic ovaries diagnosed by ultrasound versus endocrine characteristics of polycystic ovary syndrome. *Fertility and Sterility, 67*(3), 452–458. doi:10.1016/S0015-0282(97)80068-4 PMID:9091329

Vanhoecke, B. W., Delporte, F., Van Braeckel, E., Heyerick, A., Depypere, H. T., Nuytinck, M., ... Bracke, M. E. (2005). A safety study of oral tangeretin and xanthohumol administration to laboratory mice. *In Vivo (Athens, Greece), 19*(1), 103–107. PMID:15796161

Vanschoonbeek, K., Thomassen, B. J., Senden, J. M., Wodzig, W. K., & van Loon, L. J. (2006). Cinnamon supplementation does not improve glycemic control in postmenopausal type 2 diabetes patients. *The Journal of Nutrition, 136*(4), 977–980. doi:10.1093/jn/136.4.977 PMID:16549460

Varani, E. M., & Iriti, M. (2016). Odonto nutraceuticals: Pleioyropic photo therapeutic agents for oral health. *Pharmaceuticals, 9*(1), 10–13. doi:10.3390/ph9010010

Varghese, G. K., Bose, L. V., & Habtemariam, S. (2013). Antidiabetic components of Cassia alata leaves: Identification through α-glucosidase inhibition studies. *Pharmaceutical Biology, 51*(3), 345–349. doi:10.3109/13880209.2012.729066 PMID:23137344

Veltman-Verhulst, S. M., Boivin, J., Eijkemans, M. J., & Fauser, B. J. (2012). Emotional distress is a common risk in women with polycystic ovary syndrome: A systematic review and meta-analysis of 28 studies. *Human Reproduction Update, 18*(6), 638–651. doi:10.1093/humupd/dms029 PMID:22824735

Venkatachalam, T., Kumar, V. K., Selvi, P. K., Maske, A. O., Anbarasan, V., & Kumar, P. S. (2011). Antidiabetic activity of Lantana camara Linn fruits in normal and streptozotocin-induced diabetic rats. *Journal of Pharmacy Research, 4*(5), 1550–1552.

Verhaegen, A. A., & Van Gaal, L. F. (2017). Drug-induced obesity and its metabolic consequences: A review with a focus on mechanisms and possible therapeutic options. *Journal of Endocrinological Investigation, 40*(11), 1165–1174. doi:10.100740618-017-0719-6 PMID:28660606

Verma, K., & Jameel, K. (2012). Studies on traditional treatment of thyroid by the tribals of Chitrakoot district, Uttar Pradesh. *International Journal of Scientific Research (Ahmedabad, India), 3*, 2319–7064.

Verma, R. K., & Paraidathathu, T. (2014). Herbal medicines used in the traditional indian medicinal system as a therapeutic treatment option for overweight and obesity management: A review. *International Journal of Pharmacy and Pharmaceutical Sciences, 6*, 40–47.

Verma, S., & Singh, S. P. (2008). Current and future status of herbal medicines. *Veterinary World, 1*(11), 347–350. doi:10.5455/vetworld.2008.347-350

Veronese, N., Solmi, M., Caruso, M. G., Giannelli, G., Osella, A. R., Evangelou, E., ... Tzoulaki, I. (2018). Dietary fiber and health outcomes: An umbrella review of systematic reviews and meta-analyses. *The American Journal of Clinical Nutrition, 107*(3), 436–444. doi:10.1093/ajcn/nqx082 PMID:29566200

Vilhena, R. O., Figueiredo, I. D., Baviera, A. M., Silva, D. B., Marson, B. M., Oliveira, J. A., Peccinini, R. G., Borges, I. K., & Pontarolo, R. (2020). Antidiabetic activity of *Musa x paradisiaca* extracts in streptozotocin-induced diabetic rats and chemical characterization by HPLC-DAD-MS. *Journal of Ethnopharmacology, 254*, 112666. doi:10.1016/j.jep.2020.112666 PMID:32084552

Vingtdeux, V., Dreses-Werringloer, U., Zhao, H., Davies, P., & Marambaud, P. (2008). Therapeutic potential of resveratrol in Alzheimer's disease. *BMC Neuroscience, 9*(S2), S6. doi:10.1186/1471-2202-9-S2-S6 PMID:19090994

Vingtdeux, V., Giliberto, L., Zhao, H., Chandakkar, P., Wu, Q., Simon, J. E., ... Davies, P. (2010). AMP-activated protein kinase signaling activation by resveratrol modulates amyloid-β peptide metabolism. *The Journal of Biological Chemistry, 285*(12), 9100–9113. doi:10.1074/jbc.M109.060061 PMID:20080969

Vinolo, M. A., Rodrigues, H. G., Nachbar, R. T., & Curi, R. (2011). Regulation of inflammation by short chain fatty acids. *Nutrients, 3*(10), 858–876. doi:10.3390/nu3100858 PMID:22254083

Visser, W. E., Jansen, J., Friesema, E. C., Kester, M. H., Mancilla, E., Lundgren, J., van der Knaap, M. S., Lunsing, R. J., Brouwer, O. F., & Visser, T. J. (2009). Novel pathogenic mechanism suggested by ex vivo analysis of MCT8 (SLC16A2) mutations. *Human Mutation, 30*(1), 29–38. doi:10.1002/humu.20808 PMID:18636565

Vivekananthan, D. P., Penn, M. S., Sapp, S. K., Hsu, A., & Topol, E. J. (2003). Use of antioxidant vitamins for the prevention of cardiovascular disease: Meta-analysis of randomized trials. *Lancet, 361*(9374), 2017–2023. doi:10.1016/S0140-6736(03)13637-9 PMID:12814711

Vlietinck, A., Pieters, L., & Apers, S. (2009). Legal Requirements for the Quality of Herbal Substances and Herbal Preparations for the Manufacturing of Herbal Medicinal Products in the European Union. *Planta Medica, 75*(7), 683–688. doi:10.1055-0029-1185307 PMID:19204891

Voigt, K. (2006). Our look at global burgeoning Asian herbal industry. *The Wall Street Journal, 6*(11), 2006.

Vuddanda, P. R., Chakraborty, S., & Singh, S. (2010). Berberine: A potential phytochemical with multispectrum therapeutic activities. *Expert Opinion on Investigational Drugs, 19*(10), 1297–1307. doi:10.1517/13543784.2010.517745 PMID:20836620

Vuksan, V., Sievenpiper, J. L., Koo, V. Y., Francis, T., Beljan-Zdravkovic, U., Xu, Z., & Vidgen, E. (2000). American ginseng (Panax quinquefolius L) reduces postprandial glycemia in nondiabetic subjects and subjects with type 2 diabetes mellitus. *Archives of Internal Medicine, 160*(7), 1009–1013. doi:10.1001/archinte.160.7.1009 PMID:10761967

Vuksan, V., Sievenpiper, J. L., Xu, Z., Wong, E. Y. Y., Jenkins, A. L., Beljan-Zdravkovic, U., Leiter, L. A., Josse, R. G., & Stavro, M. P. (2001). Konjac-mannan and American ginseng: Emerging alternative therapies for type 2 diabetes mellitus. *Journal of the American College of Nutrition, 20*(5, supplement), 370S–380S. doi:10.1080/07315724.2001.10719170 PMID:11603646

Vuksan, V., Sung, M. K., Sievenpiper, J. L., Stavro, P. M., Jenkins, A. L., Di Buono, M., Lee, K.-S., Leiter, L. A., Nam, K. Y., Arnason, J. T., Choi, M., & Naeem, A. (2008). Korean red ginseng (Panax ginseng) improves glucose and insulin regulation in well-controlled, type 2 diabetes: Results of a randomized, double-blind, placebo-controlled study of efficacy and safety. *Nutrition, Metabolism, and Cardiovascular Diseases*, *18*(1), 46–56. doi:10.1016/j.numecd.2006.04.003 PMID:16860976

Vyas, N., Gamit, K., & Raval, M. (2018). Male infertility: A major problem worldwide and its management in Ayurveda. *Pharma Science Monitor*, *9*, 1.

Walker, A. W., Ince, J., Duncan, S. H., Webster, L. M., Holtrop, G., Ze, X., ... Flint, H. J. (2011). Dominant and diet-responsive groups of bacteria within the human colonic microbiota. *The ISME Journal*, *5*(2), 220–230. doi:10.1038/ismej.2010.118 PMID:20686513

Wallerath, T., Deckert, G., Ternes, T., Anderson, H., Li, H., Witte, K., & Förstermann, U. (2002). Resveratrol, a polyphenolic phytoalexin present in red wine, enhances expression and activity of endothelial nitric oxide synthase. *Circulation*, *106*(13), 1652–1658. doi:10.1161/01.CIR.0000029925.18593.5C PMID:12270858

Wang, X. (2014). Fruit and vegetable consumption and mortality from all causes, cardiovascular disease, and cancer: systematic review and dose-response meta-analysis of prospective cohort studies. *BMJ*, *349*(3), g4490–g4490. Available at: https://www.bmj.com/cgi/doi/10.1136/bmj.g4490

Wang, X. (2015). EGCG Enhances Cisplatin Sensitivity by Regulating Expression of the Copper and Cisplatin Influx Transporter CTR1 in Ovary Cancer. Academic Press.

Wang, D. X., Zou, Y. J., Zhuang, X. B., Chen, S. X., Lin, Y., Li, W. L., Lin, Z. Q., & Lin, Z. (2017). Sulforaphane suppresses EMT and metastasis in human lung cancer through miR-616-5p-mediated GSK3β/β-catenin signaling pathways. *Acta Pharmacologica Sinica*, *38*(2), 241–251. doi:10.1038/aps.2016.122 PMID:27890917

Wang, G. J., Anderson, A. R., Graham, M. G. III, Chu, M. C., Sauer, M. V., Guarnaccia, M. M., & Lobo, R. A. (2007). The effect of cinnamon extract on insulin resistance parameters in polycystic ovary syndrome: A pilot study. *Fertility and Sterility*, *88*(1), 240–243. doi:10.1016/j.fertnstert.2006.11.082 PMID:17296187

Wang, J., Fivecoat, H., Ho, L., Pan, Y., Ling, E., & Pasinetti, G. M. (2010). The role of Sirt1: At the crossroad between promotion of longevity and protection against Alzheimer's disease neuropathology. *Biochimica et Biophysica Acta (BBA)-. Proteins and Proteomics*, *1804*(8), 1690–1694. doi:10.1016/j.bbapap.2009.11.015 PMID:19945548

Wang, J., Ho, L., Zhao, W., Ono, K., Rosensweig, C., Chen, L., ... Pasinetti, G. M. (2008). Grape-derived polyphenolics prevent Aβ oligomerization and attenuate cognitive deterioration in a mouse model of Alzheimer's disease. *The Journal of Neuroscience*, *28*(25), 6388–6392. doi:10.1523/JNEUROSCI.0364-08.2008 PMID:18562609

Wang, J., Kim, B., Han, K., & Kim, H. (2017). Ephedra-Treated Donor-Derived Gut Microbiota Transplantation Ameliorates High Fat Diet-Induced Obesity in Rats. *International Journal of Environmental Research and Public Health*, *14*(6), 555. doi:10.3390/ijerph14060555 PMID:28545248

Wang, L., Ma, R., Liu, C., Liu, H., Zhu, R., Guo, S., Tang, M., Li, Y., Niu, J., Fu, M., Gao, S., & Zhang, D. (2017). Salvia miltiorrhiza: A Potential Red Light to the Development of Cardiovascular Diseases. *Current Pharmaceutical Design*, *23*(7), 1077–1097. doi:10.2174/1381612822666161010105242 PMID:27748194

Wang, M., Chen, D. Q., Wang, M. C., Chen, H., Chen, L., Liu, D., Zhao, Y. Y., & Zhao, Y.-Y. (2017). Poricoic acid ZA, a novel RAS inhibitor, attenuates tubulo-interstitial fibrosis and podocyte injury by inhibiting TGF-β/Smad signaling pathway. *Phytomedicine*, *36*, 243–253. doi:10.1016/j.phymed.2017.10.008 PMID:29157821

Wang, P., Henning, S. M., Heber, D., & Vadgama, J. V. (2016). Sensitization to docetaxel in prostate cancer cells by green tea and quercetin. *The Journal of Nutritional Biochemistry*, *26*(4), 408–415. doi:10.1016/j.jnutbio.2014.11.017 PMID:25655047

Wang, Q. Z., Wang, D. F., Liu, H. L., Feng, D. J., Wang, H. H., & Guo, Z. B. (2013). Effects of extracts from Liuwei dihuang Pill on the proliferation of mouse Sertoli cells. *Lishizhen Med Mat Medica Res*, *24*, 1363–1365.

Wang, T., Choi, R. C., Li, J., Li, J., Bi, C. W., Zang, L., Liu, Z., Dong, T. T., Bi, K., & Tsim, K. W. (2010). Antihyperlipidemic effect of protodioscin, an active ingredient isolated from the rhizomes of Dioscorea nipponica. *Planta Medica*, *76*(15), 1642–1646. doi:10.1055-0030-1249960 PMID:20509104

Wang, X., Ouyang, Y., Liu, J., Zhu, M., Zhao, G., Bao, W., & Hu, F. B. (2014). Fruit and vegetable consumption and mortality from all causes, cardiovascular disease, and cancer: Systematic review and dose-response meta-analysis of prospective cohort studies. *British Medical Journal*, *349*(jul29 3), g4490. doi:10.1136/bmj.g4490 PMID:25073782

Wang, Y., Campbell, T., Perry, B., Beaurepaire, C., & Qin, L. (2011). Hypoglycemic and insulin-sensitizing effects of berberine in high-fat diet- and streptozotocin-induced diabetic rats. *Metabolism: Clinical and Experimental*, *60*(2), 298–305. doi:10.1016/j.metabol.2010.02.005 PMID:20304443

Wang, Z., Zou, J., Cao, K., Hsieh, T.-C., Huang, Y., & Wu, J. M. (2005). Dealcoholized red wine containing known amounts of resveratrol suppresses atherosclerosis in hypercholesterolemic rabbits without affecting plasma lipid levels. *International Journal of Molecular Medicine*, *16*(4), 533–540. PMID:16142383

Wani, J. A., Achur, R. N., & Nema, R. K. (2011). Phytochemical screening and aphrodisiac property of *Asparagus racemosus. International Journal of Pharmaceutical Sciences and Drug Research*, *3*, 112–115.

Wargovich, M. J., Morris, J., Brown, V., Ellis, J., Logothetis, B., & Weber, R. (2010). Nutraceutical use in late-stage cancer. *Cancer and Metastasis Reviews*, *29*(3), 503–510. doi:10.100710555-010-9240-5 PMID:20714787

Wartofsky, L., & Van Nostrand, D. (2016). *Thyroid cancer: a comprehensive guide to clinical management*. Springer. doi:10.1007/978-1-4939-3314-3

Watanabe, N., Narimatsu, H., Noh, J. Y., Yamaguchi, T., Kobayashi, K., Kami, M., Kunii, Y., Mukasa, K., Ito, K., & Ito, K. (2012). Antithyroid drug-induced hematopoietic damage: A retrospective cohort study of agranulocytosis and pancytopenia involving 50,385 patients with Graves' disease. *The Journal of Clinical Endocrinology and Metabolism*, *97*(1), E49–E53. doi:10.1210/jc.2011-2221 PMID:22049174

Watzl, B., Girrbach, S., & Roller, M. (2005). Inulin, oligofructose and immunomodulation. *British Journal of Nutrition*, *93*(S1), 49–55. doi:10.1079/BJN20041357 PMID:15877895

Weinkauf, M. & Dreyling, M. (2015). *Vardenafil, a clinically available phosphodiesterase inhibitor, potentiates the killing effect of EGCG on CLL cells*. Academic Press.

Weisberg, S. P., McCann, D., Desai, M., Rosenbaum, M., Leibel, R. L., & Ferrante, A. W. Jr. (2003). Obesity is associated with macrophage accumulation in adipose tissue. *The Journal of Clinical Investigation*, *112*(12), 1796–1808. doi:10.1172/JCI200319246 PMID:14679176

Weiss, R. E., Weinberg, M., & Refetoff, S. (1993). Identical mutations in unrelated families with generalized resistance to thyroid hormone occur in cytosine-guanine-rich areas of the thyroid hormone receptor beta gene. Analysis of 15 families. *The Journal of Clinical Investigation*, *91*(6), 2408–2415. doi:10.1172/JCI116474 PMID:8514853

Wenzel, E., Soldo, T., Erbersdobler, H., & Somoza, V. (2005). Bioactivity and metabolism of trans-resveratrol orally administered to Wistar rats. *Molecular Nutrition & Food Research, 49*(5), 482–494. doi:10.1002/mnfr.200500003 PMID:15779067

Westerterp, K. R. (2004). Diet induced thermo- genesis. *Nutrition & Metabolism, 1*(1), 5. doi:10.1186/1743-7075-1-5 PMID:15507147

Whelan, K. (2019). *Artificial Pancreas—The Future for Diabetes Treatment? – Medical Expo e-Magazine.* Retrieved 29 February 2020, from http://emag.medicalexpo.com/artificial-pancreas-the-future-for-diabetes-treatment/

Whitten, P. L., & Naftolin, F. (1998). Reproductive actions of phytoestrogens. *Bailliere's Clinical Endocrinology and Metabolism, 12*(4), 667–690. doi:10.1016/S0950-351X(98)80010-4 PMID:10384819

WHO, World Health Organization. (2007). Indicators for assessing infant and young child feeding practices part 1 definition. Washington, DC: World Health Organization. Dept. of Child and Adolescent Health and Development.

WHO, World Health Organization. (2009). *Infant and young child feeding: model chapter for textbooks for medical students and allied health professionals.* Geneva: World Health Organization.

WHO, World Health Organization. (2020). *Malnutrition.* https://www.who.int/news-room/fact-sheets/detail/malnutrition#:~:text=47%20million%20children%20under%205,%2D%20and%20middle%2Dincome%20countries

WHO, World Health Organization. (n.d.). *Breastfeeding.* https://www.who.int/health-topics/breastfeeding#tab=tab_1

WHO. (2001). *Legal status of traditional medicine and complementary/alternative medicine: a worldwide review.* WHO.

WHO. (2006). *Probiotics in Food - Health and nutritional properties and guidelines for evaluation.* Available from: http://www.fao.org/tempref/docrep/fao/009/a0512e/a0512e00.pdf

WHO. (2014). *About Diabetes.* World Health Organization.

Whorwell, P. J., Altringer, L., Morel, J., Bond, Y., Charbonneau, D., O'Mahony, L., Kiely, B., Shanahan, F., & Quigley, E. M. M. (2006). Efficacy of an encapsulated probiotic Bifidobacterium infantis 35624 in women with irritable bowel syndrome. *The American Journal of Gastroenterology.* Advance online publication. doi:10.1111/j.1572-0241.2006.00734.x PMID:16863564

Wichtl, M. (2004). Herbal drugs and phytopharmaceuticals: a handbook for practice on a scientific basis (No. Ed. 3). Medpharm GmbH Scientific Publishers.

Wijarnpreecha, K. (2019). Obesity and Risk of Small Intestine Bacterial Overgrowth: A Systematic Review and Meta-Analysis. *Digestive Diseases and Sciences.* PMID:31605277

Wiklund, P. (2016). The role of physical activity and exercise in obesity and weight management: Time for critical appraisal. *Journal of Sport and Health Science, 5*(2), 151–154. doi:10.1016/j.jshs.2016.04.001 PMID:30356545

Wildman, R. E. C. (2016). Handbook of Nutraceuticals and Functional Foods. Handbook of Nutraceuticals and Functional Foods, Second Edition. https://doi.org/ doi:10.1201/9781420006186

Wildman, R. E. C. (2007). *Nutraceuticals and functional foods.* New York: CRC Press.

Willcox, M. L., Graz, B., Falquet, J., Diakite, C., Giani, S., & Diallo, D. (2011). A reverse pharmacology approach for developing an anti-malarial phytomedicine. Malaria Journal. https://doi.org/ doi:10.1186/1475-2875-10-S1-S8

Wirksamkeit. (2007). *Ayurveda bei chronischen Erkrankungen. Systematische Analysen klinischer Ayurveda-Studien.* Essen: KVC.

Witt, C. M., Michalsen, A., Roll, S., Morandi, A., Gupta, S., Rosenberg, M., Kronpass, L., Stapelfeldt, E., Hissar, S., Muller, M., & Kessler, C. (2013). Comparative effectiveness of a complex Ayurvedic treatment and conventional standard care in osteoarthritis of the knee – study protocol for a randomized controlled trial. *Trials*, *14*(1), 149. doi:10.1186/1745-6215-14-149 PMID:23701973

Wolfram, S. (2007). Effects of green tea and EGCG on cardiovascular and metabolic health. *Journal of the American College of Nutrition*, *26*(4), 373S–388S. doi:10.1080/07315724.2007.10719626 PMID:17906191

Wolf, W. M., Wattick, R. A., Kinkade, O. N., & Olfert, M. D. (2018). Geographical Prevalence of Polycystic Ovary Syndrome as Determined by Region and Race/Ethnicity. *International Journal of Environmental Research and Public Health*, *15*(11), 2589. doi:10.3390/ijerph15112589 PMID:30463276

Wolters, M., Ahrens, J., Romaní-Pérez, M., Watkins, C., Sanz, Y., Benítez-Páez, A., ... Günther, K. (2019). Dietary fat, the gut microbiota, and metabolic health - A systematic review conducted within the MyNewGut project. *Clinical Nutrition (Edinburgh, Lothian)*, *38*(6), 2504–2520. doi:10.1016/j.clnu.2018.12.024 PMID:30655101

Wong, K. V. (2012). Nutritional perspective about prostate cancer disparity between the west and the rest of the world. *Food Science and Technology Letters*, *3*(1), 14–19.

World Health Organisation. (2000). *General guidelines for methodologies on research and evaluation of traditional medicine*. World Health Organisation.

World Health Organisation. (2000). *Global Strategy on Diet Physical Activity and Health*. World Health Organization.

World Health Organization (WHO). (2003). *Traditional Medicine*. Report by the Secretariat. A 56/18. https://extranet.who.int/iris/restricted/handle/10665/78244

World Health Organization. (2000). *Obesity: Preventing and managing the global epidemic*. Technical report series No.894, Geneva: WHO.

World Health Organization. (2002). *Traditional Medicine in Asia*. WHO Regional Publications.

World Health Organization. (2011). *Global recommendations on physical activity for health*. WHO.

World Health Organization. (2018). *Diabetes*. Available from [https://www.who. int/news-room/fact-sheets/detail/diabetes

Wu, G. D., Chen, J., Hoffmann, C., Bittinger, K., Chen, Y.-Y., Keilbaugh, S. A., ... Lewis, J. D. (2011). Linking long-term dietary patterns with gut microbial enterotypes. *Science*, *334*(6052), 105–108. doi:10.1126cience.1208344 PMID:21885731

Wu, J., Pan, Z., Wang, Z., Zhu, W., Shen, Y., Cui, R., Lin, J., Yu, H., Wang, Q., Qian, J., Yu, Y., Zhu, D., & Lou, Y. (2012). Ginsenoside Rg1 protection against beta-amyloid peptide-induced neuronal apoptosis via estrogen receptor alpha and glucocorticoid receptor-dependent anti-protein nitration pathway. *Neuropharmacology*, *63*(3), 349–361. doi:10.1016/j.neuropharm.2012.04.005 PMID:22534050

Wu, L., Guo, L., Liang, Y., Liu, X., Jiang, L., & Wang, L. (2015). Curcumin suppresses stem-like traits of lung cancer cells via inhibiting the JAK2/STAT3 signaling pathway. *Oncology Reports*, *34*(6), 3311–3317. doi:10.3892/or.2015.4279 PMID:26397387

Wu, Q.-J., Wu, L., Zheng, L.-Q., Xu, X., Ji, C., & Gong, T.-T. (2016). Consumption of fruit and vegetables reduces risk of pancreatic cancer: Evidence from epidemiological studies. *European Journal of Cancer Prevention*, *25*(3), 196–205. doi:10.1097/CEJ.0000000000000171 PMID:26075658

Wu, S. Y., Cohen, R. N., Simsek, E., Senses, D. A., Yar, N. E., Grasberger, H., Noel, J., Refetoff, S., & Weiss, R. E. (2006). A novel thyroid hormone receptor-beta mutation that fails to bind nuclear receptor corepressor in a patient as an apparent cause of severe, predominantly pituitary resistance to thyroid hormone. *The Journal of Clinical Endocrinology and Metabolism, 91*(5), 1887–1895. doi:10.1210/jc.2005-2428 PMID:16464943

Wu, W., Yin, D., Yang, W., Kan, Q., Liu, Z., Ren, X., Zhai, C., & Zhang, S. (2014). Chinese herbal medicines for benign thyroid nodules in adults. *Cochrane Database of Systematic Reviews*, 3. doi:10.1002/14651858.CD010492.pub2 PMID:24596045

Wu, W., Zhou, Q., Zhao, W., Gong, Y., Su, A., Liu, F., Liu, Y., Li, Z., & Zhu, J. (2018). Ginsenoside Rg3 Inhibition of Thyroid Cancer Metastasis Is Associated with Alternation of Actin Skeleton. *Journal of Medicinal Food, 21*(9), 849–857. doi:10.1089/jmf.2017.4144 PMID:30136914

Wu, Z.-Q., Chen, D.-L., Lin, F.-H., Lin, L., Shuai, O., Wang, J.-Y., Qi, L.-K., & Zhang, P. (2015). Effect of bajijiasu isolated from Morinda officinalis F. C. how on sexual function in male mice and its antioxidant protection of human sperm. *Journal of Ethnopharmacology, 164*, 283–292. doi:10.1016/j.jep.2015.02.016 PMID:25686781

Xiang, Y., Zhao, J., Zhao, M., & Wang, K. (2018). Allicin activates autophagic cell death to alleviate the malignant development of thyroid cancer. *Experimental and Therapeutic Medicine, 15*(4), 3537–3543. doi:10.3892/etm.2018.5828 PMID:29545880

Xia, Y., Xia, M. Z., Li, Y., Liu, S. M., Ju, Z. Y., & He, J. S. (2012). Effect of aconite cake-separated moxibustion at Guanyuan (CV 4) and Mingmen (GV 4) on thyroid function in patients of Hashimoto's thyroiditis. *Zhongguo Zhenjiu, 32*(2), 123–126.

Xia, Y., Zhao, P., Huang, H., Xie, Y., Lu, R., & Dong, L. (2017). Cryptotanshinone reverses reproductive disturbances in rats with dehydroepiandrosterone-induced polycystic ovary syndrome. *American Journal of Translational Research, 15*(9), 2447–2456. PMID:28559995

Xie, B., Waters, M. J., & Schirra, H. J. (2012). Investigating potential mechanisms of obesity by metabolomics. *BioMed Research International, 2012*(805683), 1–10. PMID:22665992

Xie, X., Li, W., Lan, T., Liu, W., Peng, J., Huang, K., Huang, J., Shen, X., Liu, P., & Huang, H. (2011). Berberine ameliorates hyperglycemia in alloxan-induced diabetic C57BL/6 mice through activation of Akt signaling pathway. *Endocrine Journal, 58*(9), 761–768. doi:10.1507/endocrj.K11E-024 PMID:21705841

Xita, N., & Tsatsoulis, A. (2006). Review: fetal programming of polycystic ovary syndrome by androgen excess: evidence from experimental, clinical, and genetic association studies. *The Journal of Clinical Endocrinology and Metabolism, 91*(5), 1660–1666. doi:10.1210/jc.2005-2757 PMID:16522691

Xiu, L., Zhong, G., Liu, D., Chen, S., Liu, H., & Chen, F. (2017). Comparative efficacy and toxicity of different species of Sargassum in Haizao Yuhu Decoction in PTU-induced goiter rats. *Evidence-Based Complementary and Alternative Medicine, 2017*, 2017. doi:10.1155/2017/3526186 PMID:28713435

Xu, Y., Ding, J., Ma, X.P., Ma, Y.H., Liu, Z.Q., & Lin, N. (2014). Treatment with Panax ginseng antagonizes the estrogen decline in ovariectomized mice. *Int J Mol Sci, 15*, 7827-40.

Xu, H. Y., Barnes, G. T., Yang, Q., Tan, Q., Yang, D. S., Chou, C. J., Sole, J., Nichols, A., Ross, J. S., Tartaglia, L. A., & Chen, H. (2003). Chronic inflammation in fat plays a crucial role in the development of obesity-related insulin resistance. *The Journal of Clinical Investigation, 112*(12), 1821–1830. doi:10.1172/JCI200319451 PMID:14679177

Xu, J., Liu, D., Niu, H., Zhu, G., Xu, Y., Ye, D., & Zhang, Q. (2017). Resveratrol reverses Doxorubicin resistance by inhibiting epithelial-mesenchymal transition (EMT) through modulating PTEN/Akt signaling pathway in gastric cancer. *Journal of Experimental & Clinical Cancer Research*, *36*(1), 19. doi:10.118613046-016-0487-8 PMID:28126034

Xu, L., Chen, S. W., Qi, X. Y., Li, X. X., & Sun, Y. B. (2018). Ginsenoside improves papillary thyroid cancer cell malignancies partially through upregulating connexin 31. *The Kaohsiung Journal of Medical Sciences*, *34*(6), 313–320. doi:10.1016/j.kjms.2017.12.006 PMID:29747774

Xu, Y., Lee, D. K., Feng, Z., Xu, Y., Bu, W., Li, Y., & Xu, J. (2017). Breast tumor cell-specific knockout of Twist1 inhibits cancer cell plasticity, dissemination, and lung metastasis in mice. *Proceedings of the National Academy of Sciences of the United States of America*, *114*(43), 11494–11499. doi:10.1073/pnas.1618091114 PMID:29073077

Yacoub, R., Nugent, M., Cai, W., Nadkarni, G. N., Chaves, L. D., Abyad, S., ... Uribarri, J. (2017). Advanced glycation end products dietary restriction effects on bacterial gut microbiota in peritoneal dialysis patients; a randomized open label controlled trial. *PLoS One*, *12*(9), e0184789. doi:10.1371/journal.pone.0184789 PMID:28931089

Yaginuma, T. I., Yasui, R., Arai, H., & Kawabata, T. (1982). Effect of traditional herbal medicine on serum testosterone levels and its induction of regular ovulation in hyperandrogenic and oligomenorrheic women. *Nippon Sanka Fujinka Gakkai Zasshi*, *34*(7), 939. PubMed

Yamamoto, Y., & Oue, E. (2006). Antihypertensive effect of quercetin in rats fed with a high-fat high-sucrose diet. *Bioscience, Biotechnology, and Biochemistry*, *70*(4), 933–939. doi:10.1271/bbb.70.933 PMID:16636461

Yan, F., & Polk, D. B. (2011). Probiotics and immune health. *Current Opinion in Gastroenterology*, *27*(6), 496–501. doi:10.1097/MOG.0b013e32834baa4d PMID:21897224

Yang, K. Pyun, & Lee. (2018). Licorice ethanol extract improves symptoms of polycytic ovary syndrome in Letrozole-induced female rats. Integrative Medicine Research, 7, 264–270. PubMed

Yang, A., Liu, B., Zhang, S., Xie, C., Li, L., & Zhou, Q. (2010). Mechanism of Wuziyanzong Pills in improvement of function of Sertoli cells in rats with insufficiency of kidney essence. *J Beijing Univ Tradit Chin Med*, *33*, 378–380.

Yang, C. S., Chen, L., Lee, M. J., Balentine, D., Kuo, M. C., & Schantz, S. P. (1998). Blood and urine levels of tea catechins after ingestion of different amounts of green tea by human volunteers. *Cancer Epidemiology, Biomarkers & Prevention*, *7*(4), 351–354. PMID:9568793

Yang, J. (2015). Effect of curcumin on Bcl-2 and Bax expression in nude mice prostate cancer. *International Journal of Clinical and Experimental Pathology*, *8*(8), 9272–9278. PMID:26464676

Yang, J. Y., Della-Fera, M. A., Nelson-Dooley, C., & Baile, C. A. (2006). Molecular mechanisms of apoptosis induced by ajoene in 3T3-L1 adipocytes. *Obesity (Silver Spring, Md.)*, *14*(3), 388–397. doi:10.1038/oby.2006.52 PMID:16648609

Yang, J., Mani, S. A., Donaher, J. L., Ramaswamy, S., Itzykson, R. A., Come, C., & Weinberg, R. A. (2004). Twist, a master regulator of morphogenesis, plays an essential role in tumor metastasis. *Cell*, *117*(7), 927–939. doi:10.1016/j.cell.2004.06.006 PMID:15210113

Yang, J., & Weinberg, R. A. (2008). Epithelial-mesenchymal transition: At the crossroads of development and tumor metastasis. *Developmental Cell*, *14*(6), 818–829. doi:10.1016/j.devcel.2008.05.009 PMID:18539112

Yang, K., Guo, K. Q., & Wu, H. Y. (2007). Clinical effect of Prunellae Oral Liquid on goiter with different thyroid function. *Zhongguo Zhong Xi Yi Jie He Za Zhi*, *27*(1), 37–39. PMID:17302062

Yang, M. L., & Lu, B. (2018). Treatment of Goiter with Traditional Chinese Medicine Regimen Xing Qi Hua Ying Tang: A Clinical Study on 72 Patients with Multinodular and Diffuse Goiter. *Journal of Alternative and Complementary Medicine (New York, N.Y.)*, *24*(4), 374–377. doi:10.1089/acm.2017.0138 PMID:29215302

Yang, Q., Ji, M., Guan, H., Shi, B., & Hou, P. (2013). Shikonin inhibits thyroid cancer cell growth and invasiveness through targeting major signaling pathways. *The Journal of Clinical Endocrinology and Metabolism*, *98*(12), E1909–E1917. doi:10.1210/jc.2013-2583 PMID:24106286

Yang, X., Zhang, Y., Huang, Y., Wang, Y., Qi, X., Su, T., & Lu, L. (2020). Evodiamine suppresses Notch3 signaling in lung tumorigenesis via direct binding to γ-secretases. *Phytomedicine*, *68*, 153176. doi:10.1016/j.phymed.2020.153176 PMID:32045841

Yannakoulia, M., Poulimeneas, D., Mamalaki, E., & Anastasiou, C. A. (2019). Dietary modifications for weight loss and weight loss maintenance. *Metabolism: Clinical and Experimental*, *92*, 153–162. doi:10.1016/j.metabol.2019.01.001 PMID:30625301

Yarnell, E., & Abascal, K. (2002). Dilemmas of traditional botanical research. *HerbalGram*, (55), 46-54.

Yarnell, E., & Abascal, K. (2006). Botanical medicine for thyroid regulation. *Alternative and Complementary Therapies*, *12*(3), 107–112. doi:10.1089/act.2006.12.107

Yashiro, T., Nanmoku, M., Shimizu, M., Inoue, J., & Sato, R. (2012). Resveratrol increases the expression and activity of the low density lipoprotein receptor in hepatocytes by the proteolytic activation of the sterol regulatory element-binding proteins. *Atherosclerosis*, *220*(2), 369–374. doi:10.1016/j.atherosclerosis.2011.11.006 PMID:22153697

Yatsunenko, T., Rey, F. E., Manary, M. J., Trehan, I., Dominguez-Bello, M. G., Contreras, M., ... Gordon, J. I. (2012). Human gut microbiome viewed across age and geography. *Nature*, *486*(7402), 222–227. doi:10.1038/nature11053 PMID:22699611

Yavari, M., Rouholamin, S., Tansaz, M., Bioos, S., & Esmaeili, S. (2014). Sesame a treatment of menstrual bleeding cessation in iranian traditional medicine: Results from a pilot study. *Shiraz E Medical Journal*, *15*(3). Advance online publication. doi:10.17795emj21893

Yavari, M., Rouholamin, S., Tansaz, M., Bioos, S., & Esmaeili, S. (2016). Sesame a Treatment of Menstrual Bleeding Cessation in Iranian Traditional Medicine: Results From a Pilot Study. *Shiraz E Medical Journal*, *5*(3), 114–121.

Yen, C. H., Lai, C. C., Shia, T. H., Chen, M., Yu, H. C., Liu, Y. P., & Chang, F. R. (2018). Gynura divaricata attenuates tumor growth and tumor relapse after cisplatin therapy in HCC xenograft model through suppression of cancer stem cell growth and Wnt/β-catenin signalling. *Journal of Ethnopharmacology*, *213*, 366–375. doi:10.1016/j.jep.2017.07.019 PMID:28729225

Yen, S. S. (1980). The polycystic ovary syndrome. *Horumon To Rinsho*, *12*(2), 177–207. doi:10.1111/j.1365-2265.1980.tb02132.x PMID:6772357

Ye, X., Brabletz, T., Kang, Y., Longmore, G. D., Nieto, M. A., Stanger, B. Z., & Weinberg, R. A. (2017). Upholding a role for EMT in breast cancer metastasis. *Nature*, *547*(7661), E1–E3. doi:10.1038/nature22816 PMID:28682326

Ye, Z., Chen, D., Zhong, J., Zhang, Y., Zhang, W., & Wang, G. (2013). Effect of Jiawei Wuzi Yanzong decoction on sperm quality and hormone level. *World Chin Med*, *8*, 626–629.

Yi, J.-L. (2015). Myricetin and methyl eugenol combination enhances the anticancer activity, cell cycle arrest and apoptosis induction of cis-platin against HeLa cervical cancer cell lines. *International Journal of Clinical and Experimental Pathology*, *8*(2), 1116–1127. https://www.ncbi.nlm.nih.gov/pmc/articles/PMC4396221/ PMID:25972998

Yildiz, B. O., Bozdag, G., Yapici, Z., Esinler, I., & Yarali, H. (2012). Prevalence, phenotype and cardiometabolic risk of polycystic ovary syndrome under different diagnostic criteria. *Human Reproduction (Oxford, England), 27*(10), 3067–3073. doi:10.1093/humrep/des232 PMID:22777527

Yilmaz, M., Bukan, N., Ayvaz, G., Karakoç, A., Törüner, F., Cakir, N., & Arslan, M. (2005). The effects of rosiglitazone and metformin on oxidative stress and Homocysteine levels in lean patients with polycystic ovary syndrome. *Human Reproduction (Oxford, England), 20*(12), 3333–3340. doi:10.1093/humrep/dei258 PMID:16123091

Yin, J. L., Xu, Y., & Wu, B. (2013). Wuziyanzong compound relieves oxidative stress injury and inhibits the apoptosis of Sertoli cells. *J Natl Androl, 19*, 257–261. PMID:23700734

Yin, J., Xing, H., & Ye, J. (2008). Efficacy of berberine in patients with type 2 diabetes mellitus. *Metabolism: Clinical and Experimental, 57*(5), 712–717. doi:10.1016/j.metabol.2008.01.013 PMID:18442638

Yin, J., Xing, H., & Ye, J. (2008). Efficacy of Berberine in Patients with Type 2. *Diabetes & Metabolism, 57*(5), 712–717. PMID:18442638

Yokozawa, T., Kim, H. Y., Cho, E. J., Choi, J. S., & Chung, H. Y. (2002). Antioxidant effects of isorhamnetin 3,7-di-O-β-d-glucopyranoside isolated from mustard leaf (*Brassica juncea*) in rats with streptozotocin-induced diabetes. *Journal of Agricultural and Food Chemistry, 50*(19), 5490–5495. doi:10.1021/jf0202133 PMID:12207497

Younis, N., Soran, H., & Farook, S. (2004). The prevention of type 2 diabetes mellitus: Recent advances. *QJM, 97*(7), 451–455. doi:10.1093/qjmed/hch077 PMID:15208433

Yuan, C. S., Mehendale, S. R., Wang, C. Z., Aung, H. H., Jiang, T., Guan, X., & Shoyama, Y. (2004). Effects of Corydalis yanhusuo and Angelicae dahuricae on cold pressor-induced pain in humans: A controlled trial. *Journal of Clinical Pharmacology, 44*(11), 1323–1327. doi:10.1177/0091270004267809 PMID:15496650

Yuan, H., Ma, Q., Ye, L., & Piao, G. (2016). The traditional medicine and modern medicine from natural products. *Molecules (Basel, Switzerland), 21*(5), 559. doi:10.3390/molecules21050559 PMID:27136524

Yue, G. P., Chen, Q., & Dai, N. (1996). Eighty-seven cases of male infertility treated by bushen shengjing pill in clinical observation and evaluation on its curative effect. *Chin J Integr Tradit West Med, 16*, 463–466. PMID:9387745

Yue, Z., Zhang, L., Li, C., Chen, Y., Tai, Y., Shen, Y., & Sun, Z. (2019). Advances and potential of gene therapy for type 2 diabetes mellitus. *Biotechnology, Biotechnological Equipment, 33*(1), 1150–1157. doi:10.1080/13102818.2019.1643783

Yu, J., Ren, P., Zhong, T., Wang, Y., Yan, M., Xue, B., Li, R., Dai, C., Liu, C., Chen, G., & Yu, X. F. (2015). Pseudolaric acid B inhibits proliferation in SW579 human thyroid squamous cell carcinoma. *Molecular Medicine Reports, 12*(5), 7195–7202. doi:10.3892/mmr.2015.4418 PMID:26460192

Yu, M., Bardia, A., Wittner, B. S., Stott, S. L., Smas, M. E., Ting, D. T., Isakoff, S. J., Ciciliano, J. C., Wells, M. N., Shah, A. M., Concannon, K. F., Donaldson, M. C., Sequist, L. V., Brachtel, E., Sgroi, D., Baselga, J., Ramaswamy, S., Toner, M., Haber, D. A., & Maheswaran, S. (2013). Circulating breast tumor cells exhibit dynamic changes in epithelial and mesenchymal composition. *Science, 339*(6119), 580–584. doi:10.1126cience.1228522 PMID:23372014

Yu, R., Kim, C. S., Kwon, B. S., & Kawada, T. (2006). Mesenteric adipose tissue-derived monocyte chemoattractant protein-1 plays a crucial role in adipose tissue macrophage migration and activation in obese mice. *Obesity (Silver Spring, Md.), 14*(8), 1353–1362. doi:10.1038/oby.2006.153 PMID:16988077

Yu, X. M., Phan, T., Patel, P. N., Jaskula-Sztul, R., & Chen, H. (2013). Chrysin activates Notch1 signaling and suppresses tumor growth of anaplastic thyroid carcinoma in vitro and in vivo. *Cancer, 119*(4), 774–781. doi:10.1002/cncr.27742 PMID:22991264

Zahra, A., Ayoob, R., Mohsen, M., Masih, H., & Mahmoud, R. (2018). A review on role of medicinal plants in polycystic ovarian syndrome: Pathophysiology, neuroendocrine signaling, therapeutic status and future prospects. *Middle East Fertility Society Journal*, *23*(4), 255–262. doi:10.1016/j.mefs.2018.04.005

Zamiska, N. (2007). Dueling Therapies-Is a Shotgun Better Than a Silver Bullet? *Wall Street Journal,* p. B1.

Zang, M., Xu, S., Maitland-Toolan, K. A., Zuccollo, A., Hou, X., Jiang, B., Wierzbicki, M., Verbeuren, T. J., & Cohen, R. A. (2006). Polyphenols stimulate amp-activated protein kinase, lower lipids, and inhibit accelerated atherosclerosis in diabetic ldl receptor-deficient mice. *Diabetes*, *55*(8), 2180–2191. doi:10.2337/db05-1188 PMID:16873680

Zanini, S., Marzotto, M., Giovinazzo, F., Bassi, C., & Bellavite, P. (2015). Effects of dietary components on cancer of the digestive system. *Critical Reviews in Food Science and Nutrition*, *55*(13), 1870–1885. doi:10.1080/10408398.2012.732126 PMID:24841279

Zare, R., Nadjarzadeh, A., Zarshenas, M. M., Shams, M., & Heydari, M. (2019). Efficacy of cinnamon in patients with type II diabetes mellitus: A randomized controlled clinical trial. *Clinical Nutrition (Edinburgh, Lothian)*, *38*(2), 549–556. doi:10.1016/j.clnu.2018.03.003 PMID:29605574

Zeinab, F., Siavash, F., Mahdi, S., & Reza, G. (2017). Nutritional management in women with polycystic ovary syndrome: A review study. *Diab Met Syndr: Clin Res Rev, 11*(S1).

Zeisel, S. H. (1999). Rehulations of "Nutraceuticals". *Science*, *285*(5435), 1853–1855. doi:10.1126cience.285.5435.1853 PMID:10515789

Zemel, M. B. (2005). The role of dairy foods in weight management. *Journal of the American College of Nutrition*, *24*(6), 537S–546S. doi:10.1080/07315724.2005.10719502 PMID:16373953

Zhang, Y. J., Gan, R. Y., Li, S., Zhou, Y., Li, A. N., Xu, D. P., Li, H. B., & Kitts, D. D. (2015). Antioxidant phytochemicals for the prevention and treatment of chronic diseases. Molecules. https://doi.org/ doi:10.3390/molecules201219753

Zhang, Y., Ma, S.W.J. & Xie, H.L.J.Y.S. (2014). *Laboratory investigation EGCG inhibits properties of glioma stem-like cells and synergizes with temozolomide through downregulation of P-glycoprotein inhibition.* Academic Press.

Zhang, C., Lv, B., Yi, C., Cui, X., Sui, S., Li, X., Qi, M., Hao, C., Han, B., & Liu, Z. (2019). Genistein inhibits human papillary thyroid cancer cell detachment, invasion and metastasis. *Journal of Cancer*, *10*(3), 737–748. doi:10.7150/jca.28111 PMID:30719173

Zhang, D., Liu, B., Cao, B., Wei, F., Yu, X., Li, G. F., & Wang, P. L. (2017). Synergistic protection of Schizandrin B and Glycyrrhizic acid against bleomycin-induced pulmonary fibrosis by inhibiting TGF-β1/Smad2 pathways and overexpression of NOX4. *International Immunopharmacology*, *48*, 67–75. doi:10.1016/j.intimp.2017.04.024 PMID:28476015

Zhang, H., & Chen, J. (2018). Current status and future directions of cancer immunotherapy. *Journal of Cancer*, *9*(10), 1773–1781. doi:10.7150/jca.24577 PMID:29805703

Zhang, H., Wei, J., Xue, R., Wu, J.-D., Zhao, W., Wang, Z.-Z., Wang, S.-K., Zhou, Z.-X., Song, D.-Q., Wang, Y.-M., Pan, H.-N., Kong, W.-J., & Jiang, J.-D. (2010). Berberine lowers blood glucose in type 2 diabetes mellitus patients through increasing insulin receptor expression. *Metabolism: Clinical and Experimental*, *59*(2), 285–292. doi:10.1016/j.metabol.2009.07.029 PMID:19800084

Zhang, J. Y., Xue, H. Y., Su, J., Zuo, Y. H., Fan, X. Q., & Cheng, Y. Q. (2015). Clinical effects of tanshinone on polycystic ovary syndrome patients with hyperandrogenism. *Guangxi Medical Journal*, *37*, 767–769.

Zhang, J., Tian, X. J., Zhang, H., Teng, Y., Li, R., Bai, F., & Xing, J. (2014). TGF-β–induced epithelial-to-mesenchymal transition proceeds through stepwise activation of multiple feedback loops. *Science Signaling*, *7*(345), ra91–ra91. doi:10.1126cisignal.2005304 PMID:25270257

Zhang, J., Wider, B., Shang, H., Li, X., & Ernst, E. (2012). Quality of herbal medicines: Challenges and solutions. *Complementary Therapies in Medicine*, *20*(1-2), 100–106. doi:10.1016/j.ctim.2011.09.004 PMID:22305255

Zhang, L., Cheng, X., Gao, Y., Bao, J., Guan, H., Lu, R., Yu, H., Xu, Q., & Sun, Y. (2016). Induction of ROS-independent DNA damage by curcumin leads to G2/M cell cycle arrest and apoptosis in human papillary thyroid carcinoma BCPAP cells. *Food & Function*, *7*(1), 315–325. doi:10.1039/C5FO00681C PMID:26442630

Zhang, L., Cheng, X., Gao, Y., Zheng, J., Xu, Q., Sun, Y., Guan, H., Yu, H., & Sun, Z. (2015). Apigenin induces autophagic cell death in human papillary thyroid carcinoma BCPAP cells. *Food & Function*, *6*(11), 3464–3472. doi:10.1039/C5FO00671F PMID:26292725

Zhang, L., Cheng, X., Xu, S., Bao, J., & Yu, H. (2018). Curcumin induces endoplasmic reticulum stress-associated apoptosis in human papillary thyroid carcinoma BCPAP cells via disruption of intracellular calcium homeostasis. *Medicine*, *97*(24), e11095. doi:10.1097/MD.0000000000011095 PMID:29901626

Zhang, Y. J., Deng, G. F., Xu, X. R., Wu, S., Li, S., & Li, H. B. (2013). Chemical components and bioactivities of cape gooseberry (*Physalis peruviana*). *International Journal of Food Nutrition and Safety*, *3*, 15–24.

Zhang, Y., Feng, F., Chen, T., Li, Z., & Shen, Q. W. (2016). Antidiabetic and antihyperlipidemic activities of Forsythia suspensa (Thunb.) Vahl (fruit) in streptozotocin-induced diabetes mice. *Journal of Ethnopharmacology*, *192*, 256–263. doi:10.1016/j.jep.2016.07.002 PMID:27377336

Zhang, Y., Liu, Y., Wang, T., Li, B., Li, H., Wang, Z., & Yang, B. (2006). Resveratrol, a natural ingredient of grape skin: Antiarrhythmic efficacy and ionic mechanisms. *Biochemical and Biophysical Research Communications*, *340*(4), 1192–1199. doi:10.1016/j.bbrc.2005.12.124 PMID:16406237

Zhang, Y., Li, X., Zou, D., Liu, W., Yang, J., Zhu, N., Huo, L., Wang, M., Hong, J., Wu, P., Ren, G., & Ning, G. (2008). Treatment of type 2 diabetes and dyslipidemia with the natural plant alkaloid berberine. *The Journal of Clinical Endocrinology and Metabolism*, *93*(7), 2559–2565. doi:10.1210/jc.2007-2404 PMID:18397984

Zhang, Y., Li, Y., Mao, X., Yan, C., Guo, X., Guo, Q., Liu, Z., Song, Z., & Lin, N. (2016). Thyroid hormone synthesis: A potential target of a Chinese herbal formula Haizao Yuhu Decoction acting on iodine-deficient goiter. *Oncotarget*, *7*(32), 51699–51712. doi:10.18632/oncotarget.10329 PMID:27384475

Zhang, Y., Shen, N., Qi, L., Chen, W., Dong, Z., & Zhao, D. H. (2013). Efficacy of Schizandra chinesis polysaccharide on cyclophosphamide induced dyszoospermia of rats and its effects on reproductive hormones. *Chin J Integr Tradit West Med*, *33*, 361–364. PMID:23713251

Zhang, Y., Sun, B., Huang, Z., Zhao, D. W., & Zeng, Q. (2018). Shikonin Inhibites Migration and Invasion of Thyroid Cancer Cells by Downregulating DNMT1. *Medical Science Monitor*, *24*, 661–670. doi:10.12659/MSM.908381 PMID:29389913

Zhang, Z., Auyeung, K. K. W., Sze, S. C. W., Zhang, S., Yung, K. K. L., & Ko, J. K. S. (2020). The dual roles of calycosin in growth inhibition and metastatic progression during pancreatic cancer development: A "TGF-β paradox". *Phytomedicine*, *68*, 153177. doi:10.1016/j.phymed.2020.153177 PMID:32106002

Zhan, Y., Chen, Y., Liu, R., Zhang, H., & Zhang, Y. (2014). Potentiation of paclitaxel activity by curcumin in human breast cancer cell by modulating apoptosis and inhibiting EGFR signaling. *Archives of Pharmacal Research*, *37*(8), 1086–1095. doi:10.100712272-013-0311-3 PMID:24318305

Zhao, J. (2007). *Nutraceuticals, nutritional therapy, phytonutrients and phototherapy for improvement of human health: A perspective on Plant Biotechnology Application*. Bentham Science Publishers. http://www.benthamscience.com/biot/samples/biot1-1/Zhao.pdf

Zhao, J. (2008). Nutraceuticals, Nutritional Therapy, Phytonutrients, and Phytotherapy for Improvement of Human Health: A Perspective on Plant Biotechnology Application. *Recent Patents on Biotechnology*. Advance online publication. doi:10.2174/187220807779813893 PMID:19075834

Zheng, C. (2016). Synergistic effects of curcumin and bortezomib on multiple myeloma cells. *International Journal of Clinical and Experimental Medicine*, *9*(11), 21787–21793.

Zheng, G., Sayama, K., Okubo, T., Juneja, L. R., & Oguni, I. (2004). Anti-obesity effects of three major components of green tea, catechins, caffeine and theanine, in mice. *In Vivo (Athens, Greece)*, *18*(1), 55–62. PMID:15011752

Zheng, X., Carstens, J. L., Kim, J., Scheible, M., Kaye, J., Sugimoto, H., & Kalluri, R. (2015). Epithelial-to-mesenchymal transition is dispensable for metastasis but induces chemoresistance in pancreatic cancer. *Nature*, *527*(7579), 525–530. doi:10.1038/nature16064 PMID:26560028

Zhong, C., Qu, C., Wang, B., Liang, S., & Zeng, B. (2017). Probiotics for Preventing and Treating Small Intestinal Bacterial Overgrowth: A Meta-Analysis and Systematic Review of Current Evidence. *Journal of Clinical Gastroenterology*, *51*(4), 300–311. doi:10.1097/MCG.0000000000000814 PMID:28267052

Zhong, D., Wu, C., Zeng, X., & Wang, Q. (2018). The role of gut microbiota in the pathogenesis of rheumatic diseases. *Clinical Rheumatology*, *37*(1), 25–34. doi:10.100710067-017-3821-4 PMID:28914372

Zhou, J., Zhou, S., Tang, J., Zhang, K., Guang, L., Huang, Y., Xu, Y., Ying, Y., Zhang, L., & Li, D. (2004). Protective effect of berberine on beta cells in streptozotocin- and high-carbohydrate/high-fat diet-induced diabetic rats. *European Journal of Pharmacology*, *606*(1-3), 262–268. doi:10.1016/j.ejphar.2008.12.056 PMID:19374872

Zhou, Q.-M., Sun, Y., Lu, Y.-Y., Zhang, H., Chen, Q.-L., & Su, S.-B. (2017). Curcumin reduces mitomycin C resistance in breast cancer stem cells by regulating Bcl-2 family-mediated apoptosis. *Cancer Cell International*, *17*(1), 84. doi:10.118612935-017-0453-3 PMID:28959140

Zhou, S. H., Deng, Y. F., Weng, Z. W., Weng, H. W., & Liu, Z. D. (2019). Traditional Chinese medicine as a remedy for male infertility: A review. *The World Journal of Men's Health*, *37*(2), 175–185. doi:10.5534/wjmh.180069 PMID:30644235

Zhou, Y., Tang, J., Du, Y., Ding, J., & Liu, J.-Y. (2016). The green tea polyphenol EGCG potentiates the antiproliferative activity of sunitinib in human cancer cells. *Tumour Biology*, *37*(7), 8555–8566. doi:10.100713277-015-4719-x PMID:26733173

Zhu, H., Cheng, H., Ren, Y., Liu, Z. G., Zhang, Y. F., & De Luo, B. (2012). Synergistic inhibitory effects by the combination of gefitinib and genistein on NSCLC with acquired drug-resistance in vitro and in vivo. *Molecular Biology Reports*, *39*(4), 4971–4979. doi:10.100711033-011-1293-1 PMID:22160570

Zhu, J., & Wen, K. (2018). Astragaloside IV inhibits TGF-β1-induced epithelial-mesenchymal transition through inhibition of the PI3K/Akt/NF-κB pathway in gastric cancer cells. *Phytotherapy Research*, *32*(7), 1289–1296. doi:10.1002/ptr.6057 PMID:29480652

Zmora, N., Suez, J., & Elinav, E. (2019). You are what you eat: Diet, health and the gut microbiota. *Nature Reviews. Gastroenterology & Hepatology*, *16*(1), 35–56. doi:10.103841575-018-0061-2 PMID:30262901

Zou, X., Liang, J., Sun, J., Hu, X., Lei, L., Wu, D., & Liu, L. (2016). Allicin sensitizes hepatocellular cancer cells to anti-tumor activity of 5-fluorouracil through ROS-mediated mitochondrial pathway. *Journal of Pharmacological Sciences, 131*(4), 233–240. doi:10.1016/j.jphs.2016.04.017 PMID:27177453

Zubair, H., Azim, S., Ahmad, A., Khan, M. A., Patel, G. K., Singh, S., & Singh, A. P. (2017). Cancer chemoprevention by phytochemicals: Nature's healing touch. *Molecules (Basel, Switzerland), 22*(3), 395. doi:10.3390/molecules22030395 PMID:28273819

Zuo, J., Guo, Y., Peng, X., Tang, Y., Zhang, X., He, P., & Xu, D. (2015). Inhibitory action of pristimerin on hypoxia-mediated metastasis involves stem cell characteristics and EMT in PC-3 prostate cancer cells. *Oncology Reports, 33*(3), 1388–1394. doi:10.3892/or.2015.3708 PMID:25571882

Zygmunt, K., Faubert, B., MacNeil, J., & Tsiani, E. (2010). Naringenin, a citrus flavonoid, increases muscle cell glucose uptake via AMPK. *Biochemical and Biophysical Research Communications, 398*(2), 178–183. doi:10.1016/j.bbrc.2010.06.048 PMID:20558145

About the Contributors

Ruby Alexander-Lindo is a Senior Lecturer in the Department of Basic Medical Sciences (Biochemistry Section), Faculty of Medical Sciences, The University of the West Indies, Mona Campus, Kingston 7, Jamaica.

Melisa Anderson is a Lecturer in the School of Allied Health and Wellness, College of Health Sciences, University of Technology, Kingston 7, Jamaica.

Lennox Anderson-Jackson holds the Caribbean Diploma in Diagnostic Radiological Science from the University of the West Indies Mona, Kingston, Jamaica; A Bachelor of Science degree with honors in Diagnostic Medical Sonography from Weber State University in Ogden, Utah, USA; A Master of Science degree in Counselling and Consulting Psychology from the International University of the Caribbean, Kingston, Jamaica. Presently Mr. Anderson-Jackson is pursuing the MPhil / PhD in Chemical Pathology at the University of the West Indies, Mona, Kingston, Jamaica. He has over 29 years of experience in the field of radiological science and has worked in 4 countries including Jamaica, United States of America, Cayman Islands and Anguilla. He worked in several Government hospitals and Private hospitals and clinics in Jamaica including: Kingston Public Hospital (1991), Bustamante Hospital for Children, Cornwall Regional Hospital, Montego Bay Hospital, Radiology West (2003-2013), Royale Imaging Centre (2009-2013) and Reddy's Medical Centre. He also worked as a Clinical Ultrasound Instructor at the School of Medical Radiation Technology, University of the West Indies, Mona, Jamaica in collaboration with Michner Institute in Canada (2004-2008). Mr. Anderson-Jackson is presently the CEO and chief Medical Ultrasound Practitioner and Radiographer at the LYL Ultrasound Centre in Lucea, Hanover, Jamaica. He is a member of Who's Who amongst Students of American Universities and Colleges (Edition 1999). He was also a nominee for Crystal Crest Scholar of the year for Weber State University (1997). A Member of the Profession Supplementary to Medicine, Jamaica. He has been involved in some published articles as author and co-author. Mr. Anderson-Jackson was honoured in 2011 with the Distinguished Alumni Award by the Rusea's Old Student Association (ROSA) for achievements in the field of Science and Research.

Vikas Bansal, born in Dhuri (India) in 1983, received his Master's degree in Food Engineering & Technology in the year 2010 from SLIET (Sant Longowal Institute of Engineering & Technology, Longowal, India). In 2006, after completion of a Bachelor's degree in Food Engineering, He joined Supreme Agro Foods Pvt Ltd., Where he served as a Dairy Chemist. With five years of dairy industry experience, in the year 2013, he joined Shoolini University, Solan, where he served as Assistant Professor for three years. He has guided many graduate and postgraduate students and published research papers in National and International Journals. At present, Mr. Vikas Bansal working as Assistant Professor in the Department of Food Technology, School of Engineering & Technology, Jaipur National University, Jaipur, India. His research interest includes new product development and food powders. He has published many papers in this field. Mr. Vikas Bansal is a Life member of many Professional bodies like AFSTI, ISoFE, BRSI and reviewer of many National and International research journals.

Alexandra Bernardo is an Associate Professor IUEM, Physical-Chemistry PhD, Chemistry and Biotechnology BSc, Vice-Coordinator of the Clinical Nutrition Master degree, Health Environmental Researcher, Director of the document analysis office of the Forensic and Psychological Sciences Laboratory Egas Moniz.

Donovan McGrowder holds Bachelor of Science (Honours) and Doctor of Philosophy (PhD) degrees in Biochemistry and Chemistry, and Biochemistry respectively from the University of the West Indies, Mona, Kingston, Jamaica. Dr. McGrowder also holds a Master of Science degree from University of Westminster, London, UK and a Master of Arts in Psychology and Counselling from St. Stephens College, Alberta Canada. He also has post-graduate training and experience in Clinical Biochemistry and Molecular Biology. Dr. McGrowder joined the staff of The University of the West Indies, Mona in 2001 as Research Fellow in the Department of Basic Medical Sciences – Biochemistry Section and was promoted to Lecturer in 2003 and Senior Lecturer in 2009. He is also Consultant of Chemical Pathology at the University Hospital of the West Indies. He is Fellow of the Institute of Biomedical Science, UK, Fellow of the Royal Society of Tropical Medicine and Hygiene, UK, and Member of the Institute of Health Promotion and Education, UK.

Fabian Miller is a Lecturer, Researcher and the Head of Department of Physical Education at The Mico University College; he has participated in research in the Medical field and Sport Science field. He has worked on research in sport services in the CARIFORUM region which aim was to establish regional policies for sport services for the member states involved and to establish sport services as a viable industry in the region. His current research is aimed to establish Biological Passports of College/University Athletes who compete in Sprinting and Long Distance events. Mr. Miller also published peer reviewed journal articles and book chapters. He co-authored the manuscript titled "Prostate Specific Antigen Testing in a Tertiary Teaching Hospital" and co-authored the book chapter titled "Dietary Antioxidants in the Chemoprevention of Prostate Cancer. Mr. Miller is a graduate from G.C Foster College where he completed a Diploma in Education and a Bachelors Degree in Physical Education and Sport, he went on to pursue and complete his Masters of Science in Physical Education at The University of Technology, Jamaica and he is currently a PhD student in Biotechnology, Faculty of Science and Technology, University of the West Indies, Mona. Mr. Miller is a board member of the Social and Human Sciences Advisory Committee of Jamaica National Commission for UNESCO (Period of 2016-2019).

Zakir Mohammad is a Research Officer (Unani) & Assistant Professor in the National Research Institute of Unani Medicines for Skin Disorders under CCRUM, ministry of AYUSH Govt. of India, New Delhi, where he has been a Research officer since 2013 and faculty member since 2016. He was an Assistant Professor in Ayurvedic and Tibbia College and Hospital, Karol Bagh, New Delhi from 2010-2013. Zakir has completed his M.D (Ilmul Advia) at Aligarh Muslim University, Aligarh and his undergraduate studies from the same university. His research interest lies in area of Pharmaceutical of alternative medicine, Biotechnology, Pharmacy and Clinical trial of Unani drugs. He has worked in interdisciplinary Biotechnology Unit of AMU, Aligarh as Senior Research Fellow (SRF) from 2008-2010. He is supervising three Post graduate scholar while one PG scholar has completed work under his guidance. He has also supervising seven scholars as co-supervisor. Zakir has attended 19 conferences, 13 workshops on different topics and published 17 research and review papers in reputed journal. He has attended three Continuing Medical Education (CME) for teachers. He has completed three clinical trial studies on Unani Pharmacopoeial validation and drafted three clinical trial protocols. He has convened six Institutional Ethics committee meetings of the institute during 2013-2016.

Yogesh Murti is presently working as Assistant Professor, (Pharmaceutical Chemistry) at the Institute of Pharmaceutical Research, GLA University, Mathura (UP). He has published 30 Research and 25 Review Articles in International and National repute Journals. He has cosupervised 10 M Pharm students. He is guiding PhD students. He is also life member of many professional bodies like IPA, APTI, IPGA, ISTE, CSI, etc. and Nominee of IAEC nominated by CPCSEA.

Chukwuemeka Nwokocha is a Senior Lecturer in the Department of Basic Medical Sciences (Physiology Section), Faculty of Medical Sciences, The University of the West Indies, Mona Campus, Kingston 7, Jamaica.

Monica Premi is presently working as Assistant Professor in the Department of Food and Nutrition Science at Manipal University, Dubai. Dr Monica is a food technologist with a special interest in nutraceuticals and functional foods. She has acquired proficiency in the field of food processing through his experience in the food industry, research, and teaching by working for more than 10 years. She has published more than 10 research papers in national and international journals and has written several book chapters also. Monica acquired her bachelor degree in Food Technology from Rajasthan university, and her master's and Ph. D degree in Food Engineering and Technology from SLIET, Longowal, Punjab.

Sowmya Rao, an Indian with a PhD in Food Science and Nutrition, has been pursuing her interests in the field of Food and Nutrition since 17 years. Her passion in teaching grew since her childhood with family and teachers inspiring her to pursue a career in teaching and research. She has attended many seminars, workshops and presented her research work in conferences. She has to her credit, research articles published in scientific journals in the field of food science, clinical and community nutrition, and food microbiology. Public speaking is her strength, and she has delivered talks on nutrition in seminars and community gatherings as invited speaker. She was a part of shows conducted by South Indian television channels - Zee and Colors Kannada in India, leading a role as a Nutritionist, creating awareness and advising people on food and nutrition.

Raghunath Satpathy received his M.Sc in Botany (with specialization in Biotechnology) from Berhampur University science, India; (Post M.Sc.) Advanced P.G Diploma in Bioinformatics from University of Hyderabad and M. Tech. degree in Biotechnology from VIT University, Vellore India. He was awarded the degree for the doctor of philosophy (PhD) in Biotechnology by Sambalpur University, Odisha India. Currently he is working as an Assistant professor in the School of Biotechnology, Gangadhar Meher University, Samabalpur, Odisha, India. He is having more than 11 years of experiences in both teaching and research. He has authored many national and international journal papers and book chapters to his credit. In addition to this Dr. Satpathy is associated with many professional bodies and he is the recipient of many academic and research awards.

Pushkar Singh Rawat has awarded PhD from the Department of Biochemistry, University of Lucknow, Lucknow. He has completed his M.Sc in Biochemistry from the Department of Biochemistry, University of Lucknow, Lucknow. He has University Gold Medalist in Graduation. He has qualified ASRB NET, Uttarakhand State Eligibility Test (USET), Himachal Pradesh State Eligibility Test (HPSET) & Chhattisgarh State Eligibility Test (CGSET). He has also selected for the prestigious ICMR SRF fellowship. His areas of expertise are Biochemical toxicology and Clinical Biochemistry. He has more than 5 years of research experience. He likes to write on several emerging research contents.

Bhupesh C. Semwal is an Assistant Professor M.Pharm (GLA University, Mathura) He is accomplished as a teacher & researcher in the field of Pharmacology. He has more than twelve years of teaching as well as research experience. He authored more than 15 research articles in several national and international journals. He also attended UGC sponsored workshop and given presentation in more than 15 national and international conferences in India and abroad. He has completed his B. Pharm in 2004 and M. Pharm in 2006 in Pharmacology. Even he has guided more than 20 post graduate students.

Ashish Shukla is working as Junior Research Fellow (JRF) in Department of Medicine, Institute of Medical Science, BHU. I also worked in IIT-Mandi from 12/02/2019 to 30/06/2019 where my work was focused on Immuno-modulation of T.solium. I have expertise in PCR, gene cloning and Western blotting.

Ana Rita Silva has a Bachelor in Nutrition Sciences (2011) in Instituto Universitário Egas Moniz (IUEM) and in IUEM; Master in Clinical Nutrition (2014) in IUEM; PhD student in Clinical Nutrition in Faculdade de Ciências da Nutrição e Alimentação da Universidade do Porto (FCNAUP). Clinical Practice in Clinical Nutrition, since 2011. Oral and Poster communications in scientific meeting. Paper and book chapter published in scientific journal.

Maria Leonor Silva has a Bachelor in Nutrition and Food Engineering (2007) in Instituto Universitário Egas Moniz (IUEM) and Bachelor in Nutrition Sciences (2009) in IUEM; Master in Food Safety and Public Health (2009) in IUEM; PhD in Clinical Nutrition in the University of Central Lancashire, Preston (2011). Assistant lecture, since 2008. Clinical Practice in Clinical Nutrition, since 2009. Researcher in a Scientific Project, since 2008; Oral and Poster communications in scientific meeting. Paper and book chapter published in scientific journal. Scientific committee member of scientific meeting. PhD and Master degree supervisor.

Shalini Singh is completed her PhD from the Department of Biochemistry, University of Lucknow, Lucknow. She has qualified GATE and ASRB NET examination. She has also University Gold Medalist and selected for the prestigious DST INSPIRE fellowship. She is a passionate researcher in the area of Molecular biology, Microbiology and Enzymology. She has published various book chapters and research papers in many national and international journals. She has also presented her research findings in national and international conferences.

Sonia Singh is an Assistant Professor M.Pharm (GLA University, Mathura) ORCID number: https://orcid.org/0000-0003-1503-2745 She had an experience of about 12 years of teaching in the GLA University, Mathura. She has written about more than 20 papers, including review and research in the field of herbs and pharmacognosy. She also attended many national workshops. She has completed her graduation in pharmacy in the year of 2005 and post-graduation in 2008 from Rajiv Gandhi Institute of Health Science, Karnataka. Now She is pursuing her PhD from GLA University, Mathura U.P.

Shyam Sundar's pioneering work on rapid rK39 strip test resulted in the global application of this tool for the diagnosis of kala-azar, and it is being used in the national programmes of India and several countries of the world. He described several breakthroughs in the treatment of kala-azar, and developed first orally effective drug "miltefosine" for the treatment of VL. Miltefosine was used for the Kala-azar Elimination Programme in India, Nepal and Bangladesh, and now it is being used worldwide. He led the pivotal paromomycin trial, based on which the drug was approval by the Government of India. He has also done excellent work on lipid associated amphotericin B. His work with single dose liposomal amphotericin B is considered as a major breakthrough and has earned worldwide acclaim. This single dose regimen is now the most preferred according to WHO recommendations, and it is being used in the control programmes in India, Nepal & Bangladesh. Dr Shyam Sundar first to successfully conduct multidrug therapy of VL, and these regimens are also approved by WHO as the second most preferred regimen. Combination of paromomycin and miltefosine is also being used at primary health centers by the National Control Programme.

Bui Thanh Tung received his PhD in Pharmacology from the Seville University, Spain in 2014. Then he worked in School of Medicine and Pharmacy, Vietnam National University Ha Noi as lecturer. In 2018 he was pointed as Associate professor. His main research focuses on medicinal plants for the treatment of various diseases such as diabetes, Alzheimer, cancer… His special interest is on the development of new drugs from Vietnamese natural resources. He writes and presents widely on issues of natural products, bioactive compounds and their pharmacological activities.

Lowen Williams is a Graduate student who is pursuing PhD studies in the Department of Biotechnology, Faculty of Science and Technology, The University of the West Indies, Kingston 7, Jamaica, West Indies.

Cameil Wilson-Clarke is a Lecturer in the Department of Basic Medical Sciences (Pharmacology &Pharmacy Section), Faculty of Medical Sciences, The University of the West Indies, Mona Campus, Kingston 7, Jamaica.

Index

A

B

C

D

L

M

N

O

P

Q

R

S

T

W

www.ingramcontent.com/pod-product-compliance
Lightning Source LLC
LaVergne TN
LVHW080531300926
849162LV00007B/1582
9781799848080